OXFORD SPECIALTY TRAINING

How to pass the MRCS OSCE

Volume 1

OXFORD SPECIALTY TRAINING

How to pass the MRCS OSCE

Volume 1

EDITED BY

Pradip K. Datta

Christopher J. K. Bulstrode

Vasha Kaur

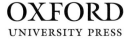

OXFORD
UNIVERSITY PRESS

OXFORD
UNIVERSITY PRESS

Great Clarendon Street, Oxford OX2 6DP

Oxford University Press is a department of the University of Oxford.
It furthers the University's objective of excellence in research, scholarship,
and education by publishing worldwide in

Oxford New York

Auckland Cape Town Dar es Salaam Hong Kong Karachi
Kuala Lumpur Madrid Melbourne Mexico City Nairobi
New Delhi Shanghai Taipei Toronto

With offices in

Argentina Austria Brazil Chile Czech Republic France Greece
Guatemala Hungary Italy Japan Poland Portugal Singapore
South Korea Switzerland Thailand Turkey Ukraine Vietnam

Oxford is a registered trade mark of Oxford University Press
in the UK and in certain other countries

Published in the United States
by Oxford University Press Inc., New York

© Oxford University Press 2011

British Library Cataloguing in Publication Data
Data available

Library of Congress Cataloging in Publication Data
Data available

Typeset by Glyph International, Bangalore, India
Printed in Great Britain
on acid-free paper by
Ashford Colour Press Ltd, Gosport, Hamshire

ISBN 978-0-19-958299-0

10 9 8 7 6 5 4 3 2 1

Oxford University Press makes no representation, express or implied, that the drug
dosages in this book are correct. Readers must therefore always check the product
information and clinical procedures with the most up-to-date published product
information and data sheets provided by the manufacturers and the most recent codes of
conduct and safety regulations. The authors and the publishers do not accept responsibility
or legal liability for any errors in the text or for the misuse or misapplication of material in
this work. Except where otherwise stated, drug dosages and recommendations are for the
non-pregnant adult who is not breast-feeding.

Foreword

The Objective Structured Clinical Examination is now in its third year as part of the MRCS examination. The name means what it says. There should be no unfair variation in questioning and the topics tested in each session must be the same for all candidates. This does not mean that the standard of the examination is any different from the previous free questioning nor is the syllabus narrower.

While focussed on the type of testing found in the OSCE stations, this book is in fact a comprehensive textbook, incorporating basic science and clinical surgery, not in a didactic way, but presenting real life practical scenarios. The authors present their experience in a highly practical way. Do not be put off by the apparent stress on 'communication skills'. This may be the spirit of the age but this book also gives young doctors and even medical students plenty of relevant facts to communicate!

Candidates for the MRCS and others studying this book will not only learn enough to pass the examination but will also be equipped with the basic knowledge to start their careers as specialist trainees.

John Black
March 2010

Preface

The diploma of Fellow of the Royal College of Surgeons (FRCS) of Edinburgh, England, Glasgow, and Ireland was replaced by the Collegiate Membership of the Royal College of Surgeons (MRCS). The MRCS went through various phases of change. In due course this gave way to the Intercollegiate MRCS in an attempt to make the examination uniform throughout all the Royal Colleges of Surgeons. The methods of testing were similar to the FRCS—vivas followed by clinical examination. The candidate had to be successful in the vivas to proceed to the clinicals.

The Intercollegiate MRCS (IMRCS) replaced the Collegiate MRCS. This was far more structured both in the vivas and the clinicals with the addition of a 'Communication Skills' component in the clinical section. The candidate could pass the 'Communication Skills' and the 'Clinical' parts separately, being able to bank success in one of the sections having to re-sit only the unsuccessful section.

In the autumn of 2008 the second part of the MRCS examination was held as an Objective Structured Clinical Examination (OSCE) for the first time. This replaced the vivas, clinicals, and communication skills (all of them put together) of the old examination. The present examination tests the knowledge, ability, deductive powers, clinical diagnostic ability, and communication skills of a doctor about to enter surgical training. It has been described as 'a day in the life of a first year specialist training (ST1) doctor'.

The Intercollegiate Surgical Curriculum Programme (ISCP) is an integral part of surgical training. Recognizing this, the two volumes of this series are designed to reflect the syllabus and curriculum across the nine specialities as set out in the ISCP. The books aim to consolidate the trainee's learning by highlighting essential topics in the syllabus with a multitude of examples. This will not only help the trainee excel in the MRCS OSCE examination but also provide a firm foundation for tomorrow's surgeons.

This book is aimed at the FY2 and ST1 doctor who proposes to embark on a surgical career and has already completed the MCQs and is preparing for the OSCE. It deals with each of the 18 9-minute stations; 18 stations are manned and there are 2 rest stations. Most readers would have been through an OSCE examination during their undergraduate days. Whilst the format remains the same, the MRCS OSCE expects the candidate to be aware of more details providing answers with a surgical slant. This book is the ideal preparation for this purpose.

The surgical trainee should be aware that the vast majority of medico-legal problems in the National Health Service stem from poor communication, particularly when things do not go according to plan. The general public accepts that a surgeon is only human and therefore is apt to make the occasional mistake for which they are prepared to forgive. Forgive they will not, if the surgeon avoids communicating with the patient or the relatives, as often happens, when something has gone wrong. Therefore, this volume deals with communication skills in various forms which a trainee may come across from time to time and helps the candidate through this section of the examination.

Although this book is primarily aimed for the trainee on the threshold of a surgical career sitting the MRCS OSCE examination, it is hoped that the final year medical student with a surgical bent aspiring to more than a mere pass in the examination will also find this book very worthwhile.

Pradip K. Datta MBE, MS, FRCS
Christopher J.K. Bulstrode MCh, FRCS (Tr & Orth)
Vasha Kaur MBChB (Hons), MRCS

Acknowledgements

In 2008 the MRCS examination (Intercollegiate Membership of the Royal College of Surgeons) was changed completely. The new design is based on the latest educational theories, and relies heavily on Objective Structured Clinical Examinations (OSCEs). The curriculum is also very different. There is now much more emphasis on testing communication skills.

Chris Reid, Commissioning Editor for medicine at Oxford University Press, had the foresight to see instantly that a new book was needed to help Basic Surgical Trainees prepare for this novel method of assessment. Within months he had assembled a team of writers willing to take on the challenge. We are all grateful to him for this initiative.

Once the proposal was accepted, Katy Loftus took over the reins as Project Manager and steered the task to completion. She has done a huge amount of work to bring all the contributors together, go through the manuscript with a fine-toothed comb, and keep every one of us on our toes. Her patience with the 'herd of cats' that formed the writing team was finely balanced with her determination to keep the project moving forward swiftly. To her we owe a debt of immeasurable gratitude.

There is a massive wealth of experience amongst the contributors who range from senior retired professors and examiners to young trainees embarking on their careers. To all of them we record our thanks not only for their thoughtful contributions, but also for their promptness when manuscripts have been returned for amendments. Our grateful thanks also to Dr Nic Williams for her efficient copy-editing. Finally, to Siân Jenkins, Assistant Production Editor, we are grateful for her overseeing the project to fruition on time.

Finally, we sincerely thank Mr John Black, President of the Royal College of Surgeons of England, for his Foreword.

P.K.D.
C.J.K.B.
V.K.

Image acknowledgements

We thank Mr P W Fisher, Consultant Surgeon, Wick, for image 6.57; Department of Radiology, Raigmore Hospital, Inverness, for Figures 6.62 and 6.66; CMRI, Kolkata, India, for Figure 6.68; Department of Surgery, MAMC, New Delhi, for Figure 6.69; Department of Surgery, Gandhi Medical college Hospital, Hyderabad, India, for Figure 6.73; and Dr Richard Weller, Consultant Dermatologist, Royal Infirmary Edinburgh, for images 21.2 and 21.9.

Contents

List of contributors

Professor Anthony Angel BSc, PhD

Emeritus Professor of Physiology, University of Sheffield
Examiner, Royal College of Surgeons of Edinburgh

Chapters 24, 26, 28, and 30

Christopher J. K. Bulstrode MCh, FRCS (Tr & Orth)

Professor and Honorary Consultant Orthopaedic Surgeon,
University of Oxford, Member of Council, Royal College of Surgeons of Edinburgh

Chapters 10, 11, 12, 19, 20

Pradip K. Datta MBE, MS, FRCS(Ed, Eng, Irel, Glasg)

Honorary Consultant Surgeon, Caithness General Hospital
Member of Council, Royal College of Surgeons of Edinburgh

Chapters 6, 13, 14, 15, 16, 25

Vasha Kaur MB ChB (Hons), MRCS

Specialty Trainee in General Surgery, London Deanery

Chapters 5, 9, 17, 21, 23

Professor Pawanindra Lal MS, MNAMS, DNB, FRCS (Ed & Glasg), FRCS(Eng)

Professor of Surgery, Maulana Azad Medical College, New Delhi, India
Examiner, Royal College of Surgeons of Edinburgh

Chapters 4, 7, and 8

Dr Ian Leeuwenberg MBChB

Specialty Trainee in Anaesthesia, South East Scotland

Chapter 2

Dr Alistair May MBChB, FCARCSI, FRCA

Specialty Trainee in Anaesthesia, West of Scotland

Chapter 2

Mr Iain Nixon FRCS(Ed) (ENT and Head & Neck)

Specialist Registrar, West of Scotland Rotation
Clinical Research Fellow, Head & Neck Surgery
Memorial Sloan Kettering Cancer Center, New York

Chapters 1, 3, and 18

Professor William F.M. Wallace BSc, MD, FRCP, FRCA, FCAI, FRCS(Ed)

Professor Emeritus of Applied Physiology, Queen's University, Belfast
Examiner, Royal College of Surgeons of Edinburgh

Chapters 22, 27, 29, and 31

Introduction

Christopher J. K. Bulstrode

The MRCS is one of the major post-graduate examinations, a useful qualification for entry into many specialties, not just surgery. Like other clinical examinations, Objective Structured Clinical Exams (OSCEs) have come to dominate its format. OSCEs are no more difficult than other types of assessment; they just require a slightly different approach. This book is designed to give you the facts, concepts, and skills that you need to pass this examination. However, this book is also devoted to OSCE scenarios of the type you are likely to face on the day of your test. To get yourself comfortable with OSCEs, you can test yourself on these scenarios and then you can turn to the answer section to see whether you have covered the key points which are being looked for by the examiner. We have also included one or two OSCEs which are written out in full with the actual dialogue which might take place in a good viva. This is to give you an idea of how it might all sound (when it is going well).

The unique feature of this book is that it is designed to work with you, to help you get comfortable with the OSCE exam format in the MRCS and ensure that you pass!

Fixed action patterns

Some actions such as greeting the patient/actor, washing hands, etc. are common to many OSCE stations. These need to be practised so often that you don't even have to think to remember to do them. They should also be so slick that the examiner's first impression of you (a critical moment) is that you are a calm, well practiced, professional.

Dress

To keep abreast of guidelines regarding modern infection control practices, a standard dress code is advised for the day. This would not require any change in the dress between stations. The dress requirements should follow this pattern: arms to be bare below the elbow and no jewellery on hands or wrists with the exception of wedding rings. Wear a conventional, white or light-coloured, short-sleeved shirt/blouse open at the neck, or a long-sleeved shirt/blouse with sleeves rolled up. Candidates who wish not to conform to this dress code for religious/cultural reasons are advised to read up the section on 'dress code' in 'Candidate instructions and guidance notes'. Smart polished footwear is expected. Get your hair cut and make sure it is tidy and tucked away. Remove designer stubble, and if you insist on a beard ensure that it is tidily trimmed.

Jewellery and scent

Do not wear heavy or gaudy jewellery and please go light on the scent. Both can be distracting to an examiner in a confined space and contribute nothing to their impression of you as a professional.

Equipment

You need an alcohol wash bottle for washing your hands. There should be one available but nevertheless it is probably best to have your own. You should probably also bring your own stethoscope and tendon hammer, although these too should be available on the table in the station.

Timing

Arrive very, very, early. If public transport lets you down it is only you who suffer, and if you arrive with only minutes to spare you will be flustered. Your performance will suffer and your image as a calm professional will be damaged.

Smile and eye contact

Engage eye contact and smile at everyone. In some cultures it is slightly rude to engage eye contact, but as a professional in British culture you are expected to do so.

Timing

You will be given 9 minutes at each station. It is difficult for you to estimate time in an OSCE station but if it appears that you have completed your task before the bell rings, do not worry. That is exactly what the examiners hope and expect. If you have not already done so you should summarize what you have done/found against the task you were set. So you might say 'I was asked to take a history relating to peripheral vascular disease, and I have covered the following areas…'. If there is still time after you have done this then you should look the examiners in the eye, smile and say that you believe you have finished. If the examiners want to clarify anything then they may do so at this stage. Otherwise they will thank you and let you go.

If you run out of time, do not try to persevere. Just engage eye contact, smile, and explain in one swift sentence what you would have done next. Nothing more will be allowed, or listened to. If you persist it will only annoy the examiners, and encourage them to give you a lower mark. You will not run out of time if you have practised that skill many times before.

Waiting outside the station

When waiting outside each station, it is normal to have a card describing first the scenario and then the task which you are going to be expected to perform. Read the scenario and the task twice, then THINK 'Why have they set this scenario, and this task?'. The answer to this question is the 'Learning Objective' of that station and will be the foundation around which the examiner's mark sheet is written. Read the scenario and task one more time to make sure that you have got the Learning Objective correct. Satisfied? Good. Now you need to make a mental list of the tasks you need to perform to demonstrate this Learning Objective, and the best order for performing them. In reality you are creating your very own 'examiner's mark sheet' and if you have got things right, it should exactly match the examiner's sheet. Finally, revise the fixed action patterns of the start (introductions and hand-washing) and the end (summarize and think), and it will be time to go in.

Entering the station

The examiners should introduce themselves and check your number. Smile and engage eye contact. As soon as this is completed, wash your hands (using the handwashing gel that you have with you) then carefully look all around the room for props. These will be such things as a glass of water for checking swallowing when examining a lump in the neck, tendon hammer, ophthalmoscope, etc. There should not be any props there which you do not need but all those which you should be using should be immediately visible to you. This is therefore a chance to check your plan of tasks.

The patient

Your introduction to the patient should be swift. Give your name, explain what you have been asked to do, and then ask their permission to proceed. Most experienced patients will start disrobing or whatever is required of them before you even ask, so a moment's hesitation at this stage does no harm, and may even give you a clue what to do next. Don't forget to thank the patient at the end, and make sure that they are comfortable. Some candidates ask the patient if there are any other points they would like to mention (when taking a history), or problems they would like to show (in examination). This is a good way of checking that you have not missed anything out, and is good professional practice.

Talking during a viva

Most examiners like you to talk during an OSCE station, but not to them! They are supposed to be invisible, and if you continuously talk to the examiner while looking for confirmation that you are on the right track, all you will succeed in doing is convincing them that you are too unsure of what you are doing to be marked as professionally competent. By all means describe what you are doing (especially if you are using a system) but talk quietly and clearly to yourself as if your well-organized mind is talking out loud. Do also talk to the patient explaining what you are doing next just as you would in a clinic. In communication skills viva stations, all your talking will be to the patient, and it is these stations which require the most practice.

If the examiner speaks

Examiners are not supposed to speak during an OSCE. If they do, stop at once and listen very carefully indeed. It usually means that you are doing something very wrong, but that the situation is salvageable and you need to take immediate action. It may be that you have misread the scenario/task sheet, or that you have misheard the patient or misinterpreted the physical sign. Review whatever it is they have questioned, assuming that your last interpretation was wrong. If you discover your mistake, apologize, and quickly restart. It is not too late to put things right.

Don't panic or give up

It is unprofessional to panic or to give up, so if you do either of these then you really deserve to fail. However badly you think that things are going, the examiners want you to pass and if they can possibly salvage your marks they will do so. However, they need your help so you need to get the best rack of marks that you possibly can.

Rest station

There are two rest stations. We would suggest that they should be used as such—to have a rest, both mental and physical. Try and relax during this enforced rest period of 10 minutes. There may be daily newspaper for you to read. One thing certainly you should never do during this time is to dwell upon a station that you have finished which in your mind has not gone well. Forget that completely and look forward.

The marking system*

Each station has a total of 20 marks. In addition each candidate is given a separate, overall global rating (global examiner judgement) for the station based on the assessment of the candidate's overall performance. In stations with two examiners there will be an agreed rating which is as follows:

- Fail
- Borderline fail
- Borderline pass
- Pass

Marks out of a maximum of 20 plus the global examiner judgement for each of the 18 stations are checked and the performance at individual stations analysed.

'Using the contrasting groups method of standard setting analysis a mark out of the maximum 360 available' is calculated as the minimum pass mark. In addition to achieving the overall pass mark, candidates must also achieve separately a minimum mark in each of the four broad content areas to pass Part B MRCS OSCE. The four areas are:

- Anatomy and surgical pathology (four stations)
- Clinical and procedural skills (six stations)
- Communication skills (five stations)
- Applied surgical science and critical care (three stations)

All 18 stations are manned.

(*Examiner guidance notes: MRCS Part B (OSCE) Examination. April 2010.)

Help others

When you have passed the exam, give others exam practice so that they too can pass the exam first time.

PART 1
SURGICAL SKILLS AND PATIENT SAFETY

Section 1 **Peri-operative care**

Introduction

This section will prepare the candidate to confidently face the stations dealing with physiology, critical care, and pre-operative assessment. It deals with all the aspects in the care of a surgical patient. Uneventful recovery after an operation is dependent upon recognizing comorbidities in a patient and taking proper steps to ensure smooth recovery. Such an assessment is more important in the emergency situation.

A basic knowledge of anaesthetics helps the surgical trainee whose duty it is to have performed the necessary investigations both in the emergency and elective situations. Local anaesthetic is administered by the surgeon and therefore knowledge on this is important.

Once the patient is in the operating theatre, efficient teamwork should ensure that surgery is being performed under optimum safety. Attention to detail regarding the use of diathermy, tourniquets, and laser should ensure their safe use.

In this day and age, minimal access surgery is the most sought after approach. The surgical trainee must be aware of the basic principles and the pitfalls that accompany such surgical techniques. Finally, post-operative care and knowledge on how to prevent and deal with complications should be the remit of the trainee surgeon as he/she would be the first person on the scene of a complication.

Pre-operative diagnosis is dependent upon appropriate investigations. A large number of images are shown in the form of a self-assessment exercise—an ideal tool for the OSCE stations.

Chapter 1 **Pre-operative assessment and preparation of the surgical patient**

This chapter teaches you pre-operative assessment. There will be a station with one examiner who will ask you to examine a patient (who may be an actor or a proper patient) with regard to a particular system such as respiratory or cardiovascular, and stratify the patient's risk with regard to an operation that the patient is due to undergo. You are advised to give a running commentary as you go along in your examination. Finally classify the patient according to the ASA (American Society of Anesthesiologists) scoring system.

Introduction: the pre-operative anaesthetic clinic

During pre-operative assessment you will aim to determine the medical status of the patient and arrange investigations to quantify risk or identify areas where optimization of medical conditions may improve outcome. A patient does not need to be completely fit to undergo an operation under anaesthetic. It is only necessary for all possible risk factors to be discovered and their severity measured as far as possible. A treatment plan should then be put into place which reduces those risks to a minimum. Then and only then can a rational decision be made as to whether the benefits of surgery outweigh the risks and therefore whether surgery should go ahead.

History

You will need to know if the patient has had a previous anaesthetic and whether they or any other member of their family have had any problems with an anaesthetic. You also need to know what medications they are on and whether they have any allergies. In children it is also useful to know whether they had any problems at or around birth or any subsequent hospital admissions.

At this point you may need to make a decision as to whether their medications should be discontinued over the period of surgery or whether they need to be continued by a different route (e.g. changing oral tablets to intravenous (IV) injection).

Examination

Examination will include assessment of the neurological, cardiac, and respiratory systems. Particular attention will be paid to the anatomy of the upper airway to identify patients in whom endotracheal intubation may be difficult. Around 5% of cases without a history of difficult intubation will involve difficulty with mask or endotracheal intubation.

Predictors of the difficult intubation include age >55 years, body mass index (BMI) >26, a history of snoring, immobility of the neck, an interincisor distance of <4cm a significant overbite (where the upper incisors extend significantly anterior to the lower incisors), an inability to shift the lower incisors in front of the upper incisors, and a short thyromental distance (the distance between the thyroid cartilage and anterior mandible).

The amount of posterior pharynx visible pre-operatively correlates with the difficulty of intubation and is described by the Mallampati classification (Table 1.1). This is based on the structures visualized with maximal mouth opening and tongue protrusion in the sitting position.

No single test will sufficiently predict the difficult airway. A combination of the Mallampati score and thyromental distance has been shown to be the most useful bedside test, although even this only has a sensitivity of around 36%. For this reason a careful history and examination should be performed and the anaesthetist will still be vigilant when performing instrumentation of the airway.

Pre-operative investigations

The traditional approach to pre-operative investigation is currently under review. Pre-operative surgical patients often undergo radiological, cardiological, biochemical, and haematological testing. The information from such tests can be used to support a current course of management, to alter management, to

Table 1.1 The Mallampati classification

Class	Visible structures
1	Soft palate, tonsillar pillars, uvula
2	Soft palate, tonsillar pillars, portion of uvula
3	Soft palate, base of uvula
4	Hard palate only

assess risk, to predict post-operative complications, to establish baselines for future comparisons, and for opportunistic screening unrelated to surgery.

More recently it has been recognized that no *routine* laboratory tests are required for the pre-anaesthetic evaluation of patients, and that clinicians should order tests when the results may influence decisions regarding risks and management of anaesthesia and surgery.

A NICE (National Institute of Health and Clinical Excellence) guideline does not support the use of routine chest X-ray in patients unless undergoing cardiovascular surgery. Electrocardiography was recommended in the elderly and those with a history of cardiovascular comorbidities. A full blood count was recommended when the risk of significant blood loss was high. Assessment of renal function was recommended in patients with cardiovascular or renal comorbidity or those undergoing extensive surgery.

Cardiopulmonary exercise testing

Cardiopulmonary exercise (CPEX) testing aims to provide a combined assessment of heart and lung function. In patients undergoing major surgery (particularly vascular), CPEX testing can be used to predict poor outcome. The test is carried out by recording electrocardiogram (ECG) activity, oxygen uptake, and carbon dioxide output in patients first at rest and then during graded exercise on a bike. The anaerobic threshold (AT) is a measure of when the patient converts from aerobic to anaerobic metabolism. Fitter patients will have a higher AT and may be at lower risk of complications.

Fitness for surgery

Surgery constitutes a physiological challenge for the body. The impact of this depends on the nature of the intervention. The extremes range from minor skin surface surgery to major intrathoracic intervention (Table 1.2).

Physiological reserve is the ability to withstand and compensate for both internal and external stresses. A way of determining physiological reserve is to quantify how much a person can increase their level of activity over and above that required for the tasks of daily living. Young, fit people will be able increase their level of activity 15–20-fold. With ageing, physiological reserve decreases and elderly people may have almost none at all. Many patients learn to compensate for this loss of fitness by limiting and adapting the way they carry out their activities. Often this change is very gradual and patients may not even themselves be aware of it. This can easily lead to misconceptions about patients' fitness unless the assessing clinician is alert to this possibility.

When discussing levels of activity and categorizing patients in terms of fitness it is often useful to quantify it using the term metabolic equivalents or METs: 1 MET is equivalent to $1kcal.kg^{-1}.h^{-1}$ and is approximately equivalent to the energy expended at rest (or oxygen consumption $3.5ml.kg^{-1}$). Table 1.3 shows some examples of activities with METs.

A number of systems are available for categorising patients according to levels of fitness but one of the most ubiquitous is the American Society of Anaesthesiologists' (ASA's) physical status classification system (Table 1.4). It is based on the patient's pre-operative state and although widely used it has many limitations: the definitions are vague leading to inter-clinician variability; it does not take account of the patient's age, smoking status, obesity, pregnancy or the nature of the surgery. In addition, although it is often used to predict risk it is not intended for that purpose.

Table 1.2 Grades of surgery (NICE: Preoperative Tests 2003)

Grade 1 (minor)	Excision skin lesion, drainage of breast abscess
Grade 2 (intermediate)	Inguinal hernia, varicose veins, tonsillectomy, knee arthroscopy
Grade 3 (major)	Total abdominal hysterectomy, endoscopic resection of prostate, lumbar discectomy, thyroidectomy
Grade 4 (major+)	Total joint replacement, thoracic surgery, colonic resection, radical neck dissection, cardiovascular surgery, neurosurgery

Table 1.3 Examples of activities with METs

MET	Approximate level of activity
1	Sitting at rest
2	Household walking, washing, dressing
4	Climbing stairs, golf
6	Dancing, doubles tennis, mowing lawn
8	Bicycling (moderate effort), football
>10	Running up stairs, boxing, squash

Table 1.4 The ASA physical status classification system

Class	Description	Mortality (%)
1	A normal healthy patient	0.1
2	A patient with mild systemic disease	0.2
3	A patient with severe systemic disease	1.8
4	A patient with severe systemic disease that is a constant threat to life	7.8
5	A moribund patient who is not expected to survive without the operation	9.4
6	A declared brain-dead patient whose organs are being removed for donor purposes	n/a

Pre-operative management in special circumstances

Cardiovascular disease

Ischaemic heart disease is important to identify at the pre-operative visit. It results from an imbalance between myocardial oxygen demand and supply. Although factors such as hypoxia, hypotension, and anaemia can underlie ischaemia, the most common cause is a reduction in the luminal area of the coronary arteries due to atherosclerosis.

There has been a lot of interest in devising ways to predict risk of cardiac events in non- cardiac surgery.

Lee's Revised Cardiac Risk Index uses six factors:

1 High-risk surgical procedures
2 History of ischaemic heart disease
3 History of congestive heart failure
4 History of cerebrovascular disease
5 Pre-operative treatment with insulin
6 Pre-operative serum creatinine >177 μmol.L^{-1}

The number of points can then be used to calculate the risk of cardiac events (Table 1.5) which includes: myocardial infarction (MI), pulmonary embolism (PE), ventricular fibrillation, complete heart block, and cardiac arrest.

Patients in the high-risk group may be further stratified using stress ECGs or dipyridamole thallium imaging. It is unclear whether the high-risk subgroup would benefit from pre-operative cardiac procedures such as percutaneous coronary intervention (PCI) or coronary artery bypass grafting (CABG).

Management of patients with ischaemic heart disease should continue during the peri-operative period. The withdrawal of beta blockers or antihypertensives can result in increased sympathetic activity, leading to an increased myocardial oxygen demand and ischaemic damage. Isolated hypertension (<180/<110) is not thought to affect surgical outcome.

Table 1.5 Risk of cardiac events using Lee's Revised Cardiac Risk Index

Points	Class	Risk
0	I	Very low: 0.4%
1	II	Low: 0.9%
2	III	Moderate: 6.6%
>3	IV	High: 11%

Table 1.6 Indications for implantable cardiac pulse generators

Pacemaker	ICD
Diseases of impulse formation	Ventricular tachycardia
Diseases of conduction	Ventricular fibrillation
Long QT syndrome	Brugada syndrome
Hypertrophic obstructive cardiomyopathy	Arrhythmogenic right ventricular dysplasia
Dilated cardiomyopathy	Long QT syndrome
	Hypertrophic cardiomyopathy

Implantable cardiac pulse generators

The original battery-operated cardiac pacing devices were introduced in the 1950s. As electronic and battery technology has improved devices have been miniaturized and are now complex programmable devices. There are two broad categories of pulse generators: pacemakers and implantable cardioverter defibrillators (ICDs).

Modern devices, palpable in a pectoral pocket, are extremely reliable, however they can fail. Malfunction rates of around 1% for pacemakers and 2% for ICDs are reported and probably underestimate the problem. For this reason devices should be under review at least annually.

Patients who have such an implantable device often have significant comorbidities in addition to abnormalities of cardiac rhythm (Table 1.6). Pre-anaesthetic management of the patient includes optimization of these conditions as well as assessment of the device.

During pre-anaesthetic assessment, the device will be evaluated to identify the type, battery status, and current program. The need for re-programming of the device will depend on the specific device, the current program, and the nature of surgery. The patient should be assessed for their underlying rhythm and rate. This will generally be done by a cardiologist or pacemaker service, who will also address reprogramming if required in the post-operative period.

Pre-operative planning should include attempts to minimize the use of electro-surgery. Monopolar devices are more likely to cause problems than bipolar. The most common problem encountered is a ventricular oversensing, leading to pacing inhibition.

If monopolar electrosurgery has to be used, the current return pad should be placed to ensure that the current path does not cross the pacing system.

Note: MRI scanning is contraindicated by most device manufacturers.

Respiratory disease and smoking

Both general anaesthesia and surgery have effects on the respiratory system.

Surgical trauma may lead to an increase in airway tone and reactivity. Patients undergoing thoracic or upper abdominal surgery are at particular risk due to diaphragmatic dysfunction. Following laparotomy, the functional residual capacity is reduced to around 50% of normal, and takes 12 weeks to recover.

Post-operative pulmonary complications occur in up to 30% of surgical patients. Risk factors include: cigarette smoking, pre-existing pulmonary conditions, emergency surgery, surgery lasting >3 hours, and upper abdominal or thoracic procedures.

Pre-anaesthetic testing in patients with lung disease may be used to diagnose previously occult chronic disease, but pulmonary function tests do not allow patient risk stratification and should be used selectively. Arterial blood gas analysis also does not improve risk assessment and since the need for supplemental oxygen therapy depends on post-operative hypoxia, baseline testing is rarely indicated.

Cigarette smoking leads to chronic lung disease which in turn increases the risk of post-operative pulmonary complications. Smokers have reduced tissue oxygen delivery, poorer wound healing, and reduced resistance to infection. They are also more likely to have serious comorbidities such as ischaemic heart disease and emphysema. It is always worthwhile counselling people about smoking cessation as even stopping for 24 hours prior to surgery is beneficial.

- Half-life of carboxyhaemoglobin is 4 hours when breathing air
- Within 12–24 hours the systemic effect of nicotine is greatly reduced
- Within 6–8 weeks ciliary function is restored, and sputum production is significantly reduced

Recognition of pre-existing lung disease and optimization in the pre-operative period should be routine. Poorly-controlled asthmatics risk bronchospasm, sputum retention, atelectasis, infection, and respiratory failure during anaesthesia and surgery. The history will give the most information about how well they are managing their asthma—a useful measure is the peak flow test.

Patients with obstructive sleep apnoea should be identified, as pre-surgical treatment can optimize cardiorespiratory function, and non-invasive ventilator devices (such as continuous positive airway pressure ventilators) should be available in the post-operative period.

Endocrine disease, including diabetes

Endocrine disease encountered in the pre-operative assessment may be the primary indication for surgery, a cofactor in the disease being treated, or be unrelated to the procedure.

Over 50% of patients with diabetes mellitus will need surgery at some point during their life. The post-operative recovery period is extended by 50% in diabetics and this patient group has a mortality rate five times that of the non-diabetic population. Morbidity and mortality result from end-organ damage as a result of both micro- and macroangiopathy, and from impairment of leucocyte function. Good long-term diabetic control will determine the degree of organ dysfunction encountered in the surgical patient. Tight glycaemic control during the peri-operative period is the aim in management of diabetics, and this can be best achieved using a multidisciplinary approach.

During the anaesthetic assessment, particular attention will be paid to cardiac, renal, neurological, and peripheral vascular disease. A positive 'prayer sign' (inability to approximate fingers and palms with fingers extended) may be an indicator of joint rigidity, signifying a difficult intubation. Investigations including electrocardiography, blood electrolytes, creatinine, and HbA1c and orthostatic blood pressure testing to detect autonomic dysfunction should be considered routine. More invasive testing such as stress echocardiography or coronary angiography should be considered in diabetics who present for vascular surgical procedures.

On the day of surgery, diabetics should be scheduled first on the list in an attempt to minimize the disruption of their diabetic regimen. Patients managed on oral regimens should be advised to omit their dose on the day of surgery. Metformin carries the risk of lactic acidosis and should be withheld for 24 hours before surgery restarting around 48 hours post-operatively. These patients can be maintained on short-acting insulin preparations during the peri-operative period.

Patients who depend on insulin should lower their dose the night before surgery to prevent hypoglycaemia related to fasting and will require an insulin regimen over the peri-operative period which should be directed by regular monitoring of blood glucose levels.

Diabetics are at a higher level of risk for peri-operative myocardial and cerebrovascular ischaemia. They are also more susceptible to infection, lower extremity ulceration ileus, and poor wound healing. All of these factors make surgery on the diabetic high risk, and all attempts should be made to maintain normal blood glucose levels throughout the peri-operative period, returning patients to their pre-operative diabetic regimen as soon as the nature of the surgery and anaesthesia allows.

Hyperthyroidism results in effects throughout multiple systems. Cardiac and renal dysfunction can result from abnormal levels of circulating thyroid hormone due to alterations in systemic vascular resistance and the renin–angiotensin–aldosterone system. The most feared complication is 'thyroid storm', which is usually seen in patients with undiagnosed hyperthyroidism. The condition occurs in the first 48 hours after surgery and is characterized by hyperthermia, tachycardia, and delirium. Treatment includes beta-blockade, antipyretics and thionamides. Mortality rates are high (up to 75%) and these patients should be managed in a critical care environment.

Hypothyroidism is relatively common, affecting around 1% of patients. Again, effects can be wide ranging but cardiorespiratory depression can lead to hypoxaemia. Myxoedema coma is a rare condition that can affect hypothyroid patients in the post-operative period. It results in hypothermia, bradycardia, heart failure, and hypopnoea. Treatment involves rehydration, systemic steroids, and thyroxine replacement. The mortality rate is reported to be as high as 80%.

Clinical signs of thyroid dysfunction are subtle. During pre-operative assessment symptoms such as lethargy, fatigue, heat intolerance, depression or anxiety, and signs such as tachycardia, atrial fibrillation, tremor, and hoarseness should alert the clinician to the possibility of thyroid disease. Levels of thyroid stimulating hormone and thyroid hormones (T_3 and T_4) are diagnostic and should be treated prior to elective surgery.

Neurological diseases

Peri-operative management of patients with disease of the central nervous system requires an understanding of the relationship between mean arterial pressure (MAP), intracranial pressure (ICP), cerebral blood flow (CBF), and the cerebral metabolic rate of oxygen consumption. Assessment of ICP in the pre-operative period is difficult as symptoms are vague, and signs such as papillo-oedema do not manifest acutely. Imaging with computed tomography (CT)/magnetic resonance imaging (MRI) may reveal mass lesions or midline shift.

Intracranial procedures may require specific conditions, for example, cerebral aneurysm surgery requires a stable blood pressure especially during the stress produced by laryngoscopy and intubation.

Inhalational anaesthetics cause cerebral blood vessel dilatation and a drop in cerebral vascular resistance, in turn leading to an increase in CBF. In contrast, propofol reduces CBF and ICP and may lower MAP so reducing cerebral perfusion pressure.

During the recovery period from surgery on the central nervous system, pain, straining, and coughing should be minimized to reduce a swinging blood pressure and ICP which can lead to bleeding at the operative site.

Victims of head trauma are at particular risk. Opioid medications can decrease ICP, but their sedative effects can lead to an increased P_aCO_2 causing vasodilation and a raised ICP. Fluids must also be used carefully to maintain MAP whilst avoiding fluid overload which can result in cerebral oedema.

Hepatobiliary disease and alcohol excess

The liver synthesizes albumin and coagulation factors, metabolizes drugs, and has a role in glucose homeostasis. Dysfunction of this organ therefore has wide-ranging effects on both the anaesthetic and the surgical procedure.

When regional techniques are inappropriate, general anaesthetic doses must be reduced and the choice of agent will depend on the clearance mechanisms for these drugs. Patients with cirrhosis, for example, can have low plasma cholinesterase activity sensitizing them to the effects of non-depolarizing muscle relaxants.

Halothane hepatitis is a rare condition which may have an immunological basis related to multiple exposures to the volatile anaesthetic.

Biliary disease can affect hepatic function, but it is more commonly encountered as a surgical indication, particularly in relation to laparoscopic cholecystectomy. During laparoscopic procedures, abdominal insufflations can impede ventilation and venous return. Use of the reverse Trendelenburg position (feet down) clears organs from the surgical site and can improve ventilation but results in further impeded venous return. Cardiac output in this situation should be maintained by ensuring sufficient fluids to maintain intravascular volume.

Renal disease

Surgical patients are at high risk of renal injury. The reason for this is a combination of fluid shifts, haemodynamic changes, and exposure to renal toxins. Patients with existing renal disease are at most risk of further deterioration in renal function. For this reason it is important to identify such patients during pre-operative assessment.

A history of renal disease or comorbidities such as diabetes or cardiac dysfunction is important. Conditions which compromise renal blood flow render the kidney more susceptible to ischaemia and nephrotoxins.

Particular attention should be paid to the patient's volume status. Pre-operative assessment will include blood electrolytes and creatinine, a full blood count, and urinalysis. Maintaining intravascular volume during surgery preserves renal blood flow so minimizing hypoxia in the renal medulla. Diuretics are often stopped in the immediate pre-operative period as patients taking these drugs have unpredictable fluid shifts and blood loss during surgery. Most anaesthetic drugs reduce renal blood flow, increasing the need for careful monitoring of blood pressure and volume status during the procedure.

Nephrotoxins such as contrast agents and aminoglycosides should be avoided whenever possible in the patient with renal dysfunction. When the use of contrast is unavoidable, consider spacing out infusions as the degree of nephropathy is dose dependent.

Patients with renal disease are at a higher risk of infection and may have vitamin deficiencies and malnutrition, whilst uraemia impairs lymphocyte function. An increased bleeding risk is associated with chronic renal failure, particularly in the patient on dialysis. The bleeding risk affects both the surgical field and rates of peptic ulceration. Platelet dysfunction prolongs bleeding time which can be improved by treatment with DDAVP (desmopressin) or cryoprecipitate.

Rheumatoid arthritis

This chronic inflammatory condition affects multiple systems and so the effects on surgery and anaesthesia are wide ranging. Patients may present with restrictive lung disease, pleural effusions, pericarditis, and anaemia.

A specific problem that requires pre-operative consideration is atlanto-occipital instability. If the condition exists, cervical flexion can lead to compression injury of the spinal cord. Neck pain radiating from the occipital region may be an early sign of instability. If suspected, radiology including flexion/extension cervical spine films, CT, or MRI can be helpful. Irrespective of radiological evidence, care should be taken with the position of the cervical spine during surgery, anaesthesia, and any patient repositioning. If tracheal intubation is required, fibreoptic intubation with the patient awake may be the best way to minimize neck movement. Involvement of the cricoarytenoid joints may reduce the mobility of the vocal cords, making tracheal intubation more challenging.

Immunocompromised patients

Patients can be immunocompromised by drugs, such as steroids and chemotherapy, or diseases, such as diabetes, malignancy, and HIV. The immunocompromised patient will be more susceptible to perioperative infections, and may have poor wound healing.

In these patients you should check for recent treatment with immune-suppressive drugs as well as symptoms and signs of opportunistic infections. If testing for HIV is indicated then these tests should be administered by staff trained in counselling patients. Until the results are available patients should be managed as if they are seropositive to minimize the risk of cross infection.

Chemotherapy treatments have a wide range of potential side effects that can interfere with peri-operative care. These include cardiac, pulmonary, hepatic, renal, and neurotoxicity in addition to myelosuppression.

The growth in the field of organ transplantation has resulted in more patients being candidates for elective surgery. Corticosteroids were the first immunosuppressive medications used in this group. They have complex effects on the body and affect not only the immune system but also can affect mental status, glucose tolerance, and blood supply to the femoral head in the short term. Long-term effects include impaired wound healing, hypertension, and osteoporosis. Modern immunomodulatory drugs have effects on all organ systems and each patient will need to be assessed on an individual basis.

Haematological disease including hyper/hyposplenism

Patients should be assessed for frequency of infections and bleeding tendencies. A family history or recent exposure to myelosuppressive treatments may also be suggestive of possible abnormalities. Enquire about regular medications such as aspirin and non-steroidals.

Patients undergoing minor surgery with no history of bleeding disorders require no specific laboratory testing. In patients undergoing major surgery, it is not unreasonable to perform a platelet count, pro-thrombin time, and activated partial thromboplastin time. Patients with abnormal results or a history suggestive of a bleeding disorder should be referred to a haematologist for further investigation.

Haemophilia A is a hereditary deficiency in factor VIII, transmitted as an X-linked trait. Patients with a factor VIII activity under 1% are at risk from spontaneous haemorrhage. Levels over 10% are likely to be asymptomatic. All patients with this condition should be admitted to hospital for surgery and management should be coordinated with their haematologist. Treatment for haemorrhage includes simple measures such as pressure, antifibrinolytics such as tranexamic acid, and replacement of factor VIII.

Von Willebrand's disease is the most common inherited bleeding disorder and results in a reduced plasma concentration function of von Willebrand's factor (vWF). Symptoms may be mild and include bleeding from mucosal surfaces. DDAVP can be administered to raise the plasma concentration of vWF. Plasma concentrates of vWF are also available.

Hyposplenism can be encountered following multiple splenic infarctions from sickle cell disease, secondary to autoimmune destruction in diseases such as *systemic lupus erythematosus* (SLE), or in relation to treatments such as radiotherapy which can affect splenic function. These patients are at risk of overwhelming sepsis (see 'Asplenics' section).

Hypersplenism can result from infiltration, extramedullary haemopoiesis, inflammation, autoimmune processes, and from systemic or portal hypertension. Peripheral blood counts decrease as a result of increased cell destruction on the spleen.

Asplenics

Following splenectomy, patients are at risk from overwhelming sepsis and atherosclerosis.

Overwhelming infection is rare but can be rapidly fatal. Organisms that would be removed by splenic macrophages evade recognition by macrophages in the liver and lung as they circulate too rapidly through these organs. The encapsulated organisms *Streptococcus pneumoniae*, *Haemophilus influenzae* type b and *Neisseria meningitidis* are the ones most commonly involved. Trauma patients have a cumulative incidence of post-splenectomy bacterial sepsis of around 1.5% and a 50-fold greater risk of septic death than patients with an intact spleen.

Nutrition: malnourished and obese patients

Malnourished patients have been shown to have an increased risk of post-operative complications including wound problems, infections, respiratory failure, and even death. Identifying these patients is important as pre-operative nutrition can reduce these complications.

Assessment should include measurement of weight (Table 1.7), muscle wasting, loss of subcutaneous fat, oedema, and ascites. Serum albumin levels <3.5g/dl in a general surgical population is predictive of malnutrition.

Poor nutritional status is most easily addressed by giving more food (enteral feeding). Patients can be fed by IV infusion (total parenteral nutrition) and this has been shown to improve outcome, but it is not without its own risks.

Obesity is associated with comorbidities. The common ones are diabetes and cardiovascular disease, but vascular access and intubation are also likely to be more difficult. Ventilation may be difficult and arterial oxygenation tends to be lower during surgery. Rates of wound infection, PE, and sudden death

Table 1.7 Risk of health problems associated with BMI

Weight	BMI (kg/m²)	Risk of health problems
Underweight	<18.5	Increased
Normal	18.5–24.9	Least
Overweight	25.0–29.9	Increased
Obese	30.0–39.9	High

are also higher in this population. The pharmacokinetics of anaesthetic agents are altered as most are highly fat soluble, and recovery from anaesthesia is likely to be delayed.

Particularly high-risk patients may be identified from a previous history of anaesthetic problems including difficulty during intubation and intensive care admission in the post-operative period.

During surgery, an appropriate operating table must be available. Consider also that surgeries may take up to 25% longer in this patient group which has effects on management of hypothermia, fluid administration, and efficient structuring of the operating list.

Drug therapy and allergies

Both prescription and over-the-counter medications should be documented. The decision to continue medications in the immediate pre-operative period depends on the disease, the medication, the surgery, and the type of anaesthesia. Typically medications for asthma and beta blockers will be continued, diuretics and warfarin will be stopped, and diabetic medications will require specific planning.

Patients should be asked specifically about allergies and interrogated about their definition of allergy which is often very different to that of the clinician. Only around 10–20% of patients reporting penicillin allergy have a true allergy.

Patients at risk of latex allergy include those who have undergone multiple procedures, those with a history of atopy, and healthcare workers.

Malignant hyperthermia is a clinical syndrome occurring during anaesthesia with a volatile anaesthetic gas such as halothane and the depolarizing muscle relaxant suxamethonium. Uncontrolled skeletal muscle metabolism results in a rapidly rising temperature, lactic acidosis, and rhabdomyolysis. Management with dantrolene has reduced mortality to <5%.

Obstetric anaesthesia

Most patients who require anaesthetic assessment do so in relation to their pregnancy, but 2% of pregnant women undergo non-obstetric surgery during their pregnancy. Throughout pregnancy hormonal, mechanical, metabolic, and haemodynamic changes affect both mother and fetus.

There is a 40% increase in cardiac output during pregnancy. Systemic vascular resistance drops, so maintaining blood pressure. During the third trimester, the cardiac output drops due to the pressure of the gravid uterus in the inferior vena cava which can compromise venous return.

During the second trimester, functional residual capacity reduces to 80% of the non-pregnant state. This increases the risk of hypoxaemia which can develop during short apnoeic periods, such as during intubation.

It is important to remember that any woman of childbearing age could be pregnant, and a urinary pregnancy test is routine prior to elective surgical treatment in this patient group.

Paediatric anaesthesia

The specialty of paediatric anaesthesia incorporates children from pre-term neonates to full developed young adults. As children grow, their anatomy and physiology change, so affecting pre-operative considerations. Congenital abnormalities are more common in young children, with acquired conditions affecting the older age group. Families must also be considered in the pre-operative visit as the potential for significant anxiety exists, which may be transferred from parent to child.

Special pre-operative measures

Bowel preparation

Standard pre-operative preparation for lower gastrointestinal (GI) surgery includes the administration of cathartics such as polyethylene glycol solutions. These act to rid the colon of solid stool the night before surgery. This reduces the bacterial load of the colon, and so, it is hoped, decreases the post-operative infection-related morbidity. The necessity for bowel preparation is obvious for endoscopic procedures. A growing body of evidence suggests that its use before standard colonic resections, however, may not result in reduced morbidity. In addition to the questionable benefit in terms of bacterial load reduction, side effects include: electrolyte disturbance, patient discomfort, and a possible alteration in bacterial translocation.

Pre-medication

Pre-medication is given to decrease anxiety in the patient, reduce the risk of aspiration, and minimize post-operative nausea, vomiting, and pain.

Commonly used anxiolytics are the benzodiazepines which are of particular use in children. In the setting of day case surgery, anxiolytics should be used with care as they can lead to longer post-operative recovery periods and less efficient use of day bed areas. By reducing the pH of gastric contents with proton pump inhibitors, patients risk from aspiration can be reduced. Post-operative nausea is often caused by opioid use and can be controlled with antiemetics.

Antibiotic prophylaxis

Prophylactic administration of antibiotics inhibits the growth of contaminating bacteria, so reducing the risk of infection. Surgical site infections are one of the most common healthcare-associated infections, leading to greater patient morbidity, longer hospital stays, and greater costs. Giving antibiotics, however, leads to a higher incidence of resistant bacteria, and predisposes to infection with organisms such as *Clostridium difficile*. It also exposes patients to the risk of allergic reactions.

Specific guidelines exist to help clinicians choose an appropriate strategy for prophylactic antibiotic use (e.g. *Scottish* Intercollegiate Guidelines Network (SIGN) guidelines).

Deciding whether to administer antibiotics depends on patient- and procedure-based factors. Patients at particular risk from surgical site infections include those at the extremes of age, the malnourished or obese, diabetics, smokers, the immunosuppressed, those with a prolonged hospital stay, and patients with coexisting infection at other sites.

Procedure-based factors include the length of procedure, surgical technique, post-operative hypothermia, and the presence of foreign material in the surgical site. Finally, wounds may be classified as clean, clean-contaminated, contaminated, and dirty (Table 1.8).

Although decisions on prophylaxis should be made on an individual patient basis, general recommendations are that clean procedures do not benefit from prophylactic antibiotics; clean-contaminated, contaminated, dirty procedures do. Most procedures involving the implantation of foreign material also benefit from antibiotic prophylaxis. Notable exceptions include craniotomy where the effect of a post-operative infection is devastating so antibiotics are used despite no implant being used. Conversely, hernia repairs with mesh do not require antibiotics.

Venous thromboprophylaxis

Venous thromboembolism (VTE) includes deep venous thrombosis (DVT), which can be symptomatic or asymptomatic and picked up on ultrasound and PE. Ninety per cent of PEs are from asymptomatic DVTs. There are multiple risk factors for VTE (Table 1.9), with a 10-fold increased risk in the post-surgical patient over the general population.

Table 1.8 Classification of operation (from SIGN Guideline 104)

Class	Definition
Clean	Procedures without inflammation, where there is no entry to GI, genitourinary (GU), or respiratory tract
Clean-contaminated	Procedures where the GI, GU, or respiratory tract is entered without significant spillage
Contaminated	Procedures where there is inflammation but no pus, or visible contamination of the wound
Dirty	Procedures in the presence of pus, or compound injuries >4h

Table 1.9 Risk factors for venous thrombosis (from SIGN guideline 62)

Age	Exponential increase in risk with age
Obesity	3× greater risk if BMI >30 kg/m²
Previous VTE	Recurrence rate 5%/year
Thrombophilias	Low coagulation inhibitors/high coagulation factors
	Activated protein C resistance
	Antiphospholipid syndrome
	High homocysteine
Thrombotic states	Malignancy: 7× greater risk
	Heart failure/recent MI/CVA
	Severe infection
Pregnancy	10× greater risk
Hospitalization	Acute trauma, illness, or surgery 10× greater risk
Anaesthesia	2× greater risk general vs. spinal/epidural

Patients who undergo general or gynaecological surgery for >30 minutes who are over 40 years old have rates of asymptomatic DVT in the range of 25%. Following orthopaedic surgery rates of up to 50% are reported. Despite the higher rates of asymptomatic DVT in the orthopaedic group, rates of fatal PE are similar in both groups at around 0.4%.

Routine thromboprophylaxis has been shown to reduce morbidity and mortality from VTE, whereas screening for asymptomatic DVTs has been disappointing.

Methods for prophylaxis include: early mobilization following surgery, the use of compression stockings and pneumatic foot pumps, adequate hydration, and pharmacological agents. Contraindications for compression stockings include: massive leg oedema, pulmonary oedema, severe peripheral arterial disease, severe peripheral neuropathy, and dermatitis.

A number of pharmacological agents are available. Aspirin reduces VTE rates but is associated with higher rates of major bleeding. Warfarin is rarely used due to the need for daily international normalized *ratio* (INR) monitoring. Low-molecular-weight heparins have been shown to reduce VTE rates with an increase in major bleeding, but not in fatal bleeding complications. Heparin-associated thrombocytopenia is a possible complication of low-molecular-weight heparin therapy. Patients should have a baseline platelet count and monitoring if they are expected to receive treatment for 5 days or more.

All patients admitted for surgery should be risk assessed for VTE. Basic prophylaxis should be practised in all surgical patients. Pharmacological measures should be considered in all patients undergoing major procedures or those patients with multiple risk factors undergoing more minor procedures.

Pre-operative fasting (please also refer to Chapter 2)

A period of pre-operative fasting is recommended to reduce the risk of pulmonary aspiration. Other measures that can be employed to reduce the risk include: provision of pharmacological agents to modify the volume and acidity of the gastric contents, and anaesthetic techniques such as rapid sequence induction and awake endotracheal intubation.

Patients at higher risk of aspiration include those with a history of gastro-oesophageal reflux, dysphagia, GI motility disorders, difficult airways, or metabolic disorders such as diabetes. The recommended fasting times based on type of liquid times is shown in Table 1.10.

Although the use of prokinetics, H_2 antagonists, proton pump inhibitors, and anticholinergics may reduce gastric volume and acidity prior to surgery, they have not been shown to reduce aspiration risk. Their use should be restricted to those at high risk, or patients who routinely use such medication over the pre-operative period.

Table 1.10 Recommended fasting times based on ingested material

Ingested material	Minimum fasting period (h)
Clear liquid	2
Breast milk	4
Infant formula	6
Non-human milk	6
Light meal	6

Table 1.11 Recommended steroid supplementation

Minor surgery	25mg hydrocortisone at induction
Moderate–major surgery	25mg hydrocortisone at induction
	100mg hydrocortisone/day until GI function returns

Pre-operative steroid management

Patients taking corticosteroids who present for surgery require special consideration. The stress of surgery leads to a rise in endogenous steroids in the normal patient. A patient who is dependent on exogenous steroids may have depression of the hypothalamic–pituitary–adrenal axis, which prevents him/her from responding to their body's need for extra steroids during periods of stress such as surgery. These patients may develop peri-operative shock due to secondary corticosteroid insufficiency.

Patients who take a steroid dose equivalent to 10mg of prednisolone or more are recommended to receive a physiological replacement regimen (Table 1.11).

Wrong-site surgery

Doing the wrong operation, operating on the wrong patient, or on the wrong side can be termed 'wrong-site surgery'. It is said to occur even if the error is realized and the procedure is not completed. The true incidence of such wrong-site surgery is difficult to determine but studies calculate a rate of between 1 in 15,000 to 1 in 30,000 cases. This makes wrong-site surgery as common as retained foreign objects. Operating on the wrong side is the most common cause of wrong-site surgery. Other wrong-site procedures that fall outside of the definition of surgery include: radiographs of the wrong site, vascular access at inappropriate sites, and administration of contrast agents at incorrect sites. It is estimated that over a career, a surgeon who operates on bilateral structures has a 25% chance of performing wrong-site surgery.

Methods which can be used to reduce the incidence of wrong-site surgery include pre-operative verification of procedure, patient, and site, and involving the patient in the checking process. Use of standardized items such as consent forms, radiological tests, pathology reports, and blood products may help to reduce mistakes prior to all procedures. Marking the skin when there is more than one possible location for the procedure should be practised. Ideally the patient should be involved in this process also. The mark should be unambiguous, made in permanent ink, and visible even when the patient is draped. A 'time-out' should be performed immediately prior to starting surgery. This period of time should be used by the whole team to check on the patient identity, correct site, and procedure to be done.

Wrong-site surgery is rare, but there is significant risk that surgeons will make an error during their career. It is not a risk that patients should have to accept and it can be minimized by performing multiple independent verifications. The most important is the pre-operative verification, as the patient is likely to be the most reliable source of accurate information. A structured approach to risk management involving the patient in as many steps as possible should protect both the surgeon and patient from the possibility of wrong-site surgery.

Day case surgery

The great majority of patients would prefer to avoid an overnight stay in hospital if possible. Patient, surgical, anaesthetic, and administrative factors should be considered prior to deciding on the suitability of a case for day surgery. Although the initial definition of day case surgery was surgery that involved no overnight stay, many hospitals now consider a 23-hour admission as a form of day surgery. The UK government aims for >75% of elective surgery to be performed on a day case basis.

Patient factors:

- Medical fitness: patients should be ASA grade I or II (occasional grade III)
- Social circumstances:
  - Patients should have someone to care for them until they are self-caring
  - Patients should live in easy reach of the hospital
  - Patients should have access to a telephone at home

Surgical/anaesthetic factors:

- Pain: procedures that involve significant post-operative pain should not be considered for day surgery
- Transfusion: procedures that have a high risk of requiring a blood transfusion are not suitable for day surgery
- Recovery: patients unlikely to recover from the procedure or anaesthetic in time to be discharged are not suitable for day surgery.

Administrative factors:

- Facilities: a day surgery unit must have sufficient transport, pre-operative assessment, pre- and post-operative ward facilities, operating theatres, recovery areas, sitting accommodation, and reception areas
- Staff: day surgery units should be staffed with teams including consultant surgeons and anaesthetists, nursing, theatre, recovery, and administrative staff. There should be a 24-hour point of contact for patients discharged to avoid reliance on primary care
- Information: both pre-operative and post-operative information should be available to patients to prepare them for their surgery and to address issues that may be encountered on discharge. Patients should be aware of follow-up arrangements prior to discharge

The expansion of minimally invasive techniques and the use of local anaesthetic techniques has facilitated an increase in the use of day case surgery. Careful choice of anaesthetic minimizes the risk of post-operative nausea and vomiting. Multimodal balanced analgesic and anti-emetic regimens allows for faster post-operative recovery. Initially cases of >90 minutes were considered unsuitable for day case surgery, but now even procedures that take >3 hours may be considered.

Pre-operative assessment in the emergency surgical patient

Patients are at higher risk of morbidity and mortality following emergency surgery. Increasing age and ASA grade are associated with higher risks within patients who require emergency procedures. Within the first 100 days after emergency surgery the leading causes of death are malignancy, infection, and cardiac complications.

The needs of patients range from those requiring immediate life-saving intervention to those who require surgery in a matter of hours. Conditions range from acute infections, such as appendicitis, to major trauma following motor vehicle accidents. The situation in which an emergency patient is encountered can vary from the pre-hospital setting, through the emergency department, to the intensive care unit.

The goals of assessment in an emergency are no different from those in an elective setting. Assessment of the airway, chronic disease, medications, and the impact of the presenting illness must all be performed. Details of pre-morbid conditions may be available from the patient, relatives, or previous medical notes. Examination should include an assessment of the airway and cervical spine, cardiorespiratory status, and intravascular volume. Choice of investigation must be tailored to the individual situation.

The complexity of emergency surgery patients and their higher risk of post-operative complications was reflected by the National Confidential Enquiry into Peri-operative Deaths (NCEPOD) report in 2003 that supported higher levels of senior involvement in emergency cases and a move to decrease the number of procedures done out of hours.

Constructing an operating list

Designing an operating list depends on the patients and procedures expected, the time allocated for surgery and the time expected per case, the staff available, and the post-operative recovery facilities. Lists and orders may need to change at short notice depending on emergencies, patient arrival times, and unexpected events.

Competing factors will shape the final order of a daily schedule but certain principles should be kept in mind. Patients with significant comorbidities should be scheduled early in the day. This gives the longest period for recovery and allows post-operative monitoring during working hours, when staff with the highest level of experience are available. Diabetic patients will often be first on the operating list to minimize upset to their treatment regimen. Children should be prioritized as long delays will result in prolonged fasting, which is unkind to the child, and risks losing their cooperation. The uncooperative child presents a challenge to the anaesthetist. Patients with latex allergies should be scheduled first to reduce the chance of exposure to allergens. Provision for operating room cleaning should be made following cases with specific infections (methicillin-resistant *Staphylococcus aureus* (MRSA)/*Clostridium difficile*) so these cases are often done last.

Effective scheduling requires cooperation between the surgeon, anaesthetist, and nurses. Prompt starts, short turnover times, and realistic times for procedures will promote a positive atmosphere, maximize efficiency within the theatre, and minimize the cancellation of elective surgical patients. As a candidate you will be asked to make the order of an operating list which has the following operations: a diabetic foot for amputation (Type 1 diabetes), a sigmoid colectomy, a HIV patient needing laparoscopic cholecystectomy and a MRSA positive patient needing wound debridement.

Scenarios

Scenario 1

An obese 56-year-old woman with a history of hypertension for which she takes beta blockers and diuretics attends for assessment prior to elective laparoscopic cholecystectomy. On examination she has a blood pressure of 135/82. Examination of her mouth reveals her soft palate and base of her uvula. How would you grade this patient's airway and what pre-operative investigations would you request?

Scenario 2

A 62-year-old man with an implantable pacemaker is admitted as an emergency with small bowel obstruction. Following assessment, the decision is made to resuscitate him with IV fluids and take him to theatre the following day during working hours. What precautions should the anaesthetist and surgeon take in dealing with this case?

Scenario 3

A 59-year-old woman with renal failure is being investigated for a malignant mass in the neck. Following her clinic visit, arrangements are made to admit her to hospital for CT scanning and endoscopy with biopsy of a suspicious lesion in the larynx. What specific considerations need to be considered by her admitting team?

Scenario 4

A 40-year-old heavy smoker attends for inguinal hernia repair. How long should he abstain from smoking to reduce his chances of pulmonary morbidity in the post-operative period?

Scenario 5

A 43-year-old man presents for elective right nephrectomy. What measures can you take to prevent wrong-site surgery, and which methods are likely to be most effective?

Answers

Scenario 1

Patients with a BMI >26, a history of snoring, immobility of the neck, an interincisor distance of <4cm, or a significant overbite are at a higher risk of having a difficult airway. This patient is in class II of the Mallampati classification. Although no single assessment is highly sensitive and specific, a number of features in this case suggest that the securing of an airway may be difficult. In the light of this patient's known cardiovascular disease and medications affecting the renal system, an ECG and urea and electrolyte blood sample should be taken. The operation is unlikely to involve significant blood loss so many centres may not routinely order a full blood count. Chest X-ray would not be indicated unless this patient was undergoing cardiovascular surgery or there was a history of intercurrent pulmonary illness.

Scenario 2

In assessing patients with pacemakers, the anaesthetist will review the reason for the patient receiving a pacemaker as well as any related cardiovascular comorbidities. During the pre-optimization period, the device can be checked to assess the battery life, program settings, and need for reprogramming during anaesthesia.

The presence of a pacemaker is not an absolute contraindication to monopolar electrosurgery, but the surgeon should be aware of the device's position and place the current return pad as far from the device as possible. The use of bipolar diathermy is preferred if possible.

Scenario 3

Patients with renal failure are at risk of worsening renal failure due to nephrotoxic medications and contrast. Pre-operative assessment will include electrolytes and a full blood count as well as urinalysis. Contrast-enhanced CT scanning should be avoided as it risks worsening this patient's renal failure. MRI or non-contrast-enhanced CT could be considered instead. Most anaesthetic drugs reduce renal blood flow and so maintaining adequate volume status is important during the peri-operative period. During surgery, patients are at a higher risk of bleeding, and this patient is undergoing biopsy of the airway. Although bleeding is unlikely, the surgeon should be aware of the risk in the peri- and post-operative period.

Scenario 4

All patients should be advised to abstain from smoking in the pre-operative period. The acute effect of nicotine stimulation of the cardiovascular system and ciliary dysfunction improve after about 48 hours, but patients who cease smoking for 2 months prior to surgery lower their rate of pulmonary complications.

Scenario 5

Patients are at higher risk of wrong-site surgery when they present for procedures on bilateral structures such as the kidney. Surgeons are at a 25% career risk of performing wrong-site surgery so precautions are necessary. Pre-operative verification of the procedure, patient, and site are essential. Double checking clinical, radiology, and pathological results prior to a procedure is also important. The site should be marked in permanent ink so that the mark is visible following skin preparation and draping. A time-out prior to surgery should be performed, ensuring that all agree on the patient, site, and procedure. The most important person to involve in the process is the patient as they are likely to have the most accurate information.

Chapter 2 **Anaesthetics**

Contents of this chapter will help the candidate in the applied surgical science and critical—both generic and specialty—stations. In the station of clinical and procedural skills, the candidate should be prepared to explain, for example, the need to insert a central venous pressure (CVP) line or a venous cut-down may be necessary. Methods of post-operative pain relief are essential knowledge.

Grateful acknowledgement is made to Cicely Birkett-Jones for the figures and diagrams in this chapter.

Introduction

In any surgical book, a chapter on anaesthesia is an integral part. In the MRCS OSCE examination, questions pertaining to anaesthetics in the form of regional/local anaesthesia, relief of post-operative pain, and aspects of post-operative complications are often asked. This chapter will give a surgical trainee in the early years of training a comprehensive knowledge of how to look after a critically ill surgical patient with the background knowledge of the relevant physiology.

General anaesthesia

Pre-operative preparation

The aim of pre-operative assessment and preparation is to reduce peri- and post-operative morbidity and mortality. We need to identify and minimize risk, and discuss the balance of risks with the patient. Patients may have significant comorbidities; health and physiology must be optimized. Ideally patients should attend a pre-operative assessment clinic to streamline the process.

Please refer to sections 'Fitness for surgery' and 'Pre-operative management in special circumstances' in Chapter 1 for further discussion.

Fasting

The aim of fasting patients pre-operatively is to prevent vomiting/regurgitation and subsequent aspiration while anaesthetized. In elective surgery, aspiration is a rare event (approximately 1:10,000 cases) and it carries a low risk of mortality. Clinically significant aspiration is more likely to occur in emergency cases.

> **The current UK fasting guidelines are:**
> * 2 hours for clear fluids
> * 6 hours for solids and milky drinks

Despite adequate fasting the stomach will still normally contain a residual volume of 30ml. This is not usually a problem provided lower oesophageal sphincter integrity is maintained. Patients are at risk of regurgitation despite fasting in situations where this barrier is disrupted as occurs with hiatus hernia. Another example is during the second and third trimesters of pregnancy.

There are several factors which significantly decrease gastric emptying. These include:

* Pain
* Trauma
* Labour
* Opiates
* Bowel obstruction
* Acute abdomen

In these situations an empty stomach is never guaranteed and the anaesthetist may use a technique called a rapid sequence induction in order to ensure that the airway remains protected. This is discussed later in the chapter.

There is no benefit in fasting patients for longer than the recommended current guidelines and indeed patients can become significantly fluid depleted after prolonged fasts. Patients should be actively encouraged to keep hydrated with clear fluids up to 2 hours prior to the procedure.

Medication

Medications have the potential to significantly affect anaesthesia and surgery; however, most long-term medication should be continued during the admission, particularly cardiac medications and inhalers. There is evidence that beta blockers in particular should be continued as stopping them pre-operatively may lead to worse outcomes. Drugs that may need to be reviewed include:

* **ACE inhibitors and angiotensin II antagonists:** many anaesthetists will withhold these on the day of surgery as they have the ability to cause resistant hypotension

- **Warfarin:** depending on the indication for use, warfarin may need to be converted to heparin
- **Antiplatelets:** clopidogrel increases the risk of bleeding and needs to be stopped for 7 days pre-operatively if the effects are to be reversed. Clopidogrel is a contraindication to using a regional technique such as a spinal or epidural. It may not be safe to stop antiplatelet agents in patients with recent coronary stent insertions
- **Insulin and oral hypoglycaemics:** refer to local protocols
- **Steroids:** patients on long-term corticosteroids may need peri-operative supplementation due to adrenal axis suppression

As well as continuing usual medications there is the opportunity to prescribe pre-medications. Their use is now less common but may include:

- Anxiolytics
- Analgesics
- Antiemetics
- Antisialogogues

Conditions with specific anaesthetic implications

Information about previous anaesthetics is helpful, particularly with regards to problems experienced. A family history of problems is equally important. Uncommon conditions such as muscle disorders, porphyrias, and sickle cell disease have serious anaesthetic implications but are beyond the scope of this chapter.

Airway problems

Airway problems can generally be divided into two categories:

- Patients that pose a difficulty with mask ventilation (remember OBESE: **O**bese, **B**earded, **E**lderly, **S**norers, **E**dentulous)
- Patients that are difficult to intubate

It is challenging to predict with accuracy which patients are going to have a difficult airway. Most tests have poor sensitivity and specificity.
The causes of a difficult airway can usually be divided into four categories:

- Abnormal dentition
- Jaw: receding mandible, craniofacial abnormalities, facial trauma
- Joints: neck arthritis, temporomandibular joint, cervical spine instability
- Soft tissues: pregnancy, infections and abscesses of the airway, tumours, radiotherapy to the head and neck, burns, thyroid

Cardiovascular disease

Recent myocardial infarction, particularly with complications, is associated with increased risk.
Severe aortic stenosis (AS) causes a fixed cardiac output. Patients may be unable to compensate for changes in peripheral vascular resistance that may occur during anaesthesia, leading to marked hypotension and compromised coronary blood supply. Risk varies based on the severity of AS.
For patients with pacemakers it is important to establish the type and the indication for pacing. Diathermy, particularly unipolar, can interfere with the pacemaker and should be avoided where possible. Any defibrillate function should be turned off and an external pacing/defibrillation device should be readily available.
Isolated hypertension (<180/<110mmHg) is not thought to affect surgical outcome.

Respiratory disease

Poorly controlled asthmatics risk bronchospasm, sputum retention, atelectasis, infection, and respiratory failure during anaesthesia and surgery. The history will give the most information about how well they are managing their asthma, a useful measure is the peak flow test.
Smokers have reduced tissue oxygen delivery, poorer wound healing, and reduced resistance to infection. They are also more likely to have serious comorbidities such as ischaemic heart disease

and emphysema. It is always worthwhile counselling people about smoking cessation as even stopping for 24 hours prior to surgery is beneficial.

- Half-life of carboxyhaemoglobin is 4 hours when breathing air
- Within 12–24 hours the systemic effect of nicotine is greatly reduced
- Within 6–8 weeks ciliary function is restored, and sputum production is significantly reduced
- Immunological function returns to normal after 6 months

Diabetes

Poor chronic glycaemic control and peri-operative hyperglycaemia are both associated with an increased risk of surgical site infection.

Long-term complications of diabetes include:

- Ischaemic heart disease
- Cerebrovascular disease
- Renal impairment
- Peripheral neuropathy
- Autonomic neuropathy (blunted cardiovascular responses and gastroparesis)

Obesity

Obese people pose several challenges for the anaesthetist;

- Moving and positioning
- Gaining venous access or attempting regional techniques
- Difficult airway maintenance
- Reduced lung functional residual capacity and increased oxygen consumption lead to rapid desaturation
- Difficult ventilation, more likely to require intubation
- Altered pharmacokinetics
- Emergence from anaesthesia is prolonged (anaesthetic agents are highly lipid soluble)

Investigations

A thorough history and examination is the mainstay of assessing a person's fitness for surgery and should guide the need for any supplementary tests and investigations. In fit healthy patients, routine pre-operative investigations are rarely indicated as it is uncommon even for abnormal results to cause a change in management. The NICE publication *Preoperative tests: The use of routine preoperative tests for elective surgery* (2003) provides advice on the appropriateness of specific investigations depending on patient age, ASA, and grade of surgery. Most hospitals will have a local policy based on this.

Cardiopulmonary exercise testing

CPEX testing aims to provide a combined assessment of heart and lung function. In patients undergoing major surgery (in particular vascular), CPEX testing can be used to predict poor outcome. The test is carried out by recording ECG activity, oxygen uptake, and carbon dioxide output in patients first at rest and then during graded exercise on a bike. The anaerobic threshold (AT) is a measure of when the patient converts from aerobic to anaerobic metabolism. Fitter patients will have a higher AT and may be at lower risk of complications.

Day case surgery

Day case surgery, when possible, provides many benefits to patients. The UK National Health Service (NHS) is planning to achieve a target of 75% of operative procedures being done on a day surgery basis. The selection of patients suitable for day case surgery is based on social and medical factors (Association of Anaesthetists of Great Britain and Ireland (AAGBI) guidelines: *Day Surgery* (2005)):

Social factors:

- Patient should be willing for procedure to be done as a day case
- A responsible adult should be available to care for the patient at home for at least the first 24 hours

- The patient or their carer should have access to a telephone
- The patients home should be suitable for post-operative care

Medical factors:

- The patient and carer should understand the planned procedure and subsequent post-operative care
- The patient should either be fully fit or have well controlled chronic disease. Fitness should not be determined by arbitrary limits such as age or ASA. For example obesity or diabetes mellitus are not absolute contraindications to day case surgery

Risks of anaesthesia

While specific anaesthesia consent forms are not yet commonplace in the UK, the anaesthetist will have a discussion with the patient about risk and this is usually documented on the anaesthetic chart. Serious adverse effects related directly to anaesthesia are rare; the Royal College of Anaesthesia provides information for patients about risk as shown in the box.

Very common and common side effects

- Nausea and vomiting after surgery
- Sore throat
- Aches, pains, and backache
- Confusion or memory loss

Uncommon side effects and complications

- Chest infection
- Damage to teeth: 1:4500
- Awareness: 1:1000–1:14,000

Rare or very rare complications

- Equipment failure
- Damage to the eyes
- Heart attack or stroke
- Life-threatening anaphylaxis: 1:10,000–1:20,000
- Nerve damage
- Death directly related to anaesthesia 1:250,000

Intra-operative considerations

General anaesthesia is a drug-induced state that comprises loss of consciousness associated with analgesia, amnesia, muscle relaxation, and obtunded autonomic reflexes. It is the primary responsibility of the anaesthetist to maintain optimal physiology.

The first public demonstration of general anaesthesia was on 16 October 1846 at the Massachusetts General Hospital in Boston when William Morton administered ether to Gilbert Abbott. Local anaesthetics were introduced in 1877 and it was not until the 1920s that IV induction agents became available. The first muscle relaxants were introduced in the 1940s.

Conduct of general anaesthesia

Monitoring is established according to guidelines set by the AAGBI:

- Pulse oximetry
- Non-invasive blood pressure (NIBP)
- ECG
- Airway gases; O_2, CO_2, and anaesthetic vapour
- Airway pressure

The following should also be readily available:

- If muscle relaxants are used, a nerve stimulator, used to monitor the degree of muscle relaxation
- A device for measuring the patient's temperature

Flow-based cardiac output monitors (e.g. oesophageal Doppler) may be used to guide fluids and cardiovascular support in major cases.

Other considerations:

- IV access for emergency drugs
- DVT prophylaxis
- Antibiotics for surgical prophylaxis
- Optimal fluid management
- Need for invasive monitoring (e.g. arterial line)

In the UK the anaesthetist is assisted by an operating department assistant (ODP) or trained anaesthetic nurse and they are a vital part of the anaesthesia team. In many departments the anaesthetist may also be assisted by a physicians' assistant in anaesthesia—PA(A)—who can maintain anaesthesia with indirect supervision.

Induction of anaesthesia

The mode of action of anaesthetic agents is not fully understood.

The IV route is the commonest method used for induction as loss of consciousness occurs rapidly within one arm–brain circulation time (30 seconds). Propofol and thiopentone are the two main IV induction agents. Propofol is a standard drug used in day case and elective surgery where patients are adequately fasted as it has several advantages over thiopentone; it obtunds pharyngeal reflexes facilitating the use of laryngeal masks and has less of a hangover effect. Thiopentone is the classical drug for use during rapid sequence inductions as it has a more predictable and dependable onset of effect.

The inhalational route is primarily used in two situations:

- When establishing IV access prior to induction is either not possible or undesirable, i.e. with small children, needle-phobics, or IV drug users
- In situations where the airway may be difficult (spontaneous ventilation is maintained)

Sevoflurane, an anaesthetic vapour is usually used as it is non-irritant and does not have a strong unpleasant smell. The onset of anaesthesia is much slower with this route and the patient may be seen to pass through the stages of anaesthesia (described by Guedel in 1937); an initial disorientated phase, then a period of excited delirious activity before finally losing consciousness.

Ketamine can be used as an intramuscular (IM) or IV anaesthetic agent. In contrast to the other agents it has a stimulatory effect on the cardiovascular system and preserves protective airway reflexes and tone—this is valuable in battlefield situations. It may also be useful in the management of chronic pain; the main drawbacks are hallucinations, vivid dreams, and nightmares.

Rapid sequence induction

Used in patients who are at risk of regurgitation.

The patient breathes 100% oxygen from a tight-fitting facemask for at least 3 minutes. Drugs with rapid onset of anaesthesia and muscle paralysis (thiopentone + suxamethonium) are used. As the patient loses consciousness, cricoid pressure is applied to occlude the oesophagus and prevent regurgitation. Once the patient is intubated the case can proceed; however, if intubation proves impossible the relatively rapid offset of both drugs means that the patient will regain consciousness and protective airway reflexes as quickly as possible.

Muscle relaxation

Muscle relaxants can be administered for several reasons:

- Anaesthetic: facilitate intubation and ventilation, prevent coughing
- Surgical: prevent unanticipated movements in delicate surgery, surgical access

There are two main kinds of muscle relaxant; depolarizing (suxamethonium) and non-depolarizing (e.g. atracurium, vecuronium, rocuronium, and pancuronium) and they exert their effect by blocking transmission at the neuromuscular junction. Muscle relaxants have varying times to recovery and non-depolarizing drugs can be reversed from certain levels of block.

Suxamethonium apnoea

Suxamethonium is metabolized by plasma cholinesterase and its duration of effect is normally around 5 minutes. A small proportion (6%) of patients have genetic abnormalities of the cholinesterase enzyme that can lead to a prolonged duration of action of up to 8 hours. A first presentation will require the patient to be sedated and ventilated until the effects of the drug wear off. Genetic testing of family members should then be arranged and the patient may carry a MedicAlert bracelet.

Maintenance of anaesthesia

If no further drugs are administered following induction the patient will usually regain consciousness after 5–10 minutes as anaesthetic vapours are exhaled and IV agents are redistributed from their site of action. If a long-acting muscle relaxant has been given anaesthesia must continue. Anaesthesia can be maintained using an inhaled agent or an IV infusion (e.g. propofol). The main inhaled volatile agents are: sevoflurane, isoflurane, desflurane (and halothane less commonly). Nitrous oxide (N_2O) is anaesthetic and analgesic and can be used in combination with any of the above. This allows less volatile agent to be used resulting in faster emergence post-operatively.

- **Facemask:** can be used to maintain the airway either with spontaneous or hand ventilation, for longer cases it may be inconvenient
- **Laryngeal mask airway (LMA):** easy to use, muscle relaxants not required, less invasive than an endotracheal tube but does not protect against aspiration. The LMA has revolutionized difficult airway management as it may provide a patent airway in situations where intubation has failed
- **Endotracheal tube (ETT):** protects airway against aspiration, also used where access to the airway during surgery is difficult. Many different types are available; oral, nasal, cuffed, un-cuffed, reinforced, double-lumen, tracheostomy… the list goes on

---

Malignant hyperthermia (MH)

Very rare condition, often inherited, 10% mortality.

Triggers

Inhaled anaesthetic agents (not N_2O) and suxamethonium cause sustained activation of an abnormal ryanodine receptor in muscle. This leads to excess calcium release and greatly increased metabolic activity causing increased CO_2, heat and lactic acid production with sympathetic activation and acidosis.

Management

- Stop trigger agents
- Finish surgery quickly
- Dantrolene IV is the specific treatment
- Active cooling
- Treat effects of MH: hypoxia, ↑K^+, ↑H^+, arrhythmias, DIC, myoglobinaemia
- Transfer to Intensive Care Unit (ICU) post-operatively
- Counsel family about genetic testing

Depth of anaesthesia

Awareness under anaesthesia comprises a wide spectrum of situations. It ranges from a vague memory of speaking or noise to full recollection with pain. Most cases of awareness have occurred in patients who received muscle relaxants.

The anaesthetic effect of inhaled agents depends on brain concentration. The expired concentration (similar to alveolar concentration) is roughly equal to brain concentration at equilibrium. The minimum alveolar concentration (MAC) is the concentration of a particular agent that will prevent movement in response to a skin incision in 50% of anaesthetized patients. Several factors influence the amount of anaesthetic required.

- Decrease: increasing age, hypothermia, hypothyroidism, concomitant opioid and/or sedative administration
- Increase: pregnancy, long-term alcohol or opioid use, pyrexia, sympathetic stimulation (e.g. pain, anxiety)

It follows that the anaesthetist will have to titrate the dose of anaesthetic against the amount of stimulation that a patient is being subjected to. Without stimulation a patient requires very little anaesthetic to remain unconscious; the response to a sudden painful stimulus in this situation could be reflex movements, laryngospasm, or waking up. Good communication between the surgeon and anaesthetist is therefore vital to prevent mishap e.g. prior to skin incision.

The main way of monitoring depth of anaesthesia is by looking at expired anaesthetic concentration (in relation to MAC) and the level of sympathetic activity: blood pressure, heart rate, pupillary dilatation, and lacrimation. In some situations it may also be appropriate to use depth of anaesthesia monitors. These generally rely on continuous analysis of parts of the EEG obtained from scalp electrodes and can give an indication of depth of anaesthesia.

Temperature management

The NICE guideline on peri-operative hypothermia defines hypothermia as a core temperature of <36°C. Hypothermic patients undergoing surgery are at increased risk of cardiac complications, surgical site infections, and blood loss.
Heat loss:

- 40% radiation
- 30% convection
- 20% evaporation
- 10% respiration

Anaesthetized patients cannot compensate for this heat loss by shivering and in addition anaesthetic agents cause vasodilatation which transfers heat from the core to the peripheries. The patient should be normothermic upon arrival in the anaesthetic room. Radiation and convection losses can be reduced by blankets and forced air warmers while heat loss from respiration is trapped by a heat and moisture exchange device (HME) situated in the breathing circuit. In addition, IV and irrigation fluids can be warmed.

Positioning and nerve injury

Careful positioning of anaesthetized patients is essential in order to avoid injury (e.g. nerve, ocular) while still allowing adequate surgical access. All hard edges should be padded, eyes should be taped and protected from pressure, and the patient should be positioned so that joints remain in neutral positions.

Nerve injury can be due to stretching, direct pressure, hypoperfusion injuries from tourniquets, needle trauma during conduct of a regional anaesthetic, and from the surgical procedure itself. It is often impossible to determine the exact cause of a nerve injury post-operatively. This highlights the importance of documenting any pre-existing neurological deficits.

Certain positions also create other difficulties: the prone position makes access to the airway difficult, head-up positions can compromise brain perfusion and risk air embolus. Patient ventilation, both spontaneous and controlled, is mainly dependent on free diaphragmatic movement. Diaphragmatic movement is impaired in situations where intra-abdominal pressure is increased or when abdominal contents are pushed against the diaphragm (splinting). This often occurs in obese patients, in patients who are head down, in pregnancy, during laparoscopic surgery, and in prone patients if the abdomen is not allowed to move freely. Problems can occur if airway pressures become significantly raised and ventilation becomes inadequate.

Raised intra-abdominal pressure can also cause compression of the vena cava and impair venous return. Impaired venous return via Starlings mechanism of the heart will reduce cardiac output and may cause severe hypotension. This is the reason for using the left lateral tilt in pregnant patients.

Autonomic reflexes

Certain actions can precipitate marked bradycardia with hypotension or asystole especially in children and young females. It is often a vagally mediated reflex. Examples include:

- Oculo-cardiac reflex—pulling on ocular muscles during squint surgery
- Peritoneal stretching
- Cervical or anal dilation

Post-operative considerations

The recovery period following anaesthesia can be divided into three stages:

- 1st stage: until patient is awake, orientated with protective reflexes, and pain is controlled
- 2nd stage: until patient is ready for discharge from hospital
- Late stage: may take weeks for physiological and psychological recovery

Following surgery, critically ill patients are often transferred directly from theatre to the ICU. During the 1st stage of recovery all other patients should be managed in a designated area within the theatre complex. They should be cared for by trained staff on a one-to-one basis and appropriate monitoring should be continued. They often require oxygen to compensate for hypoventilation. Discharge from the recovery unit is only appropriate once the following criteria are met (AAGBI: *Immediate Postanaesthetic Recovery* (2002)):

- The patient is fully conscious and maintaining own airway
- Respirations and oxygenation are satisfactory
- The cardiovascular system is stable
- Pain and nausea are controlled
- Temperature is within acceptable limits
- Oxygen and IV therapy is prescribed where appropriate

Four levels of post-operative care are available to patients depending on nature of surgery and clinical condition;

- Level 0: normal ward care
- Level 1: acute care (ward area with critical care support)
- Level 2: HDU care (requiring continuous monitoring and/or organ support, one-to-two nursing)
- Level 3: ICU care (invasive respiratory or multi-organ support, one-to-one or higher nursing)

Discharge criteria for day case surgery

Following discharge from recovery most patients will be managed in a ward setting. They should be reviewed by the anaesthetist and surgeon prior to discharge from hospital and given clear advice about potential problems and a point of contact. Written information for general practitioners (GPs) and district nurses should be available regarding dressings, sutures, further reviews/investigations, etc. The patient should be able to eat and drink, stand and walk unaided, and have voided urine. The discharge prescription should include analgesia and antiemetics as appropriate.

Regional anaesthesia

This involves providing anaesthesia for a specific anatomical area and may be either central (spinal/epidural) or peripheral. Pre-operative management and intraoperative monitoring follow similar standards as for general anaesthesia.

Central neuraxial regional anaesthesia

Access for local anaesthetic to the spinal cord can be gained directly via cerebral spinal fluid (CSF), a spinal or indirectly by diffusion and nerve roots, an epidural (Fig. 2.1). The procedure is usually performed in the awake patient to reduce the risk of intraneural and intravascular injection and to allow assessment of block adequacy. The patient is positioned either sitting or lateral, and the procedure performed with full asepsis and local anaesthetic to skin. For a spinal, a needle is passed into the CSF space. Smaller diameter, non-cutting type needles reduce the incidence of post dural puncture headache. For an epidural, a loss of resistance technique is used to identify the epidural space and then a fine bore multi-hole catheter is fed into the space. Spinal anaesthesia has rapid onset (5–15 minutes) and short duration (1.5–2.5 hours) of anaesthesia. Epidural anaesthesia has a slightly slower onset time but the duration of anaesthesia is similar following bolus administration. The benefit of using an epidural catheter is the ability to give further boluses or run infusions of local anaesthetic for analgesia. Adding a low dose of opiate to the mixture can prolong the analgesia and has a synergistic action on anaesthesia (e.g. diamorphine 300mcg spinally or 3mg epidurally). The block (tested to cold sensation) should stretch to cover the dermatomes affected by surgery. Regional techniques may offer advantages in patients with severe respiratory disease in addition to the analgesia. Spinal and epidurals are generally avoided in patients with sepsis, coagulopathies, and thrombocytopenia.

A poorly working epidural may be worse than an alternative analgesic approach.

Complications of central neuraxial anaesthesia:

- Drug errors (epidural infusions should use unique equipment and top-ups must be by trained staff only)
- Opiate side effects (itch, nausea, urinary retention, respiratory depression—may be delayed)
- Failure of block or missed dermatome (more likely with epidurals)
- Hypotension (due to sympathetic block causing vasodilatation)
- Post-dural puncture headache (delayed, severe, persistent, and postural headache that can lead to further complications including subdural haematoma)
- Local anaesthetic toxicity (unlikely with spinal due to lower dose)
- Unanticipated high block (above T4 dermatome) resulting in respiratory and cardiovascular compromise with unconsciousness if level reaches brainstem
- Direct nerve damage

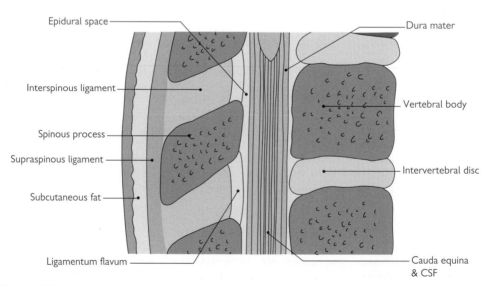

Figure 2.1 Sagittal cross section of the lumbar spine. With permission from Cicely Birkett-Jones.

- Central infection (meningitis or epidural abscess)
- Central haematoma with cord or nerve root compression

Peripheral regional anaesthesia

Specifically blocking peripheral nerves with local anaesthetic is useful when the surgery is anatomically defined (e.g. total knee replacement). The nerve can be localized with anatomy, electrical nerve stimulation, and /or ultrasound. Care is taken to avoid intraneural injection with the patient preferably awake to site the block. Local anaesthetic is administered in divided doses with intermittent aspiration to minimize risk of intravascular injection. The block may be used for one-off analgesia or a catheter may be inserted to allow continuous infusion and/or subsequent boluses. A low concentration with high volume of local anaesthetic is generally preferred to minimize motor block and maximize spread.

Examples of peripheral nerve blocks:

- Brachial plexus: interscalene approach in the neck for shoulder surgery, axillary approach for hand surgery
- Femoral: for surgery on the anterior knee
- Combined: e.g. femoral and sciatic for surgery on the ankle

---

Intravenous regional anaesthesia: Bier's block

Useful for surgery of the forearm and hand which is of short duration (e.g. manipulation of fractures).

Patients should be fully assessed pre-op and fasted.

Once ECG, NIBP, and pulse oximetry monitoring is established, IV access should be gained in both hands. A double cuffed tourniquet is then placed around the upper arm which is exsanguinated by elevation prior to cuff inflation. The cuff should be inflated to >50mmHg above systolic blood pressure (BP). Local anaesthetic is then injected into the cuffed arm (e.g. lignocaine 3mg.kg^{-1}/prilocaine 6mg.kg^{-1}). Surgical anaesthesia occurs in 5–15 minutes as local anaesthetic diffuses into the tissues and nerves.

Problems:

- Cuff discomfort can be alleviated by using the proximal cuff initially and then the distal one once the block is working
- Entonox can be added in cases where anaesthesia is insufficient

Once the procedure is complete and a minimum of 20 minutes has elapsed since injection of anaesthetic, the cuff(s) can be deflated. At this point the operator must be vigilant for signs of local anaesthetic toxicity and monitoring should continue.

Care of patients following spinal anaesthesia

Following uneventful spinal anaesthesia, the block would be expected to begin to recede at around 2 hours. Protection of the lower limbs, including joint positioning should be observed for the duration of sensory and motor block. **Motor power usually returns after sensation and proprioception is often impaired for the longest and so mobilization must be cautious even when full motor power is present.** It is important to check that full motor and sensory functions return and the patient must be able to pass urine. **Anticoagulant medications should not be given within 4 hours of administering the spinal.** If there has been a 'bloody tap' (blood staining of CSF indicates vessel trauma) then the case should be discussed with the anaesthetist before giving these medications. This is to reduce the risk of spinal haematoma development, classical symptoms of which are severe back and radicular pain.

Care of patients with epidural analgesia

Similar precautions must be taken regarding lower limb protection and spinal haematoma formation. Anticoagulant medication should not be administered within 4 hours after insertion, removal, or repositioning of an epidural catheter. The catheter should not be repositioned or removed until 12 hours after prophylactic dose low-molecular-weight heparin. Patients will usually have continuous infusions of local anaesthetic (often with an opiate) post-operatively for analgesia and they should be monitored in terms of BP/heart rate (HR)/respiratory rate (RR)/SpO$_2$/block height/pain score.

Patients in pain with an epidural infusion should be discussed with acute pain staff. They may require additional bolus top-up analgesia, addition of systemic analgesia, or repositioning/re-siting the epidural.

It would be unusual for an epidural infusion (without recent additional top-up) to cause acute hypotension and therefore another cause should be sought. Low-dose epidural infusions should not produce profound motor block (this may indicate a misplaced catheter into the CSF or an expanding epidural haematoma) and this must be reported to anaesthetic staff immediately.

Sedation

Conscious sedation means that verbal contact is maintained with the patient. The patient should be assessed and fasted as for general anaesthesia. In addition to the surgical operator, there should be a separate sedation trained person to administer the sedation and monitor the patient.

Risks of sedating a patient:

- Airway obstruction
- Respiratory depression
- Confusion and agitation
- Gastric regurgitation
- Hypotension

The secret to safe sedation is careful titration and prompt access to help in the event of an emergency. Examples:

- Midazolam bolus: $0.1mg.kg^{-1}$ starting with 1–2mg for an adult (rapid onset, minimal respiratory depression, may be reversed with flumazenil)
- Morphine: $0.1mg.kg^{-1}$ starting with 1–2mg for an adult (can be used alongside sedation for analgesia although caution as increased risk of respiratory depression)
- Propofol infusion or bolus (narrow therapeutic index between respiratory depression and sedation, suppresses airway reflexes and therefore not recommended outside experienced use)

Local anaesthesia

Mode of action of local anaesthetics

Neurons are specialized cells that transmit electrical signals (Fig. 2.2). Propagation of the electrical signal along the axon is dependent on voltage-gated sodium (Na^+) channels. At the ends of the nerve where the synapses are, transmission is via neurotransmitters. Conduction is fastest along large, myelinated nerves.

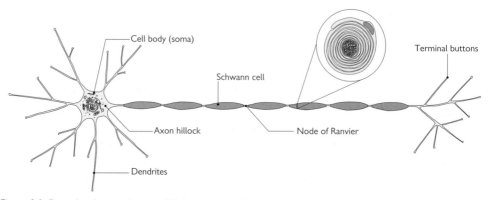

Figure 2.2 Example of a typical neuron. With permission from Cicely Birkett-Jones.

Local anaesthetics reversibly inhibit neuronal transmission by blocking Na^+ channels in the cell membrane. The Na^+ channels are blocked from within the nerve cell and therefore the anaesthetic needs to diffuse across the cell membrane in order to exert its effect (Fig. 2.3).

Local anaesthetics are weak bases. Onset of action depends on the amount of ionization of the local anaesthetic molecules. Cell membranes are impermeable to the ionized form and therefore a local anaesthetic which is highly ionized at physiological pH will take longer to diffuse into the neuron. The degree of ionization is dependent on the pH of the environment (7.4 for blood), and on the specific dissociation constant (pKa) of the local anaesthetic. The relationship between pH, pKa, and ionization can be expressed using the Henderson–Hasselbach equation;

$$pH = pKa + log\ [unionized\ form]/[ionized\ form]$$

For example, bupivacaine (pKa 8.1) is only 17% unionized at physiological pH and thus has a slow onset of action. Lignocaine on the other hand (pKa 7.9) is 25% unionized and is thus faster in onset. In acidic environments (e.g. abscesses, necrotic/infected tissue), an even smaller proportion of the drug will be in the unionized state. Local anaesthetics should therefore be administered away from these sites as they will have a minimal effect.

There are two categories of local anaesthetics based on structure: amides and esters:

- **Amides** include lignocaine, bupivacaine, ropivacaine, and prilocaine and are metabolized slowly in the liver by amidases
- **Esters** include procaine, amethocaine, and cocaine. All are rapidly metabolized in the plasma by esterases, apart from cocaine which is metabolized by the liver. One of the breakdown products is para-amino-benzoate (PABA) a compound that can trigger allergic reactions

Duration of action is determined by the degree of protein binding, rate of removal from the site of action, and total dose (Table 2.1). In highly vascular tissues the anaesthetic is rapidly transported away. Addition of vasoconstrictors (adrenaline 1:200,000 or felypressin) to the mixture reduces removal and

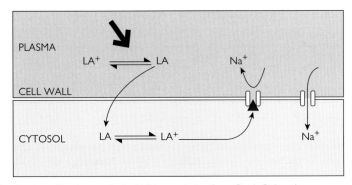

Figure 2.3 Mode of action of local anaesthetics. With permission from Cicely Birkett-Jones.

Table 2.1 Pharmacological properties of various local anaesthetics

Local anaesthetic	Onset	Duration of action	Maximum dose without vasoconstrictor	Maximum dose with vasoconstrictor
Lignocaine	Fast	Moderate	$3mg.kg^{-1}$	$7mg.kg^{-1}$
Bupivacaine	Moderate	Long	$2mg.kg^{-1}$	$2mg.kg^{-1}$
Ropivacaine	Moderate	Long	$2–3mg.kg^{-1}$	$2–3mg.kg^{-1}$
Prilocaine	Fast	Moderate	$6mg.kg^{-1}$	$8mg.kg^{-1}$
Amethocaine	Slow	Long		

prolongs action. Cocaine has intrinsic vasoconstrictive properties, and is used as a spray in ear, nose, and throat (ENT) surgery in order to provide a bloodless field; Moffat's solution. Local anaesthetic solutions containing vasoconstrictors should not be administered to tissues with an end arterial supply as ischaemia and necrosis may occur.

Lignocaine

Lignocaine is available as 0.5%, 1%, and 2% solutions with or without adrenaline (1:80,000 or 1:200,000). It is also available for topical use as a 2% gel, a 4% solution, a 5% ointment, and as a spray delivering 10mg per dose.

EMLA

EMLA stands for eutectic mixture of local anaesthetic and contains 2.5% lignocaine and 2.5% prilocaine in oil:water emulsion. The eutectic mixture allows the local anaesthetic in EMLA to remain in the non-ionized state allowing rapid absorption. EMLA should be applied under an occlusive dressing for 1–2 hours and will then provide topical anaesthesia for about 2 hours. It should not generally be applied to mucous membranes, the exception being genital mucosa where application for 15 minutes will yield 10–15 minutes of topical anaesthesia. EMLA will initially cause vasoconstriction followed by vasodilatation and may also cause local skin reactions. A breakdown product of prilocaine is o-toluidine which can cause methaemoglobinaemia. Rare cases of clinically significant methaemoglobinaemia have been reported in children.

Amethocaine

Amethocaine is available as 0.5% and 1% drops and also as a 4% gel. It has an advantage over EMLA in that a 30–45-minute application will provide anaesthesia for 4–6 hours.

Bupivacaine and levobupivacaine

Bupivacaine is available in 0.25% and 0.5% solutions. Co-administration of adrenaline does not influence the maximum safe dose. It has an increased potential for cardiac toxicity due to its high affinity for cardiac sodium channels. This has lead to the development of levobupivacaine, an enantiopure preparation of the S-isomer of bupivacaine which is less cardiotoxic. Levobupivacaine is available as 0.25%, 0.5%, and 0.75% solutions.

> **Converting from % concentration to mg.ml^{-1}**
>
> Remember: simply move the decimal point one digit to the right.
>
> For example, 1% lignocaine = 10mg.ml^{-1}.

Toxicity

If local anaesthetics enter the systemic circulation in sufficient concentrations they can affect Na+ channels in the heart and central nervous system (CNS). Whether these toxic effects will manifest themselves depends on the peak plasma concentration of local anaesthetic. Factors that influence the peak plasma concentration include:

- Vascularity of administration site
- Total dose of local anaesthetic
- Co-administration of adrenaline

The maximum recommended doses in Table 2.1 refer to local anaesthetic given subcutaneously or for peripheral nerve blocks. If inadvertently administered intravascularly, severe toxicity would occur at much lower doses. Aspirating prior to injection and after every few millilitres is therefore crucial.

Signs of toxicity

- **Mild:** light headedness, circumoral numbness, abnormal taste, tinnitus, confusion, drowsiness
- **Severe:** bradycardia, hypotension, muscle twitching, convulsions, loss of consciousness, respiratory arrest, ventricular fibrillation/tachycardia, asystole

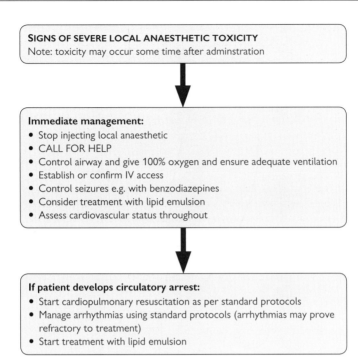

Figure 2.4 Signs of severe local anaesthetic toxicity.

Treatment of toxicity

Potentially cardiotoxic doses of local anaesthetic should only be administered in a monitored patient with IV access established. Resuscitation equipment should be immediately available. The AAGBI guidelines for the treatment of severe local anaesthetic toxicity are summarized in Fig. 2.4.

Intralipid

Intralipid 20% is a lipid emulsion indicated for treatment of local anaesthetic toxicity. The mechanism of action is unclear but it may act by binding lipophilic local anaesthetic molecules and thus removing them from the sodium channels.

1 Administer a bolus of 1.5ml.kg^{-1} and continue cardiopulmonary resuscitation (CPR)
2 Start an infusion at $15\text{ml.kg}^{-1}.\text{h}^{-1}$
3 The bolus can be repeated a further two times with 5-minute intervals
4 Double rate of infusion at any time after 5 minutes if an adequate circulation is not restored

Pain relief

Physiology of pain

Pain can be defined as an unpleasant sensory and emotional experience associated with actual or potential tissue damage. Inadequate management of pain can lead to impaired cough resulting in sputum retention, reduced mobility, and increased sympathetic tone with resultant increased myocardial oxygen demand and delayed gastric emptying.

The pain receptor is called the nociceptor, and responds to heat, mechanical, and/or chemical stimuli. Pain impulses are then transmitted to the dorsal horn of the spinal cord via either Aδ or C-fibres (Fig. 2.5).

- Aδ fibres:
  - Fast conduction ($12–30\text{m.s}^{-1}$ myelinated), 2–5µm diameter
  - Sharp, localized pain

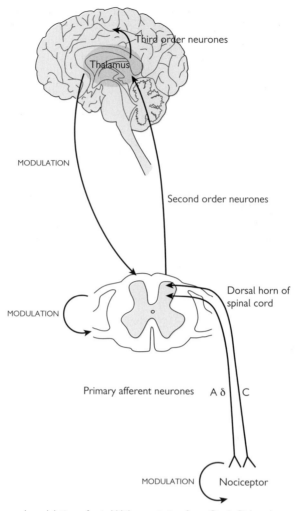

Figure 2.5 The pathways and modulation of pain. With permission from Cicely Birkett-Jones.

- C fibres:
  - Slow conduction (0.5–2m.s^{-1} unmyelinated), 0.4–1.2μm diameter
  - Dull, diffuse pain

Second-order neurons project up to the thalamus, reticular formation, nucleus raphe magnus and the periaqueductal grey area. Most of these fibres cross the midline to the contralateral side at spinal level and ascend as the spinothalamic tracts. This includes the medial spinothalamic tract which mediates the autonomic and emotional aspects of pain. Third-order neurons continue the transmission from the thalamus to the somatosensory cortex.

The perception of pain is modulated at different sites along this pathway. This allows us to target different parts of the pathway to manage pain.

Peripheral: nociceptors become sensitized following repeated stimulation; this is due to inflammatory mediators (e.g. histamine, bradykinin, prostaglandin, and leukotrienes). Sensitized nociceptors have a reduced threshold and increased frequency of firing with ectopic discharges.

There may be development of cross-talk between either sympathetic or Aβ fibres (normally fine touch sensation) and nociceptive fibres. This can result in normally non-painful stimuli being experienced as pain (allodynia).

Central: there is normally a degree of descending inhibition from the higher centres to spinal cord level (serotonin and noradrenaline-α_2 synapses). Local spinal inhibitory neurons also exist to reduce pain impulses (gamma-amino butyric acid (GABA) and glycine synapses), whereas sensitization at spinal level occurs due to N-methyl-D-aspartic acid (NMDA). NMDA mediated 'wind up' of transmission causes a continuing pain stimulus to elicit increasing pain impulses.

These complex processes may persist after the injury has healed thus leading to chronic pain.

> Chronic post surgical pain is an increasingly recognized problem. Risk factors for its development include pre-operative pain, longer duration of surgery, adjuvant chemotherapy/radiotherapy, and severity of post-operative pain.

Assessment of pain

Pain is a subjective experience and is simply what the patient says it is. Scales for assessment at the bedside vary between institutions but examples are shown here. Whichever scale is used, changes in the score are more important than absolute numbers. There should also be a target score that triggers intervention. Post-operative mobilization and physiotherapy requires effective pain control.

Verbal rating scale

Patient states a severity and it is scored 0 to 3

No pain   = 0
Mild pain   = 1
Moderate pain = 2
Severe pain   = 3

Numerical rating scale

Patient rates pain as a number between 0 (no pain) and 10 (worst ever pain).

Pain pharmacology

Paracetamol

The mechanism of action is not fully understood. It is generally a safe and effective analgesic when combined with other systemic analgesia and has relatively few contraindications. The bolus dose is 1000mg up to a maximum of 4000mg per day (or 15mg.kg^{-1} and maximum 60mg.kg^{-1} per day in patients <50kg). Hepatic toxicity can develop due to accumulation of the metabolic intermediate N-acetyl-p-benzo-quinoneimine (NAPQI) and it is therefore important to use the weight corrected dose with reduction or avoidance when there is underlying hepatic impairment (e.g. alcohol use).

Non-steroidal anti-inflammatory drugs (NSAIDs)

NSAIDs all act by inhibiting cyclo-oxygenase (COX) enzyme which under normal circumstances is responsible for production of prostaglandins and thromboxane from arachidonic acid. Prostaglandins are involved in pain and inflammation. Side effects of NSAIDs include renal impairment and fluid retention, gastric erosion, bronchospasm in susceptible patients (around 20% of asthmatics), and reduced platelet function. Newer NSAIDs that preferentially target the COX-2 isoenzyme (inducible form) may have a reduced effect on gastric mucosa but are associated with increased risk of thrombotic events.

> NSAIDs must therefore be used with caution or are contraindicated in renal failure, hypovolaemia, heart failure, active peptic ulcer disease, asthmatics sensitive to NSAIDs, and anticoagulated patients.

Opiates

The main site of analgesic action is at µ-opiate receptors found centrally and peripherally. Opiates can be administered orally, topically, subcutaneously, intramuscularly, intravenously, and via the intrathecal or epidural routes. The key to effective analgesia is dose titration. A reasonable starting dose of morphine for acute severe pain would be 0.1mg.kg^{-1} IV (e.g. 5–10mg for an adult) administered in divided doses over 5–15 minutes. Patients on long-term opiates will require a basal amount of opiate in addition, if in doubt contact the acute pain team.

Side effects are generally dose related and include pruritus, nausea, constipation, respiratory depression, urinary retention, hallucination, and sedation. **Overdose can be treated with the antagonist naloxone, usually in an initial dose of 400mcg IV (or IM).** Remember that the effects of naloxone only last for 20–30 minutes and this may well be shorter than the opiate that has been given (so there is a risk of rebound respiratory depression). An IM dose given concurrently with the IV dose prolongs the duration of reversal but close monitoring is still needed. Other opiate side effects such as pruritus and constipation may respond to low-dose naloxone without compromising analgesia. Morphine is metabolized to an active compound (morphine-6-glucuronide) which is renally excreted and therefore toxicity may occur in renal impairment.

> Morphine 10mg PO = oxycodone 5mg PO = morphine 3mg IV
>
> Fentanyl 25mcg.h^{-1} patch = morphine 60–90mg PO in 24 hours

Strong opiates are increasingly being administered via the oral route when it is available. The regimen consists of a sustained release preparation for background analgesia, combined with an immediate release preparation at a dose of around 1/4 to 1/6 of the 24-hour dose for breakthrough pain.

Codeine phosphate is a weak opiate and its effects are believed to be due to metabolism to morphine by the cytochrome P450 enzymes (CYP2D6). Some individuals with reduced CYP2D6 activity may not get adequate analgesia. Conversely, there are case reports of 'ultrarapid CYP2D6 metabolism' whereby opiate toxicity can occur with standard doses of codeine.

Tramadol is another weak opiate but also exerts its effect via modulation of serotonin and nora-drenaline neurotransmitter conduction.

Others

Nitrous oxide with oxygen (e.g. Entonox 50%) can be useful for short-term procedural pain. It has a rapid onset and offset but is relatively contraindicated in cases where it can rapidly diffuse into a confined air-space (pneumothorax, chronic obstructive pulmonary disease (COPD) with bullae, bowel obstruction, head or maxillofacial trauma) and should not be used more frequently than every 4 days (MHRA advice) due to inactivation of vitamin B12 and subsequent neurological and haematological toxic effects.

Ketamine is an NMDA receptor antagonist. It may be a useful adjunct for analgesia, sedation, or general anaesthesia via oral, IM, or IV routes.

Some analgesics may be given topically in the form of patches. The effects are systemic and the advantage is long duration of action (>24 hours with one patch). It takes time to reach the analgesic level (e.g. around 12 hours for fentanyl) and offset is even more prolonged after removal of patch. Drug delivery is dependent on local blood flow.

Management of pain

A good starting point is the World Health Organization (WHO) analgesic ladder (see Fig. 2.6). This concept emphasizes the fact that there is a ceiling effect to analgesic drugs and once ineffective, the next step should be taken. In general, non-opiates can be continued throughout whereas strong opiates usually replace weak opiates although this is not a rule.

Bearing this in mind, adequate post-operative pain management is often via a multimodal approach. This may include local or regional techniques (with or without centrally acting opiates), combined with systemic analgesia. Combining different analgesics and the use of non-opiate analgesics has greater efficacy as shown by Table 2.2.

Patient controlled analgesia (PCA)

A specialized syringe pump with pre-programmed variables allows the patient to safely self-administer analgesia.

- Bolus dose: set for intensity of pain
- Lockout period: to prevent overdose and should reflect onset time of the drug

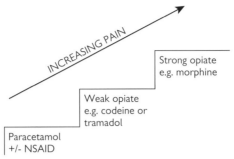

Figure 2.6 The WHO analgesic ladder. With permission from the World Health Organization: http://www.who.int/cancer/palliative/painladder/en/.

Table 2.2 Excerpt from the Oxford league table of analgesics in acute pain

Drug	NNT*
Diclofenac 100mg	1.8
Paracetamol 1g + codeine 60mg	2.2
Ibuprofen 400mg	2.5
Morphine 10mg (IM)	2.9
Paracetamol 1g	3.8
Tramadol 100mg	4.8
Codeine 60mg	16.7

*NNT (number needed to treat): number of patients who need to be treated to get 50% or greater improvement in pain, compared with placebo.

- Background infusion: useful to prevent breakthrough pain during sleep or compensate for long-term opiate use but can cause more side effects

A common example of morphine PCA for an adult would be a 1-mg bolus with 5-minute lockout and 1–2mg.h^{-1} background if required. For paediatric patients up to 50kg, 1mg.kg^{-1} of morphine can be diluted to 50ml and bolus set for 1ml (20mcg.kg^{-1}).

Patients must be monitored clinically while receiving opiate PCA, particularly respiratory rate and sedation levels. There must be a dedicated IV line with antisiphon and antireflux valves and usually a continuous infusion of fluid to ensure patency. Only the patient should administer the bolus as this is part of the safety aspect of PCA. Supplementary oxygen should be administered to compensate for hypoventilation and anti-emetic medication should be prescribed. **PCA is effective only once the patient has had analgesia titrated up to control their baseline level of pain.** A patient with a PCA and ongoing pain should be reviewed in case a change to PCA settings after reloading with analgesia is required, or alternatively a progressive cause for pain has developed (e.g. compartment syndrome, anastomotic leak). PCA can be used outside the post-operative setting, e.g. acute pancreatitis, pre-operative trauma patients, sickle cell crises (especially in paediatrics).

Non-pharmacological analgesia

- Splinting fracture
- Covering wound or burn
- Relaxation techniques—emotional state has profound effects on overall pain perception.
- Cold packs
- Heat packs
- Transcutaneous electrical nerve stimulation (TENS)
- Acupuncture

Analgesia in palliative care

The WHO analgesic ladder was developed specifically for cancer pain management. Immediate release analgesia is usually titrated to effect and then converted to a 24-hour sustained release dose with break-through doses as described earlier. In this situation, patients often become less prone to respiratory depression and nausea but constipation and hallucination can become problematic. Neuropathic pain components are often present in palliative patients and advice should be sought about the use of anti-neuropathic atypical analgesics (e.g. low-dose tricyclic antidepressants, gabapentin, and other anticonvulsants). Bone pain may improve specifically with NSAIDs and bisphosphonates (reduction in osteoclast activity). Corticosteroids reduce tissue oedema and inflammation and can improve pain experience overall.

Scenarios

Scenario 1

Situation

You are on your surgical ward assessing a 54-year-old woman for whom a laparoscopic cholecystectomy is planned for later today.

Background

She was admitted with right upper quadrant pain, nausea, and vomiting 2 days ago and her pain has now improved. Gallstones are confirmed on ultrasound and there are no signs of biliary obstruction or other complications of acute cholecystitis. Her BMI is 43 and she admits that the control of her diabetes is not good; her blood sugar is never below 11mmol.L^{-1} even after fasting.

Assessment

• What additional information do you need about her health and fitness?

Recommendation

• Should this lady proceed to surgery today?

Discussion

This lady has significant comorbidities: obesity and diabetes. You need to find out more about complications related to these to have a discussion about risk of proceeding with surgery now, versus benefit and risk of performing surgery at a later date.

You will need to get more history and organize other investigations to look for secondary complications of her diabetes and obesity, particularly ischaemic heart disease, renal impairment, and obstructive sleep apnoea. An HbA$_{1c}$ will give more information about how good her glycaemic control has been. If she has poor control then she is at risk of surgical site infection. It may be beneficial to discuss her optimization with the GP or the diabetic team first.

From the anaesthetic point of view, this lady is still vomiting and may require a rapid sequence induction along with all the airway problems associated with obesity.

Once you have all of the information you will need to discuss the case with the anaesthetist and patient and come to a decision about whether to perform the surgery today or postpone to optimize her diabetes first. She may also require post-operative critical care depending on what you find and this should be incorporated into your plan.

Scenario 2

Situation

You are called to see a 48-year-old man who is in pain on the post-operative ward

Background

He had a laparotomy with bowel resection and primary anastomosis for tumour yesterday. An epidural was inserted in theatre and he has had bupivacaine 0.125% with fentanyl 2mcg.ml^{-1} running at 10ml.h^{-1} since theatre. He was comfortable initially but developed central abdominal pain early this morning and it continues to get worse. He is not on any other analgesia and he has been hypotensive 80/45 and tachycardic 125bpm since this morning.

Assessment
- What is the differential diagnosis of the current problem?

Recommendation
- What are your priorities in his management?
- Who else do you need to speak to about your management plan?

Discussion
Pain may explain the tachycardia but this does not account for the BP; he may have a new cause for his pain. The epidural rate has not changed and so the hypotension is unlikely to be due to this. He needs a degree of resuscitation with fluid and rapid control of his pain. Following this, he should be examined and assessed for the possibility of a new surgical cause. You can give him some paracetamol and fluid bolus while you wait for the anaesthetist from the acute pain team to arrive. The anaesthetist will assess the block height and cardiovascular status and consider epidural top-up versus titrating systemic analgesia.

Scenario 3

Situation
You receive an emergency call from your post-operative surgical ward about a 72-year-old woman who is drowsy.

Background
This elderly lady had a nephrectomy for tumour yesterday and PCA morphine was established in recovery with standard settings and no background infusion. She was also given 100mg of diclofenac overnight for pain. The nurse says that her visitors have been in for the past 2 hours and they thought she was in pain and may have pressed the PCA button for her. When you see her she is snoring, with a respiratory rate of 4 and SpO2 84% and her oxygen mask is on the floor, HR 89, NIBP 120/80. She has no eye opening, withdraws to pain and is not making any verbal response.

Assessment
- What is the main problem here?
- What factors may have contributed to the problem?

Recommendation
- What is the immediate management of this situation?
- What help do you need?

Discussion
This lady has airway obstruction, hypoventilation, and reduced conscious level which can all be explained by opiate toxicity. She could have had 24mg of morphine in the past 2 hours due to her relatives administering the PCA to her. She is an elderly lady post-nephrectomy and has had an NSAID and therefore may have impaired renal function with reduced morphine clearance over the past 24 hours. This is an emergency and you need help urgently. Using an ABC approach; a simple airway manoeuvre, giving oxygen, and titrating naloxone 100–400mcg IV will improve the situation while help arrives. She may require assisted ventilation with a bag mask valve resuscitator. If there is no response to initial management then other causes must be sought. Rapidly reversing opiates can cause acute severe pain and you should be alert to this.

Chapter 3 In the operating theatre

Introduction

Surgeons strive to eradicate errors from their clinical practice. A strict system of education, training, mentorship, and practice have developed to promote excellence within the profession, helping to maintain the high standards that our patients expect. Despite this process, accidents do happen, and patients suffer because of them. As the leader of a surgical team it is often the surgeon who is expected to shoulder the responsibility.

Patient safety can be defined as the freedom from accidental injury. An error can be defined as the failure of a planned action to be completed as intended, or the use of a wrong plan to achieve an objective. Errors therefore can be split in to errors of execution or errors of planning.

Principles of safe surgery

Safe surgery requires dedicated and conscientious staff, interacting effectively to form safe clinical teams. These teams can develop systems for achieving clinical outcomes and minimizing errors. It is these systems rather than individuals acting alone that promote safe surgery. Systems constantly change and adapt within the medical setting, so safety becomes a dynamic concept. As complexity increases within the fields of investigation, diagnosis, and treatments there is increasing opportunity for error.

Not all errors result in harm, and generally large systems fail because multiple faults occur together, leading to an accident. Despite this, study of medical errors suggests that they constitute a significant problem for a modern day health care provider. It is estimated that between 44,000–98,000 patients die each year from medical errors in the USA. If these figures are correct, this makes medical error the eighth leading cause of death.

Errors can never be eliminated, in medicine as in other fields. There are steps that can be taken, however, that may help to improve safety in surgical care. Leaders should prioritize helping the staff they supervise and improving the service those staff provide. Breaking down barriers between staff and departments allows professionals throughout a team to identify areas where errors could occur, and take steps to avoid them. Training programmes that promote safety should be encouraged as a part of ongoing education. All team members should be charged with working to accomplish the goal of patient safety, as no individual can achieve it alone.

As with clinical teams, management strategies will also have an impact on medical error rates. Systems which run at full capacity will maximize economic and workload outcomes, but this may come at the cost of an increased rate of errors. A lack of hospital beds, ICU capacity, nurse staffing, surgical instruments, and resources will result in a state where all systems are running at maximum capacity. This makes accidents more likely, more difficult to detect, and more difficult to remedy. Managing the conflict between patient safety and financial concerns is important in providing effective health care in the modern environment.

Certain medical errors are more common than others. The issue of wrong-site surgery was addressed in Chapter 1. Retained items following surgery are an ongoing concern for all staff within an operating environment. A retained item refers to any surgical item found inside a patient after they have left the operating theatre. Current estimates suggest that this occurs in somewhere between 1 in 8000–18,000 cases, although that is likely to be an underestimate.

Factors which increase the risk of surgical errors are listed in Box 3.1.

The most common retained item is a surgical swab. Needles and instruments can also be left inside a patient inadvertently. Almost all retained items will require removal, with the exception of small needles

---

Box 3.1 Factors increasing the risk of surgical errors

- Emergency surgery
- Unplanned changes in the procedure
- High BMI
- Multiple surgeons and nurses involved in one procedure
- Case duration covering multiple nursing shifts

---

which have not been shown to result in morbidity. Safeguards to protect against retained items include surgical counts, thorough wound examination prior to closure, use of only X-ray detectable items in the operating room, and a post-operative debriefing. Although in themselves each measure has not been shown to reduce the incidence of retained items, the concept of introducing multiple lines of defence should help to minimize the problem.

Similar to wrong-site surgery, retained items should be considered a 'never event' in surgery, and should the patient move to legal action, proof of negligence will not be required.

In the event of such a medical error it is important that the surgeon involved is open and truthful with the patient. The error, possible causes, and steps taken to improve the system should be outlined to the patient. Such patients should not be avoided, but treated with the utmost courtesy and speed. It is in these situations where a surgeon's communication skills and bedside manner can go a long way to preventing conflict and legal proceedings.

Theatre etiquette and effective team working

The operating theatre is one of the most complex and demanding environments within healthcare. To produce safe and effective outcomes for patients, all staff involved with a case must work as a team. This team consists of surgeons, anaesthetists, nurses, and allied health professionals within the room, but also pathologists, radiologists, portering staff, and administrators working outside.

Surgeons are well placed within this team to take a leadership role. Team leaders must be proficient and respected in their primary role. They must also be approachable and fair. Leaders should be able to identify impaired members of the team, offering support and access to training as required.

Communication failure is the most common root cause of errors such as wrong-site surgery, and should be avoided if at all possible. Unfortunately the culture within the operating theatre often develops to prevent effective communication. Nursing and junior staff are hesitant to question decisions made or situations controlled by the senior medical staff. Research from the aviation industry shows that such reluctance can lead to errors, with disastrous consequences. By promoting an atmosphere where all staff are encouraged and expected to engage in such error reduction behaviour, not only can mistakes be avoided but higher job satisfaction ratings and lower sick time can be achieved.

Perceptions of teamwork often vary within surgical teams, with surgeons perceiving far higher standards than nursing staff. Surgeons consider collaboration to be good when nursing staff anticipate their needs and follow instruction. Nursing staff, however, value having their input respected. Surgeons should work to address this discrepancy and promote an atmosphere where all team members feel that their opinion counts, so they are not afraid to voice it.

During patient care, teams will come under pressure at certain predictable times, referred to as gaps. These include a nursing shift change in the operating room and patient transfer to different units within the hospital. During these times, information is passed between team members and can be lost. Teams should anticipate such gaps and consider ways to maintain high standards of information communication. Increasing use of time-outs before surgery or de-briefings after, and checklists or algorithms to encourage effective information transfer are becoming common.

Theatre design

The modern day operating theatre must balance requirements for space, storage, ease of access and cleaning, ventilation, and equipment against costs and available resources. The competing interests mean that the ideal operating theatre is impossible to design. There are important concepts, however, that are crucial to delivering an environment where surgery can be performed in a comfortable, cost-efficient, and safe environment.

Within a hospital, operating rooms should be situated in easy reach of other vital areas (Fig. 3.1).

Although most wound infections originate from the patients' own flora, airborne contaminants can cause infections. Most of these contaminants will be associated with shed squames and hairs from persons within the room. It seems reasonable therefore to take steps to reduce contamination of the operating theatre from external pathogens. Traffic patterns around the suite should be designed to minimize

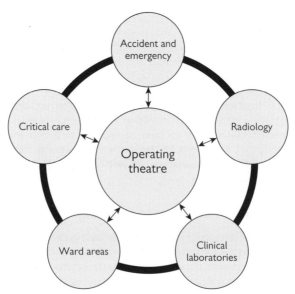

Figure 3.1 Position of an operating theatre in relation to other areas within the hospital.

the movement of personnel and equipment from the outside environment to within the operating theatre. Minimizing the number of people in the room, limiting their movement within the room and keeping the doors of the room closed all contribute to reducing bacterial contamination.

Operating rooms should be large enough to accommodate all necessary equipment and staff, whilst allowing room for movement through the space without the need for adjustments. Current recommendations suggest a size of at least 40m².

Spaces adjacent to the operating room can be used for preparation of sterile equipment, scrubbing-up, and induction of anaesthesia. Using such areas efficiently can maximize the output of the operating room by allowing preparation for the next surgery whilst the operating room itself is still being cleaned following the previous case.

Within the operating room, floors should be non-slip under wet and dry conditions. External windows allow the entry of natural light, which enhances staff morale; however, certain procedures require darkening of the room and so disadvantages can outweigh advantages. The room should be designed to be easy to clean and to avoid having ledges that can collect dust.

Most equipment used during surgical procedures should be stored elsewhere, with only equipment used in every case located within the operating room at all times. For this reason, dedicated operating rooms for specific uses such as laparoscopic surgery are ideal.

Ventilation is the most important factor in preventing surgical site infections. A positive pressure system provides air flow from the operating room out in to the surrounding area. At least 15 air changes per minute should be maintained. Most rooms use a system that provides air at ceiling level and an exhaust near the floor (Fig. 3.2). This relies on limiting the time spent with open doors. Laminar flow systems move particle-free air across the surgical field, picking up particles en route to an air filter. This more expensive method of ventilation is only considered necessary during the most high-risk operations such as joint replacements, where infections can have devastating consequences.

Surgical site preparation

Preparation of the site chosen for surgical incision should start long before the patient arrives in the operating theatre. The overall condition of the patient, including nutritional status and management of chronic diseases such as diabetes, should be optimized prior to elective surgery. Pre-existing areas of infection should be eradicated if at all possible to avoid cross contamination.

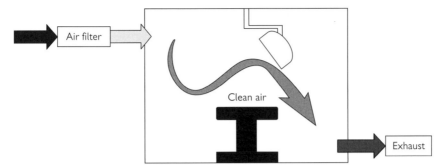

Figure 3.2 Passage of air through an operating room.

Patients may also be screened for drug resistant bacteria including MRSA. Although routine pre-operative screening has yet to be adopted, screening of high-risk patients, such as those undergoing implantation of foreign material, or those likely to be nursed in a critical care environment, should be considered.

Following admission to hospital, it seems reasonable to isolate pre-operative patients from inpatients who are at risk of carrying resistant bacteria. The use of day surgery admission areas allows for the pre-surgical patients to be prepared in an environment less likely to be colonized with such organisms.

Methods to reduce the skin's flora such as pre-operative showering with antiseptic soaps have been shown to reduce bacterial load but this has not translated into reduced post-operative infection rates. Despite the lack of evidence, it is not an unreasonable measure, particularly in patients who have been in the ward for a number of days prior to surgery.

Hair has classically been thought of as a potential source of infection as well as a hindrance to surgical technique. Many surgeons choose to remove hair around the surgical site. Hair removal can be achieved by shaving, clipping, or the use of depilatory creams. Shaving and clipping can be performed on the operating table, whereas depilatory creams take longer to have an effect. Loose hairs during a procedure can contaminate a sterile surgical field which could potentially raise the risk for post-operative wound infection.

Shaving with a sharp metal blade can cause micro-cuts which can then become colonized. There can also be an associated ooze which provides a culture medium for bacteria. The use of clippers and depilatory creams prevent such skin damage and results in lower post-operative infection rates.

Skin disinfection

A number of preparations are available for skin disinfection. These are commonly based either on iodophor, alcohol, or chlorhexidine gluconate. Despite numerous studies using different preparations, no one antiseptic has been shown to reduce post-operative infections over another.

The area of skin treated should be sufficient to include any potential incision (e.g. consider preparing the whole abdomen prior to laparoscopic abdominal surgery). The solution should be applied in concentric circles, using an applicator which is discarded following use (Fig. 3.3). Adequate time should be allowed for drying particularly when using solutions which contain alcohol and are therefore flammable.

Prior to making the incision, consideration should be given to the use of prophylactic antibiotics. This subject is covered in more detail in Chapter 1.

Scrubbing up

Joseph Lister (1827–1912) demonstrated the effectiveness of skin disinfection for reducing surgical site infections. Despite the introduction of sterile surgical gloves since this time, the importance of 'scrubbing up' is still recognized.

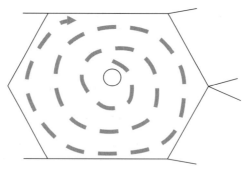

Figure 3.3 Application of skin preparation to the abdomen in concentric circles.

Around 18% of gloves are punctured following surgery which exposes the operator's skin and bacteria to the patient. This number rises to over 30% for procedures >2 hours in duration.

Indirect data has linked infectious outbreaks to the flora of contaminated surgical staff. Endocarditis following cardiac surgery has been traced to staff carriage of coagulase negative *Staphylococcus aureus* on a number of occasions. No randomized controlled trial has ever proven the need for hand preparation prior to surgery, and it is unlikely that a modern ethics committee would authorize such a trial.

The objective of skin preparation is to decrease the bacterial load by eliminating transient flora and reducing the resident flora present at the start of the procedure. The use of anti-microbial preparations should also reduce bacterial growth under the surgical glove.

The most common preparations used are chlorhexidine or povidone-iodine containing soaps. Warm water helps to make these solutions more effective, although very hot water actually breaks down protective fatty acids on the skin so should be avoided. Fingernails should be cleaned under a running tap, but the routine use of brushes on the skin should be avoided.

Alcohol-based solutions are even more effective at reducing bacterial counts. They have the added advantage of reducing rates of dermatitis amongst users. As experience with these preparations grows, they are growing in favour. They offer particular advantages in countries with limited or potentially contaminated water sources.

The time required to ensure adequate reduction in bacterial load is dependent on the product used. Most manufacturers recommend at least 3 minutes of application, although shorter exposures may be acceptable. Clinical groups that have looked that this issue report conflicting results, and tend to recommend times of 3–5 minutes.

Draping

Following skin preparation, the surgical site is isolated using sterile drapes. These prevent contact between sterile instruments and contaminated skin, protect the patient from superficial liquid spillage, and provide a working area for the surgical team. They also provide some additional warmth for the patient during the procedure. Drapes can be made from cotton or synthetic materials, and are held in place using towel clips, sutures, or an adhesive backing.

In placing drapes prior to a procedure, the surgeon should ensure that adequate exposure is achieved. The full length of the planned incision should be exposed including any extensions to the incision that may be required. Other areas that should be observed during the procedure (such as the ipsilateral facial muscles during parotid surgery) should also be considered. Access to the airway, arterial and venous catheters, and leads for cardiac and temperature monitoring should be ensured so as to cause minimal disruption to the theatre team.

The use of adhesive plastic drapes has become commonplace. These are transparent plastic drapes which adhere to the skin whilst still allowing incisions to be made accurately. They can act as a microbial barrier preventing bacteria, which remain in hair follicles and the deep layers of the skin, from entering the wound. The addition of antimicrobials to the undersurface of these drapes also has the potential to reduce bacterial contamination. A number of studies have shown the potential to reduce bacterial counts under such drapes, but as yet a corresponding reduction in wound infection rates has not been proven.

Electrosurgery

Definitions: cautery describes the conductive heating of tissue by heating an object which is then applied to a single vessel to produce haemostasis. Electrocautery describes using electricity to generate that heat and is rarely used in modern surgical practice. The term electrosurgery refers to the use of radiofrequency electricity to heat tissue.

Since William Bovie and Harvey Cushing collaborated to bring the first electrosurgical generator to the operating room in 1926, surgeons in all disciplines have realized the advantages such techniques can offer. Modern electrosurgical devices allow manipulation of the electrical energy to produce cutting, coagulating, and ablating effects whilst producing haemostasis and minimizing risk to the patient and operator.

The ideal tool for dissection in surgery would allow rapid and accurate dissection whilst providing the benefit of simultaneous haemostasis but without the risk of collateral damage. It would be cheap, reliable with a shallow learning curve, and the ability to lend itself to multiple surgical procedures.

Electrosurgical tissue effects are the result of two types of tissue destruction, boiling and coagulation. Rapid heating causes water to boil which produces steam. This in turn causes cells to burst, producing a plume of steam and cellular debris. Slow heating in comparison causes cellular proteins to coagulate prior to boiling point, which results in white desiccated tissue.

The rate of heating depends on the rate of electrical energy supplied to the tissues per unit time, described in watts. Energy effects can be controlled by varying the wattage of the electrosurgical unit, or by maintaining the wattage, but delivering the energy to a different tissue volume or for a different time. This is realized during surgery when a small piece of tissue is 'buzzed' between the limbs of a forceps in comparison to when a large piece of tissue is grasped, and the effect takes longer to achieve.

Electrical energy passes through tissue between two electrodes. So-called monopolar electrosurgery uses a hand-held electrode which delivers energy to the tissues then returns via an electrode on the patient's skin. The surface area of the hand-held electrode is very small, focusing the current density in a small tissue volume leading to marked tissue effects. The return electrode in comparison has a large surface area, so the current density is very low and tissue effects are small enough to be unnoticed. For this reason, when attaching the return electrode, the surgeon should ensure that the entire electrode is in contact with the skin. Poor electrode placement results in a lower surface area and higher tissue effects which can produce burns.

Bipolar electrosurgical units do not require a patient based return electrode as both the active and return electrodes are integrated into forceps. Tissue is grasped between the forceps and energy passes only through this volume. As there is less electrical energy passing through the patient, these devices are preferred in patients with implantable devices such as pacemakers and cochlear implants.

Although the perfect instrument has yet to be discovered many surgeons use the modern monopolar dissector as it approximates most of the features desirable in such a device.

Standard monopolar instruments have two major settings, cut and coagulate. The cutting mode delivers a continuous voltage which result in abrupt tissue heating, steam production, and tissue vaporization. The high current density at the point of contact quickly diffuses resulting in lower current density only a few cell diameters away and minimal collateral thermal damage.

In coagulation mode a higher voltage is delivered but the energy is applied for only around 6% of the time relative to the cut mode. The outcome is tissue heating and charring as a result of the slower rise in temperature. The duration of energy delivery and the voltage applied can be varied (referred to as the blend setting) resulting in tissue effects which between lie between the two extremes (Fig. 3.4).

Lasers in surgery

Laser—light amplification by stimulated emission of radiation.

Medical lasers use electromagnetic radiation with a wavelength from 200nm to >1000nm. The wavelength determines the visibility of the laser. To generate a laser beam, electrons within the laser medium are excited to a higher unstable orbit, and when they return to their initial orbit they release a photon

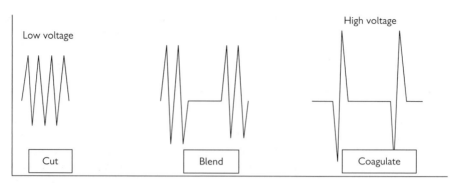

Figure 3.4 Relationship of electrosurgical settings to energy delivery.

in the process. The light produced by lasers is collimated (all photons move in a parallel direction) and monochromatic (all of one wave length).

Lasers consist of an active medium (after which the laser is named), a stimulating mechanism, and an optical chamber. Photons created by excitation of the active medium are emitted into the optical chamber which has a reflective mirror at one end and a partially reflective mirror at the other. In addition to these basic parts, lasers require a cooling system, a delivery system, a control unit, and for lasers which are not visible (carbon dioxide lasers) a second visible laser source is used as an aiming beam.

The three most common lasers in surgery are the argon laser, neodymium:yttrium-aluminium-garnet (Nd:YAG) laser, and the carbon dioxide laser.

The carbon dioxide laser has a wavelength of 10600nm. As the beam is invisible, a helium-neon laser beam is used for aiming purposes. Energy from this source penetrates to a depth of 0.2mm, and is absorbed by tissue with high water contents. Manipulation of the beam allows a fine spot to be used to make incisions, and a wider de-focused spot which can coagulate vessels <0.5mm.

The argon laser emits a green light, and penetrates 1mm. The energy at this wavelength is absorbed by haemoglobin and this laser has found use in coagulating haemangiomas.

The wavelength of the Nd:YAG laser is in the near infrared range and so an aiming beam is required. It has a deeper penetration of 3–5mm as it is poorly absorbed by water and pigment. The characteristics of this laser make coagulation possible and for this reason it has found a use in tracheobronchial lesions due to its haemostatic properties.

Lasers cause tissue destruction, and can injure the patient, surgeon, and staff within the operating theatre. The safety issues involved with using lasers require specific precautions to be taken. These include staff training, specific safety equipment and preparation of the operating theatre in which laser cases are performed.

Laser light shone directly or reflected into the eye can cause irreversible damage. All staff within the theatre must wear approved safety glasses. The patient should also be protected either with glasses or with damp eye pads. Operating room windows must be covered and non-reflective instruments should be used whenever possible to reduce the risk of inadvertent beam scatter.

The laser plume created during surgery is a result of energy contacting smoke which is created by tissue heating. This can lead to alterations in the wavelength of light and secondary emissions. The cellular debris created during procedures has given rise to concerns about fragments of viable tumour and viruses. Constant smoke evacuation and charcoal impregnated face masks should be worn to minimize these risks.

Airway fires are a problem when lasers are used in the upper aerodigestive tract. Protected endotracheal tubes, low oxygen levels, and damp drapes should be used in all cases. A syringe of water should be available to extinguish any flames in the event of an incident.

Tourniquets

Surgical tourniquets can be used to prevent blood flow to a limb, thereby providing the surgeon with a bloodless field. This technique allows faster and more precise surgery to be performed. They are most commonly used in orthopaedics and plastic surgery.

The modern tourniquet consists of three main parts: an air-tight cuff, a compressed gas source, and a microprocessor to measure and maintain the pressure within the cuff. As the cuff inflates around a limb, it compressed the soft tissues, occluding blood vessels and eventually preventing blood flow. Cuffs are wide, so dispersing the applied pressure over a large area, thus preventing tissue damage. Despite this, dry padding should always be placed between the cuff and the skin to prevent injury.

There is a well-recognized link between rising tourniquet pressures and the risk of tourniquet-related injury. The safest tourniquet pressure to use is the lowest that will stop arterial blood flow. This 'limb occlusion pressure' should be determined for each case. Prior to surgery, the cuff is inflated around the surgical limb. Arterial pulses can be palpated, or detected with a Doppler probe. The cuff pressure is then raised until the pulse can no longer be detected. Following determination of this minimum occlusion pressure, an additional pressure should be applied to accommodate physiological variations during the procedure. Although this would be the ideal, it is time consuming and often surgeons use set pressures of 100–150mmHg for convenience.

The limb should be exsanguinated prior to application of the tourniquet, to minimize blood loss. This can be achieved using a pressure bandage, or in cases of infection or tumour, where there is risk of embolization, by raising the limb for several minutes.

In prolonged cases, tourniquets should be periodically deflated. This allows the return of blood to the limb and revascularize distal tissues. Every 2 hours the cuff should be deflated for 15–20 minutes (around 5 minutes of deflation per 30 minutes of tourniquet time).

For procedures on digits, simpler methods may be employed, using the rolled finger of a rubber glove or commercially available tourniquets to occlude the digital vessels. These methods involve a narrow band around the base of the digit, and although cheap and convenient, the pressure is concentrated over a small area which puts direct pressure on digital nerves and vessels. They are well suited to rapid procedures such as simple closure of lacerations in the accident and emergency department, but should not be used for potentially prolonged surgery.

Surgical drains

The term surgical drain refers to an inert, usually plastic, device that is left in the surgical wound to drain a body cavity. Drains have been used by surgeons for many years. Their indications can be described as therapeutic or prophylactic. Therapeutic uses include draining pus from an abscess or air from the pleural cavity. Prophylactic drains can be used to reduce dead space under a flap, to drain potential blood or serous collections, or to create a controlled fistula following bile duct surgery, for example.

Drains can be further classified as open or closed. In open drainage systems, the drained fluid is exposed to the atmosphere. Closed drains prevent atmospheric exposure and can be further classified as active, where a vacuum creates suction (Fig. 3.5) and passive. Closed drains encourage an environment which favours anaerobic bacteria.

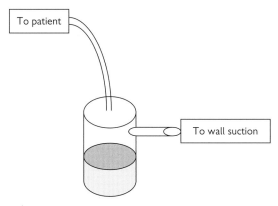

Figure 3.5 Closed, active suction.

The use of therapeutic drains following thoracic surgery or for ensuring the walls of an abscess cavity do not close over prematurely is standard practice. In these settings drains perform an important function. In the presence of a skin flap, active drains can be used to hold the skin down on to the wound bed, so preventing dead space and encouraging healing. A more recent application of active drains is their use with dressings to apply negative pressure to a wound, which can result in decreased interstitial oedema, increased perfusion, and a decrease in bacterial contamination.

It should be remembered, however, that a drain is a foreign body. As with all foreign material within the body, there is an associated risk of infection, and surrounding inflammation can irritate local structures which may result in haemorrhage or fistulation. Unsurprisingly patients do not like surgical drains, as they hinder mobility whilst *in situ* and are uncomfortable on removal.

For these reasons, the routine use of prophylactic drains is controversial in many situations. Classical teaching encouraged their use to prevent haematoma and dead-space collections, so reducing the chance for infection. Recent clinical trials in many specialties have challenged the conventional approach. They suggest that there is little evidence to support a reduction in infection, and that drains may actually lead to an increase in infection rates and duration of post-operative stay.

Thyroid surgery is a good example. One of the feared complications of thyroid surgery is post-operative haemorrhage, leading to raised pressure in the neck, venous congestion within the larynx, and subsequent airway compromise. Post-operative drainage has been considered the norm for many years. There is little evidence to support their use, however, and recent randomized controlled trials have shown that drains result in no significant difference in haemorrhage rates. As airway complications are so rare in any event, a reduction in their incidence is difficult to prove, and close post-operative monitoring remains crucial.

Choosing when to use a drain requires experience. There are both patient and disease factors to consider. Patients who are likely to bleed in the post-operative period can be good candidates for drains. Superficial, minor procedures are unlikely to require drainage, but in deep major wounds with potential or actual contamination, a drain should be considered.

Scenarios

Scenario 1

Following return of a patient to the recovery room, the scrub nurse informs you that there has been a miscount, and one swab cannot be found. What is the appropriate course of action?

Scenario 2

Whilst preparing the right leg for knee arthroscopy, the medical student mentions that she thought that the procedure was being done on the left leg. How should you proceed?

Scenario 3

An elective total hip replacement is scheduled for your afternoon theatre list; however, due to routine maintenance your normal theatre is closed. Instead your list is moved to the minor ops theatre which is available. What must you ensure prior to agreeing to the change?

Scenario 4

When planning an incision in a hair-bearing area, what is the most appropriate approach to hair removal?

Scenario 5

An 8-year-old boy with a cochlear implant is listed for emergency appendicectomy. What must be considered in terms of electrosurgery?

Scenario 6

A complex flexor tendon repair is arranged for your morning theatre list. How long can the tourniquet be allowed to remain inflated?

Answers

Scenario 1

Surgical swabs cannot be left in the patient, and must always be removed. Standard swabs contain X-ray visible material, and the radiographer should be called to image the abdomen. Assuming the swab is found on the film, and the patient is stable, plans to return to theatre to remove the swab must be made, and the patient or relatives should be informed.

Scenario 2

Communication within theatre is of utmost importance. There are a number of ways to avoid problems like this. The surgeon should have spoken to the patient prior to the procedure and marked the leg to be examined. The surgical drapes should be applied in such a way as to expose any pre-operative marking. A pre-operative 'time-out' should be performed to ensure that the team is happy that the patient and procedure have been identified correctly. The student's opinion should not be ignored, as this attitude has been shown to result in errors. The notes, consent form, and radiology should be re-checked to ensure that the correct side has been identified.

Scenario 3

The type of ventilation system installed in the minor ops theatre should be determined. Modern operating theatres have positive-pressure ventilation systems to reduce the bacterial load in the air. Orthopaedic theatres performing arthroplasty, however, use laminar flow systems which reduce the bacterial load further. General use theatres are not generally equipped with laminar flow, and so are not suited for this type of procedure.

Scenario 4

Although removing hair has never been shown to reduce the rate of infection, it can impede the surgeon, particularly during wound closure. Hair removal should be performed in advance using depilatory cream, or immediately before surgery using a shaver. Use of a razor leads to micro-cuts which can then promote bacterial colonization and increase the rate of post-operative wound infection.

Scenario 5

Cochlear implantation is a contraindication to monopolar electrosurgery. Bipolar techniques can be used. Pacemakers are a relative contraindication to the use of monopolar electrosurgical techniques, although if required, the return electrode can be placed to ensure that the current path is well clear of the device.

Scenario 6

Tourniquets should be set to the lowest pressure that occludes blood flow to the limb. This limb occlusion pressure should be determined immediately prior to each case. For prolonged surgery, the tourniquet should be deflated for 15–20 minutes every 2 hours to allow revascularization of the limb.

Chapter 4 Principles of laparoscopic surgery and endoscopic procedures

Introduction

Within the last 20 years the greatest technical advance in surgery has been the advent of minimal access surgery (MAS). This entails the use of the laparoscope. The surgical trainee should be conversant with the use of the instruments and the hazards associated with such techniques. These procedures often have a steep initial learning curve but the skills are usually transferable between different procedures. This chapter deals with the basic principles of this form of surgery.

Minimal access surgery

MAS is performed through small incisions in order to minimize the trauma of the surgical wound and has risen in popularity ever since the first laparoscopic cholecystectomy was performed by Philippe Mouret in France in 1987. All this would not have been possible without the development of technology and optics. Laparoscopic surgery today, is the culmination of the efforts of the number of pioneers in the fields of optics, instrumentation, and surgery. The word laparoscopy is derived from a Greek word *lapara,* which means 'soft part of the body between ribs and hip, flank, loin' and *skopein,* which means 'to look at' or 'to survey'.

The broad fundamental principle of MAS is to perform, as far as possible, the same operation as done in open surgery with the same anatomical landmarks and steps but with smaller access incisions for instrumentation, with the advantage of much greater magnification and lighting. For greater than 90% of the surgical procedures, these principles remain unchanged. Specific technical considerations will be discussed later in this chapter to enable the principles to be executed with success and minimal complications.

The laparoscope and its use

There are three main components in laparoscopic surgery:

1 Imaging: laparoscope or rod lens system, light source, and the camera
2 Pneumoperitoneum: insufflation of gas to create space for the operation
3 Laparoscopic instruments

Imaging

Laparoscope

This is based on the Hopkin's rigid rod lens system with a central component of series of rods of lenses interspersed with a vacuum for transmission of image proximally and a peripheral ring of optical fibres for distal transmission of light from the light cable. Delicate 3-mm, and more robust 5-mm and 10-mm laparoscopes are available with either straight or angled lenses at the tips. The angled scopes enable the surgeon to look around and over the tissues. The direction of tilt of the objective lens for an angled scope is usually opposite to the position of the light cable attachment on the circumference of the scope. Endoscopes can be of forward viewing (0°) or forward oblique direction of view (30°, 45°). The angle between the optical axis of the endoscope and the plane of the target is referred to as the optical axis-to-target view angle (Fig. 4.1).

The best task performance during endoscopic work is obtained when the optical axis-to-target view angle approaches 90° and the decrease in this viewing angle causes a significant degradation of task performance. In practice, however, only oblique viewing endoscopes or ones with flexible tips can achieve an adequate optical axis-to-target view angle approximating to 90°. For this reason, forward oblique endoscopes are preferable, despite the easier deployment of forward viewing types.

Light source and cable

Light sources consist of high-intensity bulbs filled with xenon, mercury, or halogen vapour to provide bright illumination. The most common type of light source was the halogen bulb. It is a highly efficient crisp light source with excellent colour rendering. The electrodes are made up of tungsten. They utilize

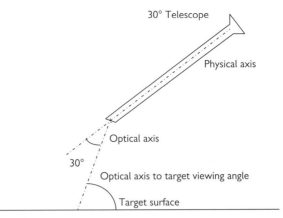

Figure 4.1 Optical viewing angles.

halogen gas that allows the bulb to burn more intensely without sacrificing its life. These lamps are cheap and can be used for laparoscopic surgery if a low budget set-up is required. However, they lack in providing the natural white light colour. The metal halide vapour arc lamp is a mix of compounds (mostly salts of rare earths and halides) and the output intensity is adjustable and can be controlled at the source. More recently, xenon lamps have been used, which give more white light.

Light is transported from the light source to the laparoscope by a cable. Light cables are flexible and have both laparoscope- and light source-specific couplers. Two types of light cable are available: **fibreoptic** and **liquid crystal gel** cable. The optical cables are made up of a bundle of optical fibreglass thread swaged at both ends. They have a very high quality of optical transmission, but are fragile. In fact, some of the fibres may break due to repeated use. The gel cables are made up of a sheath, which is filled with a clear optical gel. Theoretically they are capable of transmitting more light than optic fibres.

Cameras and monitor

High-resolution, small, and lightweight cameras are available, which are easy to handle and provide picture of optimal sharpness, high resolution, and excellent colour reproduction. Camera may be **single chip** or **three-chip**. A chip refers to a charge coupled device (CCD). Single-chip cameras process and amalgamate the three primary colours—red, blue, and green—into a single chip, while three-chip cameras have a chip for each of the three primary colours and therefore give a better definition, especially with red. The camera head is an optical/electronic interface, which is attached to the laparoscope. A standard eyepiece laparoscope requires a coupler to connect to the camera head. A video laparoscope has a camera attached directly to the lens system. The camera should be focused, and the camera should be white-balanced to optimize image colour representation. The white light is composed of an equal proportion of red, blue, and green colour and at the time of white balancing the camera sets its digital coding for these primary colours to equal proportions assuming that the target is white. The video monitor must generate a high-resolution image, a larger video screen is preferred (at least 20 inches/ 50 cm), and non-flickering medical monitors with high resolutions are preferred. A second monitor is preferable to give both surgeon and assistants a clear and comfortable view of the procedure.

The best task performance is obtained with the monitor located in front of the operator at the level of the manipulation workspace (hands), permitting 'gaze-down viewing' and alignment of the visual and motor axis and at a distance of five times the diagonal of the screen from the operator. Gaze-down viewing by the endoscopic operator allows both sensory signals and motor control to have a close spatial location and thus brings the visual signals in correspondence with instrument manipulations, similar to the situation encountered during conventional open surgery. In practice, the site of the operation determines the location of the monitor. For upper abdominal procedures, such as cholecystectomy and fundoplication, the monitor is placed near the patient's head on the right and left side respectively. During appendicectomy, the monitor is located over the right iliac fossa and the surgeon stands on the left side near the patient's hypochondrium.

Pneumoperitoneum

Insufflator

Insufflation system allows the surgeon to create a working space in the abdomen in which to see and operate. The insufflator supplies carbon dioxide to create and maintain the pneumoperitoneum. It is recommended that the intra-abdominal pressure should not rise above 12–14mmHg, to avoid compression of the inferior vena cava (IVC), with resultant decreased cardiac return. Various gases have been evaluated for laparoscopic surgery, including air, oxygen, carbon dioxide, nitrous oxide, and inert gases such as xenon, argon, and krypton. Air and inert gases are insoluble in blood and therefore carry a risk of air embolus. Oxygen is flammable and therefore is not used. The preferred agent in the majority of cases is carbon dioxide, because it is not flammable, rapidly dissolves in blood, and can be excreted by the lungs, thus greatly reducing the risk of gas embolus. The insufflation system should be continuously in direct view so the surgeon can monitor its minute-to-minute function.

Physiological changes associated with carbon dioxide pneumoperitoneum

Although a gasless approach has been described using an intra-abdominal lift, creation of the pneumoperitoneum is an essential component for laparoscopic procedures. The attraction of CO_2 as a gas for insufflation is its solubility. This speeds its elimination but increases its physiological effects. When CO_2 production exceeds its elimination, acid–base and respiratory homeostasis is disturbed.

The physiological effects of CO_2 pneumoperitoneum can be divided into two areas: (1) gas-specific effects and (2) pressure-specific effects. CO_2 is rapidly absorbed across the peritoneal membrane into the circulation. In the circulation, CO_2 creates a respiratory acidosis by the generation of carbonic acid.

Body buffers, the largest reserve of which lies in bone, absorb CO_2 (up to 120L) and minimize the development of hypercarbia or respiratory acidosis during brief endoscopic procedures. Once the body buffers are saturated, respiratory acidosis develops rapidly, and the respiratory system assumes the burden of keeping up with the absorption of CO_2 and its release from these buffers.

In patients with normal respiratory function this is not difficult; the anaesthesiologist increases the ventilatory rate or vital capacity on the ventilator. If the respiratory rate required exceeds 20 breaths per minute, there may be less efficient gas exchange and increasing hypercarbia. Conversely, if vital capacity is increased substantially, there is a greater opportunity for barotrauma and greater respiratory motion-induced disruption of the upper abdominal operative field. In some situations it is advisable to evacuate the pneumoperitoneum or reduce the intra-abdominal pressure to allow time for the anaesthesiologist to adjust for hypercarbia. While mild respiratory acidosis probably is an insignificant problem, more severe respiratory acidosis leading to cardiac arrhythmias has been reported. Hypercarbia also causes tachycardia and increased systemic vascular resistance, which elevates BP and increases myocardial oxygen demand. It is mandatory for end tidal (ET) CO_2 to be measured during all laparoscopic procedures.

The pressure effects of the pneumoperitoneum on cardiovascular physiology have also been studied. In the hypovolaemic individual, excessive pressure on the IVC and a reverse Trendelenburg position with loss of lower extremity muscle tone may cause decreased venous return and cardiac output. This is not seen in the normovolaemic patient. The most common arrhythmia created by laparoscopy is bradycardia. A rapid stretch of the peritoneal membrane often causes a vagovagal response with bradycardia and occasionally hypotension. The appropriate management of this event is desufflation of the abdomen, administration of vagolytic agents (e.g. atropine), and adequate volume replacement. CO_2 absorbed as a result of insufflation is stored until eliminated by the lungs.

Effects of carbon dioxide

CO_2 pneumoperitoneum can cause adverse cardiovascular, respiratory, and metabolic changes. In all patients, there is a 25–30% drop in the cardiac return in the first 20 minutes of a laparoscopic procedure, but most healthy patients demonstrate no ill effects.

There is, however, a risk to patients with reduced cardiopulmonary reserve. CO_2, accumulation in these patients results in decreased stroke volume and accelerated heart rate, which stresses the myocardium. Ventilation-perfusion shunts occur so that increases in arterial P_aCO_2 may not be matched by changes in the CO_2 measured in the expired gases. Patients with significant respiratory or cardiovascular disease must therefore have their arterial gases monitored.

Volume effects

The increased pressure of the pneumoperitoneum is transmitted directly across the paralysed dia-phragm to the thoracic cavity, creating increased central venous pressure and increased filling pressures of the right and left sides of the heart. If the intra-abdominal pressures are kept below 20mmHg, the cardiac output usually is well maintained. Partial obstruction of the inferior vena cava and splinting of the diaphragm become important when the procedure lasts longer than 20–30 minutes. Venous pooling in the legs may predispose to deep venous thrombosis. Diaphragmatic splinting may compromise ventila-tion, especially when there is pre-existing lung disease.

Cardiac dysrhythmias may occur during insufflation. Sinus bradycardia is most common and can be corrected by temporarily releasing the pneumoperitoneum and administering IV atropine. Other dys-rhythmias are usually secondary to reduced venous return and cardiac output with underperfusion of the myocardium.

The anaesthetist must have adequate IV access throughout a laparoscopic procedure and effective monitoring, including CVP measurement if necessary, is mandatory. Increased intra-abdominal pressure decreases renal blood flow, glomerular filtration rate, and urine output. These effects may be mediated by direct pressure on the kidney and the renal vein. The decreased renal blood flow results in increased plasma renin release, thereby increasing sodium retention. Increased circulating antidiuretic hormone (ADH) levels also are found during the pneumoperitoneum, increasing free water reabsorption in the distal tubules. Although the effects of the pneumoperitoneum on renal blood flow are immediately reversible, the hormonally mediated changes, such as elevated ADH levels, decrease urine output for up to 1 hour after the procedure has ended. Intraoperative oliguria is common during laparoscopy, but the urine output is not a reflection of intravascular volume status; IV fluid administration during an uncom-plicated laparoscopic procedure should not be linked to urine output. Because fluid losses through the open abdomen are eliminated with laparoscopy, the need for supplemental fluid during a laparoscopic surgical procedure is rare.

The haemodynamic and metabolic consequences of pneumoperitoneum are well tolerated by healthy individuals for a prolonged period and by most individuals for at least a short period. Difficul-ties can occur when a patient with compromised cardiovascular function is subjected to a long laparo-scopic procedure. It is during these procedures that alternative approaches should be considered or insufflation pressure reduced. Alternative gases that have been suggested for laparoscopy include the inert gases helium, neon, and argon. These gases are appealing because they cause no metabolic effects, but are poorly soluble in blood (unlike CO_2 and N_2O) and are prone to create gas emboli if the gas has direct access to the venous system. Gas emboli are rare but serious complications of laparo-scopic surgery. They should be suspected if hypotension develops during insufflation. Diagnosis may be made by the characteristic 'mill wheel' murmur. The treatment of gas embolism is to place the patient in a left lateral decubitus position with the head down to trap the gas in the apex of the right ventricle. A rapidly placed central venous catheter then can be used to aspirate the gas out of the right ventricle.

Gas insufflated at room temperature does not cause significant hypothermia. However, gas leakage allows water vapour to escape and there may be heat loss as latent heat of vaporization. (It is as if a wind were blowing over the exposed abdominal contents.) If the procedure is prolonged, the core tempera-ture should be monitored and hypothermia corrected.

Minimal access surgery instrumentation

The expanding range of laparoscopic procedures creates a demand for novel instruments. However, a number of basic instruments are common to all therapeutic laparoscopic procedures.

Basic instruments

A basic instrument set might consist of:

- 1 × 10-mm 0° laparoscope
- 1 × Veress needle (120mm or 150mm)
- 2 × 10-mm trocar and cannula with trumpet valve and gas inlet
- 2 × 5-mm trocar and cannula with trumpet valve and gas inlet

- 1 × 5-mm insulated grasping forceps
- 1 × 5-mm insulated grasping forceps with ratchet
- 1 × 5-mm insulated dissecting forceps
- 1 × 5-mm insulated scissors
- 1 × 5-mm reducing sleeve
- 1 × 10-mm clip applicator
- 1 × 5-mm right angled diathermy hook
- 1 × 5-mm suction/irrigator
- 1 × 10-mm retrieval forceps
- 1 × light cable
- 1 × diathermy lead
- 1 × gas lead
- 1 × cholangiography catheter

Note: try to ensure that all diathermy instruments are compatible with a single diathermy electrode fitting. Have bipolar forceps available.

Trocar and cannula

Either all metal (reusable) or all plastic (disposable) trocars and cannulae are used. Hybrid trocars made of both plastic and metal and not advisable for risk of serious diathermy injuries due to non-transmission of current to the anterior abdominal wall. Disposable cannulae for single use may be more expensive but have the advantages of being sharp and radiolucency allowing visibility through the walls. Newer trocars have non-bladed tissue separating mechanisms which cause lesser bleeding and some others allow the passage of a telescope through the trocar for direct penetration under vision.

Grasping forceps

- Used for grabbing and retracting tissues within the abdominal cavity
- May have a ratchet to keep the jaws closed
- Traumatic or atraumatic jaws
- Type used will depend on the surgery being performed

Dissecting forceps

- For spreading, separating, and dividing
- Atraumatic
- Straight or curved

Scissors

- For cutting tissue or sutures
- May be hooked, straight, curved, or micro

Suction/irrigation

Suction and irrigation systems utilize a suction/irrigation pump, which performs the dual task of negative suction to suck out fluid and also provides pressure irrigation. Some surgeons add heparin to the irrigation fluid to discourage blood clotting in the tubing system.

Additional instruments—available for particular procedures or surgeon preference:

- 10-mm 30° laparoscope—for hernias and advanced procedures
- 5-mm 0° laparoscope—for use with a 5-mm port
- 2 × 5-mm needleholders
- 1 × 10-mm retractor
- 5-mm and 10-mm Babcocks—beware! Some of these are very traumatic
- 5-mm and 10-mm bowel clamps
- Biopsy forceps

- Bipolar forceps
- Endoscopic stapling instruments
- Endoscopic retrieval bags
- Endoloops
- Desjardins stone grasping forceps

It is important for theatre staff to have a good knowledge of the instruments available within their unit. They are then able to offer assistance or guidance, especially if the unexpected occurs or the surgeon is inexperienced. For example, if the cystic duct is too wide to clip safely, an endoscopic stapling gun or endoloop might be a suitable alternative, thus avoiding conversion to an open procedure.

Selecting and purchasing instruments for MAS is complex as more than one department/specialty is involved. There are a number of manufacturers supplying instruments, each of which may have different preparation, sterilization, assembly and disassembly, cleaning, and maintenance requirements. It is therefore obviously easier for theatre staff and a better use of resources if some standardization can be agreed and maintained.

Selection of instruments will also depend on unit policy with regard to disposable equipment and the surgeon's preference.

Diathermy during laparoscopic surgery

Both monopolar and bipolar diathermy is used in laparoscopic surgery and undoubtedly, the latter is much safer since the current travels only in the tissue held in the bipolar forceps and does not travel to any other organ or part of the body. Newer vessel sealing devices like Ligasure™ etc. are applications of bipolar diathermy which can seal vessels up to 7mm in diameter by using a combination of pressure and energy. However, surgeons are more accustomed to using monopolar diathermy since there is no need to hold structures in a forceps like in bipolar and also because it is used so frequently in open surgery as well.

Use of monopolar diathermy in laparoscopic surgery needs awareness about the principles of working while using coagulation or cutting mode. Of the two, coagulation current which is generally used for **electrofulguration**, is based on using a combination of high voltage and low amperage which has the potential to damage the insulation of the working instruments and creates an electromagnetic field around the instrument which can 'jump' to another conductor in its proximity causing inadvertent injuries to structures held in the second instrument. By comparison, cutting current involves high amperage and low voltage and is inherently safer in terms of the above noted effects and is used for **electrocutting**. The most common use of diathermy is, however, **electrodessication**, which is coagulation of a vessel by holding it in a forceps and this is achieved equally well by both cutting and coagulation diathermy since this is a feature of power which is similar in both types of modes, being a product of voltage and amperage. Hence, cutting being a low voltage mode can be safer to use inside the abdominal cavity as a whole if the purpose can be achieved by doing either electrocutting or electrodessication.

Cutting mode can thus achieve the dual benefits of performing both electrocutting and electrodessication functions with much safer lower voltage requirements and thus increasing the life of hand instruments and avoiding any jump effects of current.

Inadvertent burns to the patient are a special hazard of laparoscopic surgery. There are several mechanisms:

- Burning the wrong structure
- Inappropriate or inadvertent activation of electrodes out of view
- Faulty insulation
- Instrument to instrument coupling (direct coupling)
- Retained heat
- Capacitive coupling

Burning the wrong structure

Probably the most common cause is misidentification of the structure to which the diathermy is applied.

Inappropriate or inadvertent activation of electrodes

Pressure on the footswitch leads to activation of all the active electrodes, which are connected. In open surgery, any devices, which are not in use, must not be in contact with the patient and an unused electrode should be safely stored in an insulated quiver where it will be safe if the footswitch is inadvertently activated. In laparoscopic surgery, devices connected to the diathermy generator often remain within the operating field while not in immediate use. If they are in contact with tissue when the footswitch is activated, a burn will occur. There is particular danger if the electrode is out of view at the time.

- Devices attached to the diathermy machine must not touch tissue while not in use
- It is safest to remove or disconnect devices attached to the diathermy machine when not in use
- Do not attach more than one active electrode

Faulty insulation

It is possible for burns to occur when conducting parts of instruments other than the operating electrode come into contact with the patient. In practice, this arises when there is a defect or crack in the insulation of a laparoscopic diathermy instrument, which allows current to travel to tissue as well as by the intended path from the electrode.

Abrasives used to clean laparoscopic instruments may wear away the thin insulation near the tip increasing the length of the exposed active electrode.

Raising the temperature of the bowel to 60°C for even a short time leads to denaturation of intracellular enzymes and tissue death *in situ*. Subsequent autodigestion of the necrotic tissue leads to late perforation.

Instruments are more likely to become damaged with age but you must not assume that single-use instruments are immune to this problem. The higher the effective voltage of the current being used, the more likely it is to leak.

Leakage is also more likely if the diathermy is activated when the electrode tip is distant from target tissue (open circuit activation).

- Do not use diathermy instruments, which are damaged or badly maintained
- Avoid open circuit activation

Flow of current from one instrument to another

Contact or close approximation of the active electrode and another conducting instrument can establish an unwanted and unnoticed current path. This is known as direct coupling of the current. In an open operation such contacts are easily noticed and appropriate action taken. In laparoscopy, arcing between instruments may occur outside (behind) the field of view and you may not notice anything other than that the diathermy does not work as expected at the site where you think you are applying it. Turning up the power in these circumstances can have disastrous consequences. Remember that coagulation and blend currents have a larger effective voltage, as compared to cutting current and can jump bigger gaps. Open circuit activation is particularly dangerous.

Instrument to instrument coupling is more likely with open circuit activation:

- Do not activate the diathermy unless the whole of the active electrode is in view
- Do not activate the diathermy if there is a chance that two instruments are in electrical contact or close enough for arcing to occur

Retained heat

When you have been using the diathermy for some time the tip of the active electrode becomes hot and remains so for some time. The electrode may be hot enough to damage tissue although no current is flowing.

- Do not allow a hot active electrode to touch tissue

Unintentionally high current density in pedicles

The heating effect of diathermy depends upon the current density and the resistance of the tissue. *The sight of penile necrosis on a small boy is so disturbing that most surgeons are aware of the danger of using monopolar diathermy to perform a circumcision.* The current path through the base of the infant penis is small in cross-section; the current density is high and the heating effect disastrous. The same effect can also occur when applying diathermy to a pedicled structure such as the appendix or a gall bladder freed from the liver and attached to the common bile duct by the cystic duct. The heating effect may be sufficient to cause destruction of tissue and the effects may be just as awful as penile necrosis.

Safety rule: monopolar diathermy should be avoided on organs attached by small pedicles to important structures.

Capacitive coupling

Finally, there is the more difficult concept of capacitive coupling. This occurs when current is transferred from insulated active electrode to the nearby conductive instrument. This is probably very rare and only occurs in special circumstances.

There are two ways to avoid capacitive coupling. When using a diathermy instrument through a trocar, either:

• Use a non-conducting trocar; with electroshield system. The system measures and shunts all capacitive current to the generator plate avoiding the transfer of current to biological tissue, or
• If you use a metal trocar, it should make a good electrical contact with the abdominal wall for current to be dispersed

Also, avoid open circuit activation and avoid using high-voltage diathermy currents in non-contact mode (e.g. fulguration) as it can lead to direct coupling of the instruments or even laparoscope when it touches the active electrode. The charged instrument can inadvertently transfer the charge to the tissue it comes in contact with and damage it.

Newer energy sources

Argon Enhanced Coagulation and Cutting: Argon is an inert, non combustible gas which is heavier than air and nitrogen. Argon is easily ionized by radio-frequency current and is used as a bridge between the electrode and the tissue to achieve more effective coagulation. It also decreases smoke, odour, blood loss and rebleeding.

Ultrasonic Energy or Harmonic Scalpel™: This device uses high frequency oscillations at 55,000/sec (ultrasonic energy) at the tip of the instrument transmitted from the ceramic crystal in the hand portion.

This mechanical high frequency vibration produces local heat up to 80° C in comparison to 300–400° C in conventional diathermy. Up to 3–5 mm vessels can be coagulated. Both cutting and coagulation functions can be achieved by using this ultrasonic energy thereby offering safety and ease to perform advanced laparoscopic procedures.

Theatre set-up

The positioning of all equipment must be carefully planned. Exact placement will vary depending on the procedure to be performed, the surgeon's preference, and the size of the theatre. However, some generalizations can be made. The monitors should be positioned on either side of the patient to provide a clear unobstructed view for surgeon and assistant. Ideally, the screen should be positioned directly in the surgeon's line of sight.

The insufflator should be within view of the surgeon so that he or she can always monitor the abdominal pressure. Instrument trolleys, diathermy, suction/irrigation, etc., should be positioned to allow the surgeon mobility and to give theatre staff access to equipment. Leads and cables should be positioned so that when connected, they do not become tangled or restrict the surgeon's movements. Picture interference will also be minimized if the diathermy machine is positioned away from the camera/monitors and if the diathermy instrument is not close to the camera head when in use. The diathermy and video leads should also be kept apart.

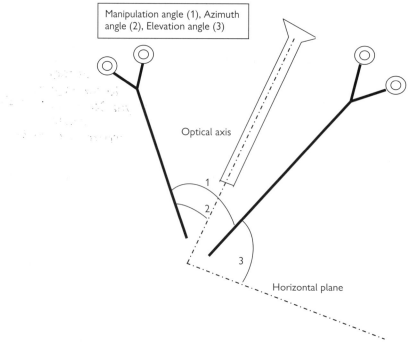

Figure 4.2 Angles governing port location.

Port placement and insertion

Port placement

For bimanual tasks, manipulation, azimuth, and elevation angles govern optimal port sites:

- Manipulation angle is the angle between the active and assisting instruments
- Elevation angle is the angle between the instrument and the horizontal plane
- Azimuth angle is the angle between instrument and the optical axis of the endoscope (Fig. 4.2)

The maximal efficiency and quality performance of intracorporeal knotting are obtained with a manipulation angle ranging between 45° and 75° with the ideal angle being 60°. A better task efficiency is achieved with an equal azimuth angle on either side of the optical port. In practice, equal azimuth angles may be difficult to achieve but wide azimuth inequality should be avoided since this degrades task efficiency. When a 30° manipulation angle is imposed by the anatomy or build of the patient, the elevation angle should also be 30° as this combination enables the shortest execution time and allows an acceptable level of performance. Likewise with a 60° manipulation angle, the corresponding optimal elevation angle, which yields the shortest execution time and an optimal quality of performance, is 60°. Thus within the range of angles that ensure adequate task efficiency, a good rule of thumb is that the elevation angle should be equal to the manipulation angle.

On planning port location, an adequate intracorporeal instrument length should be obtained. This depends on the size of the patient and the site of the operation. The intra-:extracorporeal shaft ratio for optimal task performance is 2:1.

The ports for instruments (active and assisting) and the endoscope should be inserted so that the instrument and endoscope should be aligned in the same direction. The surgeon must avoid operating against the endoscope/camera as this produces a mirror image and makes manipulations extremely difficult.

Pneumoperitoneum

To create a working space in the abdomen, pneumoperitoneum is established through an open or closed technique. Though air was the first gas used to produce pneumoperitoneum, it has largely been abandoned for the risk of air embolism and supporting combustion.

Access or placement of the first port

There are two techniques for creation of pneumoperitoneum:

1 Closed technique
2 Open technique

No single access technique has emerged as the safest and best technique. The open method is safest and is increasingly being accepted as best practice. Many surgeons prefer to have both methods available for use when appropriate.

Closed technique

This involves a Veress needle which is a spring-loaded central slim trocar; the needle traverses the rectus sheath and enters the peritoneum. The inner trocar retracts as the needle encounters resistance and springs back on entering the peritoneal cavity. This spring-loaded mechanism has to be confirmed to be in working order each time before use.

Usually a vertical or transverse stab incision is made deep inside the inferior aspect of the umbilicus. It overlies the area where skin, deep fascia, and parietal peritoneum meet at the thinnest point in the abdominal wall. The patient is placed in a Trendelenburg position of 20–30°. The surgeon and assistant lift up the anterior abdominal wall on either side of the umbilicus to create negative pressure within the abdominal cavity.

The Veress needle is then inserted, initially perpendicular to the abdominal wall, and advanced until it penetrates the linea alba and peritoneum. There is usually a distinct 'give' as the needle enters the peritoneum. It is now that damage to underlying structures can occur. The needle is to be advanced under careful control, held in the sensitive pinch grip between forefinger and thumb, like a pen or a dart, to feel the way through the layers.

A number of tests can be performed in sequence to confirm proper placement of the needle.

1 **Saline drop test**: a drop of saline is placed on the hub of the needle and the abdominal wall is lifted up. If correctly sited, the drop gets sucked inside due to the negative pressure of the intraperitoneal cavity
2 **Aspiration test**: a syringe filled with saline connected to the Veress needle is used. Drawing back should draw air or clear fluid into the syringe and not bile, blood, or bowel contents
3 **Negative pressure test**: the insufflation tubing from the insufflator should next be connected to the Veress needle. Monitoring the peritoneal pressure prior to any insufflation at this point will reveal a slight negative pressure easily accentuated by abdominal wall elevation
4 **Early insufflation pressures**: the next clue to correct positioning is monitoring of the insufflation pressure which should not exceed 8mmHg at 11L/min. The static pressure must not exceed 3mmHg. Pressures of >15mmHg with a low or no flow of gas indicate incorrect needle tip position
5 **Volume test**: in the average adult the volume required to distend the peritoneum adequately, and which creates a pressure of 8–10mmHg, is about 2.5L of gas. If this is extraperitoneal then it will often be accompanied by asymmetric anterior abdominal wall distension

If the abdominal cavity is well distended, the peritoneal contents should fall away from the abdominal wall. However, insertion of the first port in the closed method remains one of the most dangerous procedures in laparoscopy and has been reported to cause both visceral and vascular injuries.

The port is inserted with great circumspection. The body of the device is held in the palm while an index finger extended along the insertion tube will act as a guard to prevent more than a centimetre or so of the sharp end entering the peritoneal cavity.

The site for insertion of the first trocar, which holds the laparoscope, is usually around the umbilicus. In patients likely to have adhesions, the risk and severity of organ trauma is reduced if a 5.5-cm cannula is inserted in the first instance and an initial scan of the underlying omentum, bowel, and retroperitoneum is made to exclude injury. Once the surgeon is satisfied with the position and absence of iatrogenic damage, the small cannula is replaced by an 11-mm cannula using the trocar dilation system. All secondary ports are introduced under direct vision.

Usually an intraumbilical incision is used for insertion of a Veress needle but for the very obese, for some advanced upper abdominal procedures, and where there are pre-existing abdominal wall scars, other access points may be used, such as the left hypochondrium.

Open method of inserting the first port

Open laparoscopy is favoured for all cases by many surgeons who prefer not to insert a sharp instrument where they cannot see. Open access is recommended to all surgeons where there are scars in the abdominal wall close to the site of insertion of the laparoscope.

A 1–2-cm intraumbilical vertical incision is deepened down to the linea alba which is incised between stay sutures. The peritoneum is exposed and an incision made into it under vision. A finger may then be inserted to sweep away adhesions. A blunt-tipped trocar is then inserted which will not penetrate structures attached to nearby scars. A supraumbilical incision may be preferable in case of a pre-existing infraumbilical scar.

Another method of open abdominal access is by making a horizontal infraumblical incision (smiling incision) of 1–2cm. The junction of umbilical pillar with linea alba, the thinnest part of the abdominal wall, is dissected. Once the junction is displayed, a vertical 10-mm incision is made, half on the umbilical pillar and half on the linea alba, while the upward (skyward) traction on the pillar is maintained at all times. The traction is a key step because it lifts the anterior abdominal wall upward, thereby making this procedure safer. In other methods, there is a tendency to dig deeper and deeper, pressing the abdominal wall towards the vertebral column, which is hazardous. More than half the time the peritoneal cavity is opened by this incision itself. In other cases, the two edges of the linea alba are held with an Allis forceps and an artery forceps, and the peritoneum is seen below. This area is then held with a pair of artery forceps and incised under vision. The cannula is inserted, and a horizontal mattress skin suture is applied at the umbilicus to prevent any gas leakage. If a self-retaining balloon trocar is used, this suture is unnecessary. The technique was described first by the author nearly 10 years ago and is now the preferred mode of laparoscopic access for a number of surgeons with a low complication rate.

Complications in port insertion

Bleeding from port site, usually manifests itself as a continuous stream of blood dripping from one of the trocars, and/or as blood seen on the surface of the abdominal viscera or omentum. Abdominal wall haemorrhage may be controlled with a variety of techniques, including application of direct pressure with the operating port, open or laparoscopic suture ligation, or tamponade with a Foley's catheter inserted into the peritoneal cavity.

The risk of visceral injury remains during insertion of the Veress needle as well as the first trocar since both are blind manoeuvres, and even with extreme care, accidental puncture of a hollow viscus is still possible. If aspiration of the Veress needle returns yellowish or cloudy fluid, the needle is likely in the lumen of the bowel. Due to the small calibre of the needle itself, this is usually a harmless situation. Simply remove the needle and repuncture the abdominal wall. After successful insertion of the laparoscope, examine the abdominal viscera closely for significant injury.

Removal of ports

All ports should be removed under direct laparoscopic vision to be sure that there is no bleeding from portholes. The last port should be removed slowly with the laparoscope inside the port to be sure that there is no bleeding.

Closure of port sites

It is recommended to close all port sites ≥10mm to avoid later hernias. Most surgeons advocate formal closure of deep layers with interrupted synthetic absorbable or non-absorbable suture (usually using a

J-needle) with separate skin closure. Take care not to pick up small bowel in the closing stitch. A number of port closure devices are also available to achieve this under direct vision. Five-millimetre port sites do not require closure of the abdominal wall and simply need skin closure.

Endoscopic surgery

Flexible endoscopy is an important development in the area of diagnosis and therapy of the aerodigestive tract. Two types of flexible endoscopes are currently used, and they transmit the image differently. The fibreoptic endoscope has two fibreoptic bundles, one bundle of fibres carries light into the examined organ, and a second bundle transmits the image from the organ interior to the viewing optic. The image produced by a fibreoptic endoscope is composed of a multitude of images transmitted by each individual fibre. The fibres break frequently and the quality of the image produced goes down.

On the other hand, videoendoscopy applies video technology to endoscopy, with significant improvements in image quality and endoscope durability. Light is transmitted to the tip of the endoscope through a fibreoptic bundle, as in a fibreoptic endoscope. However, the viewing fibreoptic bundle is replaced with a chip camera, placed at the tip of the endoscope. This chip carries a digital image back to a video processor, which displays an image on a colour monitor.

Flexible endoscopes provide one or more instrument channels (2–3mm) for passage of diagnostic and therapeutic instruments as well as for suctioning. Air and water insufflation channels permit distention of the bowel and cleaning of the lens.

Upper GI endoscopy and colonoscopy and sigmoidoscopy are commonly performed in the outpatient department for diagnostic and therapeutic purposes in specially designed rooms for this purpose under light sedation. A number of surgical procedures have been described using endoscopy and may require the patient to be admitted. Commonly performed procedures include endoscopic banding for variceal haemorrhage, endoscopic control of bleeding peptic ulcers, endoscopic gastrostomy and jejunostomy. Other procedures performed include sphincterotomy, pancreatic pseudocyst drainage, mucosectomy or endoscopic mucosal resection (EMR), endoscopic submucosal dissection (ESD), endoscopic muscular dissection (EMD), tumourectomy, and transanal endoscopic microsurgery (TEM), endoscopy surgery for gastroesophageal reflux, etc. One of the potential roles of endoscopy is in NOTES or the natural orifice transluminal endoscopic surgery that is described below.

Endoscopy, both diagnostic and therapeutic has a huge role in GU surgery—in the kidney, ureter, bladder, prostate, and urethra. Further details are beyond the scope of this chapter.

SILS (single incision laparoscopic surgery)

SILS is a rapidly evolving field as a bridge between traditional laparoscopic surgery and NOTES. The procedure is performed through a single incision and has the advantages of reducing postoperative pain and virtually scarless surgery. SILS violates the standard principle of triangulation of surgeon's hands in laparoscopic surgery and requires a lot of un-learning and re-training. Although all types of procedures have been performed using SILS, this technique still remains under evaluation for lack of long term benefits.

NOTES (natural orifice transluminal endoscopic surgery)

NOTES is yet another controversial advance in MAS that has opened doors to closed spaces via natural routes. NOTES is performed through one of the natural orifices, i.e. mouth, anus, or vagina. These procedures are performed via the transgastric, transcolonic, and transvaginal routes. The first cholecystectomy has already been performed using NOTES procedure and the procedure is drawing the interest of both surgeons and endoscopists.

Endoscopic ultrasonography (EUS)

The ability to image the GI tract with endoscopically-placed ultrasound transducers represents a major advance in endoscopic imaging. EUS combines endoscopy and high-frequency ultrasound, incorporating a small ultrasonic transducer into the tip of endoscopes. Low-frequency transducers allow imaging of tissue up to 5–6cm from the transducer but are limited by relatively low resolution. In contrast,

Table 4.1 Indications for EUS

Diagnostic	EUS guided intervention
• Staging of malignant masses of the upper GI tract (oesophagus and stomach)	• Needle aspiration of masses and nodes adjacent to the upper GI tract
• Diagnosis of submucosal lesions	• Needle aspiration of pancreatic masses
• Upper GI anastomotic stricture	• Celiac neurolysis for pain of pancreatic cancer
• Mediastinal mass (nodes, cysts, masses)	
• Staging of malignant pancreatic-ampullary masses	
• Diagnosis of a suspected pancreatic mass	
• Diagnosis of common bile duct stones	
• Diagnosis of islet cell tumours, including gastrinomas	
• Evaluation of pseudocysts to aid in the placement of a stent	
• Staging of rectal cancer	
• Evaluation of anal sphincter	

high-frequency transducers are often used in miniprobes because they provide high-resolution imaging of structures within 1–2cm. The miniprobes are designed to provide detailed imaging of mucosal lesions, morally-based malignancies, and the wall structure of the upper GI tract. For the upper GI tract, mostly oblique-viewing endoscopes are generally used. For colorectal EUS, rigid probes for the rectum and a flexible forward-viewing echocolonoscope are available. EUS generates ultrasound either mechanically or electronically, depending on the type of instrument used. The electronic technique potentially allows the incorporation of (colour) Doppler ultrasound, which allows for additional processing and post-processing functions. On ultrasound images, hypoechoic structures are darker than the surrounding tissue, and hyperechoic structures are lighter than their surroundings. Fluids such as pleural effusion and blood are extremely hypoechoic (black). Lymph nodes are suspicious for malignancy when they have a hypoechoic structure, sharp edges, and a round shape. Benign lymph nodes are hyperechoic, with unclear edges and a long, narrow, draped, or triangular shape. There are various applications of EUS and it can be used either for diagnostic or even for the purpose of guided intervention (Table 4.1).

Chapter 5 **Post-operative care of the surgical patient**

Please note that there is no separate section on Scenarios for this chapter. Scenarios pertaining to this chapter will be found in Chapters 25–32.

This chapter will help you answer oral questions in the station on 'Applied surgical science and critical care'. These questions will be in the generic section. The scenarios will overlap with questions in the 'Communication skills specialty' station where you may be given a post-operative problem to solve.

Introduction

Post-operative recovery is an essential component of successful surgery. By the same note, the ability to manage patients competently post-operatively is an essential component of a successful surgeon.

Post-operative care begins as soon as the operation is complete and the patient leaves the operating theatre for the recovery area. It continues throughout the patient's in-hospital stay and extends to the post-discharge period until the patient is completely convalesced and has resumed their usual daily activities.

Optimal post-operative care is largely pre-emptive rather than therapeutic. Regular clinical assessment, selective monitoring, and timely intervention are key to an uncomplicated and comfortable recovery. These measures will also allow the surgical team to recognize and treat complications/potential complications early to prevent deterioration.

Immediate post-operative care

At the end of the operation, once the anaesthetic agent has been discontinued/reversed and the patient is haemodynamically stable, conscious, and responding to simple commands, the patient can be transferred, with their operation note, post-operative instructions, and anaesthetic chart, to the recovery room for further monitoring. Here, the patient will receive one-to-one or one-to-two level care. Alternatively, some patients may be transferred directly to a critical care unit post-operatively.

For most patients, recovery from anaesthetic is uneventful. However, if complications do occur they can be life threatening (e.g. airway obstruction, haemorrhage). The aim of transferring patients to the recovery area is to facilitate:

- Regular monitoring of the patient's respiratory, cardiovascular, and conscious state:
  - ♦ All patients must have a patent airway and should be on supplemental oxygen
  - ♦ Patients will be attached to continuous monitors—ECG, pulse oximeter—with set limits. Any recordings outside these limits will trigger an alarm
  - ♦ All observations of vital signs, including BP readings, should be recorded intermittently, usually every 5 minutes in the first 30 minutes and, if the patient remains haemodynamically stable, every 15 minutes subsequently until the patient is transferred out of the recovery area
  - ♦ Note sedation score and manage as appropriate
  - ♦ Ensure adequate rate of IV fluids and adequate urine output
  - ♦ Temperature—avoid hypo- or hyperthermia
- Symptom control:
  - ♦ Optimize analgesia in the early post-operative period—patients should be asked about their pain score and given analgesia to control pain. Patients requiring opioid analgesia should not be transferred to a ward setting for at least a further 30 minutes post-administration
  - ♦ Manage post-operative nausea and vomiting (PONV) with anti-emetics and if possible, identify and treat the cause of PONV
- Assessment of:
  - ♦ Surgical site and drain sites—ensure no overt bleeding, adequate closure, patent drain tubing
  - ♦ Evidence of any inadvertent injury—e.g. nerve injury from positioning
- Early recognition and management of complications in an appropriately equipped setting. Recovery areas should be staffed and equipped to deal with emergencies

Although immediate post-operative care is largely provided by recovery nurses, it is important to be aware of the role of the recovery team in your patient's journey to recovery. In addition, if there are any immediate complications, particularly if surgically relevant, you may be contacted for advice or review.

The length of time a patient stays in the recovery area depends on the length and type of surgery, type of anaesthesia, haemodynamic stability, and level of consciousness. Established criteria for discharge, such as the modified Aldrete score (Table 5.1), can be used to determine fitness for discharge to the next level. The modified Aldrete score scores patients from 0–2 in five categories—respiratory status, oxygen saturations (originally colour), circulation, consciousness, and mobility. A score of >8/10 is needed for safe discharge.

Table 5.1 Modified Aldrete score

Criteria	Score 0	Score 1	Score 2
Respirations	Apnoea	Dyspnoea	Breathes, coughs freely
Oxygen saturations	<92% on supplemental O_2	>92% on supplemental O_2	>92% on room air
Circulation/ BP	BP ± 50mmHg pre-operative value	BP ± 20--50mmHg pre-operative value	BP ± 20mmHg pre-operative value
Consciousness	Non-responsive	Wakens with stimulation	Awake and orientated
Movement	No spontaneous movement	Moves 2 limbs spontaneously	Moves 4 limbs spontaneously

Table 5.2 Post-anaesthesia Discharge Scoring System (PADSS)

Criteria	Score 0	Score 1	Score 2
Stable vital signs (BP and HR)	>40% from pre-operative baseline	Within 20–40% of pre-operative baseline	<20% of pre-operative baseline
Ambulation	Unable to ambulate	Requires assistance	Steady gait, no dizziness (or at pre-operative level)
Nausea and vomiting	Persistent despite repeated treatment	Managed with IM medication	Managed with oral anti-emetics
Pain—well controlled with analgesia and consistent with the procedure	No		Yes
Surgical	>3 dressing changes	1–2 dressing changes required	Does not require dressing change

Day surgery patients

In recent years, particularly with the advent of MAS, day surgery has been expanding both in terms of the procedures available and spectrum of patients who are suitable for day surgery procedures. To qualify for day surgery, appropriate patient selection is paramount. Similarly, patients being discharged from the day surgery unit have to meet specific criteria before being allowed home. The Post-anaesthesia Discharge Scoring System (PADSS) was developed to aid in this process (Table 5.2). Patients must have a score of at least 9/10 to qualify for discharge.

In addition, patients should also meet the following criteria before being discharged:

1 Conscious and alert—orientated to time, place, and person
2 Able to urinate asymptomatically
3 Have a responsible adult to take them home and to stay with them for 24 hours
4 Medication—understand verbal and written instructions provided:
  a Oral analgesia
  b Anti-emetics
  c Laxatives—particularly if patients are taking opioid-based analgesia
  d Antibiotics
5 Aftercare—understand the information provided on the following:
  a Normal symptoms to anticipate
  b 'Abnormal' symptoms and what to do if they occur
  c Wound care—verbal and written instructions for wound care post-discharge (suture removal, dressing change, when to shower)
  d Resuming normal activities

 e Driving
 f Information about follow-up (if any)
6 Emergency contact number supplied

Ensure that the patient and carer understand the information that they have been given and feel confident about managing at home.

> If a patient does not meet the discharge criteria and you feel the patient would not be safe at home, that patient must be admitted. A smooth uncomplicated discharge, even if protracted, is far preferable to a re-admission due to a failed discharge aiming to meet targets.

General post-operative care—the platinum 24 hours

Regular monitoring in the first 24 hours after surgery is essential as patients can develop life-threatening complications during this early period. Thirty per cent of post-operative emergencies occur within the first 6 hours of surgery and include complications involving:

- Airway/pulmonary function
- Cardiovascular system
- Fluid derangement (including haemorrhage)

Once patients are transferred from the recovery area to the ward the team taking over their care should reassess the patient. This initial assessment will determine how frequently reassessments are required. Patients with abnormal variables or severe pain must be managed and reassessed more frequently until stable and comfortable.
Initial ward assessment should include:

- History:
  - Background—diagnosis, past medical and drug history
  - Intra-operative details—operation note, post-operative instructions, anaesthetic chart
- Regular monitoring of vital signs:
  - Usually every 15–30 minutes for the first 1–2 hours, then hourly for the first 4–6 hours depending on the type of surgery.
  - Any deviation from accepted parameters should necessitate attention and appropriate management
- Assess respiratory status:
  - Breath sounds, chest excursion, and adequate cough
  - Encourage deep breathing exercises, incentive spirometry
- Note sedation score and Glasgow Coma Scale (GCS) score
- Regular (every 1–2 hours) monitoring of specific areas:
  - Vascular surgery—assess the circulatory status of the affected area
  - Neurosurgery—assess the neurological status of the affected area
- Monitor fluid balance every 1–2 hours:
  - Rate of IV fluids
  - Urine output: in patients who are not catheterized and who have not passed urine for 6–8 hours post-operatively despite judicious IV fluids, do a bladder scan and consider catheterization if in retention
- Aim for normothermia
- Symptom control:
  - Optimize analgesia:
    - Assess patient's score and manage as appropriate
    - Ensure that patients with PCA are familiar with the device
    - Good pain control is essential for deep breathing, expectoration and mobilization
  - Manage PONV with antiemetics

- Assessment of surgical site and drain sites: ensure no overt bleeding, adequate closure and patent tubing
- Early mobilization:
    ◆ At least sitting up in bed within 6–8 hours of surgery
    ◆ Mobilize to the toilet

*It is also imperative to identify patients at risk of deterioration for frequent assessment in the early post-operative period. These patients include those who have had:

- Extremes of age
- Emergency surgery
- High-risk surgery—e.g. cardiac surgery
- Patients with ASA grade 3—multiple comorbidities
- Patients with cardiorespiratory disease
- Patients requiring critical care admission post-operatively (particularly unplanned critical care admission)

General ward care

Monitoring during a patient's inpatient stay is vital to:

- Assess progress
- Identify and manage potential complications early
- Commence discharge planning

Effective pre-operative patient education has a positive impact on post-operative recovery. If patients are aware of what to expect, their post-operative recovery tends to run a smoother course and they are also more likely to comply with breathing exercises and early mobilization.

During the post-operative phase, patients should have their observations checked every 2–4 hours initially, and every 6–8 hours thereafter if they remain clinically stable. Daily review on the morning and evening ward rounds should focus on some or all of the following areas. Ensure you have a nurse with you.

1 Important developments since last review—remember to ask the **patient**!
2 Check vital signs:
    a Oxygen saturations and respiratory rate
    b Heart rate and BP
    c Temperature
    Note any deviation, even if still within normal limits, as this may be an early manifestation of a post-operative complication.
3 Pain control:
    a Pain score
    b Change in pain—improvement/deterioration, new type of pain
    c Appropriate analgesia—step-down, step-up
4 Nausea and vomiting:
    a Ensure anti-emetics are prescribed
    b Identify and manage cause if possible
5 Neurological symptoms:
    a Anxiety
    b Disorientation
    c Lethargy
    *Check—is your patient receiving a sedative? Are they hypoglycaemic?
    Monitor changes in neurological function as this is often an early manifestation of a post-operative complication, especially in the elderly.
6 Targeted examination:
    a Operative site and relevant system

    b Respiratory system including adequacy of cough, sputum inspection. Encourage deep breathing exercises, sitting upright, incentive spirometry. Listen to their chest. Physiotherapy is paramount especially in patients with poor respiratory effort or those who are unable to expectorate

    c Cardiovascular system

    d Abdominal examination—tenderness, distension, bowel sounds, passage of flatus or faeces, vomiting/nasogastric (NG) output

7 Wound inspection:

    a Inspect for evidence of infection—tenderness, swelling, erythema

    b Wound integrity—dehiscence

    c Suture or clip removal

8 Tubes (including cannulae, central or arterial lines), drains and catheters:

    a Monitor output—colour and volume

    b Remove as soon as practicable—patient comfort, prevent infection

9 Fluid balance—match input to output:

    a Input—enteral, intravenous

    b Output—urine output, GI losses (including NG tube, stoma, vomitus, and faeces, especially if diarrhoea), abdominal drains, pyrexia

10 Blood glucose monitoring—especially in diabetic patients

11 Nutrition—start early:

    a Monitor intake versus requirements (diet sheet)—use high-caloric supplements if needed

    b Involve your dietitian

    c Use enteral route where possible—associated with fewer complications, augments gut barrier function

    d If prolonged starvation anticipated, use a NG or nasojejunal (NJ) tube for feeding or insert a feeding jejunostomy tube at time of surgery

    e Total parenteral nutrition—use only if enteral route cannot be used

12 Venous thromboembolism prophylaxis:

    a Thrombo-embolus deterrent (TED) stockings

    b Low-molecular-weight heparin (LMWH)

    c Early mobilization

    d Examine for signs and symptoms of a DVT and PE

13 Drug chart:

    a Monitor necessity and duration of treatment, e.g. antibiotics, PCA

    b Convert to oral as soon as possible

    c Restart patient's regular medications

14 Investigations—review results and manage as needed. Monitor trends rather than definite values:

    a Blood tests—full blood count (FBC), urea and electrolytes (U&Es), liver function tests (LFTs), C-reactive protein (CRP), clotting

      i If low haemoglobin (Hb):

        1 Presume surgical bleeding

        2 Check haematocrit for dilution

        3 Check urea for upper GI bleed/peptic ulcer disease

        4 Consider transfusion especially if Hb <8, patient symptomatic or has ischaemic heart disease

      ii Raised inflammatory markers—white cell count (WCC), CRP

      (Note: inflammatory markers will be raised in the immediate post-operative period. Look for trends)

        1 Look for other signs of sepsis

        2 Look for potential cause of sepsis

      iii Monitor electrolytes

      iv Check clotting, especially in patients

        1 Receiving therapeutic anticoagulants—e.g. warfarin

        2 Undergoing invasive procedures—e.g. radiologically guided drains, central venous lines

    b Other investigations
       i Radiology
      ii Microbiology
    iii Pathology
    iv Special tests—ECG, arterial blood gas (ABG)
15 Plan:
    a Problem list and management
    b Discharge planning

Specific issues in post-operative care

Globally, up to one in every six patients will develop a complication post-operatively. As this is a common issue in surgical practice it will be a common OSCE station. The focus of the OSCE can range from minor problems such as nausea to major life-threatening complications such as PE. You may be asked to assess and manage patients with general complications which may occur after any operation or complications specific to the procedure the patient has had. Early recognition and management is essential to excelling in this station (and in preventing patient deterioration).

One clue to the diagnosis of post-operative complications is **timing**. Specific complications occur at specific phases in the post-operative period as detailed below:

- Immediate—within 24 hours of surgery
- Early—during the post-operative in-hospital stay or within 30 days of surgery
- Late—after discharge form hospital or more than 30 days after surgery

Note: if a patient becomes unwell in the post-operative period, it is most likely related to the procedure. Assume this is the case until proven otherwise.

Below are examples of common post-operative complications and management of each.

Post-operative pyrexia

Post-operative pyrexia is a common problem after surgery. Here is a guide on how to approach an OSCE station on post-operative pyrexia.

1 Timing:
- First 24 hours—common:
  - Systemic response to trauma—does not require treatment
  - Pre-existing infection, release of abscess causing septicaemia
  - Drug /transfusion reaction
  - Other medical problems—thyroid storm, Addisonian crisis, alcohol withdrawal, malignant hyperthermia
- Days 1–3:
  - Atelectasis
  - Chest infection
  - Phlebitis secondary to cannula site infection
  - Infected haematoma
- Days 4–7:
  - Chest infection
  - Wound infection
  - Intra-abdominal sepsis—collection, anastomotic leak
  - Urinary tract infection
- Days 7–10:
  - Chest infection
  - Wound infection
  - Urinary tract infection
  - Intra-abdominal sepsis—collection, anastomotic leak
  - DVT/PE
- Drug/transfusion reaction (including to blood products) can occur at anytime

2 Type of surgery—may predispose the patient to specific infections/risks:
  - E.g. urinary sepsis after urological procedures, DVT/PE after long bone surgery
3 Full history and clinical examination—look for other clinical signs:
  - General—rigors, tachycardia, hypotension, feeling unwell, rash
  - Respiratory system—cough, sputum, RR, O_2 saturations, chest examination
  - Wound infection—erythema, purulent discharge, dehiscence
  - Abdominal examination—distension, tenderness, paucity of bowel sounds, vomiting or high NG aspirates, diarrhoea
  - Urinary system—dysuria, smelly urine, urinalysis
  - Calf pain or tenderness
  - Examine all line sites and remove or replace where possible—central lines, peripheral cannulae, urinary catheters, drain sites
4 Is it due to an infection?
  - Look at pattern of pyrexia- persistent, swinging (suggests collection or abscess), one-off, relation to medication or infusion
  - Inflammatory markers—rising
5 Investigations—will depend on the likely cause discerned clinically:
  - Septic screen—blood cultures, sputum culture, urine culture (if positive urinalysis), line tip cultures, stool culture
  - Chest x-ray (CXR)
  - ECG
  - ABG
  - Imaging (depending on other clinical signs)—V/Q scan, abdominal ultrasound scan (USS) or CT scan
6 Management—depends on the cause:
  - Replace fluids—IV or enterally (patients fluid requirement increase when pyrexial)
  - Treat infection—appropriate antibiotics (after septic screen):
    ◆ Extra care in patients where infections can have disastrous consequences—patients at risk of endocarditis, patients with prosthetic material e.g. joint replacements
    ◆ Don't forget—you can always get advice from your micro-biologist
  - Stop offending drugs/infusion where possible
  - Treat DVT/PE

Post-operative haemorrhage

Post-operative haemorrhage can potentially, although rarely, be life-threatening if significant and a methodical approach to management is essential. Bleeding is usually covert and concealed within body cavities. Even with well-placed drains, post-operative haemorrhage rarely presents with overt signs and hence an astute clinical examination is vital in assessing patients post-operatively. Here is a guide on how to approach the assessment and management of post-operative haemorrhage OSCE station.

Post-operative haemorrhage may be:

- Arterial:
  - ◆ E.g. from loose arterial ties, from vascular anastomosis, inadvertent injury to arteries or solid organs
  - ◆ Usually rapid, bright red (depends on oxygenation), pulsatile bleeding
- Venous:
  - ◆ More common
  - ◆ E.g. from loose ligatures, opening of venous channels, solid organ trauma
  - ◆ Usually low pressure, dark red (depends on oxygenation), non-pulsatile
- Can be large volume—obscures view, can be difficult to control

Post-operative bleeding is usually classified into:

- Primary haemorrhage:
  - ◆ Immediate—intra-operative or immediate post-operative bleeding
  - ◆ Usually the result of unsecured vessels or bleeding from solid organs during the operation

- ◆ May necessitate return to theatre if uncontrolled
- ◆ E.g. bleeding from inferior epigastric artery from port-site in laparoscopic surgery
- Reactionary haemorrhage:
  - ◆ Within the first 24 hours
  - ◆ Usually venous bleeding—presumably from vessels that were not well secured intra-operatively or dislodgement of a clot
  - ◆ As a result of increase in patient's BP and cardiac output post-anaesthetic and with IV fluid
- Secondary haemorrhage:
  - ◆ Usually within the first fortnight
  - ◆ Most commonly due to infection of the operative site causing erosion into a blood vessel, clot disintegration, or erosion of a ligature

> Remember: post-op bleeding may also occur at a site remote from surgery, e.g. post-operative haematemesis secondary to NSAID use or a stress ulcer.

Patients at particular risk of bleeding (where possible optimize/reverse pre-operatively):

- Coagulopathy
- Platelet disorders
- Anaemia
- Anticoagulation therapy
- Antiplatelet agents
- Recent blood transfusion
- Disseminated intravascular coagulation (DIC) secondary to sepsis
- Steroid use, NSAID use

Assessment

1 History:
  - Details of surgery—read the operation note, review the anaesthetic chart
  - Events since surgery
  - Past medical history
  - Drug treatment
2 Clinical examination:
  - Vital signs—note trends
  - Focused examination—wounds, dressing, drain output, operation site
3 Investigations:
  - Recent blood results—Hb level and trends, urea (raised in upper GI bleeds), clotting
  - Consider imaging—CT ± angiography

Management—twofold

1 Resuscitation (as needed):
  - Large calibre IV access. (Do not try to insert central venous catheter for resuscitation in an unwell patient.)
  - Blood tests—FBC, U&Es, coagulation, cross-match
  - IV fluid bolus especially if patient tachycardic, hypotensive, oliguric
  - Fluid balance chart (catheterize if hypotensive, tachycardic, or oliguric)
  - Stop/reverse offending drugs where possible—aspirin, clopidogrel, warfarin
  - Blood transfusion to maintain Hb (have a lower threshold for transfusion in patients with ischaemic heart disease)
    - ◆ *Check patient's wishes (Jehovah's witness, personal preference, etc.)
  - Correct coagulopathy—vitamin K, fresh frozen plasma (FFP), clotting factors
  - Consider advice from Haematology, ITU
2 Identify and control bleeding:
  - If superficial or easily accessible, apply direct pressure/packing

- If persistent bleeding, the wound or operative site may need to be explored. This may be done under local anaesthetic (on the ward or in theatre) or general anaesthetic (in theatre)
- For persistent internal bleeding, consider:
  - ◆ Radiologically guided embolization
  - ◆ Re-operation
- For patients with GI bleeding, consider:
  - ◆ Endoscopy
  - ◆ Omeprazole infusion

Note: bleeding in confined spaces. If a patient develops a haematoma within a confined space, it will exert pressure on surrounding structures and this can lead to significant complications. Urgent surgical decompression may be warranted. Examples of this include:

- Haematoma post neck/thyroid surgery can lead to airway obstruction
- Large haematoma after limb surgery can lead to compartment syndrome (especially if a cast is on)
- Haematoma after formation of a flap can lead to ischaemia and flap failure

Venous thromboembolism (see Chapter 19)

Venous thromboembolism is discussed in detail in Chapter 19. A summary is provided here.

In the post-operative period patients are at higher risk of developing DVT and PE due to a combination of factors which include

- Prolonged intra-operative time
- Intra-operative venous stasis
- Surgical trauma
- Relative thrombocytosis in the post-operative period
- Poor mobility in the post-operative period
- Advanced age
- Obesity
- Malignant disease
- Inflammatory conditions
- Pelvic or hip surgery or varicose vein surgery
- Previous history of DVT/PE or pro-coagulant condition
- Steroid use including the contraceptive pill

Peri-operative measure to reduce this risk include

- TEDs
- Pneumatic compression boots intra-operatively
- LMWH
- Early mobilization

Presentation and diagnosis

- DVT (Wells Score—see Chapter 19):
  - ◆ May be asymptomatic
  - ◆ Pyrexia
  - ◆ Swollen, warm leg (compare to other side)
  - ◆ Calf tenderness
  - ◆ Duplex Doppler ultrasonography
- PE:
  - ◆ Patients may present with collapse or shock (embolism affecting >25% of pulmonary vasculature). Most PE deaths occur within 2 hours of event
  - ◆ Pyrexia
  - ◆ Pleuritic chest pain
  - ◆ Dyspnoea, tachypnoea
  - ◆ Tachycardia, hypotension, elevated jugular venous pressure (JVP)

- ECG (to rule out other causes of chest pain)—normal or right heart strain (S1, Q3, T3 is rarely seen and is not specific for PE)
- CXR (to rule out other causes for symptoms)—often normal, oligaemia, wedge infarction, pleural effusion
- V/Q scan—reliably excludes PE in patients with low probability
- CT pulmonary angiogram (CTPA)—first-line investigation

D-dimer test is only useful in patients with low probability of DVT/PE. A negative test reliably excludes DVT/PE. However, a positive D-dimer does not prove anything. Remember, D-dimer is also raised after trauma including surgery.

Management

- Immediate resuscitation as needed
- In patients with a high probability of PE/DVT—commence treatment with LMWH and warfarin immediately. Continue LMWH until international normalized ratio (INR) therapeutic
- Use caution in patients immediately post-operative as bleeding in these patient may have serious consequences. Seek advice from the Haematologist
- See Chapter 19 for further details

Wound complications

Wound complications can be classified into:

- Early complications:
  - Surgical site infection (see Chapter 17)
  - Wound dehiscence
- Late complications:
  - Scarring (see Chapter 21)
  - Incisional hernia

Wound dehiscence

Although wound dehiscence is an uncommon post-operative complication affecting <3% of all abdominal operations, it has major sequelae with a protracted recovery, high morbidity and mortality of around 12–30%. Hence it is important to be able to recognize and manage this complication in the acute setting.

Risk factors which contributes to the development of wound dehiscence include:

- Wound infection—most important factor
- Emergency surgery—three times more common in emergency surgery than elective operations
- Poor surgical technique—small (e.g stitches that are <1cm from edge when performing mass closure in the abdomen) bites, superficial bites (not including fascial layers), excessive stitch interval, too much tension, absorbable sutures, poor knotting
- Malnutrition—hypoproteinaemia, vitamin C deficiency
- Immunosuppression/steroid use
- Poor blood supply—arteriopath, inotropic support, previous scar, radiotherapy, smoking
- Raised intra-abdominal pressure—ascites, ileus, severe coughing or straining of abdominal wall muscles
- Coexisting disease—malignancy, jaundice, diabetes, renal failure, obesity, anaemia
- Advanced age

Wound dehiscence is a surgical emergency and is classified as:

- Superficial—disruption of skin and subcutaneous tissue—this requires urgent wound care but is not usually an emergency
- Deep—disruption of the deep layers only (skin and superficial tissue remains intact)
- Full thickness—disruption of all layers of the abdominal wall including fascia which often results in evisceration of intra-abdominal contents

*Always assume the defect involves the entire length of the wound

Clinical features
- Usually occurs within 7–10 days post-operatively
- May be heralded by sero-sanguinous discharge
- Usually painless, unless infected
- Open wound with visible underlying structures (superficial—visible fascia; full thickness—visible viscera)

Management—initial
- Ensure patient well resuscitated—IV access, systemically stable
- Allay anxiety (especially if there is evisceration of bowel loops)
- Analgesia, if needed
- Antibiotics, if evidence of wound infection
- If superficial wound dehiscence:
  - Open the wound to allow any pus to drain
  - Washout and pack the wound with absorbent dressing (e.g. Sorbsan)
- If full thickness with evisceration (immediate action needed):
  - Return intra-abdominal contents into abdomen
  - Apply sterile dressing over wound
  - Apply warm moist dressings over area
  - Keep patient nil by mouth (NBM) in anticipation of theatre
  - Ensure patient well resuscitated
  - Inform your seniors

Management—definitive:
- Provide nutritional support
- Treat infection/manage comorbidities affecting healing
- Eliminate necrotic debris/maintain optimal environment for granulation and epithelialization
- Superficial:
  - Regular wound washout and packing
  - Consider vacuum assisted dressings for large defects
- Full thickness:
  - Mainstay of management is immediate return to theatre for reclosure of the abdominal wall with retention sutures/deep tension sutures
  - If reclosure inappropriate (critically ill patient, wound infection, intra-abdominal sepsis), consider:
    - Conservative management (leave laparostomy to heal by secondary intention)
    - Delayed primary closure when patient's condition improves
  - Temporary measures include open packing with retention sutures that can be gradually tightened, zipper closure devices, Velcro closure devices that can be gradually tightened, Bogota bag closure (using a 3L NaCl bag), vacuum-assisted closure devices and synthetic or biosynthetic mesh sutured to either skin or fascia. This allows the general condition of the patient to improve before definitive closure is attempted
  - Most surgeons plan a second look within 48–72 hours and definitive closure (if appropriate) within 7–10 days

Incisional hernia

Incisional herniae are a late complication of fascial disruption and complicate 10–15% of abdominal and pelvic wounds. Midline wounds are more commonly affected compared to muscle splitting or transverse incisions. The sac is usually formed of peritoneum and scar tissue and typically contains omental fat or bowel as it herniates through the fascia and muscle layer. They are uncommon outside the abdomen and pelvis.

Risk factors which predispose to the development of an incisional hernia are wound dehiscence and the factors which predispose to wound dehiscence (see pg 77). In addition, patients who regularly strain their abdominal wall muscles—heavy labour, constipation, chronic cough, obstructive urinary symptoms—are at greater risk of developing an incisional hernia.

Although, incisional herniae can present at anytime in the post-operative period, >50% of incisional herniae are present within 6 months of the precipitating operation and almost 97% are present within the first 5 years.

Clinical features

- Incisional herniae vary in size from small defects to those that involve the entire length of a laparotomy wound. The risk of strangulation is higher in herniae with narrow defects
- Present as a bulge, which may reduce spontaneously when supine, in the anterior abdominal wall in close proximity to the previous wound. Often increases in size with time. Some hernias remain permanently herniated and adherent to the anterior abdominal wall
- Usually asymptomatic but patient s may describe a 'heaviness' if large
- May become painful if it strangulates
- Imaging (USS, CT) may help confirm diagnosis, delineate the anatomy of the defect

Management—can be challenging

- Surgical repair:
  - Small defects can be repaired with a simple suture repair or a Mayo repair but typically a tension-free mesh repair is employed
  - Open or laparoscopic repair
  - Laparoscopic—smaller incisions, less pain, avoids re-incising through the weakened scar tissue, allows visualization of the entire length of scar without the need for a large incision, allows identification and repair of other defects simultaneously

Cardiac complications

Cardiac complications are not uncommon in the post-operative period. If you are faced with this situation in an OSCE (and in real life) it is imperative that you identify and manage the patient urgently as any delay could lead to catastrophic consequences.

Acute coronary syndrome (ACS)/myocardial infarction (MI)

Patients at risk—take a history:

- Patients with history of cardiac disease—ischaemic heart disease, angina, previous MI, poor left ventricular function, arrhythmia, hypertension
- Recent MI—surgery within 3 months of an MI, increases risk of a peri-operative MI to 25%. Ideally wait 6 months before elective surgery
- Major surgery—especially vascular or cardiothoracic surgery
- Poor post-operative management—fluid overload, hypotension, anaemia, not receiving anti-anginals post-operatively

Presentation—perform a cardiovascular and respiratory examination

- Typically early post-operative period, peak on 2nd to 4th post-operative day
- Central chest pain which may radiate to the jaw or patient's left arm
- May be silent—especially in diabetics
- May be associated with sweating , hypotension, dypnoea, nausea

Diagnosis

- 2 out of 3 of:
  - Typical history
  - ECG changes
  - Cardiac enzyme rise

*Consider other causes of chest pain—chest infection, PE, pneumothorax, musculoskeletal pain, gastro-oesophageal reflux, pericarditis, intra-abdominal cause.

Investigations and immediate management

- Sit patient up, attach monitors—oxygen saturations, HR, RR, BP, temperature
- High-flow oxygen
- ECG—ST elevation, Q wave, T-wave inversion (normal in 20%)
- IV access—take blood for FBC, U&Es, troponin, glucose, G&S. *Repeat troponin 12 hours after onset of pain
- MONA:
  - ◆ Morphine—5–10mg IV with anti-emetic
  - ◆ Oxygen
  - ◆ Nitrate—sublingual glyceryl trinitrate (GTN) (if not hypotensive)
  - ◆ Aspirin—300mg
- Beta blockers (if no contraindications, e.g. asthma, heart failure)
- LMWH
- Ensure pre-operative anti-anginal medication is restarted
- Cardiology advice urgently

Cardiac failure

Cardiac failure is defined as an inadequate cardiac output and BP for the body's requirements. Cardiac failure may be classified as:

- Low-output failure—ejection fraction <35%:
  - ◆ Pump failure—ischaemic heart disease, inadequate filling, inadequate heart rate
  - ◆ Excessive preload—fluid overload, mitral regurgitation
  - ◆ Excessive afterload—hypertension, AS
- High output failure—sepsis, hyperthyroidism, Paget's disease

During the peri-operative period, a number of factors may cause patients to develop acute cardiac failure or exacerbation of chronic cardiac failure. These include:

- Fluid overload
- Myocardial infarction
- Arrhythmias
- Sepsis
- Anaemia

Clinical features—perform a cardiovascular and respiratory examination

- Dyspnoea, tachypnoea, orthopnea, bibasal crackles
- Tachycardic, hypotensive, raised JVP, 3rd heart sound
- Pale, sweaty, peripheral oedema

Investigation and immediate management

- Sit patient up, attach monitors—oxygen saturations, HR, RR, BP, temperature
- High-flow oxygen
- IV access and bloods—FBC, U&Es, LFTs, cardiac enzymes, brain natriuretic peptide (BNP)
- ABG
- ECG—may show evidence of hypertrophy or ischaemia
- CXR (ABCDE):
  - ◆ **A**lveolar oedema
  - ◆ Kerley **B** lines
  - ◆ **C**ardiomegaly
  - ◆ **D**ilated upper lobe vasculature
  - ◆ Bilateral pleural **E**ffusions
- Morphine—5mg IV slowly with antiemetic
- Furosemide—40–80mg IV slowly

- Nitrates—GTN spray sublingually (if not hypotensive)
- Urgent advice from cardiology
- Consider starting nitrate infusion, further doses of furosemide
- If patient not improving, consider ITU review re: inotropes, invasive monitoring

Arrhythmias—atrial fibrillation (AF)

AF is common in the post-operative period affecting >30% of patient after cardiac surgery and >5% of patients after non-cardiac surgery.

Precipitating factors

- Advanced age
- Sepsis—most common cause, any source can potentially cause AF
- Hypotension, dehydration
- Electrolyte—especially Na^+, K^+, Mg^{2+}—or metabolic derangement
- Hypoxia
- Anaemia
- Pain
- Comorbid condition—MI, PE, cerebrovascular accident (CVA)
- Patients with pre-existing cardiac disease (ischaemic heart disease, valvular disease, heart failure), hyperthyroidism, alcohol abuse

Clinical features—perform a cardiovascular and respiratory examination

- Most often seen in the early post-operative period, days 1–4
- Patients are usually asymptomatic or may describe chest pain, palpitations, dyspnoea, clamminess
- Usually tachycardic (but may have a normal heart rate), hypotension
- ECG—irregularly irregular heart rate with absent P waves which have been replaced by fibrillation waves

Management of new onset (< 48 hours) post-operative AF

- Treat the underlying cause—treat infection, correct electrolyte derangement, optimize hydration, treat hypoxia, correct anaemia
- Attach monitors—oxygen saturations, HR, RR, BP, temperature
- High-flow oxygen
- If patient is haemodynamically unstable (hypotensive, pulmonary oedema):
  - ◆ Start heparin—prevent atrial thrombosis
  - ◆ Seek cardiology advice re: urgent DC cardioversion
- If patient haemodynamically stable with HR >90bpm:
  - ◆ Cardioversion (seek cardiology advice):
    - ▪ DC cardioversion
    - ▪ Pharmacological—beta blocker, calcium channel blocker, amiodarone
- If patient haemodynamically stable with HR <90bpm:
  - ◆ No further treatment needed (besides correcting underlying cause)
  - ◆ Most patients recover spontaneously within 24 hours

Respiratory complications

Respiratory complications are a common cause of post-operative morbidity in the post-operative period as a result of surgery itself, general anaesthetic, post-operative pain, and decreased mobility in the post-operative period.
   Contributory factors include:
- Pain—inability to breathe deeply, diaphragmatic splinting
- Inability to expectorate secretions

- Anaesthetic—impairment of cilia function
- Sedation
- Abdominal distension/obesity hypoventilation syndrome
- Loss of elastic recoil—elderly, smokers
- Pre-existing respiratory disease—asthma, COPD

Atelectasis/pulmonary collapse

Atelectasis is alveolar collapse due to airway obstruction with bronchial secretions. Often mild and self-limiting but can be widespread if not managed well.

- Atelectasis usually occurs within the first 24 hours
- Leads to increase work of breathing, poor gas exchange, hypoxia, predisposition to infection
- Patients may exhibit dyspnoea, tachypnoea, tachycardia, dullness at the bases with diminished breath sounds, mild pyrexia

Management/prevention

- Encourage breathing exercises/coughing to expectorate
- Early mobilization
- Good pain control
- Chest physiotherapy
- Avoid sedation in the post-operative period
- Treat cause of abdominal distension
- Humidified oxygen if hypoxic
- If patient hypoxic, tachypnoeic and tiring, consider positive pressure ventilation (CPAP) or endotracheal intubation. Seek ITU review

Respiratory tract infection

May progress from atelectasis or develop *de novo*. Usually develops after day 4.

Presentation

- Cough, purulent sputum—send for culture
- Dyspnoea, tachypnoea
- Bronchial breath sounds, diminished air entry
- Pyrexia
- ABG—hypoxia, respiratory acidosis
- Consolidation on CXR

*Aspiration pneumonia occurs as a result of inhalation of gastric contents (especially in non-starved patients undergoing emergency intubation). It is fatal in almost 50% of patients and requires urgent treatment with IV antibiotics, bronchial aspiration, steroids and positive pressure ventilation (if needed).

Management

- Manage as for atelectasis
- Humidified oxygen
- Antibiotics—while awaiting MC&S (microscopy, culture, and sensitivity) results, treat as for hospital acquired pneumonia, use local antibiotic guidelines:
  - *If aspiration pneumonia suspected—add metronidazole to antibiotic regimen
- If patient hypoxic, tachypnoeic and tiring, consider positive pressure ventilation (CPAP) or endotracheal intubation. Seek ITU review

ARDS and respiratory failure is discussed in Chapter 26.

Gastrointestinal complications

Post-operative nausea and vomiting (PONV)

PONV can be a very distressing complication of surgery. It is a common complication and affects >50% of patients to varying degrees. In the early post-operative period it may be caused by:

- General anaesthetic agents
- Gastric distension (during intubation)
- Other medication—e.g. opiates, antibiotics
- Paralytic ileus
- Sepsis

It is important to manage PONV promptly as persistent PONV can lead to other complications:

- Aspiration pneumonia
- Limited oral intake—medication, nutrition
- Electrolyte and acid-base derangement
- Wound dehiscence
- Incisional hernia

Management

- NG tube insertion
- Anti-emetic:
  - ◆ Prescribe regular and PRN antiemetics
  - ◆ Combine different classes of antiemetics for optimal function

Paralytic ileus

Paralytic ileus is due to hypomotility of the GI tract with ensuing accumulation of gas and fluid within the bowel loops resulting in abdominal distension.

It is commonly seen in the post-operative period (occurs after abdominal and extra-abdominal surgery) as a result of:

- Handling of bowel intra-operatively
- Prolonged exposure and drying of bowel loops (cover bowel loops with moist swabs intra-operatively)
- Post-operative immobility
- Hypoxia/hypotension
- Electrolyte or metabolic derangement
- Drug induced—general anaesthetic, opiates, anticholinergics
- Intra-abdominal sepsis
- Retoperitoneal collection
- Neurosurgical procedures

Clinical features

- Nausea and vomiting—usually after oral intake has commenced
- Anorexia
- No flatus or faecal output
- Painless abdominal distension—different form mechanical obstruction
- Paucity of bowel sounds—different from mechanical obstruction
- AXR—distended loops of bowel with no transition point

Management—usually self-limiting

- Bowel rest—NBM or sips as tolerated
- NG tube to empty the stomach (drip & suck)

- Ensure patient is well-hydrated (3rd space loss with fluid sequestration around inactive bowel loops)
- Correct electrolyte derangement
- Improve mobility
- Avoid opiate analgesia (where possible)
- Repeat abdominal X-ray (AXR)
- If not resolving within 48 hours—look for alternative cause (mechanical obstruction, iatrogenic bowel injury, anastomotic leak). Consider performing a CT scan or barium enema to exclude mechanical obstruction

Mechanical bowel obstruction

*It is important to differentiate mechanical obstruction from ileus as the management is different.

Causes

- Adhesions—can occur anytime after abdominal surgery, may form within the first 24 hours. Patients usually present with intermittent episodes of bowel obstruction months or years after surgery
- Hernia—internal hernia, incisional hernia, parastomal hernia

Clinical features

- Cardinal features of bowel obstruction:
  - Colicky abdominal pain
  - No passage of flatus or faecal output
  - High-pitched bowel sounds
  - Abdominal distension—more pronounced in distal obstruction
  - Nausea and vomiting—more pronounced with proximal obstruction
- Examine for hernia—wound, parastoma, hernial orifices
- AXR/CT—distended loops of bowel with transition point

Management

- Treat as for ileus—bowel rest, drip, and suck
- Adhesional small bowel obstruction should be treated expectantly as it usually resolves spontaneously. Consider surgery if not settling
- Bowel obstruction secondary to intra-abdominal hernia is unlikely to settle with conservative management and usually requires surgical management

Neurological complications

Post-operative confusion

Post-operative confusion or an altered mental state is a common complication. Patients may present with:

- Obvious signs—agitation, disorientation, uncooperative behaviour, hallucinations, personality change
- Subtle signs—inactivity, slowed thinking, quietness, labile mood, restlessness

Causes

Common causes of post-operative confusion include:

- General anaesthetic—most patients are briefly confused after general anaesthetic. This should wear off as the effects of the anaesthetic agent wears off
- Medication—opiate analgesia, benzodiazepines, other sedatives, anticholinergics, anticonvulsants
- Sepsis—any source including chest, urinary, intra-abdominal, wound infection
- Alcohol/drug withdrawal
- Hypoxia/hypercarbia
- Hypoglycaemia
- Hypotension—poor cerebral perfusion

- Pain
- More common in the elderly—especially in patients with cognitive impairment
- Electrolyte or metabolic derangement
- Acute neurological event—infarction, haemorrhage, fall

Management
- Reverse treatable causes:
  - ◆ Manage hypoxia/hypercarbia/hypoglycaemia/hypotension (if present)
  - ◆ Stop potentially offending medication
  - ◆ Treat sepsis
  - ◆ Manage alcohol/drug withdrawal appropriately (e.g. use chlordiazepoxide reducing regimen in patients with alcohol dependence)
  - ◆ Optimize analgesia
  - ◆ Correct electrolyte or metabolic derangement
- Reassure and re-orientate patient
- Assess for an acute neurological event—perform a full neurological examination, consider CT head
- Avoid sedation unless patient's behaviour is putting themselves or others in danger

Cerebrovascular accident (CVA)/transient ischaemic attack (TIA)

CVAs affect 3–5% of patients undergoing cardiac or vascular surgery (e.g. carotid endarterectomy) and are significantly less common in patients undergoing non-cardiac/vascular surgery. Risk factors include

- Increasing age
- Peri-operative hypotension (especially sudden drops in BP) causing cerebral hypoperfusion
- Cerebral haemorrhage—deranged coagulation
- Previous history of CVAs or TIAs
- Atherosclerosis—e.g. carotid artery disease
- Atrial thrombus
- AF
- Mechanical heart valve
- Hypertension
- Smoking

Clinical features
- Focal neurological deficit—perform a full neurological examination to establish diagnosis, define areas affected
- CVAs tend to progress in a stepwise fashion over hours to days before becoming established. If the deficit resolves within 24 hours—TIA
- Prompt CT scan (or MRI if brain stem lesion suspected) to rule out or confirm haemorrhagic stroke (it is important to differentiate haemorrhagic and ischaemic strokes as the management differs between the two)

Initial management
- Ensure patient is haemodynamically stable. Monitor oxygen saturations, RR, HR, BP, and temperature
- High-flow oxygen
- IV access and blood tests—FBC, U&Es, LFTs, clotting, glucose
- Prevent hypotension. Allow permissive hypertension (cerebral perfusion)
- NBM until gag reflex established and swallow deemed safe
- If haemorrhagic cause has been ruled out, give patient:
  - ◆ Aspirin
  - ◆ Dipyridamole (once ischaemic cause confirmed)
- If hemorrhagic cause confirmed—consider evacuation
- Refer to stroke unit

Genitourinary complications

Urinary retention

Post-operative urinary retention is common especially after groin, pelvic, or perineal surgery or spinal anaesthesia. It is most often seen in elderly male patients. Post-operative pain, effects of anaesthesia, effects of other drugs (e.g. anticholinergics), immobility, difficulty initiating micturition lying or sitting in bed, constipation, and pre-existing prostatic disease may also contribute to the development of post-operative urinary retention.

Clinical features

- Inability to micturate
- Dribbling, poor stream
- Suprapubic distension/discomfort (suprapubic dullness to percussion)

Management

- Manage precipitating factors—optimize pain control, avoid offending drugs, encourage mobility, treat constipation
- Check renal function
- Catheterize if conservative measures fail and patient in discomfort
- Trial without catheter (TWOC) after 12 hours—avoid prolonged catheterization where possible

Urinary tract infection (UTI)

UTIs are most commonly seen after bladder instrumentation (urological procedures, indwelling catheters—especially if prolonged) or gynaecological surgery. It is most commonly seen in females.

Clinical features

- Dysuria, frequency, urgency, haematuria, offensive smell, dribbling
- Loin pain, pyrexia
- Urinalysis—positive for nitrites, leucocytes

Management

- Send specimen for MC&S
- Remove catheter as soon as possible
- Ensure patient well-hydrated
- Empirical antibiotic treatment—trimethoprim, nitrofurantoin, ciprofloxacin, augmentin—while awaiting MC&S

Fluid balance (also see Chapter 24)

Fluid management in the post-operative period is aimed at keeping the patient normovolaemic and should be reviewed regularly. Both dehydration and fluid overload can have serious consequences. It is vital that you are able to assess a patient's fluid balance status. Below is a step-by-step guide for assessing fluid status (Table 5.3).

1 Note history:
  a Clinical notes—admission history, past medical history (heart failure, chronic kidney disease)
  b Operation and anaesthetic chart—any inadvertent ureteric injury, intra-operative fluid balance, duration of surgery, period of hypovolaemia
2 Focused examination—general status:
  a Does the patient look unwell? Are they alert and orientated? Are they thirsty?
  b Note vital signs—oxygenation, RR, HR, BP (lying and standing), CVP (note trend with fluid challenge)
  c Examine mucous membranes, skin turgor, capillary refill, temperature, JVP, quality of pulse
  d Look for evidence of pulmonary oedema, peripheral oedema
  e Abdominal examination—palpable bladder

Table 5.3 Clinical features of fluid status

Condition	Hypovolaemia	Euvolaemia	Fluid overload
Peripheral temperature	Cool	Normal	Cool
Capillary refill	Delayed	Normal	Delayed
Skin turgor	Poor	Normal	Normal
Mucous membranes	Dry	Moist	Moist
JVP	Low	Not raised	Raised
BP	Low	Normal	Low
Quality of pulse	Tachycardic, thready	Normal	Tachycardic, normal or thready
Chest auscultation	Normal	Normal	Crackles
Peripheral oedema	No	No	Yes
CVP change with fluid challenge	Transient or no rise, <3mmHg	Rise by 3–5mmHg	Sustained rise of >5mm Hg

3 Monitor losses—as accurately as possible
  a Urine output—aim for at least 0.5ml/kg/h in an adult (1ml/kg/h in a child)
  b GI output—vomiting, diarrhoea, stoma losses, fistulae
  c Other losses—bleeding (inspect operation site, colour of drain output, haemoglobin level and change), drain output, '3rd space' losses, insensible losses, pyrexia (increases fluid requirements by 500ml/day/1°C rise in temperature in a 70-kg adult)
4 Monitor intake—aim to match losses as closely as possible. Intake = 3L maintenance fluid + extra losses/day:
  a Enteral—oral or NG/NJ feed, NBM
  b Parenteral—IV fluid (crystalloid vs. colloid), TPN, medication
5 Review:
  a Recent biochemistry—urea, creatinine, sodium, potassium
  b Arterial blood gas result—assess their acid-base status
  c Review their drug chart—diuretics, nephrotoxic drugs

Clinical features of fluid status is summarized in Table 5.3.
Post-operative oliguria can be classified into

- Pre-renal—inadequate renal perfusion, e.g. hypovolaemia, shock
- Renal—intrinsic kidney damage, e.g. acute tubular necrosis, glomerulonephritis,
- Post-renal—urinary tract obstruction, e.g. enlarged prostate, ureteric injury (solitary kidney)

In the post-operative period, hypovolaemia is the most common cause of oliguria. If, from your initial assessment, you suspect a patient has a pre-renal cause of oliguria, management should include the following:

- Ensure patient is haemodynamically stable—regular monitor oxygen saturations, RR, HR, BP, and temperature
- Ensure patient is catheterized and monitor urine output:
  ◆ *Check that catheter has been flushed and bladder scans confirms empty bladder
- IV access and bloods—FBC, U&Es, LFTs, clotting, G&S
- ABG—assess acid–base balance
- Fluid challenge with colloid and note change in HR, BP, and urine output
- Consider inserting a central venous catheter if patient stable (to guide fluid resuscitation)
- If little improvement:
  ◆ Consider further fluid challenge
  ◆ Discuss patient with your registrar

♦ Organize renal ultrasound
♦ Organize critical care review and transfer to HDU setting re: renal replacement therapy

Thermoregulation

This topic is included in this chapter because pyrexia is one of the commonest post-operative complications encountered in the patient.

In the human, a warm-blooded animal, the temperature of the central core (brain, thorax, and abdomen) of the body is maintained at a constant level. The temperature of the skin is variable. Therefore, the skin plays a major role in thermoregulation. It does so by variations in the blood flow brought about by the sympathetic nervous system and hormonal activity (secretion of adrenaline), both under the control of the hypothalamus.

What is the examiner looking for?

The question on 'thermoregulation' may be asked in the oral examination station dealing with 'Applied surgical science and critical care'. The examiner wants to know if the candidate is aware of:

• The basic physiology of temperature regulation
• Clinical signs of pyrexia
• The cause of pyrexia in a particular patient
• The broad principles of management

Physiology of temperature regulation

A constant body temperature (37°C or 98.4°F) is the outcome of a balance between heat gained and heat lost. This is regulated by a centre in the hypothalamus as:

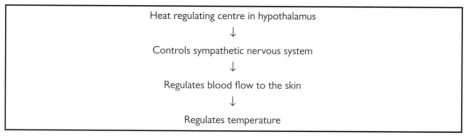

Heat regulating centre in hypothalamus
↓
Controls sympathetic nervous system
↓
Regulates blood flow to the skin
↓
Regulates temperature

Heat is gained by metabolism from oxidation of foodstuffs, muscular activity, and hot environmental temperature. Heat is lost from skin by radiation, conduction and convection, expired air, and from urine and faeces. In increased heat production, the sweat glands, under the control of the sympathetic nervous system, have an important function in heat loss by evaporation of water from the skin. Thus the sequence of events is: reduced sympathetic tone → dilatation of blood vessels → rise of skin temperature → secretion of sweat → heat loss. When the atmospheric temperature is higher than body temperature, sweating and the evaporation of sweat is a very efficient method of cooling the body provided the surrounding air is dry. In humid atmosphere, the sweat does not evaporate, causing relatively lower temperatures to be uncomfortable.

If there is diminished heat production or in a cold atmosphere, exercise increases heat production by increasing metabolism. If no voluntary exercise is done, then involuntary exercise takes place in the form of shivering. The sequence of events here is: reduced heat production → stimulates cold sensitive cutaneous nerve endings → sends impulses to hypothalamus → increases sympathetic tone and stimulates production of adrenaline → constricts cutaneous blood vessels → lowers heat loss from skin.

Abnormalities of thermoregulation

Reduced temperature

Humans at the extremes of age are most vulnerable to changes in environmental temperature. In hypothermia a hot bath is an effective way of bringing the temperature to normal. In clinical practice, prevention of hypothermia is paramount. Babies during operation should always be wrapped up carefully to prevent heat loss during operation. The same applies to adults during a long operation especially where the abdomen will be open for a lengthy period causing heat loss from exposed peritoneum and gut; the patient should be put on a warm water blanket. Patients with trauma in the accident and emergency department should be covered in a space blanket during resuscitation. Prolonged hypothermia may cause organ dysfunction from vasoconstriction.

Increased temperature

Toxins from bacteria act on the temperature regulating centre in the hypothalamus causing pyrexia. Any insult to the body (e.g. infection, trauma) causes increase in sympathetic tone as a part of the 'flight or flight' response causing cutaneous vasoconstriction. Heat is gained by shivering which in these circumstances is called rigor; hence the cold, clammy skin of a patient in shock. Fever may be a clinical presentation of certain malignancies. Adenocarcinoma of the kidney is known to present as 'pyrexia of unknown origin' presumably due to absorption of necrotic products; urothelial cancer also can present as repeated attacks of fever from *Escherichia coli* infection.

A potentially fatal condition seen in military recruits and young athletes and those not used to high ambient temperatures, is heat stroke from hyperpyrexia. This occurs from excessive muscular exertion particularly in high atmospheric temperatures. There is hyperpyrexia, dehydration, electrolyte disturbances, metabolic acidosis, rhabdomyolysis, confusion, coma, circulatory collapse, acute respiratory distress syndrome (ARDS), and acute renal failure leading to multiple-organ failure.

Malignant hyperpyrexia is the result of a genetic disorder of the skeletal muscle. The condition is of primary interest to the anaesthetist because the condition can be triggered by suxamethonium and certain anaesthetic agents. A description of this condition is beyond the scope of this book. Any known sufferer (or a first-degree relative of a sufferer) should carry a card warning of the possibility of this condition in case the person should require an emergency anaesthetic.

For clinical scenarios of pyrexia please refer to Chapter 25.

Chapter 6 Imaging in surgery

Introduction

Once you enter certain stations, the examiner will show you images or pictures. You will be asked specific questions pertaining to the picture/image. Do not start talking straightaway. You should allow yourself a latent period of some 30 seconds, even if you know the answer.

Take a deep breath to relax and formulate the answer in your mind on the following lines:

- What image is it?
- What are the findings?
- What is the diagnosis?

Start as follows: 'This is a barium study (meal/enema), intravenous urogram, angiogram, ultrasound, CT scan, ... showing........

Some of the images are supplemented with blood results to give the reader a comprehensive understanding of the subject. It is unlikely that in the examination, you will be shown images and blood results together. The blood results will help in the other stations such as in 'applied surgical science and critical care'.

All the images and pictures have been classified according to systems.

Gastroenterology

Questions

Figure 6.1

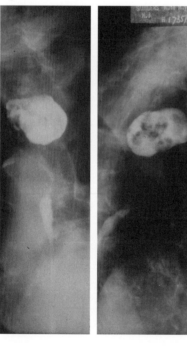

1 What X-ray is this?
2 What are the X-ray findings?
3 What is the diagnosis?
4 What is the clinical presentation of this condition—mainly symptoms?
5 What are the long-term complications?
6 What is the treatment?

Figure 6.2

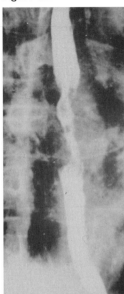

1 What is this X-ray?
2 What are the X-ray findings?
3 What is the diagnosis?
4 What are the symptoms and signs?
5 What other investigations should be done?
6 What are the methods of treating this condition?

Figure 6.3

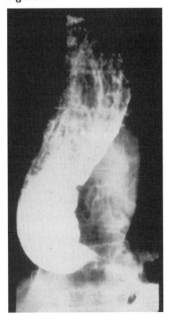

1 What X-ray is this?
2 What are the X-ray findings?
3 What is the diagnosis?
4 What are the clinical features?
5 What is the differential diagnosis?
6 What is the treatment?
7 What is the complication of surgical treatment?

Figure 6.4

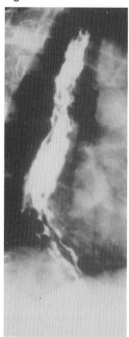

1 What does this barium swallow show?
2 What is the diagnosis?
3 What are the methods of presentation of this condition?
4 What physical findings may you find?
5 What is the next investigation?
6 What biochemical abnormalities do you expect to find?
7 What are the methods of treating this condition?

Figure 6.5

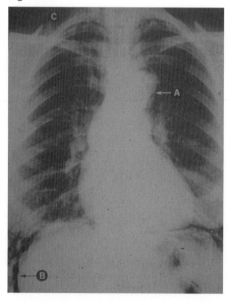

1 What are the findings in this plain X-ray of chest?
2 What is the diagnosis?
3 What is the clinical presentation?
4 What is the differential diagnosis?
5 What is the next imaging technique to be done?
6 What is the treatment?

Figure 6.6

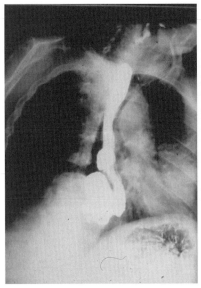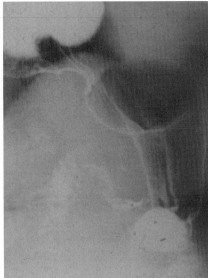

1 What are the findings of this barium swallow and meal?
2 What is the diagnosis?
3 What is the clinical presentation?
4 What are the various types of this condition?
5 What other investigations can be done in this condition?
6 What are the long-term complications of this condition?
7 How do you treat this condition?

Figure 6.7

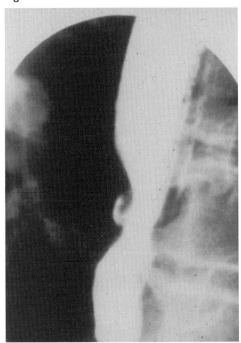

1 What are the findings of this barium swallow?
2 What is the diagnosis?
3 What is the definition of the condition?
4 What are the complications of this condition?
5 What is the treatment for this condition?

Figure 6.8

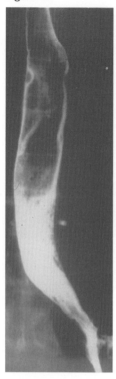

1 What are the findings in this barium swallow?
2 What is the diagnosis?
3 What symptoms would this condition produce?
4 What syndrome is associated with this condition?

Figure 6.9

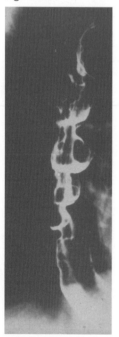

1 What X-ray is this and what are the findings?
2 What is the diagnosis?
3 What are the presenting symptoms?
4 What is the differential diagnosis?
5 How would you confirm the diagnosis?
6 What is the treatment?

Figure 6.10

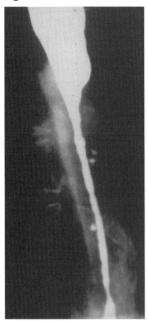

1 What are the findings in this barium swallow?
2 What is the diagnosis?
3 What will the history be?
4 What is the treatment?
5 What is the long-term complication?

Figure 6.11

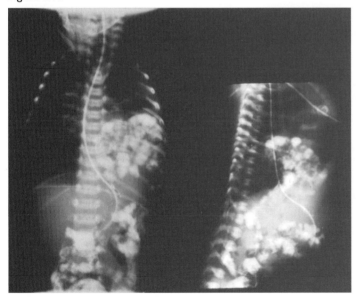

1 What X-ray is this?
2 What are the X-ray findings and what is the diagnosis?
3 What is the acid–base disturbance?
4 What is the treatment?
5 What is the prognosis?

Figure 6.12

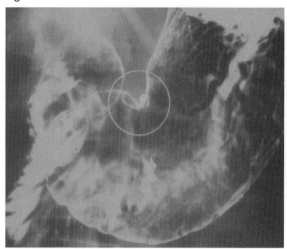

1 In this barium meal of stomach, what is seen in the middle of the circle?
2 What is the radiological diagnosis?
3 What are the subsequent relevant investigations?
4 What are the complications of this condition?
5 How would you treat this condition?

Figure 6.13

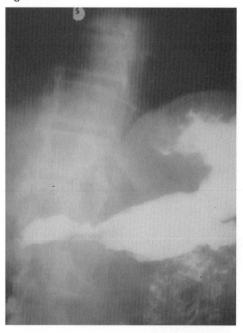

1 What are the findings of this barium meal of the stomach?
2 What is the diagnosis?
3 What are the next investigations and their findings?
4 Is there a proven cause for this condition?

Figure 6.14

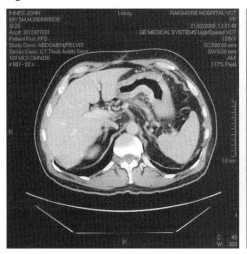 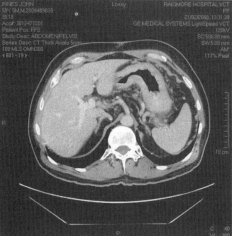

1 What is this imaging technique and what are findings?
2 What is the diagnosis?
3 What is the prognosis?

Figure 6.15

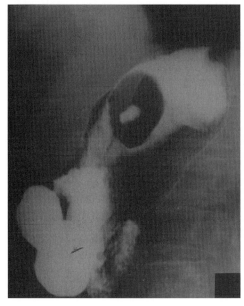

1 What does this barium meal of stomach (oblique view) show?
2 What is the diagnosis?
3 How does this condition most commonly present?
4 How is it most often diagnosed?
5 What is the treatment?

Figure 6.16

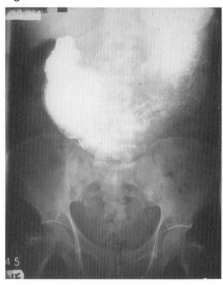

1 What are the findings in this barium meal of stomach? What is the diagnosis?
2 This patient's blood results are as follows:

>PO₂:	12kPa	Serum K:	2.5mmol/L
PCO₂:	5kPa	Serum Na:	128mmol/L
ph:	7.48	Serum Cl:	94mmol/L
HCO₃:	34mmol/L	Urea:	10mmol/L
Hb:	1g/L	Creatinine:	140mmol/L

What is the acid–base disturbance?
3 What clinical condition may occur as a result of this acid–base disturbance?
4 What is the clinical presentation?
5 What is the overall management?

Figure 6.17

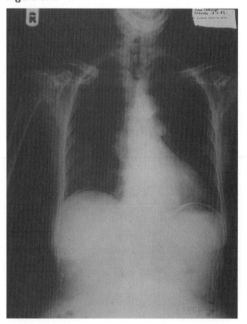

1 What does this plain X-ray of chest show?
2 What is the diagnosis and the commonest cause?
3 What are clinical features of presentation?
4 What is the overall management?

Figure 6.18

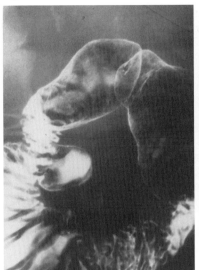
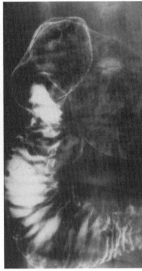

1 What does this barium meal show and what is the diagnosis?
2 How is this condition most often diagnosed?
3 What are the different types of this condition?
4 How may this condition be clinically significant?

Figure 6.19

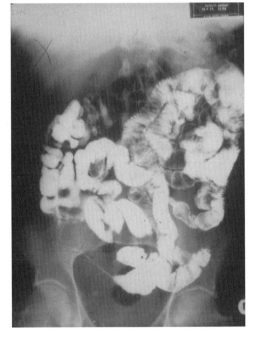

1 What does this barium meal and follow through show?
2 What is the diagnosis?
3 How would this patient present clinically?

Figure 6.20

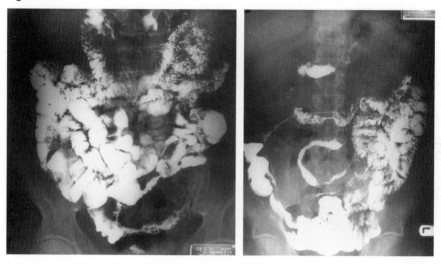

1 Enumerate the radiological findings in these two barium meal and follow through pictures
2 What is the diagnosis?
3 What complications of this condition are shown in these images?

Figure 6.21 (see also Colour Plate 1)

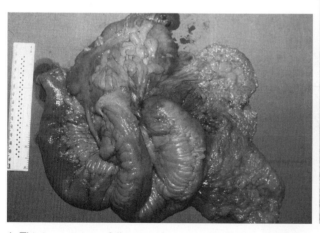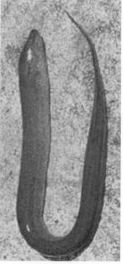

1 This is a specimen following what operation? What are the macroscopic findings and the diagnosis?
2 What are the complications of this condition?

Figure 6.22 (see also Colour Plate 2)

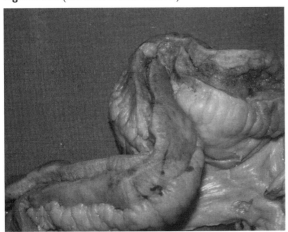

1 In this opened-up specimen of the terminal ileum what are the findings?
2 What is the diagnosis?
3 What are the histological findings of this condition?
4 What is the overall management of this condition?

Figure 6.23

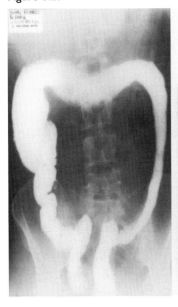
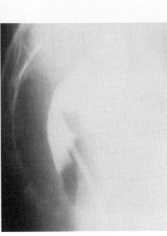

1 These are two views of a barium enema. What are findings? What is the diagnosis?
2 How do these patients present?
3 What is the next relevant investigation?
4 What is the overall management?

Figure 6.24

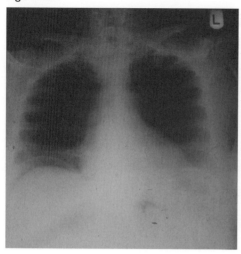

1 This patient suffered from bloody diarrhoea with mucus on and off for 3 years. She has been on systemic steroid treatment and mesalazine. She was admitted as an emergency with acute abdominal symptoms. What does the X-ray show and what is the diagnosis?
2 What should be the management now?
3 What are the complications of this condition?

Figure 6.25

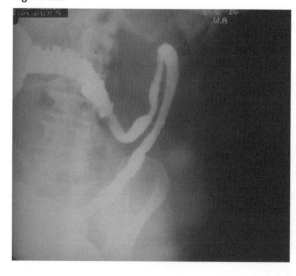

1 This is a barium enema focusing on the left colon. What are the findings?
2 What is the diagnosis? What is the differential diagnosis?
3 What are the methods of presentation of this condition?
4 What comorbid condition may accompany this condition?

Figure 6.26

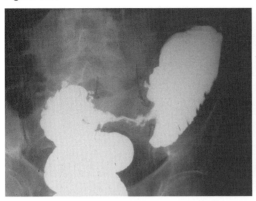 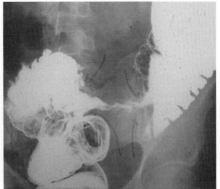

1 What are the findings in this barium enema showing the sigmoid colon?
2 What would be the differential diagnosis?
3 What should be the next relevant investigations?

Figure 6.27

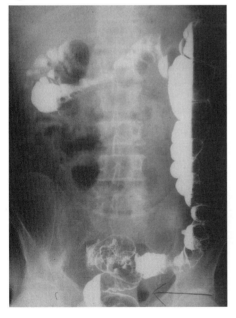

1 What does this barium enema show? What is the arrow in the bottom right hand corner pointing to?
2 What is your diagnosis?
3 What pathological conditions can cause this clinical presentation?
4 What are the presenting symptoms?

Figure 6.28

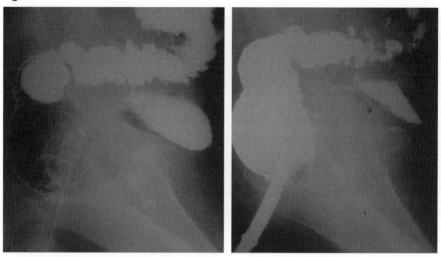

1 What is this X-ray, what are the findings, and what is the diagnosis?
2 What is the clinical presentation?
3 What are the subsequent investigations?
4 What is the management?

Figure 6.29

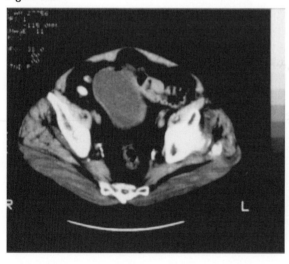

1 What is this investigation?
2 What does it show?
3 What is the diagnosis?

Figure 6.30

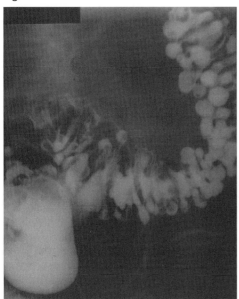

1 What is this investigation, what are the findings and the diagnosis?
2 What are the complications of this condition?
3 What causes this condition?
4 What is the underlying pathology?

Figure 6.31

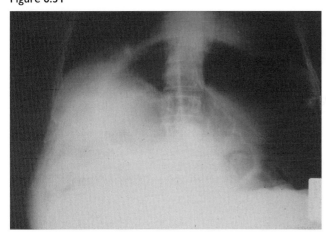

1 What are the findings and diagnosis in this plain X-ray of the abdomen?
2 How does this condition present?
3 What is the management?
4 Where else can this condition occur?

Figure 6.32

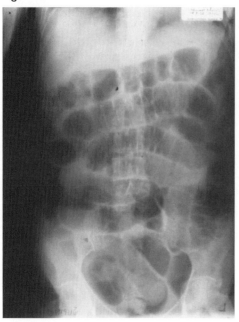

1 What are the findings in this plain abdominal X-ray?
2 What is the diagnosis?
3 What is the clinical presentation?
4 Where would you look for as a cause for this condition?
5 Outline the overall management?

Figure 6.33

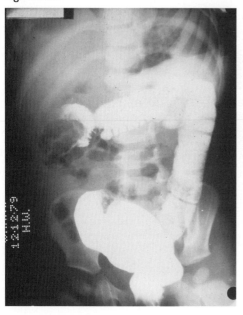

1 In this barium enema what are the findings and the diagnosis?
2 What is the clinical presentation?
3 What is the underlying pathology?
4 What are the options of treatment?
5 Can any other investigation be done for this condition?
6 Can this condition occur in an adult? If so, how?

Figure 6.34

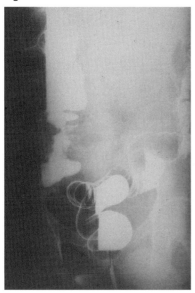

1 This is a barium enema concentrating on the ascending colon. What are findings and the diagnosis?
2 How do these patients present?
3 What investigations would you do next?
4 What is the definitive treatment?

Figure 6.35

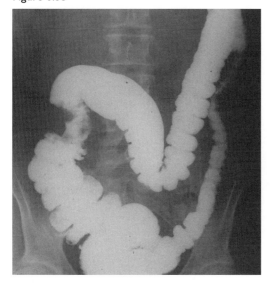

1 What are the findings and diagnosis in this barium enema?
2 What would have been the clinical presentation of this patient?
3 What would be the definitive treatment?

Figure 6.36

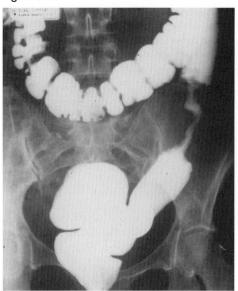

1 What are the findings and diagnosis on this barium enema?
2 How do these patients present?
3 What are the next investigations?
4 What would be the definitive treatment?

Figure 6.37 (see also Colour Plate 3)

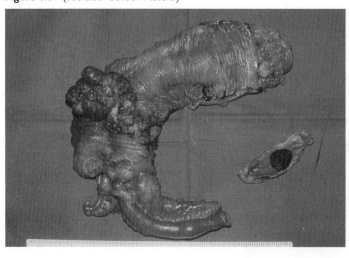

1 These are two specimens removed at the same operation. What operations have been done?
2 What pathology is seen in the larger specimen?
3 How do you stage this condition post-operatively?
4 Does the staging have any relevance to the post-operative treatment? If so, what?

Figure 6.38

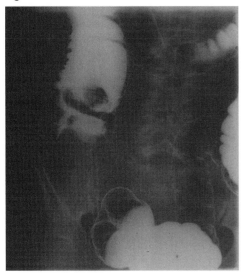

1 What does this barium enema show? Give the diagnosis.
2 After thoroughly investigating, what would be the definitive surgical treatment?
3 When doing the operation for this condition what structures should you be very careful not to damage?

Figure 6.39 (see also Colour Plate 4)

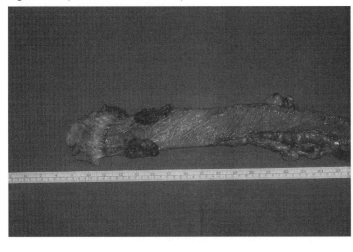

1 This is a specimen following what operation?
2 How often is this operation done for this condition?
3 In advanced inoperable cases, what palliation is done?

Figure 6.40

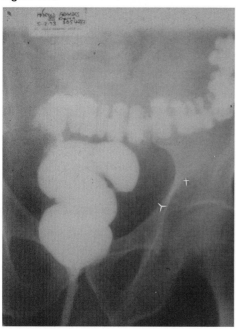

1 What does this barium enema show? What is the diagnosis?
2 What are the next investigations?
3 What adjuvant treatment may be used in advanced cases?
4 What would be the definitive surgical treatment in these cases?

Answers

Figure 6.1

1 These are two pictures of a barium swallow—oblique and lateral views
2 The findings show barium arrested in a globular space in the lower neck and upper chest. Barium is trickling down the oesophagus with some barium regurgitating into the trachea
3 The diagnosis is a pharyngeal pouch (Zenker's diverticulum)
4 Patients present with symptoms of aspiration pneumonia due to regurgitation of food, waking up in the middle of the night due to spillage of food into the tracheobronchial tree from the pouch and foetor
5 The long-term complications are lung abscess due to undiagnosed repeated aspiration pneumonia and dysplasia causing squamous cell carcinoma
6 The treatment is Dholmann's endoscopic stapling diverticulotomy usually carried out by an ENT surgeon. An open excision is a second alternative

Figure 6.2

1 This is a barium swallow focusing on the middle one-third of the oesophagus
2 There is an irregular narrowing of the middle one-third of the oesophagus with typical 'shouldering'
3 The diagnosis is carcinoma of the oesophagus
4 Patients present with dysphagia of short duration with food sticking in the mid-retrosternal region, regurgitation with bouts of chest infection, and weight loss. On examination there is obvious evidence of weight loss and in advanced cases hepatomegaly and/or left supra-clavicular lymph nodes may be present due to secondaries
5 Oesophagogastroduodenoscopy (OGD). During OGD, endoluminal ultrasound (EUS) followed by biopsy. This is followed by CT scan of chest and abdomen. If these investigations indicate a resectable growth, then laparoscopic ultrasound is done to look for peritoneal secondaries

6 In resectable growths: two-stage Ivor Lewis operation or transhiatal oesophagectomy is done. In irresectable growths self-expanding metallic stents are inserted with adjuvant radiotherapy or chemotherapy

Figure 6.3

1 This is a barium swallow
2 It shows a hugely dilated oesophagus containing a large amount of food residue with a smooth tapered lower end giving the picture a bird beak appearance
3 The diagnosis is typical of achalasia of cardia
4 Patients present with dysphagia of long standing with greater difficulty with swallowing liquids, regurgitation with chest infections, and some weight loss
5 The differential diagnosis is peptic stricture and carcinoma
6 Balloon dilatation may be tried. But the definitive treatment is laparoscopic Heller's cardiomyotomy. The procedure can also be done thoracoscopically, by an open operation through the abdomen or chest
7 The complication of Heller's cardiomyotomy is gastro-oesophageal reflux for which some surgeons combine the procedure with an anti-reflux operation

Figure 6.4

1 This shows irregular filling defects within the wall of the oesophagus affecting most of the oesophagus with marked involvement of the lower end
2 The diagnosis is oesophageal varices
3 Most of these patients present with acute haematemesis and melaena. Some of them present with features of liver failure resulting from prolonged alcohol abuse
4 One may find ascites, caput medusa, palmar erythema, and in advanced cases foetor hepaticus and flapping tremor
5 OGD besides all the usual blood tests
6 Severely deranged LFTs, anaemia
7 As an emergency: endoscopic rubber band ligation or injection; in severe haemorrhage oesophageal tamponade with Sengstaken–Blakemore tube may be tried for 24 hours. TIPSS (transjugular intra-hepatic porto-systemic stent shunt) is a good alternative if available. In the long-term patient should be put on beta blockers

Figure 6.5

1 A shows air in the mediastinum. B shows air in the abdominal subcutaneous space. C shows subcutaneous air in the right side of neck.
2 The diagnosis is rupture of the oesophagus—Boerhaave's syndrome or spontaneous rupture of the oesophagus
3 These patients present with sudden onset of severe retrosternal pain radiating to the upper abdomen and neck and features of shock with subcutaneous emphysema
4 The differential diagnosis is myocardial infarction, pulmonary embolus, rupture of thoracic aorta, dissecting aneurysm
5 Contrast-enhanced CT (CECT) scan of chest
6 If the patient presents within 12 hours, a left lower thoracotomy is done to close the perforation followed by a gastrostomy to prevent reflux and a feeding jejunostomy. If the patient arrives late, then the treatment is insertion of intercostal tubes to treat mediastinitis, antibiotics, and delayed thoracotomy

Figure 6.6

1 This picture shows a part of the stomach has rolled up into the right side of chest, a part remains below the left dome of diaphragm and the gastro-oesophageal junction in the left chest. There is an epiphrenic diverticulum at the lower end of the oesophagus
2 The diagnosis is a mixed type of hiatus hernia—rolling and sliding

3 They present with features of gastro-oesophageal reflux disease (GORD): heartburn, regurgitation, odynophagia, and sometimes dysphagia

4 There are 3 types: sliding (almost 90%), rolling, and mixed

5 OGD and biopsy to exclude dysplasia; 24-hour pH monitoring, oesophageal manometry, Bernstein's acid perfusion test

6 Anaemia, dysplasia leading to carcinoma, Barrett's oesophagus, stricture

7 Medical treatment with drugs and lifestyle changes are tried first. If this is not successful and the patient develops increasing grades of dyplastic changes, antireflux operation is carried out by the laparoscopic route. Nissen's total or partial fundoplication is done

Figure 6.7

1 This shows a smooth stricture of the oesophagus. Within the stricture is a typical ulcer crater

2 This is a Barret's oesophagus with a Barrett's ulcer. In this condition the squamo-columnar junction is at least 3cm from the gastro-oesophageal junction; thus the oesophagus is shortened. Nowadays a 'short-segment Barret's' where the columnar epithelium is <3cm is also recognized

3 The complications are carcinoma, haemorrhage and stricture. It has a 30 times greater chance of developing adenocarcinoma. The risk of cancer increases with the increased length of the columnar-lined oesophagus. Often the cancer is multifocal. Severe haemorrhage is another complication which can occur from a Barrett's ulcer

4 The treatment is that of GORD. Medical treatment in the form of high dose proton pump inhibitor (PPI) is tried. This may be combined with endoscopic ablation of the Barrett's mucosa with laser, photodynamic therapy, argon-beam plasma coagulation, and endoscopic mucosal resection. Laparoscopic antireflux operation remains the surgical treatment of choice

Figure 6.8

1 There is lack of peristalsis, stricturing of the lower oesophagus with inflammatory changes

2 This is a case of scleroderma. There is normal peristalsis in the upper one-third and minimal peristaslis in the lower two-thirds

3 The symptoms are of GORD

4 The syndrome associated with this is called CREST syndrome: **c**alcinosis, **R**aynaud's, o**e**sophageal dismotility, **s**cleroderma, and **t**elangiectasis

Figure 6.9

1 This is a barium swallow showing hyperperistalsis of the entire oesophagus

2 The diagnosis is diffuse oesophageal spasm, nutcracker oesophagus, or presbyoesophagus

3 Patients complain of retrosternal chest pain with dysphagia

4 The differential diagnosis is angina. Indeed patients have been known to have had coronary angiography that turned out to be normal.

5 Endoscopy (sometimes normal) and oesophageal manometry helps—the latter showing a large number of high-amplitude contractions

6 The treatment is mainly medical—calcium channel blockers and nitrates. In a very small number of patients a long oesophageal myotomy has been tried with not a great deal of success

Figure 6.10

1 This shows a long relatively smooth stricture with proximal dilatation

2 This is a corrosive stricture

3 In an attempt at self-harm an adult may ingest sodium hydroxide or sulphuric acid, or an accidental ingestion by a child. There will be severe dysphagia in late cases

4 This should be managed by an expert upper GI surgeon. Early OGD of the entire oesophagus and stomach is carried out. Some advocate the use of steroids followed by early regular endoscopic dilatation. There is extensive mucosal damage in 50% of patients. Elective resection with colonic replacement should be considered after 3 months

5 The long-term complication is squamous cell carcinoma which has been estimated to be <5% as a lifetime risk

Figure 6.11

1 These are two pictures of barium meal and follow through carried out through a NG tube in a neonate
2 This shows a congenital diaphragmatic hernia in the left posterolateral side of the chest. The diagnosis is often made prenatally
3 The neonate has severe respiratory acidosis from pulmonary hypoplasia
4 The treatment is respiratory stabilization by the neonatal intensivists. If they can be stabilized, then the diaphragmatic defect can be repaired
5 30% of the neonates die from this condition due to respiratory failure from irreversible pulmonary hypoplasia

Figure 6.12

1 There is a small amount of barium sticking out from the middle of the lesser curve as a crater
2 This is a benign gastric ulcer
3 OGD and biopsy; serology for *Helicobacter pylori*; rapid urease test for *H. pylori*
4 Perforation, haemorrhage, cicatrization causing an hour-glass stomach, malignancy
5 If it is proven to be a benign gastric ulcer, medical treatment with PPI, eradication of *H. pylori* with amoxycillin and clarithromycin

Figure 6.13

1 This shows the entire stomach to be extremely contracted. The entire lesser and greater curves are grossly irregular
2 The diagnosis is linitis plastica
3 OGD: this will show a very small stomach which typically cannot be distended with air. Biopsies need to be taken with special biopsy forceps so as to get very deep bites as the pathology is submucosal. A CT scan will show a grossly thickened and contracted stomach
4 Untreated *H. pylori* is a causative organism

Figure 6.14

1 This is a CT scan with contrast in the stomach. The stomach shows gross uniform thickening of the entire stomach wall
2 The diagnosis is linitis plastica or lymphoma
3 If it is linitis plastica, the prognosis is dismal as patients will die of the disease for which there is no treatment

Figure 6.15

1 The barium meal shows a smooth filling defect with the upper part of the body of the stomach. In the middle of the filling defect there is a fleck of barium
2 The smooth filling defect denotes a benign lesion and the streak of barium denotes an ulceration in the middle of the lesion. This is a leiomyoma of the stomach which is a submucosal benign tumour which has ulcerated through the mucosa
3 It presents with acute upper GI haemorrhage—haematemesis.
4 It is most often diagnosed on OGD carried out for acute haematemesis
5 The treatment is wide local excision

Figure 6.16

1 This shows a massively distended stomach with a large amount of food residue. There is a smooth sharp cut off at the pyloroduodenal junction. The diagnosis is gastric outlet obstruction (GOO). In view of the huge dilatation and the smooth distal cut-off, the GOO is due to duodenal ulcer that has cicatrized causing severe degree of duodenal ('pyloric') stenosis. The acid–base disturbance is one of hypochloraemic, hypokalaemic metabolic alkalosis
2 Long-standing metabolic alkalosis can cause tetany

3 The clinical presentation consists of incessant non-bile stained vomiting, the vomitus containing old food residue; gross dehydration as seen by dry tongue, loss of skin turgor and sunken eyes; visible gastric peristalsis; succussion splash

4 The overall management consists of:
- Rehydration with normal saline with added potassium
- Stomach wash to empty food residue
- OGD to exclude malignancy
- Balloon dilatation can be tried in very early cases
- Operation of gastrojejunostomy

Figure 6.17

1 This shows free gas under both domes of diaphragm of which the gas under the right dome is more significant because it is in the peritoneal cavity whilst the gas under the left dome is in the fundus of the stomach

2 The diagnosis is perforation of a hollow viscus, the most common cause being a perforated duodenal ulcer

3 The clinical presentation is: sudden onset of severe epigastric pain radiating to the entire abdomen and back; tachycardia; thoracic respiration and tachypnoea; board-like rigidity of the abdomen; obliteration of the liver dullness

4 The overall management consists of:
- IV analgesia
- NG suction
- IV fluids
- Laparotomy after optimization—midline incision, suck the peritoneal fluid, isolate the perforation on the anterior wall of the first part of the duodenum, close it with interrupted Vicryl sutures with a patch of omentum
- Thorough peritoneal lavage
- Close the abdomen

Figure 6.18

1 It shows an outpouching on the medial side of the second part of the duodenum which is a congenital duodenal diverticulum

2 It is most often diagnosed as an incidental finding at OGD

3 There are two types: congenital which is usually silent, and acquired as a result of a long-standing duodenal ulcer

4 It may be clinically significant because it may cause problems when doing an endoscopic retrograde cholangiopancreatography (ERCP) and endoscopic papillotomy

Figure 6.19

1 This is a barium meal and follow through of the small bowel and proximal ascending colon showing a very narrowed terminal ileum in the right lower quadrant—typical of a 'String sign of Kantor'

2 The diagnosis is regional ileitis or Crohn's disease

3 This patient would present with altered bowel habit in the form of alternating constipation and diarrhoea, colicky abdominal pain denoting symptoms of distal small bowel obstruction; there may be a mass in the right iliac fossa; in addition there may be features of any of the complications (see below)

Figure 6.20

1 This is a series of barium meal and follow through showing: various strictured segments of small bowel, mucosal fissuring with radiating spicules, cobblestone mucosa intraluminally, loops of small bowel stuck to one another (entero-enteric fistula) and skip lesions

2 This is very typical of Crohn's disease showing most of the radiological features of this condition

3 The complications shown are strictures and internal fistulae

Figure 6.21

1 This specimen shows: loops of ileum, ascending colon and appendix. Therefore this is a right hemicolectomy. The macroscopic findings of this specimen are: grossly thickened loops of ileum likened to 'an eel in rigor mortis' (hence the picture of an eel), gross oedema of mesenteric fat, over-riding of ileum with mesenteric fat and loops of ileum stuck together as a fistula. (Resected specimen of Fig. 6.20.)

2 The complications of Crohn's disease are:
   • Local
   • Distant (or metastatic)

Local complications:
• Fistulae:
  ◆ External:
    ▪ Entero-cutaneous/colocutaneous
    ▪ Entero-vaginal/colovaginal
    ▪ Perianal
  ◆ Internal:
    ▪ Entero-enteric
    ▪ Enterocolic
    ▪ Enterovesical/colovesical
• Abscesses
• Stricture
• Carcinoma
• Haemorrhage
• Perforation
• Toxic megacolon

Distant complications:
• Infected:
  ◆ Skin: pyoderma gangrenosum, erythema nodosum
  ◆ Eyes: keratitis/episcleritis
  ◆ Joints: septic arthritis
  ◆ Septicaemia
  ◆ Psoas abscess
• Non-infected:
  ◆ Polyarthropathy
  ◆ Venous thrombosis
  ◆ Physical retardation
  ◆ Hepatobiliary disease—gallstones; sclerosing cholangitis
  ◆ Ureteric strictures

Figure 6.22

1 This opened up specimen of terminal ileum shows: gross thickening of the bowel wall from transmural inflammation, very strictured lumen, apthoid and serpiginous ulcers in the mucosa, cobblestone appearance from oedematous mucosa between ulcers

2 The diagnosis is Crohn's disease

3 The histological findings are of: transmural inflammation with lymphocytes and plasma cells affecting all layers, non-caseating granuloma and Langhans and foreign body type giant cells. Granulomas are seen in about 60–70% of patients

4 The overall management of Crohn's disease is medical: systemic and local steroids, azathioprine, infliximab for perianal fistula, metronidazole and meticulous attention to nutritional deficiencies. Surgical treatment should be reserved for complications and is tailored according to the needs of the patient. The procedures available are: localized resections. strictureplasty, balloon dilatation, and exteriorization. Surgery should be as conservative as possible

Figure 6.23

1 The picture on the left is an anteroposterior (AP) view and on the right is a lateral view of the pre-sacral area. The AP picture shows: complete lack of haustrations, hose-pipe appearance of the colon, markedly contracted colon, and backwash ileitis. The lateral view shows classical increase in the pre-sacral or retro-rectal space. These appearances are pathognomonic of severe complete ulcerative colitis

2 95% of these patients present electively with bloody diarrhoea with mucus. There may be several such loose motions a day with lower abdominal pain and weight loss; 5% of these patients may present as an emergency with acute fulminating symptoms of severe bloody diarrhoea and marked prostration

3 The next relevant investigation is to do a full colonoscopy and biopsies to confirm the diagnosis by the presence of crypt abscesses and disease confined to the mucosa and submucosa. The biopsy should also exclude dysplasia and malignancy, particularly in disease of >10 years

4 The mainstay of management is medical: systemic steroids and mesalazine, local steroid enemas; blood transfusion may be necessary. Surgery is reserved for complications—either acute such as perforation or toxic megacolon or chronic such as severe symptoms, malignancy, or severe dysplasia

Figure 6.24

1 The plain abdominal X-ray shows free gas under the right dome of the diaphragm denoting perforation of a hollow viscus. In view of the history, the diagnosis is perforation of the large bowel from acute ulcerative colitis

2 This is a desperate surgical emergency which carries a high mortality. The patient requires urgent resuscitation followed by emergency laparotomy. At operation the procedure of choice would be subtotal colectomy with terminal ileostomy with the anorectal stump closed off as a Hartmann's procedure. The patient will need to be cared for in the ITU. Once the patient has recovered, several months later the patient should be reassessed for the possibility of an ileo-anal pouch procedure

3 The complications are:
   - Local:
     - Toxic megacolon
     - Perforation
     - Massive haemorrhage
     - Benign stricture
     - Inflammatory polyposis
     - Carcinoma
     - Anal fissure/abscesses
   - Systemic:
     - Arthritis
     - Ankylosing spondylitis
     - Erythema nodosum/pyoderma gangrenosum
     - Episcleritis
     - Sclerosing cholangitis
     - Stomatitis
     - Oesophagitis

Figure 6.25

1 This shows a narrow contracted left colon with loss of haustrations and thumb-printing proximal to the splenic flexure. The more proximal colon has normal haustrations

2 The diagnosis is ischaemic colitis. The differential diagnosis is segmental ulcerative colitis

3 These patients may present electively with left-sided abdominal pain with blood-stained diarrhoea; some may present with colicky left-sided abdominal pain due to subacute obstruction

from a stricture; a small proportion may present as an emergency with features of gangrene of the left colon

4 Most of these patients have myocardial ischaemia

Figure 6.26

1 The sigmoid colon shows an irregular stricture with small diverticulae in the distal part of the stricture

2 The differential diagnosis is firstly carcinoma and secondly diverticular stricture

3 The next investigation is to do a flexible sigmoidoscopy and biopsy. Colonoscopy would not be successful because it would not negotiate the stricture. This should be followed by a CT scan. (*It turned out to be a diverticular stricture.*)

Figure 6.27

1 This barium enema shows a pocket of air in the pelvis next to the rectum (pointed to by the arrow), the air being outside the rectum

2 The air is in the urinary bladder denoting a vesicocolic fistula

3 The common pathological conditions causing a vesicocolic fistula are: diverticular disease of colon, colorectal carcinoma, and Crohn's colitis

4 The usual clinical presentation is one of repeated attacks of urinary tract infection, ascending pyelonephritis, pneumaturia, and passing very foul-smelling urine from faecaluria

Figure 6.28

1 This is a barium enema showing saw-toothed appearance of the sigmoid colon (typical of diverticular disease) with a barium-lined track entering a globular space also outlined by barium. The diagnosis is diverticular disease with a vesicocolic fistula and the urinary bladder outlined with barium

2 This patient presented with severe recurrent urinary tract infections. Following the barium enema he passed barium in his urine

3 CT scan to show air in the urinary balder; colonoscopy and biopsy to exclude an unsuspected carcinoma; some may do a cystoscopy to see air bubbles coming from an inflamed are in the fundus

4 After thorough bowel preparation, a one-stage sigmoid resection is carried out; the affected segment is pinched off the bladder, resected with end-to-end anastomosis; the hole in the bladder is closed leaving an indwelling catheter for a week

Figure 6.29

1 This a CT scan of the pelvis

2 This shows the urinary bladder in the centre with a pocket of air inside at the fundus. This is the best investigation to show air in the urinary bladder

3 Vesicocolic fistula

Figure 6.30

1 This is a barium enema showing multiple outpouchings of the colonic wall typical of diverticular disease of the colon

2 The complications of diverticular disese are:
   - Stricture mimicking carcinoma
   - Acute diverticulitis
   - Diverticular abscess
   - Perforated diverticulitis causing faecal or purulent peritonitis
   - Fistulae: colo-enteric, colovesical, colocutaneous, colovaginal
   - Severe haemorrhage

3 Having long-standing low-residue diet

4 Due to a low-residue diet, there is an increase in intracolonic pressure. This causes the mucosa to herniate out at the point of maximum weakness in the bowel wall. This is the site of entry of the

vessel where the actual diverticulum occurs. This is an acquired diverticulum and therefore consists of mucosa and serosa only

Figure 6.31

1 This plain abdominal X-ray shows a huge dilated bowel without any haustrations. There is a loop of large bowel with faeces (transverse colon) just below the dilated bowel. The bowel is so dilated that the domes of the diaphragm are elevated. The diagnosis is volvulus of the sigmoid colon

2 These are elderly patients who present with acute-on-chronic large bowel intestinal obstruction. There is constipation, abdominal pain, and distension of the left side of abdomen; rectal examination shows a hollow, ballooned rectum

3 Resuscitation with analgesia, IV fluids, insertion of a catheter; a CT colonography confirms the diagnosis. If there are no signs of strangulation, deflation by a colonoscope or flexible sigmoidoscope is attempted first. If it is unsuccessful or if there are signs of strangulation, laparotomy, excision of the segment with a Hartmann type resection is carried out

4 Volvulus can also occur in the caecum and transverse colon

Figure 6.32

1 This shows distended small bowel in the centre of the abdomen. There is valvulae conniventes in the upper part denoting jejunal obstruction and in the lower part there is featureless bowel which is distended ileum. The bowel lops are separated by fluid

2 The diagnosis is distal small bowel obstruction as both jejunum and ileum are distended

3 Patient would present with colicky abdominal pain, central abdominal distension, constipation, and faeculent vomiting. The patient would be very dehydrated with sunken eyes, dry tongue, and loss of skin turgor

4 One should look for an irreducible lump in the groin particularly below the inguinal ligament and lateral to the pubic tubercle (incarcerated femoral hernia) or look for the scar of a previous laparotomy. The other causes are a carcinoma of the caecum or rarely gallstone ileus

5 The management consists of: vigorous resuscitation with IV fluids, analgesia, NG suction, indwelling catheter followed by laparotomy

Figure 6.33

1 This barium enema shows a complete block of barium just distal to the hepatic flexure. The deformity at the site of obstruction is like a crab claw. Note that the patient is a child as seen by the pelvic bones and upper ends of femur. The diagnosis is ileo-caeco-colic intussusception

2 The child presents with colicky abdominal pain. The mother says that during an attack of pain, he / she pulls the arms and legs up. The child's nappy may have red staining from blood-stained mucus which is described as red-currant jelly stools. Abdominal examination may show an empty right iliac fossa with a sausage-shaped mass in the upper abdomen

3 In children the underlying pathology is hypertrophy of Payer's patches in the terminal ileum brought on by dietary changes causing infection. Macroscopically there are two parts of the intussusception – the outer part of bowel which is called the intussusceptum and the inner invaginated part called the intussuscepiens

4 The initial treatment is hydrostatic decompression which is usually successful within the first 12 hours. If unsuccessful, laparotomy and manual reduction has to be done

5 Nowadays the diagnosis is confirmed by an ultrasound

6 This condition can occur in an adult. It would then be due to a polypoid carcinoma acting as the lead point for an intussusception. The patient would present with acute intestinal obstruction and would require an urgent gastrografin enema followed by an emergency hemicolectomy

Figure 6.34

1 This shows an apple-core deformity (an irregular stricture) in the caecum. The diagnosis is carcinoma of the caecum

2 Patients with carcinoma of the caecum can present as an emergency or electively. As an emergency they present with acute distal small bowel obstruction due to the caecal growth obstructing the ileocaecal junction. The other emergency presentation is when the patient masquerades as 'acute appendicitis' because of obstruction of the base of the appendix with the cancer. The elective presentation is the result of iron deficiency anaemia because of chronic blood loss from the carcinoma—thus the patient complains of tiredness, malaise and undue shortness of breath. Examination may show a mass in the right iliac fossa. The elective presentation is the result of iron deficiency anaemia because of chronic blood loss from the carcinoma—thus the patient complains of tiredness, malaise, and undue shortness of breath.

3 The investigations to be done after a barium enema shows a carcinoma of the caecum are: all routine blood tests; CECT scan to assess local spread and exclude a synchronous carcinoma. Some may do a full colonoscopy for the same reason and get a histological diagnosis. Some surgeons may deem a full colonoscopy unnecessary. An ultrasound of the abdomen to exclude liver secondaries and a CXR to exclude lung secondaries are carried out

4 The definitive treatment is a right hemicolectomy

Figure 6.35

1 This shows an irregular filling defect in the distal ascending colon just proximal to the hepatic flexure—typical of a plypoid carcinoma

2 As a barium enema has been carried out, this patient would have presented as an elective patient with features of anaemia—undue shortness of breath and malaise. On abdominal examination there would be a mass in the right side of the abdomen

3 The definitive treatment would be an extended right hemicolectomy

Figure 6.36

1 The barium enema shows a long, irregular stricture with shouldering just distal to the splenic flexure, typical of a tubular carcinoma

2 These patients may present as an emergency with acute closed-loop large bowel intestinal obstruction. Electively they would present with increasing constipation, having to take increasing amounts of laxatives to open the bowels and dark red rectal bleeding. They may also have colicky abdominal pain from subacute obstruction

3 The subsequent investigations should be: flexible sigmoidoscopy and biopsy, CECT scan, ultrasound of the abdomen and CXR, routine blood tests including carcino-embryonic antigen

4 The definitive treatment is radical left hemicolectomy

Figure 6.37

1 Right hemicolectomy as one can see ileum, the appendix, and the ascending colon; and cholecystectomy (incidental)

2 The bowel specimen shows a polypoid carcinoma of the caecum

3 The post-operative staging of colorectal carcinoma is by Dukes' staging which is as follows:
- Stage A: growth limited to the rectal wall 15%
- Stage B: growth extends to the extra-rectal tissues 35%
- Stage C: secondaries in the regional lymph nodes 50%
- Stage C1: involvement of pararectal lymph nodes
- Stage C2: involvement of nodes along the blood vessels
- Stage D: this was not described by Dukes. It indicates distant metastases usually hepatic

4 The post-operative staging would help to decide on adjuvant chemotherapy. Stage C and high-grade Stage B patients are offered chemotherapy

Figure 6.38

1 The barium enema shows an irregular filling defect in the caecum with non-filling of the proximal caecum. The diagnosis is polypoid carcinoma (this is the barium enema of the specimen in Fig. 6.37)

2 The definitive surgical treatment would be a right hemicolectomy

3 While doing a right hemicolectomy, the surgeon should be careful about not damaging the right gonadal vessels, right ureter, and the duodenum

Figure 6.39

1 This is a large bowel specimen showing skin at the left edge. Therefore the operation done is an abdomino-perineal excision for carcinoma of the rectum

2 This operation is done in 11%. Most patients with rectal carcinoma have a sphincter preserving operation

3 In inoperable cases, palliation is best achieved by radiotherapy with insertion of a self-expanding metallic stent in cases of impending obstruction. A loop colostomy can also be done

Figure 6.40

1 The barium enema shows a 'napkin-ring' appearance in the recto-sigmoid junction typical of an annular carcinoma

2 Sigmoidoscopy and biopsy. Although a colonoscopy is indicated to exclude a synchronous lesion, it would not be feasible as the colonoscope will not pass through the carcinomatous stricture. A CECT scan and MRI are done to assess accurately local spread. An ultrasound of the liver and CXR with routine blood tests would complete the investigations

3 In advanced cases, pre-operative adjuvant radiotherapy to downstage the tumour is carried out

4 The definitive surgical treatment would be anterior resection with total mesorectal excision

Urology

Questions

Figure 6.41

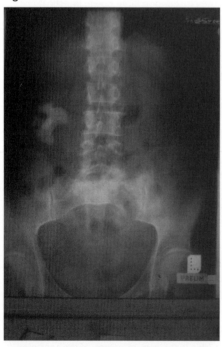

1 What type of an X-ray is this, what is the finding and what is the diagnosis?

2 How does this condition present?

3 What would be the treatment?

Figure 6.42

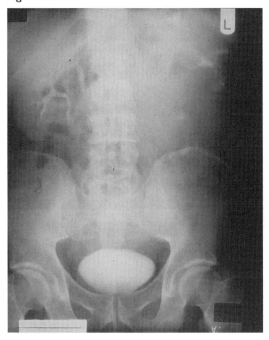

1 What are the findings in this IV urogram (IVU)?
2 What is the diagnosis?
3 What are the methods of presentation of this condition?
4 What are the next imaging investigations to be carried out?
5 What is the definitive treatment?

Figure 6.43 (see also Colour Plate 5)

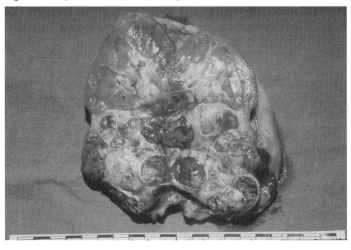

1 What is this specimen showing and what is the diagnosis?
2 What is the histological appearance?
3 What are the common methods of spread of this condition?

Figure 6.44

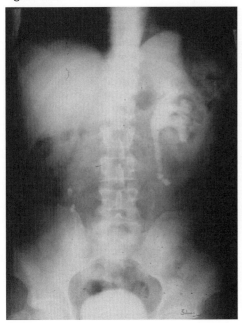

1 What is this X-ray, what is it showing and what is the diagnosis?
2 How do these patients present?
3 What is the initial treatment?
4 What is the definitive treatment?

Figure 6.45

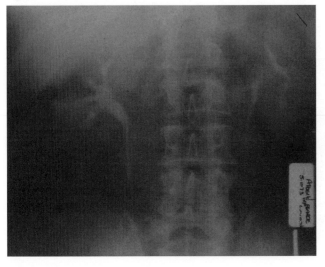

1 What are the findings in this IVU; what is the diagnosis?
2 What other imaging methods can be used to confirm the diagnosis?
3 How would such patients present?
4 What is the definitive treatment?
5 What are the approaches for such a procedure?
6 What is the usual histology? What can be a rare histology?

Figure 6.46

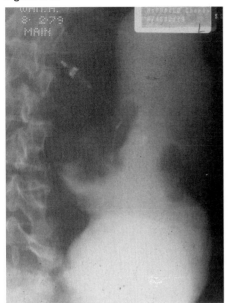

1 What is this imaging technique?
2 What are the findings and diagnosis?
3 What alternative X-ray imaging can be done to elucidate the same diagnosis?
4 Which would be a better imaging method of the two?

Figure 6.47

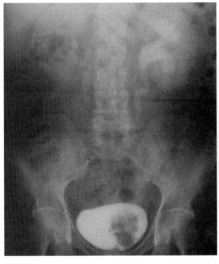 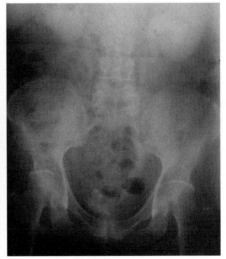

1 What are the findings in this series of IVUs; what is the diagnosis?
2 What is the presentation of this condition?
3 What is the next line in overall management?

Figure 6.48

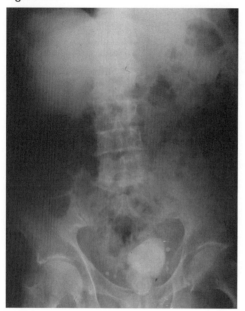

1 What X-ray is this and what is the diagnosis?
2 What symptoms does this condition produce?
3 What are the methods of treating this condition? What are the contraindications for minimal access surgery in this condition?
4 What are the complications of minimal access surgery in this situation?

Figure 6.49

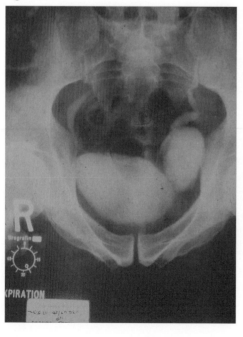

1 Give the findings in this IVU and the diagnosis
2 What causes this condition and what changes occur before it forms?
3 What are the complications of this condition?
4 How would you treat this condition?

Figure 6.50

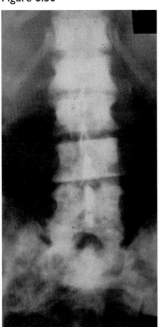

1 What are the findings in this X-ray of lumbar vertebrae?
2 What is the diagnosis?
3 What is your next line of management?
4 What will be your options of treatment in this patient?

Figure 6.51 (see also Colour Plate 6)

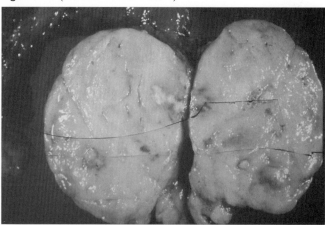

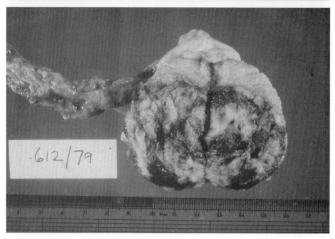

1 What is the diagnosis in these two specimens?
2 How do such patients present?
3 What investigations would you do when you suspect this condition?
4 Outline the management

Figure 6.52 (see also Colour Plate 7)

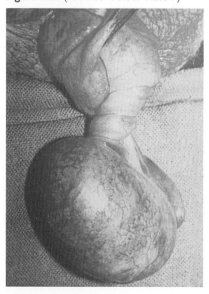

1 What is the diagnosis?
2 What is the clinical presentation?
3 What is the differential diagnosis?
4 What is the treatment?

Figure 6.53

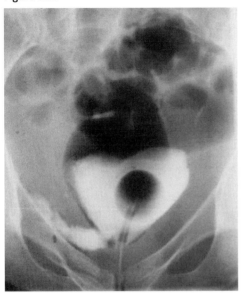

1 What X-ray is this; what are the findings and the diagnosis?
2 What are the types of this condition?
3 What is the treatment?

Answers

Figure 6.41

1 This is a plain X-ray of KUB (kidney, ureter, and bladder) area showing a radio-opaque shadow in the region of the right kidney—typical of a stag-horn calculus
2 This condition can be found incidentally. Clinically it can present with dull aching pain in the loin, attacks of urinary tract infection, and haematuria. As an emergency it can present as a pyonephrosis with marked toxicity from septicaemia and severe pain in the loin
3 If the kidney is non-functioning, nephrectomy is carried out. In a functioning kidney a combination of percutaneous nephrolithotomy (PCNL) and extra-corporeal shockwave lithotripsy (ESWL) is carried out. Before ESWL a stent is inserted in the ureter

Figure 6.42

1 This IVU shows a bifid renal pelvis on the right. On the left there is a large soft tissue shadow with irregular excretion of contrast. The urinary bladder is filled
2 The diagnosis is a left renal cell carcinoma (hypernephroma)
3 These patients may present in a variety of ways:
  • Haematuria with pain in the loin
  • Pyrexia of unknown origin
  • Hypertension
  • Polycythaemia
  • Pathological fractures of long bones or haemoptysis from lung secondaries
  • Palpable loin lump
  • In left-sided growths, recent onset of varicocoele from obstruction of the left testicular vein from growth along the renal vein
4 Ultrasound should be followed by a CECT scan
5 The definitive treatment is radical nephrectomy

Figure 6.43

1 This specimen is that of a nephrectomy with a growth in the lower part with normal kidney in the upper part. There are septa in between haemorrhagic areas of solid growth. This is typical of a renal cell carcinoma

2 The histology is adenocarcinoma with clear cells; therefore also called clear-cell carcinoma

3 This spreads predominantly by bloodstream to the long bones, lungs, and brain. The skeletal secondaries are typically pulsating because they are very vascular and osteolytic. They also spread to the hilar lymph nodes and then to the para-aortic nodes

Figure 6.44

1 This is an IVU showing the right kidney has excreted and there is delayed excretion with hold-up in the left kidney. Half-way down the left ureter there is a radio-opaque shadow causing an obstruction to the flow of contrast. The diagnosis is left hydronephrosis and hydroureter from a stone in the middle one-third of left ureter

2 These patients present with ureteric colic (wrongly referred to as renal colic). They complain of sudden onset of very severe pain originating in the loin and radiating to the groin and testis or labia. The patient writhes round in pain unable to find a comfortable position. This is one of the most painful conditions ever

3 The initial treatment is IV morphine followed by rectal diclofenac. Confirmation of the diagnosis is made by a spiral CT scan or a limited IVU

4 The definitive treatment is expectant for a stone <0.5cm. Stones >0.5cm in size are treated by ureteroscopic hydraulic lithotripsy ± stent

Figure 6.45

1 This IVU shows an irregular filling defect within the left renal pelvis. The diagnosis is a transitional cell carcinoma of the renal pelvis

2 A CECT is the next investigation of choice. The other imaging modality that can be used is a retrograde pyleogram

3 These patients complain of haematuria and pain in the loin radiating to the groin due to clot colic. They also have dull loin ache. Clinically there is usually nothing to find on examination

4 The definitive treatment is nephro-ureterectomy with excision of a cuff of the urinary bladder around the ureteric orifice.

5 Nephro-ureterectomy can be done by an open operation through two separate incisions—one in the loin for the nephrectomy and another in the lower midline for the ureterectomy. The lower incision can be dispensed with by doing the lower part through a transurethral resection (TUR) called pluck operation. Nowadays the entire procedure can be done by minimal access surgery – laparoscopic nephrectomy and ureterectomy and TUR of the ureteric orifice

6 The usual histology is a transitional cell carcinoma. Rarely there may be a squamous cell carcinoma due to squamous metaplasia from a long-standing stone or bilharzial infection

Figure 6.46

1 This shows a needle and catheter in a renal pelvis being inserted from the loin. This is called an antegrade pyelogram

2 This shows a huge renal pelvis, hydronephrosis, with a large number of irregular filling defects typical of a transitional cell carcinoma of the renal pelvis

3 The other imaging is a retrograde pyelogram

4 An antegrade pyelogram is a better imaging modality to delineate the anatomy because it can be done under local anaesthetic, there is less chance of introducing infection and the procedure can be used to decompress the kidney

Figure 6.47

1 This series of two IVU pictures shows an irregular filling defect in the left side of the urinary bladder which is obstructing the left ureteric orifice. The diagnosis is carcinoma of the urinary bladder causing left hydroureter and hydronephrosis

2 Patients present with painless, profuse, and periodic haematuria where the blood may be in the form of clots. Clinically there may be nothing to find unless the patient has skeletal secondaries

3 The subsequent management is to confirm the diagnosis and stage the disease. This is done by: CECT, cystoscopy and examination under anaesthesia (EUA) and biopsy. Treatment is instituted according to the stage (I to IV)

Figure 6.48

1 This is a plain X-ray of the bladder area showing a large radio-opaque shadow which is bi-lobed (dumbbell-shaped). It is a stone in the urinary bladder

2 This would cause suprapubic pain haematuria, repeated attacks of urinary infection, and intermittent sudden cessation of urinary stream

3 Most of the time it is ideally treated by minimal access surgery – crushing the stone using a lithotrite and then washing out the bladder. In a very large stone such as this, an open suprapubic cystolithotomy is the treatment

4 The contraindications for using minimal access surgery in bladder stones are:
  • Do not use the method in children
  • When the stone is too large
  • When there are too many stones
  • When the stone is too hard
  • In a patient with a very large prostate
  • When the stone is inside a diverticulum

5 The complications of minimal access surgery are: urethral stricture or rupture

Figure 6.49

1 This IVU shows the urinary bladder with the lower ends of both ureters. Next to the left ureteric orifice is a large cavity with contrast pushing the left ureter medially. This is typical of a bladder diverticulum

2 This condition is caused by long-standing bladder outlet obstruction. The changes that occur before a diverticulum forms are trabeculation and sacculation

3 The complications of a diverticulum are: infection, stone formation, and carcinoma

4 At the outset the inside of the diverticulum is visualized by flexible cystoscopy to make sure that there is no stone or carcinoma. The cause is treated by transurethral resection of bladder neck and prostate and the diverticulum is observed over a period of time. It is left alone if it is not causing any symptoms

Figure 6.50

1 This shows gross sclerosis of the lumbar vertebrae

2 The diagnosis is sclerotic secondaries from a carcinoma of the prostate

3 The diagnosis is to be confirmed by: transrectal ultrasound (TRUS)-guided Tru-Cut biopsy of the prostate, bone scan to see the extent of the skeletal spread, and prostate specific antigen (PSA) to help monitor the effect of treatment

4 The patient should be given a choice of bilateral subcapsular orchidectomy or chemical castration to control the disease and local radiotherapy. He may require medical treatment for symptoms from hypercalcaemia

Figure 6.51

1 These two specimens are those of orchidectomy. The upper specimen shows a large testis, solid and homogenous in appearance. This is a seminoma. The lower specimen shows a variegated appearance and is a teratoma

2 Seminoma presents at the age of 30–40 years whereas teratomas present between 20–30 years. They may present with secondaries such as an abdominal lump from para-aortic lymph node masses or a neck lump from cervical lymphadenopathy, hepatomegaly or haemoptysis. They may complain of a testicular lump which the patient might have noticed accidentally or due to a feeling of heaviness

3 On suspicion of a testicular tumour, blood must be sent for tumour markers. US of the testes and abdomen and CXR are done. This is followed by an inguinal orchidectomy with facilities for frozen section. Then a CT of the abdomen and chest are done to stage the disease. Some units may do the CT scan before the orchidectomy

4 Depending upon the type of tumour and staging (I to IV) treatment is instituted. Depending upon the staging seminomas are treated by radiotherapy and teratomas by chemotherapy

Figure 6.52

1 The diagnosis is torsion of the testis

2 The patient is a young man who presents with sudden onset of very severe suprapubic pain radiating to the groin and then the testis. On examination the testis is pulled up and palpation is impossible because of pain. The scrotum looks red

3 The differential diagnosis is:
   • Epidydimo-orchtis
   • Torsion of the hydatid of Morgagni
   • In children idiopathic oedema of the scrotum

4 The treatment is immediate exploration. The spermatic cord is untwisted and the testis is fixed to the dartos with interrupted non-absorbable sutures. The same is carried out on the opposite side

Figure 6.53

1 This is a cystogram. This shows a catheter in the urinary bladder and there is extravasation of contrast outside the bladder at the bladder neck. The diagnosis is rupture of the urinary bladder

2 There are two types of rupture of the urinary bladder—extraperitoneal (80%) and intra-peritoneal (20%)

3 Extraperitoneal rupture is treated by diverting the urine—urethral catheter in the female and suprapubic cystostomy in the male. In intraperitoneal rupture, laparotomy is done with repair of the ruptured part of the bladder with peritoneal lavage. An indwelling catheter is left in for 10 days

Hepatobiliary surgery

Questions

Figure 6.54

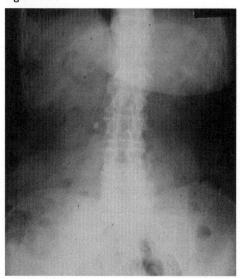

1 This plain X-ray of abdomen shows a radio-opaque shadow to the left of the L3 vertebra. However, there is some abnormality in the right upper quadrant. What is it?

2 What is this abnormality due to?

3 What are the causes of this abnormality?

4 This abnormality may be the outcome of a clinical condition that may give rise to intestinal obstruction. What would be the cause of such an intestinal obstruction?

Figure 6.55 (see also Colour Plate 8)

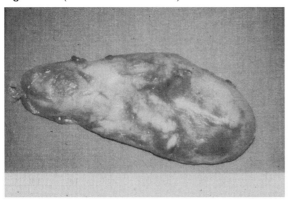

1 What is the pathology affecting this gall bladder?
2 What is the clinical presentation of this condition?
3 Outline the management of this condition

Figure 6.56

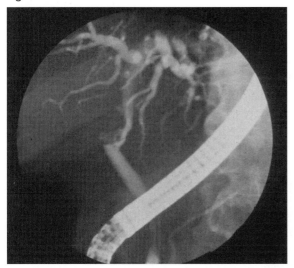

1 What is this imaging technique, what are the findings and the diagnosis?
2 How do such patients present?
3 Outline the management

Figure 6.57

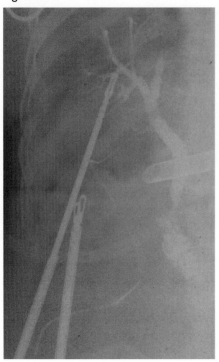

1 What is this imaging technique?
2 What are the findings?
3 Why is this imaging carried out?

Figure 6.58

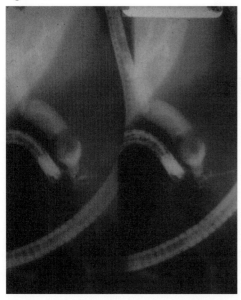

1 These two X-rays are ERCP. What are the
   findings and what is the diagnosis?
2 What is the clinical presentation of this patient?
3 What resuscitative measures would you take
   before you start to treat this patient?
4 How would you treat this patient?
5 What complication may arise from this
   situation?
6 What abdominal signs may you see in such a
   complication?
7 Outline your management of such a
   complication

Figure 6.59 (see also Colour Plate 9)

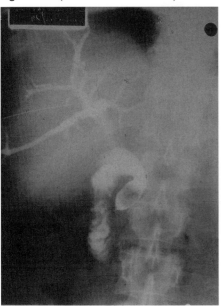

1 What is this imaging technique, what are the findings, and what is the diagnosis?
2 What precautions would you take before you perform this investigation?
3 What are the complications of this procedure?
4 What therapeutic manoeuvre can be carried out by this procedure?

Figure 6.60

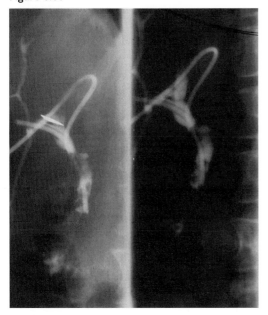

1 What is this imaging technique, what are the findings and the diagnosis?
2 How will you treat this condition?

Figure 6.61 (see also Colour Plate 10)

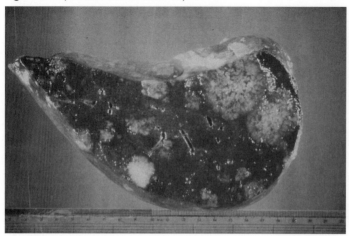

1 What is this a cut specimen of and what is the diagnosis?
2 What are the causes of this condition?
3 What imaging techniques are used to diagnose this condition?

Answers

Figure 6.54

1 There is gas in the biliary tree from a biliary-enetric fistula. Therefore the radio-opaque shadow is from a gallstone that has fistulated through to the duodenum
2 This abnormality is from a cholecystoduodenal fistula
3 The other reasons for gas in the biliary tree are:
   • Previous biliary-enetric bypass operation such as choledochoduodenostomy or choledocohojejunostomy
   • ERCP
   • Endoscopic papillotomy
   • Clostridial infection of the biliary tract

Figure 6.55

1 This gall bladder removed at open cholecystectomy shows gross distension, with fibrinous deposits with red serosa typical of acute inflammation. The diagnosis is acute cholecystitis.
2 The usual presentation is that of a female presenting with acute pain in the right upper quadrant radiating to the epigastrium, right shoulder and interscapular region. She may have fever, nausea, and vomiting. On examination she may have a temperature, may be dehydrated if she has had much vomiting; she would be tender in the right upper quadrant. When palpated at the tip of the 9th costal cartilage, there may be a catch in her breath—Murphy's sign.
3 The patient is first resuscitated with analgesia, rehydrated with IV fluids, and investigated with full haematological and biochemical investigations including serum amylase. Once the patient is stable and on antibiotics, within the next 24 hours a US of the gall bladder is carried out. If that shows stones with a normal common bile duct (CBD), a laparoscopic cholecytectomy (LC) is carried out at the same admission. If the CBD is >7mm in diameter, an ERCP or MRCP (magnetic resonance cholangiopancreatography) is done. If that shows stones in the CBD, then an endoscopic papillotomy is done followed a few days later by LC

Figure 6.56

1 This is an ERCP. It shows a normal pancreatic duct and a normal CBD. The common hepatic duct (CHD) where the cystic duct should enter is smoothly narrowed; this would be due to external compression. The intrahepatic ducts are dilated. As the narrowing is smooth and at the region of the cystic duct, there is external compression from a stone impacted in the cystic duct—Mirrizzi's syndrome

2 These patients present with biliary sepsis—pain in the right upper quadrant, fever, jaundice, and pruritis. They would be ill and may be septicaemic. There would be tenderness in the right upper quadrant and scratch marks all over the body

3 The patient is resuscitated with analgesics, antibiotics, IV fluids, and vitamin K. An US followed by ERCP confirms the diagnosis. During ERCP a CBD stent is inserted which will relieve the patient's jaundice. Once the jaundice has subsided, after about 3–4 weeks, a cholecystectomy is done, probably an open procedure.

Figure 6.57

1 This is a cholangiogram showing laparoscopic instruments in place. There is a cannula entering the cystic duct. Hence it is an operative cholangiogram (on table cholangiogram, OTC)

2 It shows a normal CBD, normal CHD, and free flow of contrast into the duodenum. There are no radio-opaque shadows. Therefore it is a normal operative cholangiogram

3 An OTC is ideally carried out during every cholecystectomy so as to delineate the anatomy of the biliary tree. It is also carried out to make sure that no unsuspected stones are present in the CBD. However, whether to do an OTC routinely or not is a controversial point

Figure 6.58

1 These ERCP pictures show a dilated lower end of CBD with a large smooth radiolucent shadow at the lower end—typical of a stone. The beginning of the pancreatic duct is also seen

2 This patient would present classically with Charcot's intermittent hepatic triad—biliary colic from the stone, intermittent jaundice due to obstruction to the flow of bile, and temperature with rigors due to ascending cholangitis; in addition there would be pruritis

3 Analgesics, antibiotics after blood is sent for culture, rehydration with dextrose-saline and vitamin K. Also acute pancreatitis must be excluded

4 Endoscopic papillotomy and stone retrieval. As the stone is quite large, endoscopic ultrasound disintegration followed by a stent insertion may be necessary

5 This situation may give rise to acute pancreatitis

6 Besides abdominal tenderness, rigidity and rebound tenderness one might see Cullen's sign (haemorrhagic discoloration around the umbilicus) and Grey–Turner's sign (haemorrhagic discoloration in the flanks)

7 The management would be:
- Resuscitation: analgesics, IV fluids, and full supportive therapy
- Investigations and stratification of the disease
- Ultrasound to look for gallstones in the gall bladder and CBD
- Manage in HDU/ITU in severe disease—CT scan to look for pancreatic necrosis
- ERCP and endoscopic papillotomy in stone in the CBD
- Laparotomy and necrosectomy in infected pancreatic necrosis

Figure 6.59

1 This X-ray is a cholangiogram showing a needle in the right upper quadrant entering the liver. It is therefore a percutaneous transhepatic cholangiogram (PTC). It shows a dilated CBD, absent gall bladder, and a radiolucent smooth shadow in the infra-duodenal part of the CBD. The diagnosis is a residual stone in the CBD

2 Patient's prothrombin studies must be checked, blood should be cross-matched, and vitamin K given.

3 The complications of this procedure are:
- Haemoperitoneum
- Biliary peritonitis
- Haemobilia

4 The therapeutic manoeuvre that can be done by this procedure is to insert a stent in a case of cholangiocarcinoma and to drain bile externally in a case of unresectable malignant obstructive jaundice where for some reason a stent cannot be inserted

Figure 6.60

1 This is a T-tube cholangiogram. It shows several radiolucent filling defects with no contrast going down into the duodenum. The diagnosis is residual stones in the CBD
2 This can be treated by endoscopic papillotomy with retrieval of the stones. The other alternative is to leave the T-tube in for 6 weeks to allow the T-tube track to mature. Then the interventional radiologist can dilate the track and remove the stones by using a flexible choledoscope or a Dormia basket—this is called the Burhenne technique

Figure 6.61

1 This is a cut specimen of the liver showing multiple nodules of various sizes and shapes. The diagnosis is liver secondaries
2 The primary may arise from anywhere in the GI tract—stomach, colon, rectum—lung, breast, malignant melanoma, pancreas
3 This is best diagnosed by US, CECT and MRI. Radionuclide studies and angiography are sometimes done for further delineation prior to resection

Vascular surgery

Questions

Figure 6.62

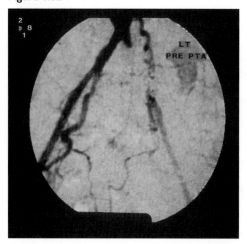

1 What is this imaging procedure, what are the findings, and what is the diagnosis?
2 When should this investigation be carried out?
3 Why is this investigation needed?
4 What should be the treatment in this case?

Figure 6.63

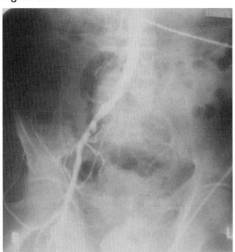

1 What is this investigation, what are the findings and diagnosis?
2 How would this patient present?
3 What comorbid conditions may be associated in this patient?
4 What surgical procedure can be carried out in the patient?

Figure 6.64

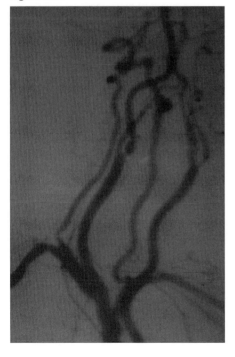

1 What is this image and what is it showing?
2 What are the presenting features of this condition?
3 What are the options of treatment?

Figure 6.65

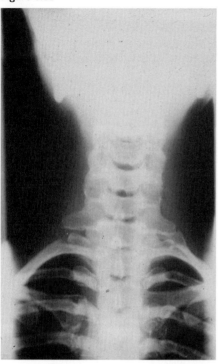

1 What X-ray is this, what is the finding and what is the diagnosis?
2 How do these patients present?
3 What structural abnormalities in this region would give rise to this condition?
4 What is the differential diagnosis?

Figure 6.66

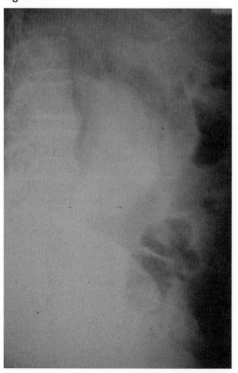

1 What is this X-ray, what are the findings and the diagnosis?
2 How do these patients present?
3 When should they be treated?
4 What are the options of surgical treatment?

Figure 6.67

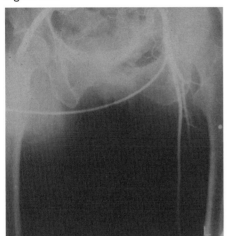

1 What is this image, what are the findings, and what is the diagnosis?
2 What is the aetiology of this condition?
3 What is the clinical presentation?
4 What is the treatment?

Figure 6.68

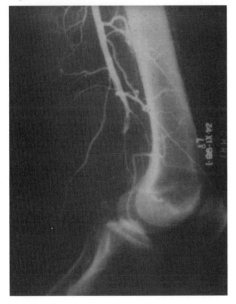

1 What is this image showing?
2 What is the presentation and differential diagnosis?
3 What should be the treatment?

Answers

Figure 6.62

1 This is a digital subtraction angiography (DSA) showing the lower end of the abdominal aorta, the right common iliac and external iliac arteries. A small part of the left common iliac is seen, most of it showing an atherosclerotic occlusion. There is some run-off in the left external iliac artery and collateral circulation

2 An angiogram should be carried out when the decision to intervene, surgically or radiologically, has already been taken on clinical grounds.

3 An angiogram is needed prior to intervention as it is the road map for the vascular surgeon or radiologist. It shows the exact site of obstruction, the length of obstruction, the number of obstructions, the collaterals, and the run-off

    4 The treatment in this patient should be percutaneous transluminal sub-intimal angioplasty (PTA) and stenting. Failing that the treatment would be aorto-iliac bypass graft

Figure 6.63

1 This is a translumbar angiogram, an investigation now obsolete as it has been replaced by DSA. It shows gross atherosclerosis of the abdominal aorta and right common and external iliac arteries with total obstruction of the left common iliac artery. The diagnosis is severe generalized atheroma of the lower limbs with complete obstruction on the left side.

2 This patient would present with critical left lower limb ischaemia—rest pain, shiny skin, lack of hair, guttering of veins, absence of pulses, dusky colouration of the limb and there may be pre-gangrene or gangrene

3 Diabetes and angina

4 This patient requires a limb salvage procedure on the left side provided there is adequate run-off. He would almost certainly have quite marked comorbid conditions. Therefore, he should have a left axillo-femoral bypass. Should his general condition allow, he could have an aorto-bifemoral bypass

Figure 6.64

1 This is a DSA of the arteries of the head and neck. It shows stenosis of the origin of the right internal carotid artery with a post-stenotic dilatation. Diagnosis is right internal carotid artery stenosis

2 Patients, who are usually heavy smokers, complain of amaurosis fugax (temporary visual loss) when the patient complains of a curtain dropping across the eye causing momentary blindness, transient ischaemic attacks (TIA) an reversible intermittent neurological deficit (RIND). On examination a carotid systolic bruit is heard. Sometimes during routine vascular clinical examination an asymptomatic bruit may be heard

3 If on investigations the stenosis is found to be >70% intervention is advisable in the form of carotid endarterectomy or PTA and stenting. In asymptomatic patients with <70% stenosis, aspirin and antifibrinolytic agent is used

Figure 6.65

1 This is an X-ray of the cervical spine showing a complete cervical rib on the left side.

2 These patients present with thoracic inlet/outlet syndrome which consists of neurological, vascular, and local symptoms. The neurological symptoms are due to compression of the lower cord of brachial plexus (C8/T1) producing pressure on the ulnar nerve with wasting of the hypothenar muscles and inability to perform finer movements of the hand. The vascular symptoms are pain on moving the arm and hand particularly abduction; in extreme cases there may be gangrene of the tips of the fingers. A systolic bruit may be heard in the supraclavicular region

3 Besides a cervical rib, the other structural abnormalities that may give rise to thoracic inlet/outlet syndrome are: a bony outgrowth from cervical rib, a prominent 7th cervical transverse process, a sharp fibrous band from the scalenus anterior muscle, a part rib with a fibrous band, and an abnormal insertion of the scalenus anterior muscle.

4 The differentail diagnosis is: cervical spondylosis, syringomyelia, progressive muscular atrophy, Pancoast tumour, ulnar nerve neuritis, and carpal tunnel compression.

Figure 6.66

1 This is a lateral view of a plain abdominal X-ray of the lumbar region. It shows a large calcified soft-tissue shadow in front of the lumbar vertebrae, the front of which are eroded. The diagnosis is an abdominal aortic aneurysm (AAA)

2 These patients may present as an emergency with leak/rupture with collapse due to features of hypovolaemic shock. Electively they would present with throbbing backache, a pulsating abdominal mass, or be discovered incidentally either during screening or on examination for some other condition. Clinical examination would reveal and expansile pulsatile mass

3 All symptomatic AAAs should be treated. Asymptomatic AAAs should be treated if they are >5.5cm in diameter

4 Intervention is by open operation or endovascular repair (EVAR). Recently it has been suggested that open operation is better in the younger patient and EVAR in the older patient because the long-term outcome of EVAR is still not known

Figure 6.67

1 This is a transfemoral angiogram with a cannula entering the left common femoral artery. It shows complete obstruction of the right common femoral artery with a calcified mass in the femoral triangle. The diagnosis is an aneurysm of the right common femoral artery

2 The aetiology may be: atherosclerosis, trauma, infection and rarely a false aneurysm from a previous graft

3 The patient presents with a pulsating mass and pain of claudication in the leg. There may be wasting of the muscles of the thigh and leg

4 Resection of the aneurysm and replacement of the artery with reversed autogenous long saphenous vein. If the long saphenous vein is not available then a synthetic graft can be used

Figure 6.68

1 This is a femoral angiogram showing a thrombosed popliteal artery aneurysm—there is no flow of contrast and a soft-tissue calcified shadow in the popliteal fossa

2 The patient presents with a painful, tender mass in the popliteal fossa and distal limb ischaemia. If it is painful, it may be confused with a popliteal abscess or if it is asymptomatic, a Baker's cyst is the differential diagnosis

3 The treatment is bypass using reversed autogenous long saphenous vein. No attempt is made to resect the aneurysm as it may be very adherent to vital nerves in the vicinity

Head and neck

Questions

Figure 6.69 (see also Colour Plate 11)

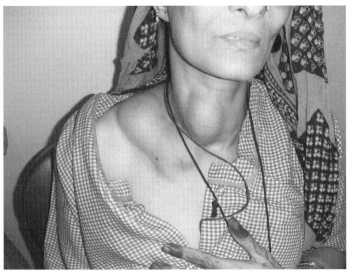

1 Describe the findings in this 40-year-old lady

2 The swelling nearer the midline moves with swallowing and has been there for 10 months. The swellings on the supraclavicular region and posterior triangle have been there for 4 months. What is your clinical diagnosis?

3 What investigations would you do now?

4 What will be the surgical treatment?

Figure 6.70

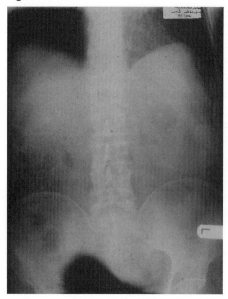

1 What are the findings in this plain abdominal X-ray?
2 What biochemical abnormality may you expect to find?
3 What would be your clinical suspicion as to the diagnosis?
4 What further specific investigations would you do?

Figure 6.71 (see also Colour Plate 12)

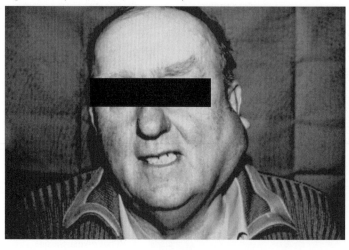

1 What are you clinical findings?
2 What is your clinical diagnosis?
3 What specific clinical test would you perform?
4 What operation would you perform for this condition?

Figure 6.72 (see also Colour Plate 13)

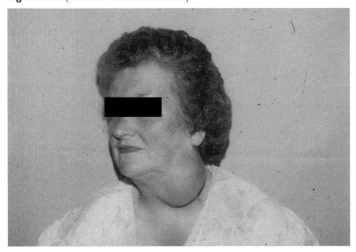

1 What are your clinical findings in this cystic swelling of 3 years' duration growing gradually?
2 What specific physical sign should be elicited? What are the 2 possible differential diagnoses?
3 What would be the surgical treatment in each case?

Figure 6.73

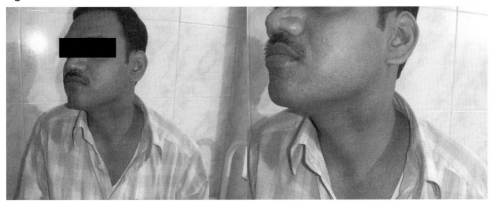

1 This is a pulsating swelling of gradual onset of 2 years' duration. What is your diagnosis?
2 What is the classical physical finding?
3 In what type of population is this condition more common and why?
4 What is the initial investigation? If you wish to operate what investigations should be done?

Answers

Figure 6.69

1 She has two separate swellings—one nearer the midline and another occupying the right supraclavicular and posterior triangles of the neck. The swellings on the lateral side are lobulated
2 As the swelling nearer the midline moves with swallowing, it is a thyroid swelling. The lateral swellings are lobulated and by the site of their location would be arising from the lymph nodes. The thyroid swelling preceded the lymph nodal swellings by 6 months. In summary, this is a 40-year-old female with a thyroid swelling on the right lobe and has subsequently developed cervical lymphadenopathy on the same side. The clinical diagnosis would be papillary thyroid carcinoma with lymph nodal metastasis

3 She should now undergo a Tru-Cut biospy or FNAC of the thyroid and lymph nodes, CT scan of the neck and CXR. Ideally the CT scan should be done before the biopsy so that the CT images are not distorted by the biopsy

4 The treatment should be total thyroidectomy (as papillary carcinoma of the thyroid is multifocal in origin) and resection of the lymph nodes in right side of the neck. Post-operatively she should be on thyroxin for the rest of her life

Figure 6.70

1 This plain X-ray of KUB area shows multiple irregular calcifications in both renal areas—bilateral nephrocalcinosis

2 The biochemical abnormality might be hypercalcaemia

3 One should suspect primary hyperparathyroidism

4 Full biochemical profile should be done; urinary calcium and phosphate; corrected serum calcium; serum parathormone; technetium 99 sestamibi scan; US of the neck for parathyroid adenoma and CT scan

Figure 6.71

1 This patient has a swelling in the left pre-auricular region about 6cm x 5cm, irregular in shape, surface is bosselated, the skin over the swelling is healthy and the ear lobe in the vicinity is distorted

2 Considering its shape, size, and site, it is a parotid tumour. The patient who is showing his teeth does not have facial nerve palsy. The clinical diagnosis is a pleomorphic adenoma, it is the commonest tumour of the parotid.

3 The specific clinical test to perform is the integrity of the facial (7th) nerve. Involvement of the facial nerve denotes a malignant tumour

4 The operation to be performed is a superficial parotidectomy in which the part of the gland superficial to the facial nerve is removed

Figure 6.72

1 This patient has a swelling on the left side of the neck on the anterior triangle about 8cm in diameter. The skin over the swelling is stretched and healthy and the surrounding area looks normal. As it is cystic in consistency and is slow growing, it is a benign swelling. Being cystic, it can be one of two conditions—a branchial cyst or a cystic hygroma

2 One should elicit transillumination as it is a cystic swelling. The two possible diagnoses are: cystic hygroma or a branchial cyst. If transillumination is positive it is a cystic hygroma; if negative it is a branchial cyst

3 Excision of the cyst. In case of a cystic hygroma there is a chance of recurrence

Figure 6.73

1 The diagnosis is a carotid body tumour

2 The classical physical finding is the mobility of the swelling—it is mobile transversely at right angles to the common carotid artery but not longitudinally

3 It is common in mountain dwellers. Because of the lack of oxygen at high altitude, the carotid sinus is stimulated causing hypertrophy of the chemoreceptors; hence called a chaemodectoma

4 The initial investigation is US. If operation is considered specialist investigations are done such as: colour Doppler scan, duplex US, and magnetic resonance angiography

PART 1
SURGICAL SKILLS AND PATIENT SAFETY

Section 2 Basic skills for the surgical trainee

Introduction

This section deals with all the skills necessary as a junior surgical trainee in the daily management of a patient on the surgical ward. This skill would be tested in the station for 'Practical surgical procedures'. The expertise that you acquired in the Basic Surgical Skills Course will be tested in this station.

You are expected to explain every step to the patient (an actor). He or she will have a plastic model strapped to his arm or leg with veins. All the necessary equipment will be on show and it will be up to the candidate to pick up the correct equipment. You may be interrupted by the examiner (a nurse examiner) who would ask you some questions. Almost every type of practical procedure has been dealt with in this section. It would be wise to practise some of these procedures on your ward if you get an opportunity.

Chapter 7 **Needles, sutures, and instruments**

This chapter is useful to the reader when he/she is in the station dealing with procedural skills and therefore ideally should be read in conjunction with Chapter 9, which deals with practical procedures. The examiner who is a nurse may ask why a particular suture or needle is being used. The techniques learnt in Basic Surgical Skills (BSS) courses are tested in this station.

Introduction

As a surgeon, it is imperative that one is conversant with the 'tools of the trade'. These are, at the most basic level, needles, sutures, and instruments. In this day and age, minimal access surgery has a major role and therefore laparoscopic instruments are dealt with elsewhere in Chapter 4. It is not possible to describe every aspect of the use of needles, sutures, and instruments. Those that are commonly used by the junior surgical trainee will be dealt with in this chapter.

Needles

Needles are necessary for the placement of sutures in tissue. Surgical needles must be designed to carry suture material through tissue with minimal trauma. They must be sharp enough to penetrate tissue with minimal resistance. They should be rigid enough to resist bending, yet flexible enough to bend before breaking. They must be sterile and corrosion resistant to prevent introduction of micro-organisms or foreign bodies into the wound.

To meet these requirements, the best surgical needles are made of high quality stainless steel, a non-corrosive material. Surgical needles made of carbon steel may corrode, leaving pits that can harbour micro-organisms. All good quality stainless steel needles are heat treated to give them maximum possible strength and ductility to perform satisfactorily in the body tissues for which they are designed.

Ductility is the ability of the needle to bend to a given angle under a given amount of pressure, called load, without breaking. If too great a force is applied to a needle it may break, but a ductile needle will bend before breaking. If a surgeon feels a needle bending, this is a signal that excessive force is being applied. The strength of a needle is determined in the laboratory by bending the needle 90°, the required force is a measurement of the strength of the needle. If a needle is weak, it will bend too easily and can compromise the surgeon's control and damage surrounding tissue during the procedure. Regardless of ultimate intended use, all surgical needles have three basic components: the attachment end, the body, and the point. The majority of sutures used today have appropriate needles attached by the manufacturer.

Swaged sutures join the needle and suture together as a continuous unit that is convenient to use and minimizes tissue trauma. Surgical needles, which are permanently swaged to the suture strand, are supplied in a variety of sizes, shapes, and strengths.

Classification of needles

Needles are classified according to shape and type of point:

- Curved or straight (Keith needle):
  - ◆ Curved: designed to be held with a needle holder, used for most suturing
  - ◆ Straight: often hand-held, used to secure percutaneously placed devices (e.g. central and arterial lines)
- Taper point, cutting, or reverse cutting:
  - ◆ Taper: for soft tissue such as GI, muscle, peritoneum, usually rounded/small holes
  - ◆ Tapercut: reverse cutting edge/taper point
  - ◆ Cutting: for skin or tough tissue (conventional, reverse, and side)
  - ◆ Blunt: liver, kidney, OB, GYN

There are two basic configurations for curved needles:

- Cutting: cutting edge can cut through tough tissue, such as skin
- Tapered: no cutting edge. For softer tissue inside the body

Anatomy of a needle (see Fig. 7.1)

The body, or shaft, of a needle is the portion which is grasped by the needle holder during the surgical procedure. The body should be as close as possible to the diameter of the suture material. The curvature of the body may be straight, half-curved, curved, or compound curved. The cross-sectional configuration of the body may be round, oval, side-flattened rectangular, triangular, or trapezoidal.

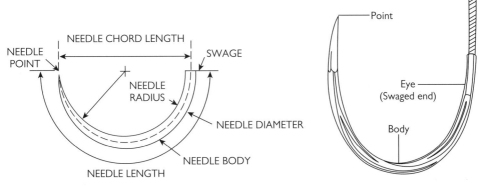

Figure 7.1 The configuration of a surgical needle.

The oval, side-flattened rectangular and triangular shapes may be fabricated with longitudinal ribs on the inside or outside surfaces. This feature provides greater stability of the needle in the needle holder.

The point extends from the extreme tip of the needle to the maximum cross-section of the body. The basic needle points are cutting, tapered, or blunt. Each needle point is designed and produced to the required degree of sharpness to smoothly penetrate the types of tissue to be sutured.

Surgical needles vary in size and wire gauge. The diameter is the gauge or thickness of the needle wire. This varies from 30 microns (0.001 inches) to 56 mil (0.045 inches, 1.4mm). Very small needles of fine gauge wire are needed for micro-surgery. Large, heavy-gauge needles are used to penetrate the sternum and to place retention sutures in the abdominal wall. Broad spectrums of sizes are available between these two extremes. Of the many types available, the specific needle selected for use is determined by the type of tissue to be sutured, the location and accessibility, size of the suture material, and the surgeon's preference.

Needle selection

In selecting a needle, the following points should be considered:

- Tissue and technique
- Alloy and coating; know packaging
- Geometry: tip is tapered, blunt, or cutting (conventional, side, or reverse)
- Body straight, half or whole
- Eye is closed, split, or swaged

Round-bodied needles

Round-bodied needles are designed to separate tissue fibres rather than cut them and are used either for soft tissue or in situations where easy splitting of tissue fibres is possible. After the passage of the needle, the tissue closes tightly round the suture material, thereby forming a leak-proof suture line which is particularly vital in intestinal and cardiovascular surgery. A summary of round-bodied needles is shown in Table 7.1.

Cutting needles

Cutting needles are required where tough or dense tissue needs to be sutured. A summary of their use are given in Table 7.2.

Sutures

Sutures can be divided into two broad groups: absorbable and non-absorbable. Regardless of its composition, suture material is a foreign body to the human tissues in which it is implanted and to a greater or lesser degree will elicit a foreign body reaction.

Table 7.1 Round-bodied needles

Needle type	Description	Typical application
Intestinal	The hole made by this needle is no larger than the diameter of the needle. The hole is then filled by the material, which reduces the risk of leakage	GI tract, biliary tract, dura, peritoneum, urogenital tract, vessels, nerves
Heavy	In some situations where particularly strong needles are required, a heavy wire diameter needle would be appropriate	Muscle, subcutaneous fat, fascia, pedicles
Blunt taperpoint	Where needlestick injury is a major concern, particularly in the presence of blood-borne viruses, the blunt taperpoint needle virtually eliminates accidental glove puncture	Uterus, pedicles, muscle, fascia
Blunt point	This needle has been designed for suturing extremely friable vascular tissue	Liver, spleen, kidney, uterine cervix for incompetent cervix

Table 7.2 Cutting needles

Needle type	Description	Typical application
Tapercut™	This needle combines the initial penetration of a cutting needle with the minimized trauma of a round-bodied needle. The cutting tip is limited to the point of the needle, which then tapers out to merge smoothly into a round cross-section	Fascia, ligament, uterus, scar tissue
Cutting	This needle has a triangular cross-section with the apex on the inside of the needle curvature. The effective cutting edges are restricted to the front section of the needle	Skin, ligament, nasal cavity, tendon, oral
Reverse cutting	The body of this needle is triangular in cross-section with the apex on the outside of the needle curvature	Skin, fascia, ligament, nasal cavity, tendon, oral

There are **two major mechanisms of absorption** resulting in the degradation of absorbable sutures:

- **Enzymatic digestion**: sutures of biological origin such as surgical gut are gradually digested by tissue enzymes
- **Hydrolysis**: sutures manufactured from synthetic polymers are principally broken down by hydrolysis in tissue fluids

Non-absorbable sutures made from a variety of non-biodegradable materials are ultimately encapsulated or walled off by the body's fibroblasts. Non-absorbable sutures ordinarily remain where they are buried within the tissues. When used for skin closure, they must be removed postoperatively.

A further subdivision of suture materials is useful: monofilament and multifilament. A monofilament suture is made of a single strand. It resists harbouring micro-organisms, and it ties down smoothly. A multifilament suture consists of several filaments twisted or braided together. This gives good handling and tying qualities. However, variability in knot strength among multifilament sutures might arise from the technical aspects of the braiding or twisting process.

Classification

- Monofilament or multifilament (braided)
- Absorbable or non-absorbable
- Natural(biological) or synthetic (man-made)

Characteristics of the ideal suture

- Minimal tissue reaction
- Smooth—minimum tissue drag

Table 7.3 Commonly used suture sizes

Bowel	2/0–3/0
Fascia	1–0
Ligatures	0–3/0
Pedicles	2–0
Skin	2/0–5/0
Arteries	2/0–8/0
Micro-surgery	9/0–10/0
Corneal closure	9/0–10/0

- Optimum tensile strength
- Non-electrolytic, non-capillary, non-allergenic, non-carcinogenic
- Non-ferromagnetic as in stainless steel sutures
- Ease of handling—pliable with minimum memory
- Knot should be secure
- Consistent and predictable performance
- Resistant to shrinking in tissues
- Consistent uniform diameter
- Sterile
- Cost effective

Size denotes the diameter of the suture material (see Table 7.3). The accepted surgical practice is to use the smallest diameter suture that will adequately hold the mending wounded tissue. This practice minimizes trauma as the suture is passed through the tissue to effect closure. It also ensures that the minimum mass of foreign material is left in the body. Suture size is stated numerically; as the number of 0s in the suture size increases, the diameter of the strand decreases. For example, size 5-0, or 00000, is smaller in diameter than size 4-0, or 0000. The smaller the size, the less tensile strength the suture will have.

Principles of suture selection

The surgeon has a choice of suture materials from which to select for use in body tissues. Adequate strength of the suture material will prevent suture breakage. Secure knots will prevent knot slippage. It is important to understand the nature of the suture material, the biological forces in the healing wound, and the interaction of the suture and the tissues.

The following guiding principles should be used for optimum suture selection.

1 When a wound has reached maximal strength, sutures are no longer needed. Therefore:
   a Tissues that ordinarily heal slowly such as skin, fascia, and tendons should usually be closed with non-absorbable sutures. An absorbable suture with extended (up to 6 months) wound support may also be used
   b Tissues that heal rapidly such as stomach, colon, and bladder may be closed with absorbable sutures
2 Foreign bodies in potentially contaminated tissues may convert contamination to infection. Therefore:
   a Multifilament sutures are avoided in a contaminated wound
   b Monofilament or absorbable sutures are preferred in potentially contaminated tissues
3 Where cosmetic results are important, close and prolonged apposition of wounds and avoidance of irritants will produce the best result. Therefore:
   a Smallest inert monofilament suture materials should be used such as nylon or polypropylene
   b Skin sutures may be avoided by using subcuticular, whenever possible

c Under certain circumstances, topical skin adhesive or skin closure tape may be used to secure close apposition of skin edges

4 Foreign bodies in the presence of fluids containing high concentrations of crystalloids may act as a nidus for precipitation and stone formation. Therefore:

a In the urinary and biliary tract, rapidly absorbed sutures are used

5 Regarding suture size:

a The finest size, commensurate with the natural strength of the tissue is preferable

b In the past, if the postoperative course of the patient was expected to produce sudden strains on the suture line, retention (tension) sutures were used for reinforcement. These were removed as soon as the patient's condition was stabilized. However, evidence in literature has shown that tension sutures are counter productive and such wounds that are difficult to appose are better treated open with secondary suturing done after the acute phase is over

For how to identify the correct suture from the pack see Fig. 7.2.

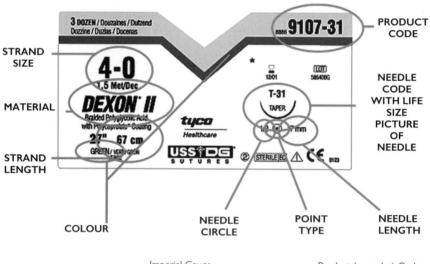

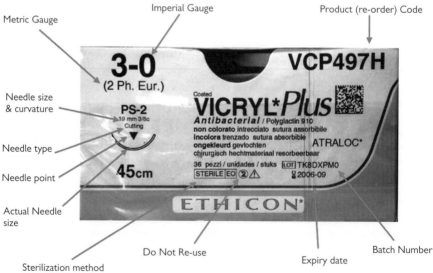

Figure 7.2 Suture packaging.

Knotting techniques

Knot tying is one of the most fundamental techniques in surgery and even then is often performed very badly. Perfecting knot tying technique will help a trainee for the rest of his/her career.

General principles of knot tying

1 The knot must be firm and should not slip
2 The knot must be as small as possible to minimize foreign material in the tissues
3 During tying the suture should not be 'sawed' as this weakens the suture
4 The suture material should not be grasped with artery forceps or needle holders except at the free end when using an instrument tie, otherwise the suture will be damaged
5 Excess tension should be avoided during tying as this could damage the structure being ligated or even cause breakage of the suture material
6 The tissue being ligated should not be torn by controlling tension when placing the knot very carefully using the index finger or thumb as appropriate

Suturing techniques

Suturing techniques cannot be accomplished in the absence of sound knowledge about the knotting techniques described in the previous section.

Basic principles

- There should be no element of tension in any anastomosis
- The needle should be inserted at right angles to the tissue and gently advanced through the tissue avoiding shearing forces
- As a rule, the distance from the edge of the wound should correspond to the thickness of the tissue and successive sutures should be placed at twice this distance apart, i.e. approximately double the depth of the tissue sutured
- All sutures should be placed at right angles to the line of the wound at the same distance from the wound edge and the same distance apart in order for tension to be equal down the wound length. The only situation where this should not apply is when suturing fascia or aponeuroses when the sutures should be placed at varying distances from the wound edge in order to prevent the fibres from splitting
- For long wounds being closed with interrupted sutures, it is often advisable to start in the middle and to keep on halving the wound
- No suture should be tied under too much tension or the subsequent oedema of the wound may cause the sutures to cut out or to develop ischaemia of the wound edge and delayed healing
- In most cases it is advisable to only go through one edge of the tissues at a time but, if the edges lie in very close proximity and accuracy can be ensured, it is permissible to go through both edges at the same time
- For elliptical wounds following lesion excision, the edges of the wound may be undermined to help closure. However, the length of the wound will need to be approximately three times the width of the wound if closure is to be safe and not under too much tension. Skin hooks may be useful to display the wound
- For skin closure where the edges should be slightly everted for optimum healing, it is essential to ensure that the subcutaneous width of the tissue bite is slightly greater than the width from the skin edge

Types of suturing

- Interrupted
- Continuous
- Mattress
- Subcuticular

Instruments

Basic instruments are essential to accomplish most types of general surgery. Most instruments used in the operation theatre are stainless steel. Gold-plated handles are used in some instruments. For hinged instruments, there are two types of joints namely the screw joint as seen in the scissors and the box joint as in a haemostat or a needle holder. The latter ensures greater security of movement without any lateral movement as may occur after prolonged use and wear in the former.

The instruments are usually constructed for the right-handed surgeons but instruments for left-handed surgeons are also available on demand. The basic design of the right-handed instrument has the right limb over the left limb when seen from the side over the joint. Even the lock design is different and a right-handed instrument has the lock on the upper limb facing the lock on the lower limb. In left-handed instruments the left limb sits over the right limb and so does the lock. However, since the left-handed surgeons get trained with the right-handed instruments during their trainee periods, the demand for left-handed instruments remains low and companies have stopped making them on a regular basis.

Instruments can be placed into one of the four following basic categories:

- Retracting and exposing instruments: these are used to hold back or retract organs or tissues to gain exposure to the operative site. They are either 'self-retaining' (stay open on their own), e.g. Travers or 'manual' (held by hand), e.g. Langenbeck
- Cutting and dissecting instruments: these are sharp and are used to cut body tissue or surgical supplies, e.g. knife, scissors
- Clamping and occluding instruments: these are used to compress blood vessels or hollow organs for haemostasis or to prevent spillage of intestinal contents, e.g. bowel clamps, artery forceps
- Grasping and holding instruments: these are used to grasp various types of organs or tissue, or to hold drapes or sponges e.g. Babcock's tissue forceps, dissecting forceps

Sterilization

All the surgical instruments are usually sterilized by autoclaving. Sharp edged instruments like scissors are not autoclaved due to the damage caused to the cutting edge and are sterilized by ethylene oxide (Et O) gas. In some developing countries, Ortho-phthalaldehyde (OPA) is used as a chemical agent especially for sharp instruments. More recently, low-temperature, hydrogen peroxide gas plasma technology has been used to sterilize all types of surgical instruments with a turnaround time varying between 30–75 minutes for various levels of sterilization. Instruments with tungsten carbide jaws are not recommended for chemical/cold sterilization.

Chapter 8 Incisions and wounds

Introduction

A **wound** is defined as an injury to the body that typically involves laceration or breaking of a membrane and damage to the underlying tissue. The spectrum of wounds seen varies from a clean incision made from a surgeon's knife to widespread damage of the tissue caused by a major trauma. Regardless of the mechanism of injury, damage to the natural structure sets in motion an interesting cascade of events that eventually lead to healing of the wound.

Classification of wounds

There is no standard classification for wounds. However, there are a number of different ways in which wounds can be classified which help in describing the wound with a view to its management and ultimate healing. The factors of greatest importance in evaluation are: the nature of the injury causing the wounds, the timing, the degree of contamination, whether acute or chronic, and the depth of injury to the skin and underlying tissues.

Type of injury is of great importance in terms of the way in which the wound will heal:

- Incised: these wounds cause little damage to surrounding soft tissue and therefore there is little disruption to blood supply. These wounds will heal quickly, usually by primary intention if sutured.
- Laceration: caused by a sharp object, however the object is not sharp enough to produce an incision and results in a wound with irregular edges. Such a wound usually needs debridement and may be closed if it presents within 6 hours of injury and with minimal contamination.
- Crushing: injuries caused by a crushing force will similarly cause immediate cell death and damage to underlying blood supply. These wounds require excision or wound debridement. There may be an element of avulsion of blood vessels and nerves which again leads to poor prognosis in terms of wound repair.
- Burns: burn wounds are classified according to their size, taking into account body surface area and the depth of injury to the skin. The surface area of the wound is important because fluid loss through the damaged epidermis may be severe.

Classification according to time

Wounds presenting in the first 6 hours of the insult are referred to as acute injury and are often described as an injury presenting in the golden period and may be closed primarily if possible after irrigation and debridement. Early wounds presenting in the first 24 hours fare better than those that present later. Infection has already established itself in wounds presenting late. It is generally not advisable to close such wounds primarily and they are sutured after serial debridement or may be left to heal with secondary intention.

Classification according to thickness

Wounds may be classified as full thickness when the whole of epidermis and dermis is involved and partial thickness when only superficial layers are involved. A full thickness wound results in a greater degree of scarring and takes a longer time to heal compared to a superficial wound.

Classification according to degree of contamination (Table 8.1)

Table 8.1 Wound classification according to degree of contamination

Class I Clean wound	An uninfected operative wound in which no inflammation is encountered and the respiratory, alimentary, genital, or uninfected urinary tract is not entered. In addition, clean wounds are primarily closed and, if necessary, drained with closed drainage. Operative incisional wounds that follow non-penetrating (blunt) trauma should be included in this category if they meet the criteria
Class II Clean contaminated	An operative wound in which the respiratory, alimentary, genital, or urinary tracts are entered under controlled conditions and without unusual contamination. Specifically, operations involving the biliary tract, appendix, vagina, and oropharynx are included in this category, provided no evidence of infection or major break in technique is encountered

Table 8.1 Continued

Class III Contaminated	Open, fresh, accidental wounds. In addition, operations with major breaks in sterile technique (e.g. open cardiac massage) or gross spillage from the GI tract, and incisions in which acute, non-purulent inflammation is encountered are included in this category
Class IV Dirty-infected	Old traumatic wounds with retained devitalized tissue and those that involve existing clinical infection or perforated viscera. This definition suggests that the organisms causing post-operative infection were present in the operative field before the operation

Acute wounds

Acute wounds heal in a predictable manner and time frame. The process occurs with few, if any, complications, and the end result is a well-healed wound. The healing of acute wounds involves a complex, dynamic, well-orchestrated series of events. A 'healed wound' is one in which the connective tissues have been repaired, the wound has completely re-epithelialized by regeneration and has regained its normal anatomical structure and function. Some wounds fail to heal in a timely and orderly manner, resulting in chronic, non-healing wounds.

Chronic non-healing wounds

Chronic wounds appear to have derangements in various stages of wound healing and have a mismatch between the appropriate levels of different growth factors. There appears to be a higher level of proinflammatory cytokines. With increased inflammation of the wound, there is less likelihood that the wound will progress to healing. The balance is shifted in favour of collagen degradation rather than collagen synthesis. Impaired healing is characterized by a failure to achieve mechanical strength equivalent to normally healed wounds. In addition, patients with compromised immune systems—such as those with diabetes, chronic steroid usage, or tissues damaged by radiotherapy—are prone to this type of impaired healing. Wounds that are chronically inflamed and do not proceed to closure are susceptible to the development of squamous cell carcinoma (Marjolin's ulcer). Conditions associated with Marjolin's ulcers are burn scar, osteomyelitis, pressure sores, venous stasis ulcers, and hidradenitis. The wound appears irregular, has overturned wound edges and a white, pearly discoloration. In patients with suspected malignant transformations, biopsy of the wound edges must be performed to rule out malignancy. The premalignant state is pseudoepitheliomatous hyperplasia. Such a carcinoma is a slow growing form of squamous cell carcinoma and has a much lower propensity for metastasis to lymph nodes due to obliteration of lymphatics by the scar tissue.

Classification of the process of wound healing (wound closure)

Primary healing (healing by first intention)

This is the best form of healing and takes place when clean wounds (surgical incisions or clean lacerations) are closed by primary suturing. There is no raw area left behind at the end of the surgical procedure. There is minimal disruption of the structure and as a result the wound heals well and scar formation is minimal. Whereas incised wounds are sutured, raw areas can be covered by skin grafts taken from donor areas. A **partial** or **split-thickness skin graft** (SSTG or a Thiersch graft) contains variable thickness of dermis and provides skin cover for resurfacing large areas of wound as a result of surgical excision or burns. SSTG donor sites heal spontaneously with cells supplied by the remaining epidermal appendages (Figs. 8.1 and 8.2). Nutrition of a STSG is derived mainly from the bed of the graft and hence needs to have a healthy granulation tissue.

   Full-thickness grafts retain more of the characteristics of normal skin, including colour, texture, and thickness, when compared with split-thickness grafts. They undergo much less contraction while healing and therefore are preferred on the face as well as on the hands and over mobile joint surfaces. Full thickness grafts derive nutrition from the edges of the graft which limits its use to cover relatively small size defects.

Secondary healing (healing by secondary intention)

This is seen in wounds that are heavily contaminated with extensive tissue destruction. The wound is allowed to heal by granulation contraction and epithelialization. This type of healing is slower and can cause contracture and scarring (Figs. 8.3 and 8.4).

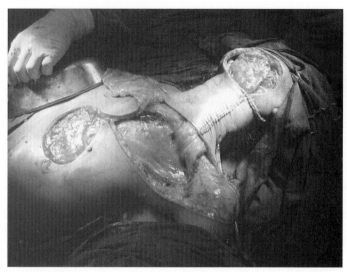

Figure 8.1 Wounds created in the operation theatre as part of the excision of oral cancer and reconstruction using fasciocutaneous and myocutaneous flaps. Note the primary closure of the neck incision of neck dissection.

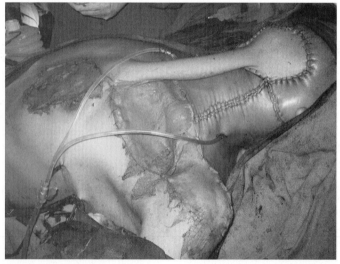

Figure 8.2 The same wound is closed primarily using primary suturing (sutures and staples) and the donor area of the flap is covered using split-thickness skin grafting leaving no raw area behind.

Delayed primary healing

This is seen in a contaminated wound, as it cannot be closed primarily because of the risk of becoming infected. The wound is sutured after a few days (delayed) after it has been debrided serially and there is no evidence of residual source of infection or dead tissue (Fig. 8.5).

Phases of wound healing (Fig. 8.6)

Healing of a wound is a well-regulated series of events that can be divided into four broad categories. Though the phases are well defined they form a continuum of wound healing process:

- Haemostasis

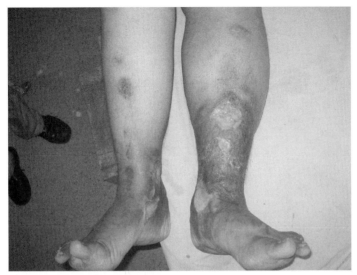

Figure 8.3 These bilateral venous ulcers need optimal wound management skills described in the section on dressings and are likely to heal with secondary intention with scarring.

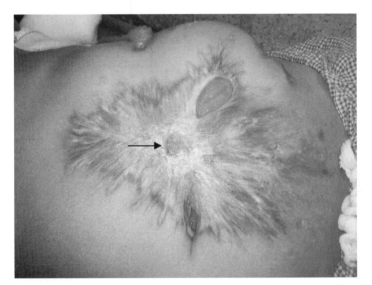

Figure 8.4 Healing by secondary intention in an infected abdominal wound after peritonitis. Note the central ulcer in the scar tissue (arrow).

- Inflammatory phase
- Proliferative phase
- Maturation and remodelling phase

Phase I: haemostasis

Injury of vasculature results in the first immediate response of haemostasis cascade that tends to control the impact of tissue injury and blood loss. Under normal circumstances, blood maintains its fluidity because of the balance of procoagulant and anticoagulant influences, including interactions at the blood–endothelium interface and many circulating factors. When a vessel is injured, tissue factor (TF) and types IV and V collagen are exposed, as a result of which platelets adhere to the site of injury and undergo a

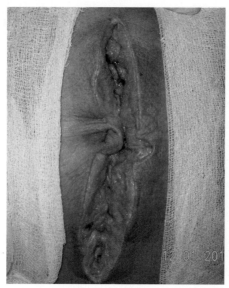

Figure 8.5 Delayed primary closure of a laparotomy wound in a case of diffuse peritonitis.

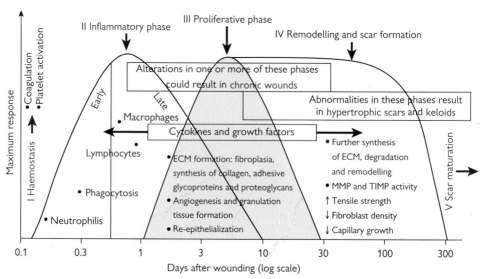

ECM: Extracellular matrix; MMP: Metalloproteinases; TIMP: Tissue inhibitors of metalloproteinases.

Figure 8.6 Phases of wound healing. From Clark RA, in: Goldsmith LA (ed.) (1991). *Physiology, Biochemistry and Molecular Biology of Skin*, vol. 1, 2nd edn., p. 577. With permission from Oxford University Press.

release phenomenon with further platelet aggregation, and thus a platelet plug is formed. The initial contact between platelets and collagen requires von Willebrand's factor (vWF) VIII, a protein that is synthesized by megakaryocytes and endothelial cells. Platelet adhesion to the endothelium is primarily mediated through the interaction between high-affinity glycoprotein receptors and the integrin receptor GPIIb-IIIa.

Vasoconstriction occurs in response to the release of vasoactive substances from platelets (e.g., thromboxane A_2 and serotonin) and endothelin from endothelial cells. Thromboxane A_2 is produced locally at the site of injury and is a very potent constrictor of smooth muscle, especially in smaller and medium-sized vessels. Larger vessels constrict in response to innervation and circulating noradrenaline.

Initial intense local vasoconstriction of arterioles and capillaries is followed by vasodilation and increased vascular permeability.

The platelets degranulate and release their alpha granules, which secrete several biologically active proteins, such as platelet-derived growth factor, insulin-like growth factor-1, epidermal growth factor, transforming growth factor-β (TGF-β), and platelet factor 4.

These proteins initiate the wound-healing cascade by attracting and activating fibroblasts, endothelial cells, and macrophages. These events also activate four major amplification systems (complement cascade, clotting mechanism, kinin cascade, and plasmin generation), which contribute to haemostasis and the subsequent stages of the healing process. However, healing can occur in wounds where there is no haemorrhage (and therefore no platelets).

The clot (comprising fibrin, fibronectin, vWF, thrombospondin) provides the provisional matrix for cellular migration. The platelets also contain dense bodies that contain vasoactive amines, such as serotonin, which causes vasodilation and increased vascular permeability, causing leakage of plasma from the intravascular space to the extracellular compartment.

Phase II: inflammation

Having achieved the first goal of haemostasis, the second phase, i.e. inflammatory phase, begins. The goal of this phase is the removal of bacteria, foreign debris, and other contaminants. Inflammation can be divided into early and late phases depending on the time and duration of response and the type of inflammatory cell involved.

In early inflammatory phase, neutrophils (polymorphonuclear (PMN) leucocytes), migrate from the surrounding microvasculature. Complement factors such as C5a and leukotriene B_4 promote neutrophil adherence and chemoattraction. In the presence of thrombin, endothelial cells exposed to leukotriene C_4 and D_4 release platelet-aggregating factor, which further enhances neutrophil adhesion. Monocytes and endothelial cells produce the inflammatory mediators interleukin-1 and tumour necrosis factor-α, and these mediators also further promote endothelial-neutrophil adherence. The increased capillary permeability and the various chemotactic factors facilitate diapedesis of neutrophils into the inflammatory site. As the neutrophils begin their migration, they release the contents of their lysosomes and enzymes such as elastase and other proteases into the extracellular matrix (ECM), which facilitates migration of the neutrophils. The combination of intense vasodilation and increased vascular permeability leads to clinical findings of inflammation, *rubor* (redness), *tumor* (swelling), *calor* (heat), and *dolor* (pain). Once in the wound environment, PMN leucocyte phagocytose bacteria and other foreign particles, and kill them by releasing degrading enzymes and free radicals derived from oxygen. The activity of PMN leucocytes usually stops within a few days of wounding (after the contaminating bacteria have been cleared). Redundant cells are cleared from the wound by extrusion to the wound surface as slough or by phagocytosis by macrophages. The main function of PMN leucocytes is to minimize bacterial contamination of the wound, thus preventing infection.

During this period, basal cells at the cut edge of the epidermis begin to exhibit increased mitotic activity. Within 24–48 hours, epithelial cells from both edges begin to migrate and proliferate along the dermis, depositing components of basement membrane as they progress.

Late inflammatory phase (days 2–3) migration of PMN leucocytes stops when wound contamination has been controlled, usually within the first few days after injury. PMN leucocytes do not survive longer than 24 hours. After 24–48 hours, the predominance of cells in the wound cleft shifts to mononuclear cells. On arriving at the wound site, blood monocytes undergo a phenotypic change to become tissue macrophages. Monocytes are attracted to the wound by a variety of chemoattractants, including complement (C5a) immunoglobulins, breakdown products of collagen elastin and cytokines. Monocytes undergo a phenotypic change to become tissue macrophages.

Macrophages are truly crucial to wound healing in that they serve to regulate the release of cytokines and stimulate many of the subsequent processes of wound healing (Table 8.2). Macrophages also induce apoptosis of PMN leucocytes and play a significant role in regulating angiogenesis and matrix deposition and remodelling.

Epithelialization begins within a few hours of wounding; a single layer of epidermal cells migrates from the wound edges to form a delicate covering over the exposed raw area, a process known as 'epiboly'.

Table 8.2 Macrophage activities during wound healing

Activity	Mediators
Phagocytosis	Reactive oxygen species
	Nitric oxide
Debridement	Collagenase, elastase
Cell recruitment and activation	Growth factors: PDGF, TGF-β, EGF, IGF
	Cytokines: TNF-α, IL-1, IL-6
	Fibronectin
Matrix synthesis	Growth factors: TGF-β, EGF, PDGF
	Cytokines: TNF-α, IL-1, IFN-γ
	Enzymes: arginase, collagenase
	Prostaglandins
Angiogenesis	Nitric oxide
	Growth factors: FGF, VEGF
	Cytokines: TNF-α
	Nitric oxide

EGF, epithelial growth factor; FGF, fibroblast growth factor; IGF, insulin-like growth factor; IFN, interferon; IL-1, interleukin-1; IL-6, interleukin-6; PDGF, platelet-derived growth factor; TGF, transforming growth factor; TNF, tumour necrosis factor; VEGF, vascular endothelial growth factor.

From Schwartz SI (2004). *Principles of Surgery*, 8th ed. New York: McGraw-Hill.

These cells undergo mitosis and migrate as a sheet, extending along the advancement edge. When advancing epithelial cells meet, further movement is halted by 'contact inhibition'.

Proliferation (day 3 to week 2)

This stage is characterized by the formation of granulation tissue, and establishes the continuity of the wound, consisting of a capillary bed, fibroblasts, macrophages, and a loose arrangement of collagen, fibronectin, and hyaluronic acid.

Fibroblasts appear after 2–4 days of wounding. They are attracted to the wound by a number of factors, including platelet-derived growth factor and transforming growth factor-β. These fibroblasts as compared to non-wound fibroblasts proliferate less, synthesize more collagen and carry out more matrix contraction. It is the interaction between the fibroblasts and the ECM that regulates further synthesis of the ECM and subsequent remodelling.

ECM stabilizes the structure and regulates the wound healing process. It consists of polysaccharide glycosaminoglycans and fibrous protein such as collagen, elastin, fibronectin, and laminin. Collagen fibres within the matrix serve to organize and strengthen it, whereas elastin fibres give it resilience and matrix proteins have adhesive functions.

Collagen appears in the wound after a period of 3–5 days. The time required for undifferentiated mesenchymal cells to differentiate into highly specialized fibroblasts accounts for the delay between injury and the appearance of collagen in a healing wound. Collagens are the most abundant family of proteins in the body. They provide strength and integrity to all tissues and so play a vital role in wound repair. Although there are at least 20 types of collagen described, the main ones of interest to wound repair are types I and III. Type I collagen is the major component of ECM in skin and bone and is the most common type of collagen. Type III, which is also normally present in skin, becomes more prominent and important during the repair process. Multiple factors can affect collagen synthesis. Vitamin C (ascorbic acid), TGF-β, insulin-like growth factor I and II increase collagen synthesis. IFN-γ decreases type I procollagen mRNA synthesis, and glucocorticoids inhibit procollagen gene transcription, thereby leading to decreased collagen synthesis.

Granulation tissue appears after 3 days and is characterized by angiogenesis. Histologically, it is denoted by proliferating fibroblasts and loops of capillaries in a loose ECM. These new vessels are oedematous due to incompletely formed interendothelial junctions and increased transcytosis. Granulation tissue bleeds easily if traumatized. Healing wounds have a moist, shiny, and reddish granulation tissue. Beefy-red and friable granulation tissue indicates poor healing.

Phase IV: maturation and remodelling

Every wound is in a continuous state of collagen synthesis and breakdown. Wound contraction occurs through the interactions between fibroblasts and the surrounding ECM and is influenced by a number of cytokines and is not completely understood. Collagen degradation is achieved by specific metalloproteinases (MMPs) that are produced by fibroblasts, neutrophils, and macrophages at the wound site. MMPs may be necessary to allow cleavage of the attachment between the fibroblast and the collagen so that the lattice can be made to contract. The fibroblast population decreases and the dense capillary network regresses. Wound strength increases rapidly within 1–6 weeks and then appears to plateau up to 1 year after the injury. As the scar matures, collagen bundles increase in diameter, corresponding with increasing tensile strength of the wound. However, these collagen fibres never regain the original strength of unwounded skin, and a maximum of 80% strength of unwounded skin can be achieved. Unlike normal skin, the epidermodermal interface in a healed wound is devoid of rete pegs, the undulating projections of epidermis that penetrate into the papillary dermis. Loss of this anchorage results in increased fragility and predisposes the neoepidermis to avulsion after minor trauma.

Local and systemic factors affecting wound healing (Table 8.3)

Wound healing is a complex procedure consisting of a series of processes regulated and also influenced at each stage by a number of factors that are both systemic as well as local. The blood supply in the lower extremity is the worst in the body; that in the face and hands is the best. In older patients healing is slower.

Excess healing (hypertrophic scars and keloids)

An example of a proliferative scar is a hypertrophic scar (HTS) or keloid. Both keloids and HTSs are characterized by excessive collagen deposition versus collagen degradation. The underlying mechanisms that cause HTSs and keloids are not known. The immune system appears to be involved in the formation of both HTS and keloids, although the exact relationship is unknown.

Table 8.3 Factors affecting wound healing

Local	Systemic
• Presence of foreign body/clot/devitalized tissue	• Advancing age
• Infection	• Obesity
• Tissue hypoxia:	• Malnutrition: deficiency of proteins, zinc, vitamins A and C
◆ Acute: vascular damage, suture tension and jaundice)	• Systemic malignancy
Chronic: radiation enteritis, diabetic microvascular disease, atherosclerosis, venous hypertension and long-term vascular damage	• Terminal illness
	• Chemotherapy/radiotherapy
	• Immunosuppressant drugs
	• Peripheral vascular disease
	• Venous oedema or lymphoedema
	• Systemic diseases (diabetes, neoplasia, uraemia)
	• Neuropathy
	• Impaired body defence

Hypertrophic scars (Fig. 8.7a) rise above the skin level but stay within the confines of the original wound and often regress over time. HTSs usually develop within 4 weeks after trauma and are independent of site, age, and race. They seldom increase in size after the first few months and usually never after the first year. They usually occur across areas of tension and flexor surfaces, which tend to be at right angles to joints or skin creases. The lesions are initially erythematous and raised, and over time may evolve into pale, flatter scars. Histologically the collagen bundles are flatter, more random, and the fibres are in a wavy pattern. HTSs are in many cases preventable by careful surgical approximation and use of pressure dressings in vulnerable wounds like burns etc. Scars that are perpendicular to the underlying muscle fibres tend to be flatter and narrower. As muscle fibres contract, the wound edges approximate if they are perpendicular to the underlying muscle.

Keloids (Fig. 8.7b) rise above the skin level as well, but extend beyond the border of the original wound into the adjoining normal skin and rarely regress spontaneously. Keloids tend to occur months to years after the initial insult, and even minor injuries can result in large lesions. They vary in size from a few millimetres to large, pedunculated lesions with a soft to rubbery or hard consistency. While they project above surrounding skin, they rarely extend into underlying subcutaneous tissues. Certain body sites have a higher incidence of keloid formation, including the skin of the earlobe as well as the deltoid, presternal, and upper back regions. Keloids are much more common in darker-pigmented ethnicities and both men and women are equally affected. Keloid formation appears to be an autosomal dominant trait with incomplete penetration and variable expression. Histologically, the collagen bundles are virtually non-existent, and the fibres are connected haphazardly in loose sheets with a random orientation to the epithelium. The collagen fibres are larger and thicker and myofibroblasts are generally absent. Intralesional steroids are recommended as first-line treatment for keloids. Surgical intervention can lead to recurrence and can have a worse result. There are fewer recurrences when surgical excision is combined with other modalities such as intralesional corticosteroid injection, topical application of silicone sheets, or the use of radiation or pressure. Surgery is recommended for debulking large lesions or as a rescue option when other modalities have failed. Intralesional injections of chemotherapeutic agents such as 5-fluorouracil have been used both alone and in combination with steroids like triamcinolone. Topical retinoids also have been used as treatment for both HTS and keloids.

Incisions

The first step of any surgery is an incision; though it may be a small step in the whole surgery, the surgeon must remember that it is one of the most important. Every incision that is made should be carefully planned so that it will cause minimal scarring and discomfort to the patient (Box 8.1).

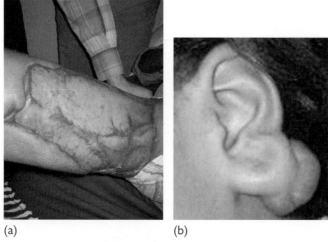

(a)　　　　　　　　　　　　　　(b)

Figure 8.7 (a) Hypertrophic scars at the graft recipient site in the thigh limited to the graft site. (b) Keloid in the pinna after ear piercing. Note the extension into the normal adjoining skin.

> **Box 8.1 Summary for incisions according to lines**
>
> - Incisions should follow wrinkle lines
> - If wrinkle lines are not readily evident, then RSTLs can be located with the pinch test
> - Circular excision can be used to determine the optimal direction of the final elliptical excision
> - Incisions and the resulting scars should never interfere with function or treatment priorities
> - Wrinkle lines and RSTLs largely coincide and should be used instead of Langer's lines

Langer's lines

Langer's lines were described in 1861 by Karl Langer, a professor of anatomy at St. Joseph's Academy in Vienna, based on his study on cadavers. It was suggested that skin incisions should be made along these lines. It was later suggested that rather than Langer's lines, surgeons should place incisions in natural **wrinkle lines**, described in 1935 by Jerome P. Webster and later elaborately by Cornelius Kraissl. It was noted later that these lines are mostly perpendicular to the muscles and therefore, in a scar placed perpendicular to the underlying muscle, collagen will be laid down in the same direction as is usual in the wrinkle lines thus allowing for optimal healing of the scar.

Relaxed skin tension lines (RSTLs), first described by Borges, follow furrows when the skin is relaxed, and are not visible like wrinkle lines. The relaxation is achieved by joint mobilization, muscle contraction, or pinching. The furrows formed with joint mobilization depend on the type of joint mobilization and are not reliable; similarly, furrows from muscle contraction depend on which muscle is contracting, and can be unreliable. Applying the pinch at a right angle to the RSTL best creates the furrows formed by pinching.

The differences between wrinkle lines and RSTLs are subtle but Langer's lines differ considerably from both. Though sited most commonly they are not always suited for incisions and surgeons rarely actually follow Langer's lines, but instead use wrinkle lines or RSTL. For example, Langer's lines on the forehead are vertical and it would be unjustified placing a vertical incision on forehead, which is placed transversely along the wrinkle lines. RSTL are followed for incisions on the face as compared to the rest of the body where wrinkle lines are preferred.

Wound management

Management of acute wounds begins with obtaining a careful history of the events and meticulous examination of the wound. A detailed clinical history should include information on the duration of ulcer, previous ulceration, history of trauma, family history of ulceration, ulcer characteristics (site, pain, odour, and exudate or discharge), limb temperature, underlying medical conditions (e.g. diabetes mellitus, peripheral vascular disease, ischaemic heart disease, cerebrovascular accident, neuropathy, connective tissue diseases (such as rheumatoid arthritis), varicose veins, DVT), previous venous or arterial surgery, smoking, medications, and allergies to drugs and dressings. Examination should assess the depth and configuration of the wound, the extent of nonviable tissue, and the presence of foreign bodies and other contaminants.

The site of the wound may aid diagnosis—diabetic foot ulcers often arise in areas of abnormal pressure distribution arising from disordered foot architecture. Venous ulceration occurs mostly in the gaiter area of the leg. Sun-exposed areas usually have more incidence of basal cell carcinoma or squamous cell carcinoma. The size of the wound should be assessed at first presentation and regularly thereafter. The outline of the wound margin should be traced onto transparent acetate sheets and the surface area estimated. Examination of the edge of the wound may help to identify its aetiology in the context of the history of the wound. For example, venous leg ulcers generally have gently sloping edges, arterial ulcers often appear well demarcated and 'punched out', an undermined edge suggests tuberculosis or syphilis, and rolled or everted edges should raise the suspicion of a malignancy. A biopsy should be taken of any suspicious wound.

The wound bed should be examined—healthy granulation tissue is pink in colour and is an indicator of healing. Unhealthy granulation is dark red in colour, often bleeds on contact, and may indicate the

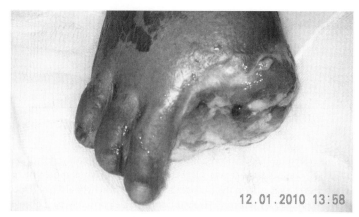

Figure 8.8 Arterial ulcer of the foot in a diabetic patient requiring serial debridements.

presence of wound infection. Such wounds should be cultured and treated in the light of microbiological results. Excess granulation or over-granulation (proud tissue) may also be associated with infection or non-healing wounds. Simple cautery with silver nitrate or topical steroid should be applied to this granulation tissue. The wound bed may be covered with necrotic tissue (non-viable tissue due to reduced blood supply), slough (dead tissue, usually cream or yellow in colour), or eschar (dry, black, hard necrotic tissue). Such tissue impedes healing. Necrotic tissue and slough may be quantified as excessive (+++), moderate (++), minimal (+), or absent (−). Examination of the surrounding skin should be carried out. Cellulitis associated with wounds should be treated with systemic antibiotics. Eczematous changes may need treatment with potent topical steroid preparations. Maceration of the surrounding skin is often a sign of inability of the dressing to control the wound exudate, which may respond to more frequent dressing changes or change in dressing type.

Local care

After examination of the wound, it should be cleansed and irrigated by a physiological solution like normal saline. Debridement (Fig. 8.8) depending upon the extent of non-viable tissue, and the presence of foreign bodies and other contaminants, should be undertaken under local anaesthesia. High-pressure wound irrigation is more effective in achieving complete debridement of foreign material and non-viable tissues. Iodine, povidone-iodine, hydrogen peroxide, and organically-based antibacterial preparations have all been shown to impair wound healing due to injury to wound neutrophils and macrophages, and thus should not be used. Antibiotic administration and tetanus prophylaxis may be needed, and planning the type and timing of wound repair should take place. In general, the smallest suture required to hold the various layers of the wound in approximation should be selected in order to minimize suture-related inflammation. Non-absorbable or slowly absorbing monofilament sutures are most suitable for approximating deep fascial layers, particularly in the abdominal wall. Subcutaneous tissues should be closed with braided absorbable sutures, with care to avoid placement of sutures in fat. Although traditional teaching in wound closure has emphasized multiple-layer closures, additional layers of suture closure are associated with increased risk of wound infection, especially when placed in fat. Drains may be placed in areas at risk of forming fluid collections. More recently, tissue glues (cyanoacrylate) have been shown to be effective for the management of short lengths of simple, linear wounds with viable skin edges.

Wound dressing

Over the past 10–15 years, the approach to a patient with a chronic wound has evolved from pure observation and topical dressing selection, into the appreciation of a complex microenvironment with numerous interdependent biochemical pathways. As the knowledge base continues to grow, so has the detail regarding which diagnostic and treatment options are available in wound care. Materials used to cover wounds have evolved from readily available materials in nature to materials specifically designed to provide particular benefits for wound healing.

The main purpose of wound dressings is to provide the ideal environment for wound healing. The dressing should facilitate the major changes taking place during healing to produce an optimally healed wound. The dressing should protect the wound from trauma and contamination by bacteria, help with absorption of the wound exudates, provide compression to assist in decreasing oedema, and yet be non-adherent. It should be non-allergic, non-irritating, safe, convenient to apply and remove, and cost-effective. Other dressings may need to provide immobilization to allow stable scar formation (i.e. bolster over a skin graft). It is important to note that not all dressings can provide all the characteristics and not all wounds require all these functions. It is essential that the choice of dressing matches the specific wound conditions.

Dressings can be classified as primary or secondary. A **primary dressing** is placed directly on the wound and may provide absorption of fluids and prevent desiccation, infection, and adhesion of a secondary dressing. A **secondary dressing** is one that is placed on the primary dressing for further protection, absorption, compression, and occlusion.

Cotton or viscose gauze dressings impregnated with saline (normal/hypertonic) or paraffin (incorporated with antiseptic or antibiotic) are generally in use. Although saline provides moisture, such a dressing adheres to the wound when the saline dries up and is traumatic to remove. Paraffin lowers the dressing adherence, but this property is lost if the dressing dries out. The hydrophobic nature of paraffin prevents absorption of moisture from the wound, and frequent dressing changes are usually needed with these types of dressing. Skin sensitization is also common in medicated types. Such dressings are mainly indicated for superficial clean wounds, and a secondary dressing may be needed.

Moisture and wound healing

One of the most significant ideas to change the nature of wound dressing materials has been the concept of moist wound healing. Moist wound healing refers to the provision and maintenance of optimal hydration of the exposed tissues in the wound as opposed to allowing or encouraging those tissues to dehydrate and dry out. The use of dressings that keep wound tissues moist has been associated with increased healing rates, improved cosmesis, reduced pain, reduced infection and reduced overall health care costs.

In cases where the wound is generating moderate to high levels of exudate, an absorbent dressing is needed. Absorbent dressings are those types that have a high capacity for capturing and holding fluid. They will require fewer dressing changes within a set period as opposed to dressings that are not as absorbent (e.g. gauze) and therefore enable undisturbed wound healing and less labour time on the part of the nurse or caregiver. Foams and calcium alginate dressings are both excellent examples of such types of dressing. In such wounds it is also important that culture and sensitivity should be performed and systemic antibiotics may be required based on the report.

When wounds are already dehydrated and therefore covered by dry, dead tissues, these tissues need to be removed to allow the wound to heal optimally. When the amount of dead tissue is not significant or when the patient is not a candidate for surgical debridement, the healthcare professional may opt for autolytic debridement. Autolytic debridement is the slow digestion of the dead cells by endogenous phagocytes and enzymes, and maintaining a moist local wound environment facilitates this process. An example of such dressings is hydrogel. The gel can cause maceration and is not to be applied to the periwound skin. Applying an amorphous hydrogel facilitates autolytic debridement of the devitalized tissue.

Type of dressing for malodorous wounds

These dressings are used in cases of fungating, infected, and gangrenous wounds, where malodour is a particular problem. They usually contain charcoal and should not be cut into because the charcoal fibres may shed into the wound, e.g. Clinisorb, Actisorb.

Antimicrobial dressings

Dressings that contain and release antimicrobial agents at the wound surface are available in the market. These dressings usually provide a continuous or sustained release of the antiseptic agent at the wound surface to provide a long-lasting antimicrobial action in combination with maintenance of a physiologically moist environment for healing. Iodine and silver have been incorporated into a wide variety of semiocclusive dressing formats such as foams, hydrocolloids, alginates, and hydrofibres.

Wound cleansers

Soaps and detergents cleanse wounds by breaking the bonds between the tissue and particles of dirt, bacteria, and other foreign material. These substances reduce the interfacial tension and hold the insoluble foreign matter in suspension so that it can be rinsed out of the wound. Compounds having this property are also called surface-active agents or surfactants.

Methods of wound cover

Wound cover can be provided in many different ways and these can be classified on the basis of their origin, as follows:

Skin cover from patient

- One of the types of primary or secondary healing discussed above
- Autografts:
  - ◆ Split-thickness skin graft
  - ◆ Full-thickness skin graft
- Combined skin and fascia: fasciocutaneous flaps—local or distant
- Combined skin, fascia, and muscle: musculocutaneous flaps—free or pedicled

Skin cover substitutes

These methods of skin cover act as biological dressings and only help to tide over a period until more skin from the same individual is available for harvesting:

- **Allografts** or **homografts**—from another individual of the same species
- **Xenografts** or **heterografts**—from another species like porcine grafts etc.

Both allografts and xenografts are biological dressings only, are ultimately rejected by the patient's immune system, and need to be removed prior to definitive wound treatment or skin grafting. While xenografts are rejected before undergoing revascularization, allografts initially undergo revascularization but are typically rejected after approximately 10 days because of the strong antigenicity of skin. One notable exception occurs in immunocompromised patients, such as burn patients, whose rejection of allografts may be delayed up to several weeks. Xenogeneic tissue such as porcine xenograft can be used as a temporary dressing for clean partial thickness wounds and has been shown to assist in re-epithelialization of large defects such as major burns by stimulating granulation tissue formation.

Cultured skin grafts

The patient's own epithelial cells may be harvested and grown in culture for use as a larger epidermal autograft, in a technique that has been applied for over 20 years. These autografts address the epidermal layer only and are typically quite thin. Cultured epidermal autografts (CEAs) such as Epicel (Genzyme Biosurgery) and Laserskin (Fidia Advanced Biopolymers) use a biopsy from the patient that is expanded via culture techniques in the laboratory setting to produce a sheet of autogenous keratinocytes for grafting.

While CEAs can ideally provide coverage of a large surface area defect using a small amount of donor tissue, this type of skin substitute has been associated with high rates of infection and graft loss, confirming the importance of the dermal layer in skin grafting. Cultured skin substitute (CSS) is composed of a CEA combined with a cultured autologous dermal layer; therefore, it addresses both the dermal and epidermal skin layers. This provides a more biologically similar material for skin replacement.

Dermal substitutes

The production of an effective replacement material for the dermis has proved more challenging given the complexity of the dermal structure, although several materials have well-documented success in this area. Substitute materials are classified based on their epidermal, dermal, or composite structure, and are further categorized by composition as acellular or cellular, and living or non-living.

Acellular dermal allografts, such as **AlloDerm** (LifeCell), are composed of cadaveric dermis that serves as a scaffold for the ingrowth of recipient tissue. AlloDerm has been studied in the repair of skin defects but has been used in multiple other applications, including reconstruction of abdominal wall and coverage of implantable prostheses. Newer acellular dermal allografts include GraftJacket (Wright Medical Technologies Inc.), NeoForm (Mentor Corporation), and DermaMatrix (Synthes Inc.), which have been studied for applications such as lower extremity, craniofacial, and breast reconstruction.

Integra (Integra Life Sciences Corporation) is an acellular dermal regeneration template that became commercially available in 1996. It is a bilaminate membrane consisting of a porous collagen layer (dermal analogue) bonded to a thin silicone layer (temporary epidermis). The dermal layer becomes revascularized and populated by cells from the patient's own underlying tissue over 7–21 days. Once this process is complete, an ultrathin split-thickness skin graft must be placed over the new dermis after removal of the silicone layer from the new dermal layer. The ultrathin graft allows for faster healing of the skin graft donor site, as well.

These dermal substitutes have been extensively studied for coverage of partial and full-thickness defects and can be permanently incorporated into the patient's new skin layers without being rejected by the patient's immune system. They also carry the advantages of immediate availability, avoidance of the risks associated with cellular allogeneic materials, the use of thinner STSGs, reduced donor site morbidity, and improved overall STSG incorporation.

Biosynthetic dressings

Several synthetic skin substitutes have become available for temporary wound coverage in preparation for definitive wound coverage.

Biobrane (UDL Laboratories, Inc.) is a biosynthetic dressing composed of a silicone membrane (the epidermal layer) coated on one side with porcine collagen and imbedded with nylon mesh (the dermal layer). When used to cover partial-thickness wounds, the mesh adheres to the wound until healing occurs below. Biobrane should be removed from any full-thickness wound prior to skin grafting.

Cellular dermal allografts are composed of a collagen or polymer-based scaffold that is seeded with fibroblasts from a donor cadaver. These products, including ICX-SKN (Intercytex Ltd.), TransCyte, and Dermagraft, have reported use in coverage of partial- and full-thickness wounds.

TransCyte (Advanced Tissue Sciences, Inc.) is a nylon mesh incubated with human fibroblasts that provides a partial dermal matrix with an outer silicone layer as a temporary epidermis. It is indicated for use in deep partial or excised full-thickness wounds prior to autogenous skin graft placement. It must be removed or excised prior to grafting full-thickness wounds.

Dermagraft (Advanced Tissue Sciences, Inc.) consists of human neonatal fibroblasts cultured on Biobrane. The neonatal fibroblasts are seeded into the nylon mesh. Approximately 2 weeks after application, the silicone membrane is removed and the wound bed grafted with a STSG. Dermagraft is a dressing and does not provide full dermal scaffolding, thus requiring standard-thickness skin grafts.

Composite allografts are bilayer products such as Apligraf (Organogenesis, Inc.), which has a dermal component comprised of bovine collagen and neonatal fibroblasts combined with an epidermal layer formed by neonatal keratinocytes, and Orcel (Ortec International, Inc.), which consists of a bovine collagen sponge coated with neonatal allogeneic keratinocytes. As allogeneic material, however, they cannot be used as permanent skin substitutes, as they will be rejected by the patient's immune system. These materials have primarily been used in the treatment of chronic wounds and donor sites. They also have reported utility when used as an overlay dressing on split-thickness skin grafts to improve function and cosmesis.

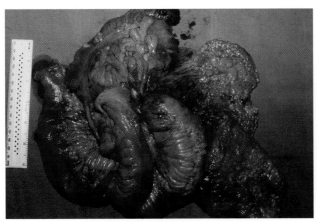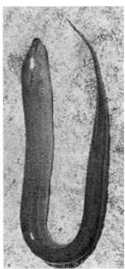

Plate 1 Also see Fig. 6.21.

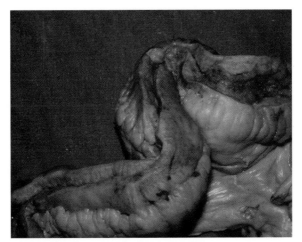

Plate 2 Also see Fig. 6.22.

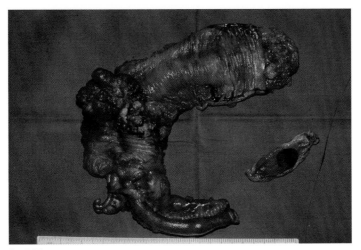

Plate 3 Also see Fig. 6.37.

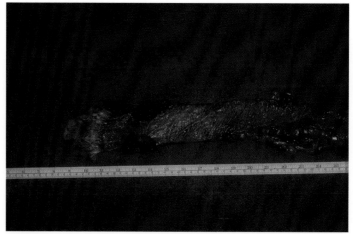

Plate 4 Also see Fig. 6.39.

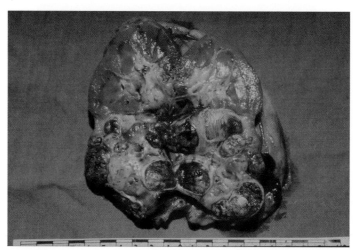

Plate 5 Also see Fig. 6.43.

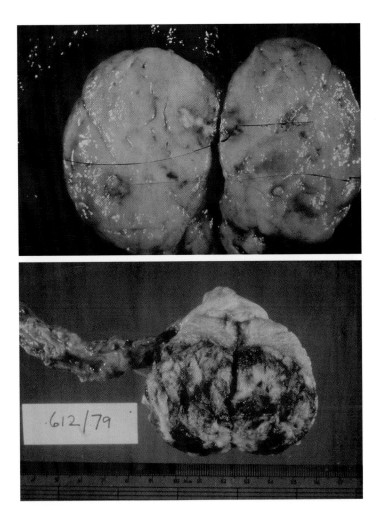

Plate 6 Also see Fig. 6.51.

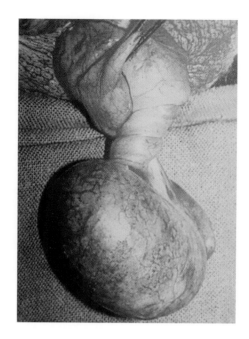

Plate 7 Also see Fig. 6.52.

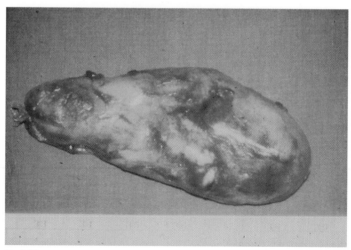

Plate 8 Also see Fig. 6.55.

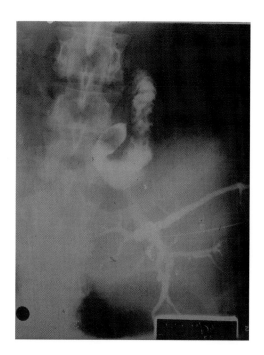

Plate 9 Also see Fig. 6.59.

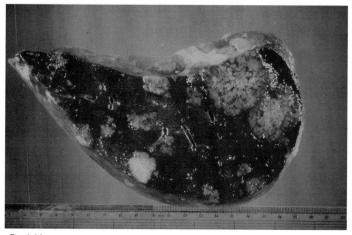

Plate 10 Also see Fig. 6.61.

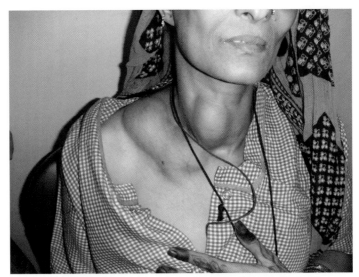

Plate 11 Photo courtesy of Mr Pradip Datta, taken with verbal consent. Also see Fig. 6.69.

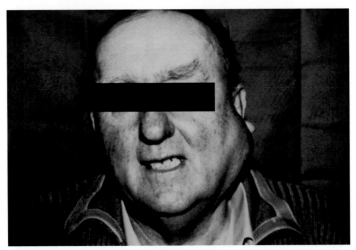

Plate 12 Photo courtesy of Mr Pradip Datta, taken with verbal consent. Also see Fig. 6.71.

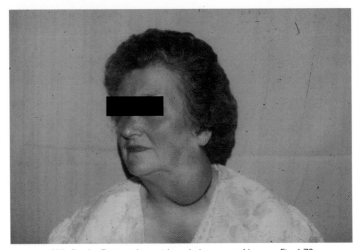

Plate 13 Photo courtesy of Mr Pradip Datta, taken with verbal consent. Also see Fig. 6.72.

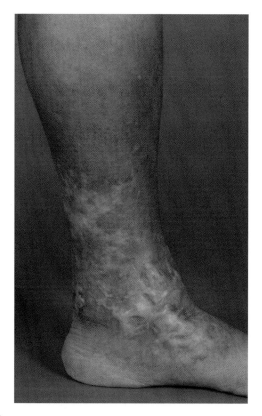

Plate 14 Also see Fig. 21.2.

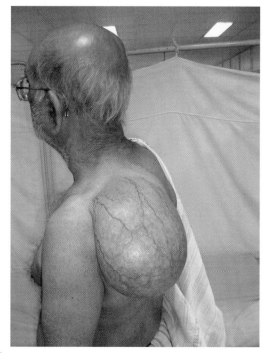

Plate 15 Also see Fig. 21.4.

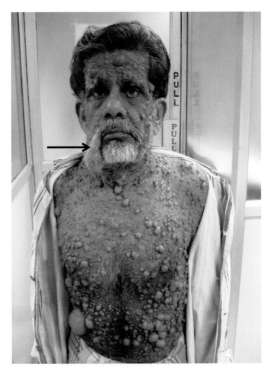

Plate 16 Also see Fig. 21.6.

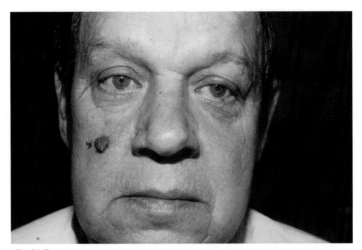

Plate 17 Also see Fig. 21.7.

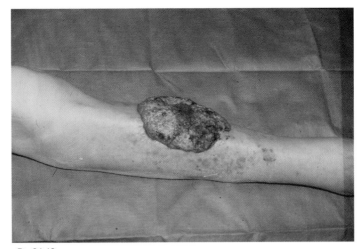

Plate 21 Also see Fig. 21.13.

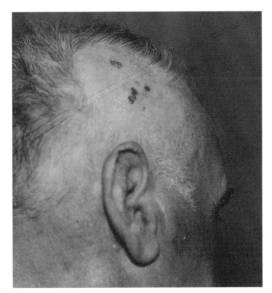

Plate 22 Also see Fig. 21.14.

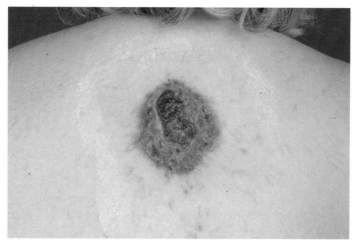

Plate 18 Also see Fig. 21.9.

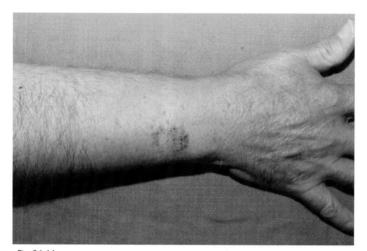

Plate 19 Also see Fig. 21.11.

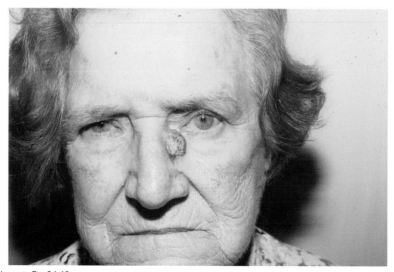

Plate 20 Also see Fig. 21.12.

Chapter 9 **Practical procedures**

Introduction

This chapter deals with routine procedures that a junior surgical trainee is expected to be able to undertake safely.

> The Clinical and Procedural Skills station tests both your ability to perform the task and your communication skills. You will likely be performing the task on a manikin but an actor will be present. You are expected to explain the procedure to the actor before you start and as you go along. Your aim here is to perform the procedure competently while ensuring that the 'patient' is comfortable and at ease throughout the procedure.

The scenarios and answers here act as a good guide to excelling in this station.

Airway and thoracic procedures

Relieving a tension pneumothorax—needle thoracocentesis and intercostal drain insertion

Tension pneumothorax is a life-threatening condition caused by air under tension within the pleural space, resulting in mediastinal displacement and cardiorespiratory compromise. This condition is discussed further in Chapter 20 on trauma. Here we will discuss the emergency procedures—needle thoracocentesis and insertion of an intercostal drain.

*Intercostal drains are also indicated in the following patients:

- Traumatic haemopneumothorax
- Pneumothorax in a ventilated patient
- Persistent/recurrent pneumothorax
- Large secondary spontaneous pneumothorax in patients >50 years
- Malignant pleural effusion
- Empyema/parapneumonic pleural effusion
- Post-thoracic surgery

Contraindications

There are relative contraindications to the procedure but tension pneumothorax is a life-threatening condition and failure to treat expectantly can result in patient death. Relative contraindications to this procedure include:

- Coagulopathy
- Previous pneumonectomy
- Underlying bullous disease
- Diaphragmatic hernia
- Cutaneous infection /disease at insertion site

Complications

- Misdiagnosis
- Misplacement
- Local haematoma
- Trauma to other structures—lung parenchyma, intercostal neurovascular bundle, heart, aorta, spleen, liver, diaphragm
- Haemathorax
- Wound infection
- Surgical emphysema

Cardiac- and vascular-related procedures

Intravenous cannulae insertion

An IV cannula is a small flexible plastic tube inserted into a patient's vein to allow the IV administration of fluids and medication. It is introduced with a trocar/needle which is removed after placement of the

Table 9.1 Different gauges of cannulae available

Colour	Gauge	Approximate max flow rate	Use
Blue	22G	1–2L/h	Small veins or in children (not for viscous fluids, e.g. blood)
Pink	20G	2–3L/h	For routine use—fluids, medications, and blood transfusion.
Green	18G	2–5L/h	For routine use—fluids, medications and blood transfusion
Grey	16G	7–11L/h	Used in theatres or emergency for rapid transfusion. Also used for peripheral administration of certain drugs (e.g. amiodarone, dopamine)
Orange/brown	14G	10–18L/h	

cannulae. There are different sizes/gauges of cannulae available (Table 9.1). Larger-bore cannulae have a faster flow rate (as per Poiseuille's law).

You can also take blood from the cannula. This should be done immediately after insertion while the tourniquet is still on.

Contraindications

It is advisable to avoid certain sites:

- Ipsilateral mastectomy/axillary node clearance
- Arteriovenous (AV) fistula (ask the patient or feel for a thrill if you have doubt)
- Overlying cellulitis/infection/burns/trauma
- Ipsilateral lymphoedema

Complications

Insertion of an IV cannula is a very common and safe procedure. Potential complications include:

- Bruising/haematoma
- Infection at entry site
- Phlebitis/thrombophlebitis
- Extravasation of infusion into tissue

Venous cutdown

Venous cutdown is an emergency procedure where a peripheral vein is surgically exposed and an IV cannula inserted under direct vision. It is used in patients in extremis to gain vascular access when IV cannulation is difficult or impossible, e.g. burns, trauma, hypovolaemic shock. The long saphenous vein is commonly used but the antecubital and femoral veins are also potential sites.

Contraindications

This is an emergency procedure. Relative contraindications include:

- Cellulitic or other cutaneous infections/disease
- Venous thrombosis
- Coagulopathy

Complications

- Cellulitis/phlebitis
- Haematoma
- Venous thrombosis
- Perforation of the posterior wall of the vein
- Injury to nearby structures—nerve or arterial transaction

Central venous catheter (CVC) insertion

A CVC is a tube which is inserted into a large vein in the neck, chest, or groin and can be used to directly measure central venous pressure. It is also used to obtain blood samples (including for mixed venous saturations), to administer drugs, fluids, or parenteral nutrition, for haemofiltration and for vascular access if a peripheral site is unavailable or unsuitable.

Contraindications

Most of these are relative contraindications which can be corrected or overcome by choosing an alternative site:

- Cutaneous infection/disease at insertion site
- Coagulopathy—reverse pre-procedure
- Distortion of anatomical landmarks, e.g. ipsilateral trauma
- Contralateral pneumothorax or haemothorax
- Uncooperative patient or patient unable to tolerate Trendelenburg position
- Patient receiving ventilator support with high positive end-expiratory pressure (PEEP)

Complications

CVC insertion is associated with the following potential complications:

- Damage to nearby structures—arterial puncture, pneumothorax, haemothorax, chylothorax, brachial plexus injury, arrhythmias
- Air embolism—maintain a Trendelenburg position
- Sepsis/phlebitis/cellulitis
- Thromboembolism
- Loss of guidewire into right atrium—keep hold of guidewire throughout procedure.

Arterial puncture and arterial cannulation

Arterial blood analysis is used to evaluate oxygen and carbon dioxide gas exchange and acid–base analysis. Arterial blood can be obtained via a direct arterial puncture or, if multiple samples are required, by inserting an indwelling arterial cannula. Indwelling arterial cannulae also provide dynamic measurement of arterial blood pressure. The radial artery is most often used but alternatives include the femoral, brachial, ulnar, or dorsalis pedis arteries. It is important to ensure good collateral circulation as there is a theoretical risk of thrombus occlusion.

For the radial artery, the collateral circulation can be assessed with Allen's test.

Allen's test—with the patient's hand elevated, apply pressure over both the ulnar and radial arteries and ask the patient to make a fist for 30 seconds. Then ask the patient to open their fist—their palm should appear blanched. While maintaining radial pressure, release the pressure over the ulnar artery, if colour returns within 7 seconds, there is an adequate collateral circulation and it is safe to proceed with arterial puncture or cannulation.

Contraindications

- Cutaneous infection/disease at insertion site—find alternative site
- Coagulopathy—reverse pre-procedure
- Insufficient collateral circulation—find an alternative site
- Proximal vascular trauma/surgery/AV shunt—find alternative site

Complications

- Infection
- Haematoma/bleeding
- Arterial occlusion/thrombosis—rarely leads to digital ischaemia
- Arterial vasospasm/vascular disease—making procedure difficult
- Rare—AV fistula formation, aneurysm, or pseudo-aneurysm formation
- For arterial cannulation:
  - ◆ Air embolism
  - ◆ Accidental administration of intra-arterial drugs–**ensure the line is appropriately labelled to avoid misidentification**
  - ◆ Kinking, blockage, or accidental decannulation of the catheter

Abdominal- and gastrointestinal-related procedures

Nasogastric (NG) tube insertion

A NG tube is a narrow-bore tube inserted through the nose into the stomach. It can be used for aspiration of stomach contents or for short- or medium-term feeding. There are basically two types of NG tubes:

- Polyvinyl chloride (PVC) tubes:
  - ◆ Usually wide-bore tubes
  - ◆ Used for aspiration of stomach contents (air, gastric secretions, bile, blood, partially digested food)
  - ◆ For short-term use (<2 weeks) as can be degraded by gastric acid
- Polyurethane (PUR) or silicone tubes:
  - ◆ Usually narrow-bore (<9F gauge) tubes—more comfortable, better tolerated by the patient
  - ◆ Used for short- or medium-term feeding up to 6 weeks—not affected by gastric acid
  - ◆ Administration of medication

Different lengths are available for adult and paediatric patients.

Contraindications

NG tubes are contraindicated or should be used with extreme caution in the following groups. Patients with:

- Maxillofacial (especially nasal) disorders, fractures, or surgery—risk of passing through the cribriform plate, resulting in intracranial penetration. In this instance, an orogastric tube may be a better alternative
- Oropharyngeal disorders, tumours, strictures, or previous surgery
- Previous laryngectomies
- Oesophageal disorders, surgery, tumours, or varices
- Base of skull fractures
- Cervical spine injuries especially C1–4—coughing or gagging during insertion may potentiate cervical injury. If NG tube has to be inserted, ensure manual stabilization of the patient's head is in place before starting

Complications

NG tube insertion is generally a safe and common procedure. However, there are a number of potential complications associated with this procedure:

- Aspiration and aspiration pneumonia (always have suction with you during the procedure)
- Discomfort/sore throat
- Nasal irritation, epistaxis
- Retro- or nasopharyngeal necrosis (rare)
- Oesophageal or stomach perforation (rare)

Proctoscopy and rigid sigmoidoscopy

Proctoscopy and rigid sigmoidoscopy are endoscopic investigations which allow direct visualization of the anal canal (with a proctoscope) or rectum up to the rectosigmoid junction (with a rigid sigmoidoscope). It is performed as part of the investigation of lower GI complaints particularly rectal bleeding and change in bowel habit. These procedures are often performed in an outpatient or ward setting and are both diagnostic (direct endoscopic visualization, access for biopsy, assess position of anorectal pathology) and therapeutic (treatment for haemorrhoids, sigmoid volvulus). It should routinely be performed prior to anorectal surgical procedures.

*Ensure you revise the anatomy of the rectum prior to performing this procedure

Contraindications

- Haemodynamically unstable patient
- Inflammation of the bowel—fulminant colitis, acute diverticulitis
- Peritonitic or suspicion of bowel perforation
- Anal stenosis or recent anorectal surgery, e.g. low anterior resection

Complications

- Uncomfortable—not usually painful. In patients with painful anorectal conditions, such as anal fissure, this examination should only be performed when the patient is anaesthetized
- Perforation
- Bleeding—especially with biopsies or therapeutic procedures. Check and correct coagulation as necessary
- Infection

Ascitic tap and drainage (paracentesis)

This procedure involves the insertion of a needle or a catheter into the peritoneal cavity to obtain ascitic fluid for diagnostic or therapeutic purposes. The fluid can then be sent for analysis to determine its aetiology. Ascitic fluid can be classified according to its serum-ascitic albumin gradient (SAAG). This is detailed further in Table 9.2.

In addition, in patients with a known aetiology, paracentesis may be carried out in patients with suspected bacterial peritonitis and to relieve symptoms in patients with massive ascites resulting in abdominal distension (therapeutic paracentesis).

Contraindications

- Coagulopathy—reverse pre-procedure
- Severely distended loops of bowel
- Pregnancy
- Abdominal wall cellulitis

Complications

Paracentesis is a safe procedure with a <1% complication rate. Potential complications include:

- Perforation of bowel or a visceral organ (liver, spleen)
  - If on aspiration the fluid is faeculent, withdraw the needle and choose another site. The patient will need to be observed for 24–48 hours for the development of peritonitis
- Bleeding /haematoma—avoid blood vessels and correct any coagulopathy pre-procedure
- Infection
- Hypovolaemia

Table 9.2 Serum-ascitic albumin gradient (SAAG) of ascitic fluid

SAAG >1.1g/dl (portal hypertension) Transudate albumin <30g/L	SAAG <1.1g/dl Exudate albumin >30g/L
Cirrhosis/alcoholic hepatitis	Peritonitis/intra-abdominal inflammation, e.g. pancreatitis, TB
Hepatic failure	Intra-abdominal/peritoneal malignancy
Portal venous thrombosis	Ischaemic/obstructed bowel
Cardiac failure	Nephrotic syndrome

Other procedures

Urinary catheterization

A urinary catheter is a tube that is inserted into the bladder to help drain urine. It may be used temporarily (e.g. patients with acute urinary retention, post-operative patients) or long term (patients with neurogenic bladder disorders such as multiple sclerosis).

There are basically three types of urinary catheters:

- Indwelling catheter (Foley)—inflatable balloon which sits in the bladder to help keep it in place. There are several subtypes with different shaped tips (Coudé or Council tip catheters) or number of ports (two-way or three-way catheters)
- Catheters for intermittent self-catheterization (no inflatable balloon)
- External/condom catheters—for incontinence in men

Here we will be discussing the insertion of Foley/indwelling catheters. These catheters are described in French (F) units and are usually between 10F and 28F (1F = 0.33mm). They can be inserted per urethram or suprapubically and may be made out of:

- Silicone latex (*check for latex allergy)—soft, usually for short-term use
- Silastic (plastic and silicone)—firmer, usually for longer-term use

Catheters may be coated with silver alloy or antibiotics to reduce infections.

Three-way catheters are larger-gauged catheters and, in addition to the two ports used for urine drainage and balloon insufflation, have an extra port which is used for irrigation. These catheters are often used in patients with haematuria to prevent clot retention.

Suprapubic catheters are used in patients when urethral catheterization is contraindicated or unsuccessful, patients with neurological conditions requiring long-term urine drainage, and, often as a last resort, in patients with incontinence.

Contraindications

Urethral catheterization is contraindicated or should be used with extreme caution in the presence of:

- Urethral trauma
- Urethral obstruction—urethral stricture, bladder neck mass
- Urethral surgery/reconstruction
- Ongoing urinary tract infection—if necessary, consider catheterizing under antibiotic cover

Suprapubic catheterization is contraindicated when:

- Bladder is undetectable clinically or ultrasonographically
- Previous lower abdominal or pelvic surgery, cancer, or radiation (at risk of adhesions)

Complications

Urinary catheterization is a common and safe procedure. However, there are a number of potential complications related to it as listed below:

- Trauma—haematuria, creating a false passage, scarring, and stricture formation
- Urinary tract infection—common
- Latex allergy (always check)
- Catheter obstruction—check for patency by flushing catheter
- Discomfort due to bladder spasm

In addition, insertion of suprapubic catheters may also be complicated by the following:

- Bowel perforation
- Entry site infection
- Entry site bleeding—check for bleeding diathesis and correct pre-procedure

Obtaining a biopsy

Taking a biopsy involves the removal of tissue for histological and/or chemical analysis by a pathologist to determine the presence or the extent of disease. There are a number of different biopsy techniques which include:

- Fine-needle aspiration cytology (FNAC):
  - ◆ Involves inserting a fine-bore needle percutaneously into a lesion to obtain cells which are then smeared and fixed onto a slide (hence technically not a biopsy as no information about tissue architecture is obtained from the cytological sample)
  - ◆ May be performed under radiological guidance
  - ◆ Often used for neck, breast, or liver lesions
- Brush cytology:
  - ◆ Involves using a special brush to collect exfoliated cells from intraluminal lesions which are then smeared and fixed onto a slide (hence technically not a biopsy as no information about tissue architecture is obtained from the cytological sample)
  - ◆ Often performed under endoscopic guidance
  - ◆ Often used for GI, bronchial, or biliopancreatic lesions
- Core biopsy:
  - ◆ Involves using a hollow needle to retrieve a core of tissue
  - ◆ May be performed under radiological guidance
- Incision biopsy (surgical biopsy):
  - ◆ Involves removal of part of a lesion for histological analysis
  - ◆ Used when a lesion is unsuitable for excision biopsy, i.e. large lesion, involves important structures
  - ◆ May be performed laparoscopically
- Excision biopsy (surgical biopsy):
  - ◆ Involves removal of an entire lesion for histological analysis
  - ◆ Often used for skin lesions—ideal for suspected melanomas
- Other methods—shave, punch, curettage:
  - ◆ Usually used for skin lesions

Complications

- Bleeding
- Insufficient sample
- False negatives or positives
- Potential spread of malignant cells

Scenarios

Scenario 1

Needle thoracocentesis

Mr Wyeth is a 35-year-old builder who has been brought in by ambulance after a 40-foot fall on a construction site. He is very agitated, dyspnoeic, tachypnoeic, tachycardic, and has tracheal deviation to the right with diminished breath sounds and hyper-resonance on the left side of his chest. You suspect a left tension pneumothorax. Demonstrate how you would proceed. Assume immediate ATLS assessment and management has already been instituted.

(This is a clinical diagnosis; do not request a CXR to confirm diagnosis.)

Scenario 2

Insertion of an intercostal drain

Mr Wyeth is a 35-year-old builder who has been brought in by ambulance after a 40-foot fall on a construction site. He is very agitated, dyspnoeic, tachypnoeic, and tachycardic with diminished breath sounds and hyper-resonance on the left side of his chest. The paramedics suspected a left-sided tension pneumothorax and performed needle thoracocentesis at the scene. You have been asked by the A&E consultant to insert a left-sided intercostal drain. Demonstrate how you would proceed. Assume immediate ATLS assessment and management has already been instituted.

(This is a clinical diagnosis; do not request a CXR to confirm diagnosis.)

Scenario 3

Insertion of an IV cannula

Ms Wright is a 36-year-old patient who has been admitted with infected hydronephrosis. The urology registrar has discussed the diagnosis with her. She needs to be commenced on IV antibiotics and the nurse has asked you to insert an IV cannula. Please demonstrate how you would proceed.

Scenario 4

Venous cutdown

You have been called to A&E for a trauma call. A young female patient, Jane Doe, has been involved in a RTA. She is maintaining her airway with an oropharyngeal tube and is tachypnoeic, tachycardic, hypotensive, with a GCS of 8/15. The anaesthetic registrar is preparing to perform an endotracheal intubation. Multiple attempts to gain venous access have failed. The patient is becoming progressively more hypotensive. You are asked to perform a venous cutdown. Please demonstrate how you would proceed.

Scenario 5

Insertion of a central venous catheter

Mr Ling is a 74-year-old gentleman who has been admitted to HDU after an emergency laparotomy and Hartmann's procedure for a diverticular perforation the day before. Over the past 4 hours he has been hypotensive despite IV fluid boluses. The HDU team feel Mr Ling would benefit from inotropic support. However, the ITU registrar has been called urgently to an ENT ward and the ITU FY2 contacts you to ask if you would mind inserting a CVC in this patient. Please demonstrate how you would proceed. The FY2 (examiner) will act as your assistant, if required.

Scenario 6

Arterial puncture

You have just been contacted by the ENT ward to review Mrs Albrecht, an 84-year-old lady, who is dyspnoeic, tachypnoeic and tachycardic 2 days post-partial laryngectomy for a supraglottic squamous cell carcinoma. Your initial assessment suggests that she may have pulmonary oedema secondary to fluid overload. You institute emergency management, send off venous blood for analysis, arrange a CXR, and would like to perform an arterial puncture for arterial blood gas analysis. Demonstrate how you would proceed.

Your instruction states that this patient has had a partial laryngectomy, hence she will not be able to communicate verbally. Be mindful of this and pay extra attention to her non-verbal cues including lip reading if possible and written communication with a notepad and pen. Be sure not to rush her and to give her enough time to ask questions and state her concerns

Scenario 7

Arterial cannulation

A 74-year-old gentleman has been admitted to ITU after an emergency abdominal aortic aneurysm repair. He is currently intubated, sedated, and is on inotropic support. He has an arterial line which was inserted in A&E when he presented as an emergency. As this was an 'unclean' emergency procedure, the ITU nursing staff have asked you to insert a new arterial cannula. Please demonstrate how you would proceed.

Scenario 8

Insertion of nasogastric tube

Mr Smith is a 76-year-old gentleman who has presented with profuse vomiting and abdominal distension.
You suspect he has small bowel obstruction and plan to insert a NG tube to decompress his stomach. Please demonstrate how you would proceed.

Scenario 9

Proctoscopy and sigmoidoscopy

You have just reviewed Mr Alphonso, a 55-year-old gentleman in outpatient clinic who has been referred by his GP with a 2-month history of painless fresh red PR bleeding and constipation. You have completed your history and examination and now would like to perform proctoscopy and rigid sigmoidoscopy to complete your evaluation. Please demonstrate how you would proceed.

Scenario 10

Ascitic tap

Mrs Jaafar is a 56-year-old woman who has presented via A&E with abdominal distension. Ultrasonography revealed the presence of ascites and these findings have been conveyed to the patient. However, the cause of the ascites is uncertain and you need to perform an ascitic tap for diagnosis. The ultrasonographer has marked an appropriate site for paracentesis. Please demonstrate how you would proceed.

Scenario 11

Therapeutic paracentesis

Mrs Jaafar is a 56-year-old patient who has recently been diagnosed with gastric cancer with peritoneal and liver metastases. She is aware of the diagnosis. Her recent staging CT, 2 days prior, demonstrated the presence of ascites. She now presents with shortness of breath, an uncomfortable tense, distended abdomen and clinical findings consistent with gross ascites. This patient needs a therapeutic paracentesis. Please demonstrate how you would proceed.

Scenario 12

Insertion of a urethral catheter

Mr Wong, a 75-year-old gentleman who suffers with benign prostatic hypertrophy, has been admitted with suprapubic pain and difficulty passing urine for the past 18 hours. On examination, he has a palpable bladder. You suspect he is in acute urinary retention. You discuss this with him and plan to insert a urinary catheter. Please demonstrate how you would proceed.

Scenario 13

Insertion of a suprapubic catheter

Mr Wong is a 75-year-old gentleman who suffers with benign prostatic hypertrophy and is known to have a urethral stricture. He presents to hospital in acute urinary retention and attempts at urethral catheterization by the Urology Registrar have been unsuccessful. It is decided that he needs a suprapubic catheter inserted and the Urology Registrar asks you to perform this procedure. Please demonstrate how you would proceed. You have a nurse (examiner) with you to help if needed.

Scenario 14

Obtaining a core biopsy of a breast lesion

Mrs Higgins is a 42-year-old lady who presents with a breast lump to the one-stop clinic. She has been seen by your consultant who asks you to perform a core biopsy of the lesion in the upper outer quadrant of Mrs Higgins' left breast. Please demonstrate how you would proceed. You have a nurse (examiner) with you to help if needed.

*Always ensure you have a chaperone

Answers

Scenario 1

- Introduction—this is an emergency. A brief introduction and explanation of procedure is sufficient:

  Hello Mr Wyeth. My name is Mr Peterson. I am one of the surgical doctors. I need to insert a small tube into the front of your chest to help you breathe better.

- Prepare your equipment:
  - ◆ Dressing pack
  - ◆ Antiseptic solution, e.g. Betadine
  - ◆ Large-bore IV cannula (14G or 16G)
  - ◆ Tape
- Prepare your patient:
  - ◆ Ensure patient is on high-flow oxygen or ventilated if necessary with continual monitoring of vital signs
  - ◆ Clinically confirm the side of the tension pneumothorax
  - ◆ If a cervical spine injury has not been excluded, keep patient in supine position with cervical spine protection (otherwise, an upright position is also appropriate)
- Prepare yourself:
  - ◆ Wash your hands
  - ◆ Put on your apron and gloves
- Insert cannula:
  - ◆ Identify the anatomical landmarks—ipsilateral 2nd intercostal space, immediately superior to the 3rd rib (to avoid injury to the neurovascular bundle) in the midclavicular line (to avoid injury to the internal thoracic artery)
  - ◆ Warn the patient you are about to start
  - ◆ Insert the cannula perpendicular to the chest wall. Continue advancing until you puncture the pleura (you feel a 'give')
  - ◆ Remove the needle, keeping the cannula in place—you will hear a hissing sound as air escapes
- Secure the cannula and tidy up:
  - ◆ Secure the cannula with a dressing at the insertion site
  - ◆ Clear your equipment
  - ◆ Wash your hands

*Needle thoracocentesis can help arrest the progression of a tension pneumothorax and may help improve cardiorespiratory function slightly but this is not the definitive treatment—this patient will need an ipsilateral intercostal drain inserted.

Scenario 2

- Introduction—this is an emergency. A brief introduction and explanation of procedure is sufficient:

  Hello Mr Wyeth. My name is Mr Peterson. I am one of the surgical doctors. I need to insert a tube into the side of your chest to help you breathe better.

- Prepare your equipment:
  - ◆ Local anaesthetic, e.g. 10ml 1% lignocaine (with adrenaline if available)
  - ◆ 10-ml syringe
  - ◆ 21G (green) and 25G (blue) needles
  - ◆ Sterile gloves and apron
  - ◆ Sterile drapes
  - ◆ Antiseptic solution, e.g. Betadine
  - ◆ Dressing, Sleek, and Tegaderm
  - ◆ Cotton gauze swabs
  - ◆ Scalpel and blade
  - ◆ Suture, e.g. 1/0 silk; instrument for blunt dissection, e.g. a curved clamp
  - ◆ Intercostal tube—a large tube, ideally between 26–32F
  - ◆ Connection tubing and connectors
  - ◆ Sealed underwater drainage system with 500ml of sterile water
  - ◆ Suction available
- Prepare your patient:
  - ◆ Ensure patient is on high-flow oxygen or ventilated if necessary with continual monitoring of vital signs
  - ◆ Clinically confirm the side of the tension pneumothorax
  - ◆ Patient in a supine patient with ipsilateral axillary area exposed (arm abducted or behind patient's head)
- Prepare yourself:
  - ◆ Wash your hands
  - ◆ Put on your gloves and gown

- Prepare the area:
  - ◆ Identify the anatomical landmark—aim for 5th intercostal space in the mid-axillary line. Safe triangle—bounded by the anterior border of latissimus dorsi, the lateral border of pectoralis major, a horizontal line through the level of the nipple with the apex below the axilla (see Fig. 9.1)
  - ◆ Clean the skin around the site with Betadine and apply sterile drapes
  - ◆ Inject local anaesthetic—initially create a subcutaneous bleb with the 25G needle, then switch to the 21G needle and anaesthetize the deeper structures, including the rib periosteum and pleura. Remember to withdraw gently before injecting to avoid injecting into any vascular structures
  - ◆ Allow the local anaesthetic a few minutes to work, then make a 2-cm incision just above and parallel to the 6th rib with your scalpel
- Insertion of intercostal drain:
  - ◆ Insert the curved clamp into the incision, walk off the top of the 6th rib, opening the clamp to spread the muscle fibres. Continue down to the pleura—once you puncture the parietal pleura you will hear a hissing sound as air escapes
  - ◆ Explore the pleural space with a finger—ensuring that there are no underlying organs which may be injured at tube insertion and to clear and adhesions
  - ◆ Using the curved clamp as a guide, advance the drain tube into the pleural space, aiming apically (basally for fluid)
  - ◆ Look for fogging of the chest tube with expiration
- Secure the tube and check tube position:
  - ◆ Connect the end of the tube to the sealed underwater drainage system. Check for bubbling of water suggesting air drainage form the pleural space
    *Do not clamp a chest drain inserted for a pneumothorax. Always keep the drainage bottle below the level of the patient's chest.
  - ◆ Secure the tube in place with sutures. Apply a dressing and tape the tube to the chest wall
  - ◆ Obtain a CXR to ensure appropriate placement of the tube and reinflation of the lung
- Tidy up:
  - ◆ Clear your equipment
  - ◆ Wash your hands
- Document the procedure in the patient's notes

Scenario 3

- Introduction:
  - ◆ Introduce yourself to the patient
  - ◆ Check the patient's details against their ID bracelet
  - ◆ Explain the procedure, the reason it is needed, risks to the patient, and gain consent (verbal consent is usually sufficient)

  Hello, Ms Wright. My name is Mr. Peterson. I am one of the ST1 surgical trainees. Before I continue can you confirm your name and date of birth for me? Thank you. As the registrar explained to you earlier, we believe you have an infection of the kidney and we need to start you on antibiotics.

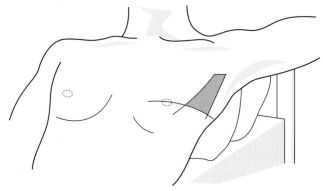

Figure 9.1 Safe triangle for intercostal drain insertion. From *Oxford Handbook of Clinical Medicine* 7 edn., Longmore et al., (2007) with permission from Oxford University Press.

For us to administer the antibiotics directly into your veins, I need to insert a cannula, which is a plastic tube, into your veins. There is a needle at the end of the tube, so you will feel a sharp pinprick as it is being inserted. We then remove the needle and secure the tube down with a dressing. It is a fairly short procedure and we perform it under clean conditions to minimize the risk of infections. Are you happy for me to proceed?

- Prepare your equipment:
  - Tourniquet
  - Alcohol swab
  - Gloves and apron
  - Cannula of appropriate size (18G or 20G)
  - Sharps bin
  - 10-ml syringe with 0.9% sodium chloride flush
  - Cannula dressing
  - Tape and cotton wool ball (in case of unsuccessful insertion)
  - Local anaesthetic cream (for phobic patients or children)
- Prepare the patient:
  - Choose an appropriate site—usually the upper limb (avoid joint flexures and dominant arm where possible). Place an absorbent layer under the arm in case of spillages. A cannula can be inserted into any superficial vein—usually in the limbs
  - Patient can be either lying down (prevents faints) or sat up in a chair
  - Apply tourniquet 5–8cm above intended insertion site
  - Rest the arm below the level of the heart and ask patient to clench and unclench their fist—feel for a palpable vein
  - Disinfect skin with the alcohol wipe. Do not re-palpate
- Prepare yourself:
  - Wash your hands
  - Put on your apron and gloves
- Insert cannula:
  - Apply traction around the skin of the chosen site
  - Warn the patient to expect a sharp scratch
  - Insert cannula—bevel up, at a 15–30° angle to the skin
  - When you see blood in the flashback chamber, advance a further 2–3mm
  - Then fix the needle and advance the cannula until it is fully inserted
  - Release the tourniquet
  - Apply digital pressure to the vein at the tip of the cannula and remove the needle completely. Dispose of it immediately in a sharps bin
- Secure the cannula:
  - Apply a cap to the hub of the cannula and release digital pressure
  - Apply a sterile, transparent, semi-permeable dressing to secure it in place
- Check position:
  - Flush the cannula with 10ml of 0.9% sodium chloride—ensure good flow. If there is a swelling or the patient complains of discomfort, the cannula has been incorrectly sited and must be removed
- Tidy up:
  - Wash hands
  - Clear your equipment
- Document procedure and planned date of change (usually 3–5 days)

Scenario 4

- Explaining the procedure in this instance is inappropriate as this is an emergency procedure in a patient who lacks the capacity to consent
- Prepare your equipment:
  - Antiseptic solution, e.g. Betadine
  - Sterile drapes
  - Sterile gloves and gown
  - Local anaesthetic, e.g. 10ml 1% lignocaine
  - 10-ml syringe and 25G needle

- ◆ Scalpel and blade
- ◆ 2 × curved mosquito haemostats/artery forceps
- ◆ Appropriate size IV cannula—18G or 16G
- ◆ Tie, e.g. 2/0 Vicryl
- ◆ Suture, e.g. 3/0 silk suture on a hand-held needle
- ◆ Tourniquet
- ◆ Appropriate resuscitative IV fluid, tubing, and connectors
- ◆ Dressing pack with scissors
- Prepare the patient:
  - ◆ Patient in supine position with the lower limb on the side concerned externally rotated slightly, if able
  - ◆ Tourniquet on proximal leg
- Prepare yourself:
  - ◆ Wash your hands
  - ◆ Put on sterile gloves and gown
- Prepare the area:
  - ◆ Identify anatomical landmarks of the long saphenous vein— 2cm anterior and superior to medial malleolus
  - ◆ Clean the area with antiseptic solution and drape with sterile drapes
  - ◆ Infiltrate the skin and subcutaneous tissue with local anaesthetic. Remember to withdraw gently before injecting to avoid injecting into any vascular structures
- Perform the cut down and cannulation:
  - ◆ Make a 2.5-cm full thickness transverse incision with the scalpel
  - ◆ Using the curved haemostats, the tissue planes are carefully dissected until the vein is identified and freed from surrounding structures for approximately a 2-cm length
    *The saphenous nerve is intimately associated with the vein—so use care when dissecting.
  - ◆ Pass a tie around the distal end of the exposed vein and ligate it. Leave the cut ends long for traction
  - ◆ Pass a tie around the proximal end of the exposed vein
  - ◆ With some traction, make a small transverse venotomy. Gently dilate the venotomy with the tip of the closed haemostat
  - ◆ Release the tourniquet
  - ◆ Introduce the cannula into the vein and advance it as far as possible to prevent dislodging
- Secure the tube:
  - ◆ Secure the cannula in place by tying the proximal ligature around the vein and cannula. Cut the long ends of the ligated ties
  - ◆ Connect the prepared IV fluid and tubing to the cannula—check for free flow of fluid through the cannula
  - ◆ Check for haemostasis and close the skin wound with sutures
  - ◆ Apply some antiseptic solution over the suture line and apply a dressing over the area
- Tidy up:
  - ◆ Wash your hands
  - ◆ Clear your equipment
- Document procedure and indication in the notes

Scenario 5

- Introduction:
  - ◆ Introduce yourself to the patient
  - ◆ Check the patient's details against their ID bracelet
  - ◆ Explain the procedure, the reason it is needed, risks to the patient, and gain consent (usually verbal consent is sufficient)

    Hello, Mr. Ling. My name is Mr. Peterson. I am one of the ST1 surgical trainees. Before I continue can you confirm your name and date of birth for me? Thank you. I have been contacted by the ITU team to insert a tube into one of the veins in your neck. Your blood pressure has been quite low the past few hours and we need to use this tube to give you some medication which will help maintain your blood pressure.

    This procedure usually lasts about 10 minutes and we will give you some local anaesthetic before we start. You will be lying at a tilt with your hand down for the entire procedure. It is a safe procedure but there is a risk of injury to the nearby structures including nerves, arteries, your heart or your lung. If we do cause a small hole in the lining of the lung we will need to insert a drain into your chest which will help drain the air or blood out. We will assess the tube daily and remove it after a few days to minimize the risk of infections. Are you happy for me to proceed?

- Prepare your equipment (take time to lay your equipment out):
  - Ultrasound probe (for internal jugular and femoral vein insertion)—with sterile bag over probe. Bag should be well filled with aqueous jelly. Also apply sterile jelly to the outside of bag before starting
  - Three- or four-lumen central venous catheter pack with three-way taps for each lumen
  - Local anaesthetic, e.g. 10ml of 1% lignocaine
  - 10-ml syringe, 21G (green) and 25G (blue) needles
  - 20-ml syringe
  - 20ml sodium chloride
  - 2/0 silk on a hand-held needle
  - Scalpel and blade
  - Antiseptic solution, e.g. Betadine
  - Sterile drape
  - Sterile gloves, gown, and mask
  - Dressing pack
  - Transparent, semi-permeable dressing
- Prepare yourself:
  - Put on your mask, wash your hands
  - Put on your gloves and gown
  - Attach the three-way taps on and flush each lumen with saline. Close the taps. Do not attach the three-way tap to the brown lumen which should be left open
- Prepare the patient:
  - Continuous monitoring with pulse oximetry and ECG trace
  - Patient lies supine and just before you start ask your assistant to tilt the bed so the patient is 15–30° head down in Trendelenburg position. If tolerated, this will keep the vein filled and help avoid air embolism
  - Turn patient's head to the contralateral side
  - Place a rolled towel under the ipsilateral shoulder to help accentuate the clavicle
- Prepare the area:
  - Identify your anatomical landmarks:
    - Internal jugular vein (IJV) catheterization should be performed with real-time ultrasound guidance. The IJV is located anterolateral to the carotid artery, within a triangle formed by the sternal and clavicular heads of sternocleidomastoid and the clavicle at the base. Aim your needle towards the opposite nipple. Ultrasonographically, the vein has a larger diameter than the carotid artery, is compressible, thin-walled, and is non-pulsatile
    - Subclavian vein (SCV) catheterization—ultrasound guidance is not used due to impedance from overlying bony tissue. The SCV lies behind the middle third of the clavicle, anterior and inferior to the artery. Aim for about 1cm below the junction between the medial and middle third of the clavicle, aiming towards the sternal notch
  - Clean the area with antiseptic solution and drape accordingly
  - Infiltrate local anaesthetic into the skin and subcutaneous tissue at the planned puncture site. Aspirate first to avoid injecting into vascular structures
- Insert CVC:
  - IJV—if right handed, use your left hand to keep your ultrasound probe in place and with your right hand insert a hollow needle and 5-ml syringe into the punctured site, aiming for the contralateral nipple and aspirating as you advance. You will see the needle ultrasonographically and use this to help you enter the IJV. You will get flashback as soon as you enter the IJV
  - SCV—as per the landmarks above, advance the hollow needle and syringe towards the clavicle. Once you hit clavicle, angle your needle below the clavicle and aim for the opposite sternoclavicular joint. Aspirate as you advance your needle and you will get flashback as soon as you enter the SCV
  - Keeping the introducer needle in place, remove the syringe and insert the guidewire down the needle, it should move down with ease. It is also visible ultrasonographically
  - *If there is any resistance, remove the guidewire, replace the syringe and aspirate to check that you are still in the vein, then try again.*

- ◆ Once about 8–10cm of wire is in, remove the needle, keeping hold of the guidewire. **Never let go of the guidewire**
- ◆ Make a 0.5-cm nick in the skin at this point
- ◆ Advance the guidewire further (watch for arrhythmias—if any, pull wire back slightly) and feed the dilator over the wire. Do not push; use a twisting motion to advance
- ◆ Remove the dilator, keeping hold of the guidewire throughout, feed the catheter over the guidewire, into the vein up to 15cm. The wire will emerge from the brown hub—remove wire. Attach three-way tap on brown lumen
- Check position and secure CVC:
  - ◆ Aspirate, flush, and close each lumen in turn
  - ◆ Suture catheter to skin and apply dressing
  - ◆ Request CXR to check position and exclude pneumothorax
- Tidy up:
  - ◆ Wash your hands
  - ◆ Clear your equipment
- Document procedure in notes and planned date of change

Scenario 6

- Introduction:
  - ◆ Introduce yourself to the patient (presumably you would have done this at the start of your assessment)
  - ◆ Check the patient's details against their ID bracelet
  - ◆ Explain the procedure, the reason it is needed, risks to the patient, and gain consent (usually verbal consent is sufficient)

    Hello, Mrs Albrecht. My name is Mr. Peterson. I am one of the ST1 surgical trainees. Before I continue can you write down your name and date of birth for me? Thank you. I need to perform a special blood test to see how well you are breathing. It will also give us information about how well your body is dealing with acid waste.

    It involves inserting a small needle into the blood vessel at your wrist. It can be slightly painful as the needle goes in but is a fairly short procedure. It is a safe procedure and we perform it under clean conditions to minimize the risk of infection. After the procedure I will apply pressure at the puncture site to avoid any bleeding. There is a small risk of the vessel becoming obstructed by a blood clot at the puncture site but this does not normally lead to any major ill effects. Are you happy for me to proceed?

- Prepare your equipment:
  - ◆ Alcohol swab
  - ◆ Gloves and apron
  - ◆ Arterial blood gas kit—pre-heparinized kit, 23G needle, cap for syringe, rubber cork for needle (to avoid re-sheathing post-procedure)
  - ◆ Sharps bin
  - ◆ Tape and cotton wool ball
  - ◆ Local anaesthetic, e.g. 2–3ml of 1% lignocaine and 25G needle
- Prepare the patient:
  - ◆ Choose an appropriate site—examine both sides and use the site which has a more easily palpable pulse
    *The radial artery lies between the tendon of flexor carpi radialis and head of radius.

    *The femoral artery lies at the mid-inguinal point—midway between the anterior superior iliac spine and the symphysis pubis.
  - ◆ Perform Allen's test to ensure adequate collateral circulation (for radial puncture)
  - ◆ Place a rolled towel under the patient's wrist to extend the wrist slightly
  - ◆ Check the oxygen concentration the patient is inhaling. Ensure that patient has been on the same concentration for at least 15 minutes—**do not take patient off oxygen to perform arterial puncture**
  - ◆ Disinfect skin with the alcohol wipe
- Prepare yourself:
  - ◆ Wash your hands
  - ◆ Put on your apron and gloves
  - ◆ Expel excess heparin from syringe

*If needed, infiltrate local anaesthetic into the skin and subcutaneous tissue at the planned puncture site. Aspirate first to avoid injecting into vascular structures.

- Perform arterial puncture:
  - ◆ Feel for the arterial pulse with two fingers of your non-dominant hand
  - ◆ Warn the patient that you are about to start
  - ◆ Hold the syringe like a pen, with the bevel facing up and aim for the point of maximum pulsation under your fingers. Advance the needle at a 45° angle until you get a flashback of blood
  - ◆ If you are in the artery, the syringe will fill up in a pulsatile manner. There is no need to pull back on the plunger

If no blood is obtained, withdraw the needle to a position just under the skin and try again. If you get non-pulsatile blood in a patient with a normal pulse pressure, try again with another syringe. The colour of the blood is not always a good guide to determine if it is arterial or venous.

  - ◆ Once you have 2–3ml of blood remove the needle
  - ◆ Apply firm pressure over the puncture site with a swab for a few minutes (you can instruct the patient to do this)
  - ◆ Using one hand, insert the needle into the cork. With the cork in place, remove the needle from the syringe and dispose of it in the sharps bin. Expel any excess air from the syringe, then cap and label the syringe
  - ◆ Noting the oxygen concentration the patient was on; take the sample to the nearest blood gas analysis machine (if there is to be a delay in analysis—keep the sample in a bag of ice)
- Tidy up:
  - ◆ Apply a dressing over the puncture site
  - ◆ Clear your equipment
  - ◆ Wash your hands
- Document your procedure:
  - ◆ Document the procedure and site
  - ◆ Attach the blood gas analysis and note the amount of supplementary oxygen the patient was on

Scenario 7

- Introduction:
  - ◆ Although an introduction is unnecessary in this scenario, ensure you are familiar with the procedure, indication, contraindications, and complications of the procedure (as stated above and detailed below)
- Prepare your equipment:
  - ◆ Antiseptic solution, e.g. Betadine
  - ◆ Sterile drape
  - ◆ Sterile gloves, gown, and mask
  - ◆ Dressing pack
  - ◆ Transparent, semi-permeable dressing
  - ◆ Local anaesthetic, e.g. 5ml of 1% lignocaine and 25G needle (if patient awake)
  - ◆ Arterial line
  - ◆ Suture, e.g. 3/0 nylon on a hand-held needle
  - ◆ Connectors, pressure bag, transducer, manometer line pre-filled with heparinized saline
- Prepare the patient:
  - ◆ Choose an appropriate site—examine both sides and use the site which has a more easily palpable pulse. Avoid the site of the previous cannulation
    *The radial artery lies between the tendon of flexor carpi radialis and head of radius.
    *The femoral artery lies at the mid-inguinal point—midway between the anterior superior iliac spine and the symphysis pubis
  - ◆ Perform Allen's test to ensure adequate collateral circulation (for radial puncture)
  - ◆ With the patient's arm extended and supported, place a rolled towel under the patient's wrist to extend the wrist slightly
- Prepare yourself:
  - ◆ Put on your mask, wash your hands
  - ◆ Put on your gloves and gown
    *If needed, infiltrate local anaesthetic into the skin and subcutaneous tissue at the planned puncture site. Aspirate first to avoid injecting into vascular structures

- Prepare the area:
  - ✦ Clean the area with antiseptic solution and drape accordingly
  - ✦ If patient awake, infiltrate local anaesthetic into the skin and subcutaneous tissue at the planned puncture site. Aspirate first to avoid injecting into vascular structures
- Cannulate the artery:
  - ✦ Feel for the arterial pulse with two fingers of your non-dominant hand and feel the direction the artery lies
  - ✦ Warn the patient that you are about to start
  - ✦ With the bevel facing up, hold the catheter in your dominant hand and aim for the point of maximum pulsation under your fingers in the direction of the lie of the artery
  - ✦ Advance the cannula at a 25–30° angle until you get a flashback of pulsatile blood. Now, keeping the needle in place, lower the cannula so it is almost parallel to skin and advance the cannula sheath over the needle into the vessel

    *Arterial cannulation can also be performed using the Seldinger technique with a guidewire
- Secure the cannula in place and check position:
  - ✦ Once the cannula is in place, remove the needle—there will be pulsatile blood from its end. You can apply pressure over the artery before removing the needle to avoid bleeding
  - ✦ Immediately connect the catheter to a manometer line which, with a transducer is connected to an onscreen display. Arterial cannulation corresponds to a pulsatile waveform with a dicrotic notch
  - ✦ Secure the cannula in place with sutures and apply a transparent dressing
- Tidy up:
  - ✦ Clear your equipment
  - ✦ Wash your hands
- Document the procedure and site

Scenario 8

- Introduction:
  - ✦ Introduce yourself to the patient
  - ✦ Check the patient's details against their ID bracelet
  - ✦ Explain the procedure, the reason it is needed, risks to the patient, and gain consent (usually verbal consent is sufficient)
  - ✦ Arrange a signal the patient can use to communicate if he/she wishes to stop (e.g. raising their hand). This gives the patient control and decreases the risk of the patient struggling during the procedure

    Hello, Mr Smith. My name is Mr. Peterson. I am one of the ST1 surgical trainees. Before I continue can you confirm your name and date of birth for me? Thank you. I understand you have been vomiting over the past few days. One of the things we do for that is to insert a tube into your nose, down the back of your throat and into your stomach to help empty your stomach. This will help stop the vomiting and decrease the risk of you aspirating your vomit which can cause a chest infection.

    It is a fairly short procedure and most people cope well with it. It can sometimes be uncomfortable and can irritate the back of your throat and make you cough. If you find the procedure too uncomfortable to continue, raise your right hand and we will stop. Are you happy for me to proceed?
- Prepare your equipment:
  - ✦ Wide-bore NG tube (alternatively, narrow bore if for feeding)— ideally, from the refrigerator as it is less flexible when cool
  - ✦ Gloves and apron
  - ✦ Non-allergic tape
  - ✦ Glass of water with straw
  - ✦ Aqueous lubricating jelly
  - ✦ Vomit bowl
  - ✦ 50-ml syringe
  - ✦ Suction
  - ✦ Collection bag
- Prepare yourself:
  - ✦ Wash your hands
  - ✦ Put on your apron and gloves

- Prepare the patient:
  - ◆ Examine the patient's nostrils for polyps/deformity. Choose a side which appears patent
  - ◆ Sit the patient up
  - ◆ Give the patient a glass of water and tell them to sip water through the straw when instructed
- Prepare the tube:
  - ◆ Measure the length from the tip of the patient's nose to their earlobe and to midway between their xiphisternum and umbilicus—note the measured length on the NG tube
  - ◆ Lubricate the gastric end of the tube
- Insert the tube:
  - ◆ Inform the patient that you are starting
  - ◆ Insert the lubricated tube into the patient's nostril with the natural curve promoting downward passage
  - ◆ Advance directly backward (not upward)—if you feel an obstruction, withdraw and try again in a slightly different direction or try the other nostril
  - ◆ When the tip is estimated to be entering the throat, rotate the tube slowly while advancing downward. Do not force the tube down
  - ◆ Ask the patient to take a few sips of water to ease passage of the tube into the oesophagus and then downward into the stomach
  - ◆ Advance the tube until the mark is reached. The stomach is about 40cm from the incisors in an adult, so the tube should be at least this far in
  - ◆ Stop the procedure and withdraw immediately if the patient starts coughing or develops any signs of respiratory distress
- Secure tube:
  - ◆ Secure the tube with tape to nasal bridge and patient's cheek
  - ◆ Connect the NG tube to a collection bag on free drainage (alternatively, tube can be spigotted)
  - ◆ Secure collection bag to patient's gown to prevent tube dislodging
- Check tube position:
  - ◆ Gently aspirate the end of the tube with a 50-ml syringe and test the aspirate for acidity with pH paper. A pH of <4 confirms gastric placement. **Note:** concurrent use of antacids/H2 antagonists/proton pump inhibitors may affect pH of gastric secretions
  - ◆ Obtain a CXR to verify position (for fine-bore tubes)
- Tidy up:
  - ◆ Wash hands
  - ◆ Clear your equipment
- Document procedure, including indication and planned date of change

Scenario 9

*Always ensure that you have a chaperone.

- Introduction:
  - ◆ Introduce yourself to the patient (presumably done at the start of the clinic appointment)
  - ◆ Check the patient's details (if in theatre for example)
  - ◆ Explain the procedure, the reason it is needed, risks to the patient, and gain consent (usually verbal consent is sufficient)

    Hello, Mr Alphonso. I now need to examine your bottom end with two small plastic tubes. This will allow me to look up the lower end of your bowel to see if there is a cause for your symptoms. The first tube is about as long as my finger and allows me to look at the anal canal. The second tube is a little longer and allows me to examine your rectum, the bottom end of the bowel. I will need to blow some air in with the second tube and you may feel the need to pass wind—this is completely normal.

    These are both safe procedures with very small risks of infection, making a hole in the bowel or causing bleeding from the bowel wall. Sometimes, if there is faecal matter in the rectum, I may not be able to see very well and may have to abandon the procedure. It is a fairly short procedure, slightly uncomfortable, but not usually painful. If it is too much to bear, let me know and I'll stop, OK? Are you happy for me to proceed? This is Nurse Beckett, she will stay with you throughout the procedure.

- Prepare your equipment:
  - ◆ Three pairs of gloves. Apron and goggles

◆ Lubricating jelly
◆ Pads—to protect surrounding from spillage
◆ Proctoscope with light source
◆ Rigid sigmoidoscope with light source and bellows. Ensure obturator is in place through the eyepiece window and the tip of the obturator emerges at the end of the scope
  *Ensure you are familiar with setting up both scopes before your exam
• Prepare your patient:
  ◆ Patient in a left lateral position with hips and knees flexed. Ask patient to bring their buttock as close to the right side of the bed as possible
  ◆ Ensure patient relaxed and comfortable—essential for successful examination
  ◆ Raise the couch to a level that is comfortable for you (warn the patient that the couch is raised, i.e. not to roll over until you lower it again)
• Prepare yourself:
  ◆ Wash your hands
  ◆ Put on gloves, apron, and goggles
• Perform the procedure:
  ◆ **Tell the patient what you are doing at every step of the procedure**—the patient cannot see you and does not know what to expect. A relaxed, well-informed, comfortable patient is essential for this procedure
  ◆ Start by inspecting the anus and surrounding area. Then perform a gentle digital rectal examination. Change your gloves
  ◆ Then using a well-lubricated proctoscope with a light source attached and obturator in place, gently insert the proctoscope fully into the patient's anal canal
  ◆ Remove the obturator and look through the scope for any obvious lesions. Examine the colour and character of the mucosa while gently withdrawing the scope
    *Do not throw the obturator away until you have completed the examination. If you need to examine a more proximal part of the anal canal, re-insert the obturator, advance the proctoscope and start again.
  ◆ Remove the proctoscope and dispose of it in a clinical waste bag. Change your gloves
  ◆ Now, using a well-lubricated rigid sigmoidoscope with light source and bellows attached and the obturator in place, gently insert the rigid sigmoidoscope into the patient's anus with your thumb over the base of the obturator. Advance only 3–4cm in the direction of the patient's umbilicus
  ◆ Remove the obturator and close the eyepiece window
  ◆ Advance the sigmoidoscope under direct vision, using the bellows to insufflate air into the rectum intermittently. Follow the natural curves of the rectum. You will find that you will now slowly be moving from pointing the scope anteriorly to pointing the scope posteriorly. At about the 12–14cm mark, aim the scope slightly anterosuperiorly
  ◆ Note the appearance of the mucosa and any lesions as you advance the scope. Note the position of any abnormalities from the anal margin using the scale on the scope
  ◆ Under direct vision, advance the scope up to 15–20cm. If the patient complains of discomfort, do not advance and begin withdrawing the scope
  ◆ Once you have inserted the scope as far as you can, gently start withdrawing the scope under direct vision. Perform the above movements in reverse and use small circular movements to try to view all four walls as you withdraw. This may reveal small lesions missed during insertion
  ◆ Remove the scope completely and dispose of it in a clinical waste bin
  ◆ Clean the perianal area, lower the examining couch and return the patient to a more comfortable supine position
• Tidy up:
  ◆ Clear the rest of your equipment
  ◆ Wash your hands
• Document the procedure, indication, extent of examination, and findings in notes. Also note how well the patient tolerated the procedure

Scenario 10

• Introduction:
  ◆ Introduce yourself to the patient
  ◆ Check the patient's details against their ID bracelet

- ◆ Explain the procedure, the reason it is needed, risks to the patient, and gain consent (usually verbal consent is sufficient)

  Hello, Mrs Jaafar. My name is Mr. Peterson. I am one of the ST1 surgical trainees. Before I continue can you confirm your name and date of birth for me? Thank you. The ultrasound scan that you had earlier demonstrated some fluid in your abdomen. We need to take a sample of that fluid for analysis to determine the cause of its presence. To do that, I need to insert a small needle into your abdominal wall under local anaesthetic and aspirate some fluid out. It is a short and safe procedure. There is a less than 1 in 100 chance of significant bleeding or making a small hole in the structures inside your abdomen such as liver or bowel. If this does occur, we will undertake the appropriate management which may include surgery. Do you have any questions? Are you happy for me to proceed?

- Prepare your equipment:
  - ◆ Local anaesthetic, e.g. 10ml 1% lignocaine
  - ◆ 1× 10-ml syringe and 1 × 20-ml syringe
  - ◆ 21G (green) and 25G (blue) needles
  - ◆ Sterile gloves and apron
  - ◆ Sterile drapes
  - ◆ Antiseptic solution, e.g. Betadine
  - ◆ Dressing
  - ◆ 18G aspiration needle (if not available use a 21G needle)
- Prepare the patient:
  - ◆ Ensure patient has emptied their bladder pre-procedure
  - ◆ Lie patient supine
  - ◆ Confirm clinically the presence of ascites over the marked site (shifting dullness)
  - ◆ If the patient has not been marked ultrasonographically, confirm the presence of ascites clinically and mark your planned site of entry, preferably in the left lower quadrant (avoids perforating an enlarged spleen or liver), usually lateral to the rectus abdminis muscle about 5cm superior to the level of the anterior superior iliac spine. Avoid sites of previous scars, stomas, or blood vessels
- Prepare yourself:
  - ◆ Wash your hands and put on your gloves and apron
- Prepare the area:
  - ◆ Clean the skin around the site with Betadine and apply sterile drapes
  - ◆ Inject local anaesthetic—initially create a subcutaneous bleb with the 25G needle, then switch to the 21G needle and anaesthetize the deeper structures including peritoneum. Remember to withdraw gently before injecting to avoid injecting any vascular structures. Continue until you aspirate a few millilitres of ascitic fluid
  - ◆ Allow the local anaesthetic a few minutes to work
- Tap the ascitic fluid:
  - ◆ Introduce the aspiration needle connected to a 20-ml syringe into the skin and subcutaneous tissue while aspirating
  - ◆ You will feel a give when you enter the peritoneal cavity and fluid should start to fill the syringe as you aspirate. Keep the needle in this position while aspirating, do not advance further
  - ◆ Once you have the desired amount (~20ml), remove the needle and apply an occlusive dressing over the aspiration site
- Tidy up:
  - ◆ Send the fluid for diagnostic evaluation (cell count, MC&S, TB culture, cytology, and biochemical analysis including protein, glucose, LDH, amylase, and tumour markers). Ensure all the specimen bottles and laboratory forms are labelled correctly with the patient's details
  - ◆ Wash hands
  - ◆ Clear your equipment
- Document procedure in notes

Scenario 11

- Introduction:
  - ◆ Introduce yourself to the patient
  - ◆ Check the patient's details against their ID bracelet

- ◆ Explain the procedure, the reason it is needed, risks to the patient, and gain consent (usually verbal consent is sufficient)

  Hello, Mrs Jaafar. My name is Mr. Peterson. I am one of the ST1 surgical trainees. Before I continue can you confirm your name and date of birth for me? Thank you. Your clinical findings and your recent CT scan suggest that you have fluid in your abdominal cavity causing you discomfort and difficulty breathing. To help with these symptoms, we need to insert a tube into your abdomen under local anaesthetic to help drain this fluid. Once the fluid has been drained, you will feel better. However, this fluid has accumulated as a result of the cancer and will most likely re-accumulate with time at which point you may need this procedure repeated.

  Once the drain is inserted we need to keep a close eye on your blood pressure and heart rate to make sure you don't lose too much fluid. We will also start an intravenous infusion to keep you well hydrated. There is a less than a 1 in 100 chance of significant bleeding or making a small hole in the structures inside your abdomen such as liver or bowel. If this does occur, we will undertake the appropriate management which may include surgery. Do you have any questions? Are you happy for me to proceed?

- Prepare for this procedure as you would for an ascitic tap. In addition, you will also need the following:
  - ◆ Bonnano catheter set—advance the outer sheath up to the end of the catheter to straighten the pig-tail out, thread the introducer (long needle) into the catheter before removing the outer sheath
  - ◆ Scalpel
  - ◆ 1/0 silk suture
  - ◆ Collection bag and tubing
  - ◆ Ensure patient has large-bore IV access
- Insert catheter:
  - ◆ Insert the catheter and introducer perpendicular to the skin at the site marked
  - ◆ With your non-dominant hand, hold on to the catheter 2–3cm from the tip and only advance the up to this point
  - ◆ Ascitic fluid should be draining freely at this point. If not, advance slightly until good flow is achieved
  - ◆ Keeping the introducer in place, advance the catheter over the introducer until it is fully inserted
  - ◆ Remove the introducer and discard it safely into a sharps bin
  - ◆ Connect the catheter to the tubing and drainage bag
  - ◆ Secure the catheter in place with sutures and dressing
- Tidy up:
  - ◆ Wash hands
  - ◆ Clear your equipment
- Post-procedure:
  - ◆ Document procedure in notes
  - ◆ Monitor volume of fluid drained—set a limit in a set time, after which time the drain should be removed, e.g. ~5L, usually within 6 hours. (This is arbitrary as there is no recognized set volume and patients may drain 10L in 2 hours.)
  - ◆ Ensure patient remains haemodynamically stable—regular monitoring, IV fluid as required
  - ◆ Use of plasma expander—e.g. 100ml of 20% human albumin per litre of fluid drained, is necessary in patients with a high SAAG. However, in patient with malignant ascites (low SAAG) there is no strong evidence to advocate this

Scenario 12

- Introduction:
  - ◆ Introduce yourself to the patient
  - ◆ Check the patient's details against their ID bracelet
  - ◆ Explain the procedure, the reason it is needed, risks to the patient, and gain consent (usually verbal consent is sufficient)

  Hello, Mr Wong. My name is Mr. Peterson. I am one of the ST1 surgical trainees. Before I continue can you confirm your name and date of birth for me? Thank you. As I explained earlier, we need to insert a tube into your bladder to help you pass urine. It is a fairly short procedure but can sometimes be a little uncomfortable going in.

  Once it is in, however, it should make you feel a lot better. The tube is inserted under sterile conditions and will be connected to a bag so we can monitor your urine output. We will start you on some tablets to help you pass urine on your own again and will remove the tube as soon as possible to reduce the risk of you developing an infection. Are you happy for me to proceed?

- Prepare your equipment:
  - Foley catheter—choose smallest size possible (usually between 12–16F)
  - Two pairs of sterile gloves and an apron
  - Sterile drapes
  - Antiseptic solution, e.g. Savlon
  - Cotton gauze swabs
  - Sterile local anaesthetic lubricant gel, e.g. Instillagel
  - Sterile water and syringe (according to size of catheter balloon)
  - Kidney dish
  - Collection bad and tubing
- Prepare the patient:
  - Absorbent pad under patient, kidney dish between patient's legs
  - Lying supine, undressed from waist down. Use a blanket to protect the patient's modesty until you are ready to start. Ensure privacy
    *Female patients should have their hips and knees flexed with their hips abducted and heels together
- Prepare yourself:
  - Put on your apron
  - Wash your hands and put on both pairs of sterile gloves
- Prepare the area:
  - Retract the foreskin (if present) and, while holding on to the penile shaft with your non-dominant hand, clean the urethral meatus and glans penis with gauze and antiseptic solution. Repeat this three times, cleaning away from the meatus each time. Place penis on a sterile gauze swab
  - Remove the 1st pair of gloves. Place the sterile drapes in place
  - Hold the penis proximal to the glans with a gauze swab and stretch the penis at a 75–90° angle. Slowly instil the local anaesthetic gel into the meatus to anaesthetize and lubricate the urethra. Wait 3–5 minutes
    *In female patient, separate the labia with your non-dominant hand and clean the meatus in a pubis-to-anus direction.
- Insert the catheter:
  - Keeping the penis in a fairly upright position, insert the catheter into the urethral meatus and advance until you feel a slight resistance
  - Straighten the penis out and continue to advance the catheter. Ensure the end of the catheter is aimed at the kidney dish to ensure urine that drains is collected
  - The catheter should slide in easily. If you feel firm resistance, try with a catheter one size larger and extra lubricant. Do not force the catheter in
    *In female patients, advance the catheter until you have urine draining, advance a further 1–2cm and inflate the balloon.
- Secure the catheter:
  - Continue to advance the catheter as far as it will go and ensure urine is draining before inflating the balloon with the appropriate amount of fluid. This is to prevent inflating the balloon while still in the urethra
  - Gently withdraw the catheter until resistance is felt—balloon resting at the bladder neck
  - Connect the end of the catheter to the collection bag and tubing
  - Replace the foreskin over the glans penis (if present)—to prevent paraphimosis
- Tidy up:
  - Wash hands
  - Clear your equipment
- Document procedure, including residual volume and planned date of trial without catheter (TWOC)

Scenario 13

- Introduction
  - Introduce yourself to the patient
  - Check the patient's details against their ID bracelet
  - Explain the procedure, reason it is needed and risks to the patient and gain consent (usually verbal consent is sufficient)

  Hello, Mr Wong. My name is Mr. Peterson. I am one of the ST1 surgical trainees. Before I continue can you confirm your name and date of birth for me? Thank you. I understand you have been having trouble passing urine and we have not been able to insert a catheter through the penis. Hence, we need to insert a catheter through the lower part of your abdominal wall into your bladder to help drain urine.

This is a fairly short procedure which we carry out under local anaesthetic and under sterile conditions. Once the tube is in, it should make you feel a lot better. We inflate a balloon at the tip of the catheter to help keep it in place and attach the catheter to a bag so we can monitor your urine output. We will give you some antibiotics at the start of the procedure to decrease the risk of infection. Although we take every care when performing this procedure, there is a risk of forming a hole in the bowel as the bowel loops can sometimes lie very close to the bladder in this position. We will be able to identify this injury during the procedure and undertake the appropriate management which may include surgery. Do you have any questions? Are you happy for me to proceed?

- Prepare your equipment:
  - Local anaesthetic, e.g. 10ml 1% lignocaine
  - 2 × 10-ml syringes
  - 21G (green) and 25G (blue) needles
  - Suprapubic catheter set—usually contains suprapubic catheter and trocar
  - Scalpel
  - Sterile gloves and gown
  - Sterile drapes
  - Antiseptic solution, e.g. Betadine
  - Cotton gauze swabs
  - Sterile water and syringe (according to size of catheter balloon)
  - Kidney dish
  - Collection bad and tubing
  - Silk suture 1/0
  - Dressing
- Prepare the patient:
  - Lie patient supine
  - Confirm the presence of an enlarged bladder clinically—distended abdomen with dullness suprapubically (ultrasonographically, if available)
  - Mark the site of planned entry—2–3 finger breadths above the symphysis pubis
- Prepare yourself:
  - Wash your hands and put on your gloves and gown
- Prepare the area:
  - Clean the skin around the site with Betadine and apply sterile drapes
  - Inject local anaesthetic—initially create a subcutaneous bleb with the 25G needle, then switch to the 21G needle and anaesthetize the deeper structures. Remember to withdraw gently before injecting to avoid injecting any vascular structures. Continue until you aspirate a few millilitres of urine
  - Allow the local anaesthetic a few minutes to work, then make a stab incision over the marked site with your scalpel
- Insert the catheter:
  - With the trocar in place, slowly advance the catheter perpendicular to the skin through the incision and subcutaneous tissue in a controlled manner. Continue until you feel a 'give'—you have entered the bladder
  - Withdraw the trocar, you should see free flow of urine. Advance the catheter further in
    *Suprapubic catheters can also be inserted with a Seldinger set (introducer needle, guidewire, dilator, and catheter)
- Secure the catheter:
  - With urine still draining into the kidney dish, inflate the balloon with the appropriate amount of fluid (as marked on the catheter port)
  - Gently withdraw the catheter until resistance is felt
  - Suture the flange of the catheter to skin
  - Connect the end of the catheter to the collection bag and tubing
- Tidy up:
  - Wash hands
  - Clear your equipment
- Document procedure, including residual volume and planned date of review/removal

Scenario 14

- Introduction:
  - ◆ Introduce yourself to the patient
  - ◆ Check the patient's details against their ID bracelet
  - ◆ Explain the procedure, the reason it is needed, risks to the patient, and gain consent (usually verbal consent is sufficient)

    Hello, Mrs Higgins. My name is Mr. Peterson. I am one of the ST1 surgical trainees. Before I continue can you confirm your name and date of birth for me? Thank you. As Mr Albert, the consultant explained earlier, we need to take a sample of tissue from this lump in your breast to send to the lab for examination under a microscope.

    To do that, I need to make a small cut on your skin, insert a special needle, and take a sample of tissue from this lump under local anaesthetic. I may need to repeat this a few times until an adequate sample has been collected. It is a short and safe procedure. It is generally painless but you may have some bruising or tenderness after the procedure. This usually settles within a day or two. Although, this is a very useful investigation, sometimes it may miss the lesion or give us an unclear result. If this is the case, we may need to take another tissue sample. Do you have any questions? Are you happy for me to proceed?
- Prepare your equipment:
  - ◆ Local anaesthetic, e.g. 10ml 1% lignocaine
  - ◆ 1 × 10ml syringe
  - ◆ 21G (green) and 25G (blue) needles
  - ◆ Sterile gloves and apron
  - ◆ Antiseptic solution, e.g. Betadine
  - ◆ Dressing
  - ◆ Scalpel
  - ◆ Tru-Cut needle
  - ◆ Formaldehyde specimen bottles
- Prepare the patient:
  - ◆ Ensure patient is lying comfortably, supine with their ipsilateral hand behind their head. The patient should be adequately exposed but use a blanket to protect their modesty until you are ready to start. Ensure privacy
  - ◆ Palpate the lump gently
- Prepare yourself:
  - ◆ Familiarize yourself with the Tru-cut needle (ideally, you should do this **before** your examination)
  - ◆ Wash your hands and put on your gloves and apron
- Prepare the area:
  - ◆ Clean the skin around the site with Betadine
  - ◆ Inject local anaesthetic into the overlying skin. Warn the patient before you start. Remember to withdraw gently before injecting to avoid injecting any vascular structures
  - ◆ Allow the local anaesthetic a few minutes to work then make a stab incision over the lesion with the scalpel (at least 6mm to allow the Tru-Cut needle in)
- Take the biopsy:
  - ◆ Palpate the lesion with your non-dominant hand and fix it between two fingers
  - ◆ With your dominant hand, insert the Tru-Cut needle into the lump. Ensure the needle is lying within the sheath before you start
  - ◆ Keeping the sheath steady with your non-dominant hand, advance the needle into the lesion (using your dominant hand) until the two hand grips touch and you hear a click
  - ◆ Now with your dominant hand, slide the sheath slowly over the needle until you hear and feel a click
  - ◆ Now withdraw the Tru-Cut needle
  - ◆ Slide the sheath off the needle and shake the needle end in the formaldehyde in the specimen bottle until the specimen is free. Inspect the specimen—if it sinks it is likely to be pathological tissue, if it floats it is likely to be fat
  - ◆ You may need to repeat the procedure a few times until you have an adequate sample. Aim for three or four specimens which sink
- Tidy up:
  - ◆ Ensure the specimen bottle and histological form is labelled correctly. Send the specimen to pathology
  - ◆ Clear your equipment including sharps appropriately
  - ◆ Wash your hands
- Document the procedure in the patient's notes

PART 1
SURGICAL SKILLS AND PATIENT SAFETY

Section 3 Evidenced-based surgical practice and professional skills

Introduction

This section prepares you in part for the stations on communication which is dealt with in greater detail in the next section. Most importantly the knowledge gained in this section would help the reader to be a good doctor in general and a good, responsible surgeon in particular. It would stand the surgeon in good stead and avoid medico-legal problems.

Chapter 10 **Clinical governance**

Introduction

Clinical governance is an essential part of a doctor's professional life, much more so for a surgeon. There-fore the surgeon in training should have a sound knowledge of all the medico-legal implications that may confront him/her. During one's surgical career, over a lifetime, it will be extremely unusual for any sur-geon not be faced with a difficult situation that may require coming up against the legal profession or the General Medical Council (GMC). This chapter helps the reader do just that.

Making mistakes

To be sued by a patient is a very hurtful experience for a surgeon. All professionals make mistakes and indeed much of our learning comes directly from reviewing errors. There is also no need for mistakes to lead to litigation. If handled properly they can be a positive learning event for the surgeon, while those harmed by the error can be left feeling that everything possible has now been done to rectify matters.

Taking a surgeon to court is only one way that a dissatisfied patient can seek resolution of a grievance. If they are successful then they will be awarded damages (money). However, this is not what most patients who have suffered harm are seeking, so litigation is avoidable in many cases.

The commonest cause of litigation, both justified and unjustified, is a breakdown in communication between the patient and the surgeon which leads to a misunderstanding. This breakdown frequently starts after a throwaway comment by another surgeon, who without thinking, or knowing the full circum-stances of the situation, may suggest to a patient that they themselves would have managed a situation or operation better. It may appear obvious to you that a colleague's treatment of a patient has been wrong or even negligent, but nevertheless you would be wise to be absolutely sure of your facts before trying to gain prestige with the patient by telling them your views. If you are wrong you will send that patient down an expensive and frustrating path, and you will have unfairly insulted a professional col-league. If you are right you still may not have done the best thing for either the patient or your colleague. Mistakes should never be covered up but there are more constructive ways of handling them than telling a patient that your colleague is incompetent.

Handling a complaint

It does not matter whether you have actually made a mistake or a patient just believes that you have, the initial response is the same.

Acknowledge

Acknowledge at once that there is a problem. The sooner you tell the patient verbally or in writing that you understand that they are not happy, the better. Delay allows grievance to fester and leaves you with unresolved anxiety. At this stage you may not know all the facts, so it is unlikely to be appropriate to offer an apology. It is therefore best just to acknowledge the situation, and explain that you are taking it seri-ously and looking in to it.

Gather information

The next stage is to try to get as much information as possible about the problem, what led up to it, what happened, and who was involved. This may include getting a description from the patient or the relative as to what they think happened, statements from any staff who were involved, and checking what was written in the notes. Once all the information is available, then a meeting needs to be set-up.

The Meeting

The meeting can be broken up in several stages.

- **Introduction** All the people present should be introduced and the reason for the meeting needs to be clearly explained
- **Listening** The next stage is an important one and involves inviting the person making the complaint to lay out fully in their own words exactly what they think happened and why they are

so dissatisfied with this. It is important not to interrupt at this stage but merely to listen careful and note down key points which need dealing with. This listening phase is very cathartic for the person complaining, and often serves to reduce the tension in the meeting

- **Clarification** Once the listening phase has been completed, it may be necessary to correct some misunderstandings or factual errors. This will require referring back to all the material obtained in the 'gathering information' phase. Frequently, through no fault of the patient, a false impression or a complete misunderstanding has arisen which can now be cleared up by reviewing the facts

- **Apology** If at this stage there remain actions or remarks which fell below the professional standard which is expected of you and your team, then a full apology for these needs to be made there and then. This apology does not include remarks like 'I am sorry that you feel this way'. This comment, which is commonly used is not an apology, it is in fact a roundabout way of saying that you do not agree with their interpretation, and can be very inflammatory. It might be thought that offering a full apology is a direct invitation to be sued, but research shows that being open about what has happened and quickly apologizing has the opposite effect, and reduces litigation. Car insurance companies advise you never to admit fault in an accident especially when you are abroad, but this is a completely different situation and does not apply to medical mistakes

- **Never again** An apology alone, however, is not enough. The most powerful tool in handling a complaint is the next phase. This is a promise to the person complaining that you are going to use this complaint to change things so that it does not ever happen again. Patients who make complaints routinely say that they realize that the clock cannot be turned back, but that they would get great satisfaction in knowing that the suffering they have gone through will improve things for others. This promise should not be made lightly, and it is mandatory that any action which is promised is indeed implemented. Some well-managed services make sure that some time after resolution of the situation, the person making the complaint is contacted to let them know that the promised action has been taken and is yielding results. Conversely a promise to improve things and then a failure to do so is likely to prove absolutely infuriating to the person complaining

- **Valuing** Some go-ahead organizations even go so far as to use complaints as a 'valuing' opportunity. Having handled the complaint in the way described above, they then go further to ask how they can try to make amends for the wrong done to their client. Most people complaining are both surprised and bowled over by this offer and may actually feel very positive towards the organization which had so irritated them originally. For example, if dealing with a patient complaining because their operation had to be cancelled at the last minute, you might ask the patient how you can try to make amends. They might ask for a firm date for their operation in the future at their convenience. Instead of just acquiescing to this, you might agree to this but also offer to send a car to fetch them into hospital and put some flowers in their room for when they arrive. The few pounds that this would cost would pale into insignificance against the thousands of pounds in legal fees that even a successfully contested claim can cost

- **Summary** At the end of the meeting, minutes need to be prepared laying out what was discussed and what actions are to be taken as a result. A copy of this needs to be send to the person complaining to make sure that they agree that this is an accurate representation of what has happened

Litigation—being sued

Most doctors will find themselves at the receiving of litigation at some stage in their careers, and some branches of surgery are especially prone to litigation, possibly because the hopes and expectations of patients are quite far removed from what surgery can actually achieve. Most litigation cases are expected, but some come out of the blue. If you suspect that a patient may be considering taking legal action, then do not put the matter to the back of your mind and hope that it will go away. Be proactive and handle the situation in the same way as you would a complaint (see above). When working in the health service you will receive legal advice and support from your Trust. They will also pay any costs or damages incurred. In return for this support, they may decide for economic or other reasons to settle cases where you are quite clear there was no breach of care. There is very little that you can do about this. 'He who pays the piper calls the tune.' The important thing is to learn from the case, and not let it destroy your faith in patients and the work that you do.

Initial stages—the writ

If a writ is taken out against you (this is the legal term for legal action being taken), then the solicitors representing the person will write to you and/or your hospital and will lay out what they think happened, where and when, and explain why they think that compensation is deserved. In the UK, your insurance (indemnity) for National Health Service (NHS) work is provided by the hospital where you work, so the hospital's legal department will handle the case for you, and you should hand any writs that you receive to them. They will ask their legal department and lawyers to handle the claim, but will ask for your help in doing this.

Statements—to settle or to defend

The legal department will first of all ask you and anyone else involved for a statement of the facts as you know them. You should tell the truth and refer to hospital notes where possible to back up your explanation. The hospital notes are critical in defending an unfair claim, and this is why writing full and clear notes is so important. The hospital's legal department will then show the claim, these statements and the hospital notes to a medical expert. This will be a consultant specializing in this branch of medicine who has experience in this type of work and s/he will prepare a report for the hospital legal department, based on this material, telling them whether this claim is reasonable or not. On the basis of this report (not just your statement), the hospital's legal department will decide whether to try to settle this claim or contest it. This decision is not yours. It is for the hospital to make. That may be very frustrating, but it is their money which is being spent, and only your dignity and reputation which are being battered. Your job is to try to learn from what has happened to try to make sure that it does not happen again.

Defence

If the hospital decides to defend the case (deny that anything went wrong), then they will prepare a document called a 'Defence' which will refute point by point the claims made by the plaintiff (the person making the complaint). There may also be requests at this stage for 'further particulars', information which is designed to provide more facts which might clarify the situation. An example of this might be a record of your experience doing that type of operation. You would be very wise to be as honest as possible about this, because if it were discovered that you were being 'economical with the truth' you might face serious action being taken against you, including being reported to the GMC.

Contemporary notes

Anything written at the time of the incident is known as 'contemporaneous notes' and carries great weight if the case comes to court. The areas where notes are often very poor are: consent, operation notes, and ward round notes. The first lesson you will learn after the first case against you is to write better notes!

Consent

The signed consent form is only a very small part of informed consent (see Chapter 11). The doctor taking consent must demonstrate that they are competent to perform the operation (even if they are not performing it), that they explained things adequately to the patient, and that the patient understood that explanation so that they could make an 'informed' decision. Claimants routinely claim that they have no memory of being consented, and the courts are currently lenient about this. However, if the court can be satisfied that 'If the patient had been properly consented, and were fully aware of the risks involved they would never have consented to surgery', then you will lose the case. This is why you must mention and record in the notes any special risks of the surgery you are planning to perform, or any factors which might make the outcome less likely to be successful than normal.

Operation notes

Similarly operation notes are critical. The more comprehensive and legible they are the better. The operation note should therefore be a carefully constructed document with a standard format (see Chapter 11), but the content should be individual to the patient, describing any point where any special actions had to be taken, and where checks were made (such as 'bleeding controlled and checked').

Ward notes

You must date and time these notes and identify yourself with your name in clear writing (not just a scrawled signature). These records are critical for you to defend your reputation, so they must be clear, comprehensive, and relevant (see Chapter 11).

Process of litigation

The process of litigation can be very time consuming but recent law has insisted that this process must not drag on unnecessarily. Therefore a patient must bring the claim within 5 years of it happening (unless there are special reasons why they could no know that they had a claim) and the whole claim must then be settled within a few years of the claim being made.

Burden of proof

British law requires that the plaintiff (the patient) has to prove that 'on balance' they have been wronged. So, the onus is very much on the plaintiff to provide the evidence needed to prove their case. This may be very difficult if the documentation needed has already been destroyed.

However, medico-legal litigation is a civil (not criminal) matter and so the burden of proof is only 'on balance', not 'beyond reasonable doubt' as is found in criminal law. This might seem to make things very easy for the patient but it is not as simple as this. The plaintiff must prove three things:

- **Breach of care** The plaintiff must convince the court that the actions by the defendants constituted a 'Breach of Care'. This means that they fell below the standard expected of a reasonable body of competent practitioners. This standard is sometimes called **Bolam proof** after the case where this was determined. For example, there is currently some dispute as to whether prophylactic anticoagulation protects patients undergoing a total knee replacement from developing significant DVT and PE. Most surgeons do give prophylactic anticoagulation but a 'respectable body of practitioners' only use foot pumps and TED stockings. If a patient who only received these last two treatments subsequently developed a fatal PE, then there would be no breach of care. If however they received no form of prophylaxis whatsoever, then it is doubtful that a respectable body of knee surgeons can be found who would support this, and so there would be a breach of care
- **Causation** Second, the plaintiff must then convince the court that something happened as a result of this breach of care. For example, if a patient was taking legal action because they had a myocardial infarct after a total hip replacement and it was noticed that the patient had not received prophylactic antibiotics before the start of surgery, there would be a 'breach of care' (they should have had antibiotics to cover the surgery), but there is no causation. The absence of the antibiotics cannot be said to have been responsible for the patient suffering a heart attack
- **Consequence** Finally, once the first two hurdles have been successfully negotiated the final requirement is that the patient must have come to harm as a result of the breach of care and the effects that it caused. So, for example if a patient inadvertently had a tourniquet cuff left on when they left the operating theatre, and the problem was only discovered and rectified in the recovery room 30 minutes later, then that is a breach of care. There is also causation in that the patient will have suffered prolonged ischaemia to that limb. However, if subsequently the limb recovered normally, then there is no consequence and so the claim will fail. If, however, the limb developed a re-perfusion injury and required decompression for a compartment syndrome then there is a consequence and damages would be payable

Damages and awarding costs

Most cases now do not come to court. Both the solicitors for the plaintiff and the defendant will have at least one medical expert who is employed to help that side to inform the court. If there is disagreement between the experts (and there frequently is) then those experts must try to resolve those differences before the trial is held. During this period of negotiation both sides will be reviewing the situation and trying to assess their chances of winning the case. They will also be discussing what damages would be payable if the plaintiff does win the case. British courts are very different from courts in the USA and do not normally award such large damages. The reason for this is that the British courts do not award punitive damages (damages aimed at punishing the defendant for bad practice), nor do they award the equivalent amount of money for 'pain and suffering' as the American courts. The British courts are mainly interested in a) potential loss of earnings (including loss of opportunity), and b) care needs. If a patient was in work and has had to give up that work as a result of the negligence then a claim will be made for their annual salary multiplied by the number of years that the plaintiff could have been expected to work. If the plaintiff is going to need help with dressing, washing, housework, etc., then this will be costed out and again multiplied by the number of years 'extra' that this would have been required. There can also be a claim for modified housing, physiotherapy, and any other needs which flow from the claim. These damages may be proportionately reduced if it is felt that that patient could perhaps have avoided some of the problems if they had behaved in a more sensible manner. For example a patient injured in a RTA who was not wearing a seat belt will have their damages reduced because, in part, their injuries were their own fault.

Once these figures for damages have been roughly calculated then the defendants (your hospital's solicitors) may decide to make an offer. If the case is unequivocal then they may offer the full sum immediately and it is likely to be accepted without the case going to court. That is then the end of the matter. If, however, there is some debate about the size of the claim, and/or there is some doubt whether the plaintiff will win then the offer may be only a proportion of what is being claimed. Once this offer has been made (paid into court) then the plaintiff is faced with a dilemma. If they accept the offer then all the expenses that they have incurred too (which may be many thousands of pounds) will be paid too. However, if they then decide to contest this case in court, the judge will not know whether any money has been 'paid in'. S/he will judge the case, decide whether negligence has been proved, and if so what damages are to be awarded. This figure is crucial. If the judge awards lower damages than that which the defendants have already offered, then the penalty for the plaintiff taking the case to court is that they must now pay the costs of both sides. As this can be a large sum of money the plaintiff may be awarded £50,000 damages, but end up with nothing at all. If however, the judge awards more than what has been paid in, then the defendant will be obliged to pay the costs of both sides. So, if they 'paid in' £40,000 and the legal fees of each side are £25,000, and the judge awards £50,000 then they will be faced with a bill for £50,000 damages plus £25,000 for each of the legal fees, a total bill of £100,000. It is therefore clear that the stakes for both sides are very high at this stage.

Legal aid and contingency

It can be seen that litigation is a very expensive business and legal fees for both sides in medical negligence frequently run into tens or hundreds of thousands of pounds. Solicitors charge by the hour and have a lot of work to do interviewing their clients, gathering information, and collating statements, and explaining what is happening to their clients. Barristers then prepare the brief (the argument on which the case will be based). They will also stand up in court and argue the case to the judge. Most patients cannot afford a solicitor's fees to draw up a claim or the barrister's charges to prepare and present the brief, nor can they afford to lose a case. There are two routes open to them. If they can demonstrate that they are quite poor and that they have a reasonable prospect of winning their case, then they will receive 'legal aid'. This means that the government will pay the cost of their legal fees to enable them to take the case forward. If however they are not poor enough for legal aid, they must either foot the cost themselves, or persuade a solicitor and barrister to take on the case on a 'contingency basis'. This means that if they lose, then the solicitor and barrister will not charge. In return for the lawyers carrying this risk, a contract will be drawn up which will give the solicitors and the barrister to take a significant proportion of the claim if the plaintiff wins.

Unrealistic expectations

Most patients say that they do not embark on the litigation for the money, and that is probably true for most at the start, but as the case drags on, it is inevitable that the plaintiff's eyes will be drawn to newspaper headlines of massive pay-outs in medical negligence cases, without realizing that these high value claims involve lifetime care (brain-damaged patients) or long-term loss of high earnings (specialist workers who cannot retrain). They also conveniently forget about costs. As a result very few medical negligence litigants end up satisfied with the outcome of the court case. Some say that all they wanted was a bit of transparency and a fulsome apology. Most say that the main hope was to use their case to make sure that no one else had to go through the suffering they had been subjected to ('never again'). Many are angry at the delays involved in processing a claim. 'Justice delayed is justice denied.' Others are struck by the unfairness of having to prove 'breach of care', 'causation', and 'consequence' before damages are payable. All are incensed by the huge costs of legal fees. It is therefore a good idea for both surgeon and patient that litigation is avoided wherever possible, and other possibilities for the patient to feel vindicated are explored.

Alternative routes which dissatisfied patients may take and serious complaints

Many patients genuinely do not want to make money out of their misfortune, and are aware that pursuing a medico-legal claim may prove deeply unsatisfactory. Trusts have therefore set up various mechanisms to enable patients to get a good 'listening to', a 'proper apology', and a promise that every effort will be made to ensure that this does not 'ever happen again'. When these complaints systems are run without delay and competently they undoubtedly benefit the patient by giving them what they want, as well as benefiting the hospital by saving on legal fees and providing a powerful source of information on how the service can be improved.

Reporting to the General Medical Council

If a patient makes a serious complaint against you, then they may decide to report you to the GMC. In this case the GMC will almost always try to refer the case back to local arbitration and complaints handling mechanisms in the first instance, as the truth is that most complaints against doctors can and should be handled locally. If however, the complaint is very serious and/or multiple and local mechanism have been exhausted or are not appropriate, then documentation will be gathered and placed with a team of doctors known as screeners. They will read through the papers and decide whether there is a case to answer under the guidelines of 'Good Medical Practice'. If they do decide that there is a case to answer, then you will be referred to the Interim Orders committee who will decide whether you need to be suspended immediately for the safety of the public and/or whether any restrictions need to be placed on what you can do (you make be required to stop doing that particular operation until the situation is resolved). You will now need to instruct solicitors to defend you (this will be a medical defence society if you are a member). The GMC will then hold a hearing, which is similar to a court case. You will be the defendant. The GMC has its own lawyers to present the case, and a panel listen to the arguments of the GMC and your side then decide on the 'balance of probabilities' whether your behaviour has fallen below acceptable levels. If it has, then they have a range of options. They can give you a warning, or they can suspend you for a period of time. This suspension may be accompanied by a requirement that you undergo some remedial training before you return to practice. Finally, they can strike you off the medical register. It is estimated that during your career one in four doctors will be reported to the GMC. However, the vast majority of cases will either be resolved locally or it will be found by the screeners that there is no case to answer.

Coroner's court

Her Majesty's coroner must be informed if there is a sudden or untoward death. In the first instance the coroner's office will decide if any action needs to be taken, and in most cases they will decide that nothing needs to be done. Nevertheless they must be informed and the decision is theirs.

If, however, there is some doubt about how the death occurred or disquiet amongst the relatives the coroner will arrange for a hearing to try to determine the cause of death. You will be required to provide a statement to the coroner about your involvement in the patient's care and the coroner will then decide whether you are required to attend the hearing. If you are required to attend make sure that you take the hospital notes with you as you may be asked to refer to these to support your evidence. It is at this moment, above all others, that you will passionately wish that you had written clearer, more frequent, and clearer notes on the progress of your patient.

The coroner will then give a judgment on what was the cause of death and whether this constituted an accident, unknown, manslaughter, or murder. The results of the coroner's judgment can be used both by you and your patient if they decide to pursue legal action.

Conflict resolution

Conflict between staff is common in a high stress environment. Once established, it can then prove very disruptive indeed to the efficient running of the department. Very few individuals actively seek conflict but the pressures of ambition and of work may lead people to say and do things, which cause upset. It is a truism that conflict can usually be traced back to one of three things—money, status, and sex. In the health service it is status, which most frequently leads to dispute.

First phase

Breakdown in communication

The seeds of conflict lie in breakdown of communication. There can be many reasons for this. It may be that someone feels that they are too busy to communicate (in other words they do not feel that communication is important). Communication may also fail when someone is doing something they are not sure their colleagues agree with. Rather than having an open discussion and risking losing the argument, they may decide to proceed without discussion and hope that the others will not notice. The other members of the team will eventually find out, and when they do, they will be upset and angry that things are being done behind their backs, and the seeds of disruption will be germinating.

Loss of respect

Once there is a breakdown in communication, misunderstandings inevitably arise. Because there is now no communication, these cannot be resolved at an early stage when it would be easy to do so (see 'Handling a complaint'). Grievance festers. Irritation becomes annoyance. Annoyance becomes rage. Anger leads to loss of respect and now individuals feel justified in doing things that they would not do to people whom they respect. The result is conflict backed by justifiable rage on both sides about how the other side has behaved.

Defusing conflict

If any attempt is to be made to resolve the conflict then both parties must want this to happen. If they are still too angry to consider trying to resolve the situation, then no attempt should be made to try to resolve the situation through a meeting of the parties. Instead a third party trusted by both sides may be needed to act as a go-between, clarifying any misunderstandings. If this phase cannot produce enough lowering of the anger levels for a meeting to be possible, then one or both parties are being unreasonable and behaving in an unprofessional way. The only way out will be for one or both parties to leave the unit.

If, however, this third party communication resolves some of the misunderstandings it should be possible for both parties to see that resolution of the conflict would be in the best interests of both parties and of the service they are trying to provide. It is at this point that a meeting between the two should be considered.

The meeting

There may need to be a series of meetings before the whole situation can be resolved, but at the first meeting there is important work to be done. The meeting will need to be chaired by someone who has the respect and trust of both sides. If the conflict is complex, then one or both of the parties may wish to have others with them to support them emotionally or with facts. If one party has more than one representative then it is best if the other party has the same. Otherwise they may feel threatened.

Purpose of the meeting and ground rules

At the start of the meeting the chair will need to summarize the reason for the meeting and then lay out and agree ground rules. The ground rules are important as without them a meeting like this can do more harm than good:

- **One at a time** The first ground rule is that only one person should speak at a time and that the chair will decide who speaks. This reduces the chance of a shouting match
- **No bad manners** The second rule is that no bad language, bad manners, shouting or rudeness and insults will be tolerated, and that the chairman has the right to terminate the meeting immediately if this occurs
- **Time out** The third rule is that either party has the right to stop the meeting at any stage if they feel that they do not want to continue

Second phase

Wish for resolution

At this stage the chair needs to check that both parties genuinely wish to seek resolution of the conflict. If there is any hesitation or qualification by either or both the meeting should be adjourned forthwith as it is doomed to fail. It may be necessary to lay out to both sides the consequences of failing to resolve the grievance. As mentioned before, this might include disciplinary action against all parties.

Grievances

Each of the parties should now be invited to lay out what they think has happened or been done that has led to the grievance. Each of the statements should be qualified at the start with 'I feel that…' or 'I believe that…'. They should not be direct accusations such as 'You said' or 'You did' as the facts of the matter have not yet been determined and so an accusation might be both unjust and inflammatory. Each person should have an opportunity to express all their grievances without any response from the other side. This is important because resolution cannot be explored until all grievances are aired.

Hidden grievances

There are almost always grievances which are too embarrassing to express, either because the person realizes that they are stupid and/or unjustified. Both parties must now be warned that these grievances must be expressed now and if they are not, then they must be dropped. New problems cannot be raised later in the process.

Third phase

Clarification

The list of grievances forms the agenda for the next part of the meeting. Each needs to be picked over to discover if this is merely a misunderstanding, due to lack of communication, or whether it is a genuine cause for annoyance. Those which are misunderstandings need the agreement of the person who misunderstood it for this item to be crossed off the list. Those in which it is agreed that there is a genuine cause for upset require an apology from the person who caused it.

There will then be left a hard-core of issues where the parties cannot agree whether there was a misunderstanding or an insult. These are usually very few in number, and it can often be agreed that now that the bulk of problems have been resolved, the remainder are not enough to be grounds for a conflict. This stage may need more than one meeting especially if time-out needs to be taken. It is at this point that negotiation becomes crucial.

Fourth phase

Emotional versus pragmatic versus logical

When discussions like this are taking place individuals tend to argue in one of three domains 'emotional', 'pragmatic', and 'rational'. Emotional arguers start their arguments with phrases such as 'I feel' and talk about principles and fairness. Pragmatic arguers use phrases like 'practical solution', 'compromise' and 'what works'. Logical arguers inevitably revert to 'what is the scientific evidence' for this. If two people in conflict are arguing in different domains (and they usually are) then both need to be drawn out of their comfort domain so that they are prepared to reconsider their position. For example, a person arguing in the emotional domain should be asked to consider the evidence (logical) or what will actually work on the ground (pragmatic). Logical people and pragmatists should be asked how they feel about the position that they are taking. When reading this you may feel that the pragmatic approach is obviously the best. This may be because the culture where you were brought up is predominantly pragmatic (British people are renowned for their pragmatism). Some claim that the French are equally famous for their logical nature, while the Germans have a strong emotional streak.

Resolution of intractable issues

One technique which can be used for intractable problems are known as Harvard negotiating rules. These are especially valuable when negotiating and no agreement can be made without coercion. The first rule is that if one side is 'compelled' to accept the terms of the other side, then they will consciously or unconsciously work to get their own back and will sour the deal in the long term. In order to get agreement from both sides it is important first to explore with both sides how far they are prepared to give ground in the hope of obtaining a settlement. If this does not resolve the situation because there is no common ground, then a good negotiator uses their imagination to find other issues over which ground can be given by each party to the other in order that both feel able to give ground on the central issue. For example, two consultants may be in conflict, and the final issue over which there is no resolution is that the senior consultant insists that he should do less 'on call' than the junior one. If he is compelled to do more on call it will be inevitable that he will not fulfil his duties properly and refuse to see his colleague's patients when he is on call etc. This will just lead to a new conflict. An alternative solution which might be acceptable to both would be the suggestion that as the young consultant has school age children, the older consultant will provide cover over Christmas and give the younger consultant first choice of holiday dates during school holidays. That is what is called a win/win solution. Both have got some important compromises, which are useful to them.

Setting up routes for good communication

If resolution has been reached, then the next stage is to put in place mechanisms to prevent a new toxic cycle of breakdown in communication. This may involve arrangements such as a weekly meeting to review issues arising in the department. If there is any likelihood that these meetings will fall into abeyance then there needs to be a mechanism put into place to ensure that this does not happen.

Scenarios

Scenario 1

One of your trainees has had a complaint made against him that he failed to come to see a patient in a timely manner when he was on call. The daughter claims that her mother was left in pain for 6 hours because he would not come to the ward to see her. This actor is your junior. Discuss with him how he should handle a complaint.

Scenario 2

You have invited a patient's daughter to a meeting to discuss a complaint that you failed to come to see her mother in a timely manner when you were on call. She claims that her mother was left in pain for 6 hours because you would not come to the ward to see her. This actor is the daughter. Carry out the initial conversation with the daughter.

Scenario 3

You have invited a patient's daughter to a meeting to discuss a complaint that you failed to come to see her mother in a timely manner when you were on call. The lady claims that her mother was left in pain for 6 hours because you would not come to the ward to see her. You have clarified the facts and apologized for the errors made that night. This actor is the daughter. Carry out the next part of a 'Complaint meeting'.

Scenario 4

There has been a row between a staff nurse on the ward and one of the FY1 doctors, and now the staff nurse has complained to sister that the doctor is rude. The doctor has gone to his consultant and complained that the staff nurse is lazy, insolent, and does not look after the patients properly. It is clear that this row has been brewing for some time and that this current spat is just the culmination of an escalating situation. You have set up a meeting between the two, which you are now going to chair. Please carry out the initial part of this meeting.

Scenario 5

There has been a row between a staff nurse on the ward and one of the FY1 doctors, and now the staff nurse has complained to sister that the doctor is rude. The doctor has gone to his consultant and complained that the staff nurse is lazy, insolent, and does not look after the patients properly. It is clear that this row has been brewing for some time and that this current spat is just the culmination of an escalating situation. You have set up a meeting between the two, where you have now reached the second phase—clarification. Please carry out this part of this meeting with the two actors here.

Scenario 6

A colleague comes to you very worried because he has just been told that he is being sued. This actor here is your colleague. Explain to him as much as you know about how litigation works

Scenario 7

A colleague comes to you to ask your advice because he has just been told that he is being reported to the GMC. This actor here is your colleague. Explain to him as much as you know about how disciplinary action at the GMC works

Answers

Scenario 1

You may want to try to put the trainee at ease a little to start with as they are likely to be distraught about a complaint especially if it is the first that they have ever received.

You then need to explain that the complaint needs to be 'acknowledged' as quickly as possible, and a decision needs to be made who will do this and what will be said (the patient needs to be assured that the complaint is being taken seriously and will be investigated immediately).

Then there needs to be a discussion about the information which needs to be gathered. Is there any record in the nursing notes when they were called, what was said, and when you attended? Was anyone else involved? What other problems were holding things up at the time, etc.?

Finally, there needs to be a discussion about whether this complaint needs a meeting or can be managed by a phone call and/or letter. If there is to be a meeting then a plan needs to be made on how that is going to be organized quickly, and who needs to be present.

Scenario 2

Welcome the daughter. Introduce yourself and everyone else in the room explaining their role and reason for being there. Make sure that the daughter understands why the meeting is being held (the complaint that it relates to) and that the purpose of the meeting is first of all transparency to clarify what happened that night, clearing up any possible misapprehensions or misunderstandings.

Listening—the daughter should now be invited to explain in full (and without interruption) what she thinks happened that night.

Clarification—with careful reference to contemporary notes (nursing and doctor's notes) clarify and explain (without being defensive) any areas where you feel the daughter might not have understood what was happening.

Apology—if there are areas where an apology is owing this should now be made without reservation. If there is still disagreement about the facts do not use the phrase 'I am sorry that you feel this way'. It is insulting and inflammatory.

Scenario 3

You now need to discuss with the patient how you plan to take action to try to make sure that anything which was unsatisfactory does not happen again. This may be achieved by improving communication

You may wish to go forward to ask how you can try to make amends to the patient and/or the daughter for what has happened. It may be that a personal letter will be all that is required, but some flowers or chocolates might help.

Scenario 4

You need to introduce yourself and check that both know why this meeting is being held.

You then need to check whether both are certain that they want to resolve this situation. If they are not sure, then you should not proceed until they are. It may help if you explain to them the consequences for each of them if the other lodges a complaint and the complaint is upheld.

Only if there is absolute agreement from both can you proceed to the next stage, which is laying out ground rules. These are that there are to be no insults. Only one person is to speak at a time, and that if either side feels that they want to stop proceedings to take a 'breather' they have only to say. Only once these are agreed can you proceed to ask each to lay out fully their grievances about the other.

Scenario 5

You have got agreement on ground rules and now need each side to lay out *all* their grievances. It should be explained to them that no new grievances can be introduced after this stage. Once all the grievances are out, it is time to discuss each and to discover whether they are a result of a misunderstanding or misinformation (clarify), or of misbehaviour, which merits an apology. If resolution on any issue cannot be obtained move into Harvard negotiating rules and find inventive options which lead to a win/win solution. Once you have got agreement on ground rules and have dealt with grievances. You now need each side to confirm that all issues are now resolved, and then makes arrangements that this cannot happen again by making sure that regular meetings take place to prevent minor irritations from growing into grievances.

Scenario 6

Explain that this happens to all of us. The hospital's legal department will ask for a statement on which to base their response to any claim. He should tell the truth about what happened and refer to any notes or records at that time to support what he believes happened. He should not try to cover things up. We all make mistakes and if a mistake has been made then it is best to be open about it.

A medical expert will read his statement and the notes and then advise whether there is a case to answer. Hospital lawyers will decide whether to fight or settle. This is not his decision and he may not agree with that decision, which may be made on financial not clinical grounds. The Hospital Trust will pay the damages. Although he should try to learn from what has happened, he should not take it too much to heart.

Scenario 7

The GMC will try to get issues sorted out locally wherever possible, so the Trust will be asked to resolve this locally using their complaint mechanisms and the Medical Director if at all possible.

Screeners will decide if complaint is severe enough to warrant investigation by GMC. If the case is though to be serious there will be a hearing, where he will have legal representation.

Chapter 11 **Consent, confidentiality, and information management**

Introduction

It cannot be emphasized enough that recording clear, concise, but comprehensive notes are the hallmark of a top professional. You may feel on many occasions that you are 'too busy' to write in the notes, but this reflects a lack of understanding of your role as a professional, which is to assess, act, and record what you have done so that others can continue your work seamlessly and at the same level. This is even more important these days, since the reduction in surgeons' working hours has made the process of handover a regular part of every day. Writing in the notes is also a good opportunity to stop and reflect on what you have done, and what needs to be done next. One of the commonest causes of severe errors in airline pilots has been shown to be the failure to pause and reconsider the information coming in before continuing along the same path.[1] Surgeons are no different in this respect.

Ward notes (mnemonic SOAP)

This is the area where a doctor's deficiencies show most clearly in the courts. Notes are too often incomplete, illegible, incorrect, and infrequent. Each time that you speak to a patient, you should try to record this in the notes. All patients should be seen at pre-admission, and on admission. So there should be notes on both these encounters. They should be seen on the same day after surgery, and at least once a day until discharge. This is the minimum set of notes required.

Structuring ward notes

The note should start with the date and time, your name in block letters, and your bleep number.

Mnemonic SOAP

A simple structure for ward notes is SOAP:

S Subjective. This is a record of how the patient feels. It might include how well they slept, whether they are feeling dry or nauseated, how bad their pain is, whether they are having problems passing water.

O Objective. This is a record of relevant observations since the last medical input. These will include basic observations if abnormal (temperature, pulse, and respiration), special observations (e.g. distal neurovascular status or volume in drains), and the results of any investigations (laboratory and imaging) which have now been received.

A Assessment. This is the conclusion, which you draw from the patient's report on their condition (S), and the results which you have to hand (O). It might simply be 'Doing fine' or it might be 'Possible wound infection'.

P Plan. This records the actions that you propose to take as a result of your assessment. This might include a wound swab, blood tests, blood cultures, and increased observations of the patient. These can be ticked in the notes, once the relevant action has been taken.

Informed consent (mnemonic LED TO REASON)

Introduction

It is a key right of the individual in a free society that, wherever possible, their wishes about how they should be treated are to be respected.

Surgery is a powerful tool for good, but can also cause harm. Surgeons must therefore obtain permission from patients before doing any operation on them, however minor. This is both a requirement in law and an integral part of practice as a good doctor.

[1] Beaty D (1991). *The Naked Pilot. The Human Factor in Aircraft Accidents*. London: Methuen.

This section discusses what needs to be done to obtain this permission and why. It also deals with some situations where obtaining the patient's permission may be complicated or impossible.

Informed consent is one grade higher than simple consent, as it means that the patient understands the key issues on which they are giving consent, not simply agreeing to something in ignorance. Clearly, it is unlikely that the patient will be able to understand all the subtleties of the information on which a rational decision can be made but the patient must be given as much information as they want, and this must be presented in a way which is clear (to them) and unbiased.

In current British practice it is not necessary for the doctor performing surgery to take the consent, but the person doing so (who may be a junior doctor) **must** be competent to perform the operation if they are to take consent.

Once again, current British law does not require that you have to tell the patient everything about the operation. Some patients become very frightened if you dwell on all the gory details of the operation and then enumerate all the complications. In fact you may actually harm them if you insist on telling them all these things against their wishes. So before you go into details, check with patient how much they already know and how much more they want to know.

If for any reason the patient is not able to give consent, then British law insists that you must act in the patient's 'best interest'.

In either case you need to record at the time (contemporary notes) what you said and did. These notes will be the cornerstone of your defence if you find yourself in court defending yourself against a patient who is claiming that you did not consent them adequately and that therefore your operation was an 'assault'.

A simple system for taking a comprehensive consent is cued by the simple acronym **LED TO REASON**:

L	Lead in.	Introduce yourself. Check the patient's name. Explain what you are doing and by what authority. Note that you should only be taking consent if you are the surgeon performing the operation, or if you are yourself also competent to do this procedure.
E	Explore.	Find out how much the patient already knows, and how much they want to know. It is pointless going over things that they already know. Equally it is unnecessarily frightening for the patient to go into lurid detail, when they would much rather not know.
D	Diagnosis.	Make sure they know the diagnosis for which the operation is being proposed.
T	Treatment.	Explain what you are proposing to do in as much or little detail as they want, using simple non-technical language. If you are working to standard guidelines then you need to confirm this. If you are not, then you need to explain how your treatment differs and why.
O	Options.	Discuss any options. This will include the option of doing nothing.
R	Results.	Explain what the outcome is going to be. (How long will it be painful? Will they be able to return to normal activities?) If there are options being discussed, then the results of these too need to be explained.
E	Eventualities.	Are there any extra things, which may need to be done? If there are extra actions which may need to be taken depending on what needs to be done, then these must be mentioned here. For example, the possibility of needing to remove the testicle in a hernia repair needs to be discussed, if only for the patient to say that under no circumstances will they allow this to happen.
A	Adverse events.	What could go wrong and what precautions are you taking to avoid these? (General such as heart attack, stroke, and embolus, local such as bleeding, and special such as damage to the ilio-inguinal nerve in a hernia operation.)

S Sound mind.   A patient can only give *informed* consent if they have a) been told the relevant information, b) taken it in, c) been able to think about it, and d) express their views. Asking the patient to feedback to you what they have understood from your discussion is a quick way of checking that they have the mental capacity to give informed consent.

O Open question.   Check to see if any clarification is needed, or doubts remain.

N Notes.   Record what has been discussed and agreed, specifically any special complications relevant to this patient which you have explained.

Consenting children—Gillick

The problem of whether children can consent to treatment without, or even against, their parents' wishes is a thorny one, which has not really been clearly laid out in British law as yet. This is because British law is based on 'precedent', in other words judgment on similar cases which have been decided before, and in the case of consent by or for children there have not been judgments by the courts on cases that will cover the major issues faced by surgeons. What is clear is that after the age of 16 years a child, is deemed an adult in terms of the law relating to consent and confidentiality, and can consent to or refuse treatment whatever their parents say. Even more importantly they can refuse to allow parents access to their notes. You would therefore be breaking the law if you discussed a young person's case with their parents in any way without their express permission. Below the age of 16 the situation becomes less clear, and the judgment on which current law is based is called 'Gillick'. There is more than one judgment on this particular case which revolves round whether a child can be prescribed the contraceptive pill against their parents' wishes, and indeed without their parents' knowledge. The short judgment by Lord Scarman is that:

> As a matter of Law the parental right to determine whether or not their minor child below the age of sixteen will have medical treatment terminates if and when the child achieves sufficient understanding and intelligence to understand fully what is proposed.

So the law as far as it has been clarified suggests that if the child is old enough to understand the issues that they are consenting to, then their wishes on consent are paramount and over-rule those of their parents. In fact, in most cases, where a major conflict has arisen, it has been between the parents and the doctors, and it has been felt that the child is not fully competent. In these circumstances the child has been made a ward of court and the court has decided on the best interests of the child.

Where informed consent is not possible—acting in best interest

If a patient is demented, confused, or unconscious, it is clear that they are not able to give an informed decision on consent. In these cases you have to act in the best interest of the patient. In other words you have to consider what you think will be best for that patient. That decision will be helped if you can gain any insight into what the patient's wishes would have been had they been able to express them. It may be advisable to seek the views of the relatives, not to hear what they think should be done, but to find out what they know about the wishes of the patient. If you are not happy that the decision being put forward by relatives of an 'incompetent' patient is not actually in that patient's best interests, then you may apply to a court to have the patient made a 'ward of court' and for the decision about their best interests to be made by that court.

Clinical trials

Research is critical to improve surgery but it is difficult to perform. We should not bring in new techniques without first testing whether they improve outcomes and/or reduce risks and complications. Many new ideas, passionately advocated by their inventors who genuinely believe in the benefits, turn out to be valueless or even harmful when checked out properly. The gold standard for determining whether a new treatment is better than what went before is a randomized controlled trial. The new treatment is compared against the current best and accepted practice. Trials are expensive and time-consuming to perform but they need very careful planning if they are not to prove valueless.

Formulating the research question

This statement is usually in the form of a 'null' hypothesis, e.g. the new X surgical approach is not better in avoiding complications than the standard Y operation. The experiment is then designed to challenge that null hypothesis:

- Inclusion criteria—these define the group from which you are going to recruit your patients and should be as wide as possible so that you can recruit adequate numbers as quickly as possible
- Exclusion criteria—if the variability of the patients in the study is large then the results will be 'confounded' by effects caused by differences between patients. Exclusion criteria are designed to remove patients whose results will not help the study. They can be extremes of age, different diagnoses, or even gender

Randomization

The way in which it is decided which treatment each patient is to receive must be completely removed (blinded) from the control of anyone involved in doing the surgery or assessing the results. This is to ensure that any chance of bias is removed,

Outcome

Similarly the people involved in assessing the results should also be 'blinded' to the treatment, which the patient has received if, once again, the chance of bias is to be removed. This is called double blinding. Ideally, only once the results of the surgery have been evaluated can the code be broken. This is very difficult in a surgical trial as the incision, or the X-ray will often give the game away.

'P' value

The statistical analysis involves testing the 'null' hypothesis which is that there is no difference between the two treatments. Actually there is always some difference but the 'p' value tells us how likely it is that this difference has occurred by chance. Usually a 'p' value of <0.05 is accepted as making it probable that we can believe that there is a real difference between the new treatment and the old, and so discard the null hypothesis.

Consent to trial

Any patient who is to be asked to enter a trial will need to have the purpose of the trial explained to them, if they are to make a rational decision whether to enter or not. They also need to be told that they are free to decline to enter the trial if that consent is indeed to be valid.

Medical records

Writing an operation note

An operation note is important because it is a unique record of what a surgeon saw and did at operation, and because it is a legal document which will be needed in a court action as a contemporary record of what happened at the time of surgery. It is also a truism that good surgeons write good operation notes.

An operation note needs to be legible. For this reason some surgeons arrange to have them typewritten. If you do this then the definitive typed note will need to be supported by a hand-written note written immediately after surgery as the recovery room staff and the ward staff will need to know at once what has happened and what is planned.

The operation note described below may appear over long, especially in relation to operation notes which you have seen written by your seniors. The reason for suggesting this is that writing an operation note in this way is a very good way of learning how to do operations well (leaving out no important steps) and is crucial for presenting descriptions of operations at exams like the MRCS. You will, however, only really be convinced of the value of a good operation note when you have to stand in Her Majesty's Coroners Court or in the High Court justifying your actions as a professional.

Structure of an operation note

Date, place, and time These need to be recorded clearly at the top of the note.

Names The name of the patient (a sticky label is best), the surgeon, the anaesthetist, and any assistants need to be written in block capital (not a signature).

Indications The patient's diagnosis and indications for surgery next need recording, e.g. osteoarthritis of all three compartments of the left knee.

Position, preparation, and anaesthetic This describes any special position used for the patient. For example, it is important to mention if a tourniquet was used, or lithotomy stirrups were used to position the patient. All devices have complications and if you note that they were used and that the appropriate protective measures were taken, then your position as a competent professional is secure. If an anaesthetist has administered a general or regional anaesthetic then this will all be covered in their notes, but if the surgeon administers local anaesthetic then this must be covered here.

Incision and exposure It is probably best not to use acronyms to describe incisions, as one person's Kocher's incision may not be the same as another. Better to describe where the incision is centred, its length, and whether it is straight or curved. Better still, draw it.

Exposure will define the structures parted, divided, or protected during the first part of the surgery. The surest way of protecting a nerve is to identify it, expose it through the length of the incision, and then protect it. For example, in the posterior approach to the hip joint the sciatic nerve is at risk. It should be identified and exposed through its length. The short external rotators should then be divided and folded back over it, so that a retractor can then be used to protect it.

Findings The findings should hopefully confirm your diagnosis but may also determine the actual procedure that you perform. Therefore the pathology found, its severity and its extent should all be recorded, as this will both justify your decision to operate and explain your subsequent care plan.

Procedure Surgeons vary in how much detail they give here but if there are critical stages where there are decisions to be made and checked, then these must be recorded. For example, it is important in surgery for a pertrochanteric fracture of the neck of femur that the guidewire lies central in the femoral neck and that the correct cannulated drill length is set. It therefore needs to be recorded that the guidewire was centrally positioned (as checked on two views of the image intensifier) and that measurement indicated that the drill should be set at X millimetres.

In a knee replacement it is critical to check that when the trial (test) implants are inserted, the knee is correctly aligned, has a full range of movement, and is stable to varus/valgus and anteroposterior draw throughout its range before the definitive implants are chosen and inserted.

Tidying up and final check If the wound is to be washed out or the tourniquet deflated and haemostasis obtained before closure or the patency of a graft tested once more, then these checks which relate to patient safety should be noted.

Closure The type and method of closure should be described. This may include the dressing if a special type was used and any final checks which are made after the drapes are removed. If a tourniquet has been used this would include noting the time that the tourniquet was deflated and the fact that the distal circulation had returned. The same distal check would be critical at the end of a vascular procedure. You should also check under the diathermy pad and over any pressure areas although neither of these need recording in the notes unless a problem is experienced.

Post-operatively Once again there is some variation in surgeon's notes here. Some will merely record 'Routine' if they have been doing the same operation in the same hospital for many years, but for a trainee surgeon this is once again an opportunity to reflect on and record who needs to know what.

- The recovery staff need to know what observations you require and how frequently. They also need to know what recording is so abnormal that it requires action and if so what action. They also need to know any special precautions that they need to take. For example, you should want the recovery staff to open up any vacuum drains at 15 minutes after the end of surgery and then to inform you if the drain fills with >500ml of blood in the first half hour. Patients who have had a hip replacement will need to be nursed with a abduction pillow between their legs to reduce the risk of dislocation

- The ward staff will need to know how often observations need to be performed, when drains and stitches need to be removed, when a check X-ray is needed, and when the patient can first get up
- If the patient is a day case, you will wish to record the criteria for discharging the patient, e.g. provided the patient's pain is adequately controlled they can go home, and need an outpatient appointment in 2 weeks

Phoning your consultant at home—the 5 Ps

Proper preparation prevents poor performance. This is a well-known adage for all professions. It also applies to ringing your consultant at home, but the 5 Ps stand for something else as well. Purpose, patient, problem, plan, purpose. If you want the correct response from your consultant when you ring him/her at home, and you want them to consider that you are behaving in a highly professional way, then you need to plan out the call before you make it, ensuring that you have all the information to hand that the consultant will need.

Purpose

The first question you need to address in your plan is the purpose of your call. Do you want your consultant to:

- 'Be aware' of what is happening, e.g. the patient they operated on today appears to have had a heart attack and has been taken over by the physicians
- Confirm that you are doing the right thing, e.g. you are giving a blood transfusion to a total hip replacement whose blood pressure and urine output has dropped a little, and who lost 800ml of blood into the drain, but has stopped draining now
- Advise you on what to do, e.g. a patient has become confused after abdominal surgery and is now pulling out all their drips and drains
- Come in to manage the case. The aortic aneurism which they repaired this afternoon has dropped their blood pressure and urine output and appears to be bleeding

Patient

The second phase of the conversation will be to give the basic details:

- Who is the patient?
- What is their age and diagnosis?
- What is to be, or has been done?

Problem

The third phase is what has now happened which has prompted this call.

Plan

What have you done so far? For example, what investigations have been sent and what results are back? What options have you considered, and what do you think are their pros and cons?

Purpose

The final task is to repeat for the consultant what it is that you are asking for, repeating the request which you made at the start of the conversation.

Referrals to another team

Referrals will usually be made by phone but when that team arrives to give their opinion it is professional courtesy to have everything ready for them. A summary note will make their job quicker and easier as well as more likely to deliver what you need.

The note should start by thanking them, and then lay out clearly what is the purpose of the referral. Do you want the patient to be taken over, or just some advice on their care? Next, the background to the problem needs to be given, providing only the information relevant to their needs. This may need careful thought as the information that they need may be very different from what we as surgeons may consider important. The results of all tests and investigations performed should then be presented with a time-line if change in condition over time is important. Investigations which have been performed but which are not yet back need noting. The outcome of any attempts at treatment and the results also need recording. A well-written referral should give all the information needed in logical order and without any extraneous information.

Discharge summaries

When you transfer the care of a patient to a medical team it is both courteous and critical that they should know what you have done and what you want them to do. The note may be short but comprehensive so that the transition of care can be seamless (see Table 11.1).

Table 11.1 The ideal succinct discharge summary

What	Example
Your name, your team. Contact details. Patient name	Dr Jones bleep 2447 ST3 to Mr Datta
	Patient: Edwin Falconer 12/8/1951
Date of discharge from where to where	6 November 2009 from Morris ward to home
What was done and when	Left cemented Exeter total hip replacement 1/11/2009
Problem	Developed atrial fibrillation post-op. Started on digoxin
What if	Fell and dislocated hip day 2. Uneventful relocation. Needs referral to the emergency department immediately if he feels it is coming out again
Review	Out patients 6 weeks. X-ray on arrival

Complex tasks

Brain death

Brain death is defined as a situation where the patient no longer has any brain function so that although they are being kept alive with the help of artificial ventilation, they are no longer a sentient human being. In order to make this decision it must be determined that there is no brain activity, and that there is no likelihood of any developing in the future. It is not the same as 'persistent vegetative state' (PVS) where the brainstem is still working even though the cerebral cortices are not. In PVS there is a small chance of recovery. In brain death there is none, provided that the tests to determine its presence have been properly performed.

Preparation

Tests for brainstem death should not be performed if there is any factor which might be suppressing the measurement of brain function. Patients who are hypothermic or under the influence of high doses of drugs such as alcohol, morphine, or barbiturates may appear to have suffered brain death when they have not. It is therefore a requirement first to make sure that the patient's core temperature is above 32°C and that there are only low levels of any drugs in their bloodstream which might suppress the measurement of brain function. Time is a second safety precaution. Brain death should not be diagnosed hastily after a major brain insult, and so it is usual to repeat all tests a further 24 hours after an initial check, just to be certain that the suppression of brain function is not transitory.

The second way of ensuring reliable diagnosis of brainstem death is the use of more than one test, all of which must point to brain death before any conclusion can be drawn.

The brainstem tests

Coma

The patient should be unresponsive to painful stimuli. Probably the best test is pressure on the supra-orbital nerve in the medial part of the supra-orbital ridge.

Brainstem reflexes

- **Pupillary reflex**—the pupil should be mid-dilated and unresponsive to light
- **Oculocephalic reflex**—the eyes should not move when the head is rolled rapidly from side-to-side
- **Vestibular reflex**—the head is raised to 30° to tilt the horizontal canal to vertical; 50ml of ice cold water is injected into the external auditory meatus and there should be no eye movements
- **Facial reflexes**—there should be no response to stimulating the cornea (with a throat swab), or applying firm pressure over the temporomandibular joint. The jaw reflex should also be absent
- **Bulbar reflexes**—there should be no cough reflex on sucking out the trachea down to the carina

Apnoea test

The patient is pre-oxygenated and then disconnected from the ventilator. If there is no sign of any attempt at breathing and the pCO_2 has reached 60, then brainstem death can be diagnosed.

Organs for transplantation

Organs can only be taken for transplantation from a patient who is legally dead. In the case of patients who are on ventilators, the diagnosis of brainstem death must be made first. Then the organs may be removed but the ventilator may be left on to maintain optimum oxygenation of organs for as long as possible. In Great Britain, permission must be sought from the next of kin for organs to be taken. The interview asking next of kin to consider allowing organ donation can be the one faint beacon of hope and light for the relatives in what may otherwise appear to be a tragic waste of a young life, so it should not be shirked.

Breaking bad news

This is a difficult and unhappy task and therefore tends to be postponed or never done at all. It is not good professional behaviour to shy away from unpleasant tasks. As a general rule they are best tackled right away. Then they no longer nag at the back of your mind as a task 'yet to be done'. Most of us find that unpleasant tasks are never quite so bad as you expect, and patients and their relatives frequently demonstrate the best of human nature when confronted by adversity.

Patients have a right to information about themselves, and just as justice delayed is justice denied, information withheld is effectively as bad as not giving it at all.

Breaking bad news is not a 'corridor conversation', so a quiet room needs to be found and adequate time set aside to discuss the situation without interruption. In order to avoid interruption phones should be switched off and bleeps should be handed to someone else to carry for the time being. If the person who is receiving the bad news is alone then it may be wise to tactfully invite them to have someone with them whom they trust. You may also wish to have someone with you who knows the patient well, such as the nurse in charge of the patient's care.

The meeting should start with introductions (as all meetings should) and an explanation of why the meeting is being held. It is then important to explore with the person (patient, relative, or both) how much they know and how much they want to know. If they are clear that they don't want to know anything more, then that view should be respected. On other occasions the patient/relative will save you the worry of telling them the diagnosis by confirming that they are pretty sure that they know anyway and that all they want is confirmation of their thoughts. However, for most the news will initially be devastating. In the first instance they are likely to go into denial so that there is little point in continuing the conversation until they have recovered from that. The second phase is usually sadness. This too needs respecting, and there is little point in giving any more information at this stage as they simply may not be able to take it in. What they may need at this stage is simple support in whatever way is possible.

The next phase of a grief reaction may be anger, and this can be directed in the most inappropriate directions. Luckily it does not usually last long, and it is finally replaced by resignation. At this stage information, advice, and support can be offered and it will be heard. It is always difficult to know what to say, and it is sometimes best to be guided by the person you are trying to help. If you listen to the cues, they will tell you want they want to know.

Scenarios

Scenario 1

This actor is going to act as your patient for the sake of this scenario; he is 70 years old and has osteoarthritis of his right hip, which is becoming increasingly painful. It has been decided to perform a standard cemented total hip replacement. Please take consent from him for this surgery. You are going to assist your consultant Dr. Y but have performed this operation yourself several times.

Scenario 2

A 14-year-old girl has a lipoma on her shoulder which is completely benign but which she finds cosmetically unacceptable. She has come to see you, without her parent's knowledge, and asked you to perform the operation. You have taken proper informed consent and she has understood the issues well and signed the consent form. Her parents have now got in touch with you having belatedly heard about what is proposed. They want to know what has been happening (their daughter refuses to talk to them) and forbid you to perform the surgery. The mother has now made an appointment to see you. Please carry out an appropriate discussion with them.

Scenario 3

An 85-year-old lady who has been in a home with dementia for some years is brought in after a fall. It is found that she has sustained a displaced fractured of femur, for which the ideal treatment is open reduction and internal fixation. The risk of mortality is probably 30% in 3 months. However, it is technically possible to treat this non-operatively but the treatment will involve a stay in hospital for many months, considerable pain, and a risk of death of probably 60% in 6 months. It is quite clear that the patient cannot give informed consent, but her daughter has come to meet you. She is the next-of-kin and she is adamant that she does not want her mother to have surgery because her father died of a heart attack after the same surgery some years before. Please carry out an appropriate discussion with her.

Scenario 4

An 18-year-old man is brought in after a high-speed RTA where he sustained multiple injuries including what subsequently turned out to be rupture of the liver and of the spleen. He was in coma secondary to hypovolaemic shock on arrival at hospital. His parents arrived at the hospital at the same time having heard that there had been a serious accident. They are implacably opposed to him being given any form of blood transfusion because they are Jehovah's Witnesses, and confirmed that their son is also a devoted Jehovah's Witness. Their religion absolutely forbids transfusion of blood. Please carry out the conversation that you would have with the parents.

Scenario 5

A 6-year-old child is brought in with what appears to be acute bowel obstruction. Her twin sister died 2 years before during surgery to try to correct a congenital malrotation of the bowel which had developed into a torsion. Since the loss of their first child the parents have become very deeply religious and are now convinced that they wish to rely on the power of prayer to cure their daughter. You have explained what you think is wrong and the consequences of not undertaking surgery as quickly as possible, but they have explained why they wish to rely on prayer. You are at an impasse. You have taken a quick break for both sides (you and the parents) to consider their position. You are now returning to the room, to continue the discussion and to reach resolution one way or the other as, unless surgery is undertaken soon, it will be too late for surgery to save her.

Scenario 6

A 25-year-old man is involved in a high-speed motorcycle accident where he sustained a tibial fracture. He subsequently develops a compartment syndrome but unfortunately the diagnosis and treatment was delayed and the decompression was not successful. After several attempts at reconstruction an amputation was performed. He was promised that the amputation would at least remove the pain, but he has been left with severe phantom pain and with a painful neuroma which has made fitting an artificial leg impossible for the moment. At the release of the compartment syndrome it appears that he suffered significant kidney damage from rhabdomyolysis and may need to go onto dialysis in the near future. The patient is very angry indeed about what has happened and is suing the driver of the car which hit him and the surgeon in charge of his case as he claims that the compartment syndrome was diagnosed late. He is also suing the surgeon who performed the amputation which appears to have left a neuroma.

He has now come to you for consideration of exploration and excision of the neuroma to try to control pain. You feel from your examination that this operation has a 70% chance of resolving the neuromatous pain and might even help the phantom pain, but could also make it worse. When you explain this to him, he states quite baldly that if he is made worse then he will start legal action against you too. Carry out the conversation that you would have with him from this point.

Scenario 7

A patient develops peritonitis following an episode of bowel necrosis with perforation. After a very stormy post-operative course where the wound became infected, the patient recovered but was left with a large and ugly incisional hernia. She has now come back to you 1 year later. Her marriage is in difficulties. She feels that this is because of the disfiguring hernia and wants you to re-operate to repair. You are aware that there will be severe adhesions and that this cosmetic operation may end up causing a new bowel perforation and at best a colostomy, at worst her death. You doubt that her difficulties with her marriage will necessarily be resolved by repair of this incisional hernia and feel that the risks of the surgery far outweigh any theoretical benefits. You have discussed this with her and sent her away to think about it. She has now returned, adamant that she wants the surgery to go ahead. You too have thought about and are even more certain than before that this surgery is not appropriate. Carry out the conversation that you would have with this patient.

Scenario 8

This telephone here is linked directly to another phone where your consultant is at home. It is 2am and you are going to phone him. At 1am you were called to the ward to see Mr Jones, a 70-year-old man, who was admitted for a total knee replacement 2 day ago and had a routine total knee first on the list yesterday. Post-operatively everything went fine. His observations during the day have been fine but he has only passed 100ml of urine all day despite having a urinary catheter in place. He seems to be becoming increasingly confused. His temperature is 38.0°C and he looks warm and flushed. Pulse is 100 and blood pressure 120/60. You have not taken down the dressing on his knee replacement as there is a strict protocol on the unit that dressings are not to be touched for 24 hours. However, the foot has normal pulses and sensation, and is not red or swollen. There is 250ml of blood in the drain. His chest is clear, ECG normal. Haemoglobin is 12, oxygen saturation is 98%, U&Es show a slightly raised creatinine, cardiac enzymes are normal, and you have sent off blood cultures. You have given a fluid challenge of 250ml of Hartmann's solution and his blood pressure has risen to 130/75. You propose start IV antibiotics, and to give analgesia, as well as putting him on oxygen and hourly observations. You don't think there is any need to put in a central line at this point but are concerned that he may be developing septic shock, and have informed the ITU outreach team who say that they will review him first thing in the morning.

Scenario 9

Write an operation note for an excision of sebaceous cyst on a patient's neck. Make up the details based on your experience

Scenario 10

A patient is 3 days post-op after a total knee replacement. You have been called to see the patient by the nursing staff because the wound is red and discharging. This is in fact an infected knee joint. Imagine what you might find when seeing the patient then write this up as a 'Ward Note'

Scenario 11

Write a discharge summary for a patient who has had a motorcycle accident on 10 April 2009 where he sustained an open left tibial fracture which was washed out and closed primarily and then fixed with a locked intramedullary nail. No post-operative problems apart from a low-grade pyrexia.

Scenario 12

You have admitted a 16-year-old patient who slipped backwards on some icy steps and hit his head. He was deeply unconscious on arrival and required endotracheal intubation. CT scan showed generalized brain contusion and multiple haemorrhages. He was admitted to the ICU 7 days ago but has shown no sign of recovery. The actor here is the patient's father who now knows that there is no hope of any recovery. Please explain to him the tests which now need to be done to determine brain death.

Scenario 13

You have admitted an 18-year-old patient who took an overdose of tricyclics 10 days ago, and has shown no sign of recovery. The tests for brainstem death have now been performed twice and there is no sign of any brain activity. You have arranged for his mother (Mrs. Jones) to come to see you (his father died of a stroke 2 years ago) to discuss switching off the ventilator and the possibility of removing organs for transplantation. You have already explained about the brainstem tests and now need to break the bad news, as well as discuss the possibility of organ transplantation

Scenario 14

You are performing a double blinded randomized controlled trial of open repair of the ruptured tendo Achilles comparing nylon and with wire. Mr Johnson has just ruptured his tendo Achilles playing squash, and is suitable for entry into the trial. He knows that he has ruptured the tendon, and that you are doing a trial comparing wire with nylon. Please carry out the conversation you would have with him inviting him to be part of the trial.

Answers

Scenario 1

- Introduction and explain authority to take consent
- Give a clear and full explanation of what is to happen and common complications
- Describe the likely outcome
- List extra things which might need to be done
- Check understanding and for questions. Listen to patient's queries

You should use LED TO REASON for this.

Lead-in 'Good morning, my name is Dr X, can I please check your name?' … 'Thank you. I would like to take informed consent from you. I will be assisting my consultant Mr Y but I would like to confirm to you that I am competent to do this surgery myself and therefore am competent to take consent.'

Explore 'Before I start, can I just check with you how much you already know about this operation, and how much detail you would like me to go into, when explaining things to you?'…

Diagnosis 'You have osteoarthritis of the hip as I am sure you know. This means that the surface of the joint is worn out, so you are getting pain and stiffness.'

Treatment 'We are proposing to replace the surface of your hip joint with an artificial hip. This means an operation of around one and a half hours where the lower part of your body will be asleep. The anaesthetist will explain how this works to you. You, yourself can be awake or asleep during this time, and you need to tell the anaesthetist which you would prefer. We will make a cut here on the outside of your hip, split the muscles beneath and then remove the top of the femur. We will then clean out the arthritis from the joint and fit in the artificial hip joint. We will give you pain relief through the following night through a drip, and then get you up the following morning. This is a standard plan for your problem and we are using a well-proven design of hip replacement. You should go home in 4 to 5 days.'

Options 'We have really explored all other options of treatment with you. Pain-killers are no longer controlling your pain, and I am afraid that this pain and stiffness will only get worse over time. However you do not have to have this surgery. The choice is yours, and you have an absolute right to decide to delay your surgery or even not to have surgery at all.'

Result 'When you wake up from the surgery, you should already be almost pain free. You will go home once you are safe on stairs. Initially you will be on crutches but we would hope that within weeks you will be walking without a stick and then be completely pain free. These hip replacements should now last 15 to 20 years, and when it does it can be replaced.'

Eventualities 'If there is a lot of bone damage in your hip, we may need to build up certain areas with extra bone, but we can use some of the bone that we normally remove, when fitting the hip, so this does not need to concern you.'

Adverse events 'There are of course things which may go wrong, and with your permission I would like to run through these with you now. This is a major operation and so there is a very small risk—less than 1%—that you might suffer a heart attack, a stroke, or a clot on the lung and indeed this might be fatal. However, we are going to do everything to avoid these. You will have a consultant anaesthetist to look after you. If there any problems then we will move you immediately to the Intensive Care Unit. We are also going to thin your blood a little to avoid you from developing clots which might go to your lung. If you lose a lot of blood then we have blood ready for transfusion. Infection of the hip can also be a problem but we are going to protect you with antibiotics before we start the surgery and we will be using a super-clean operating theatre so the risk is less than 1%. There may be a problem with dislocation of the new hip, but we will be using a cushion between your legs to prevent your legs from crossing, and all our nurses are trained to move you in a way which keeps this risk to a minimum. Even so, about 1 in 20 hip replacements does jump out of joint after surgery, and if it does then we will simply put it back. It is not always possible to equalize your leg lengths, but we will do our best to do so. If there is some difference which is troubling you, then we will fit you with a shoe raise to correct this. Finally there is a small risk that the nerve behind the hip will be stretched or bruised at the time of surgery. This happens in about 1 in 20 cases but it normally gets better over a period of months.'

Sound mind 'Can I just check with you what you have understood that we have discussed?'... 'If I could just clarify that point for you.'

Open question 'Now, have you got any questions whatsoever on what we have discussed and what we are planning?'

Notes 'I am now going to record in the notes the key points of our discussion under the headings of LED TO REASON.'

Scenario 2

- Introduction
- Explain what is proposed and why
- Explain that it is quite reasonable to do this as it is low risk
- Explain law relating to Gillick
- Negotiate, do not confront

In this case it seems that the child is 'Gillick competent'. In other words according to Lord Scarman's judgment, the daughter is mature enough to understand the issues involved so the powers that her parents have to overrule her wishes have finished. However, it would clearly be much better for the girl and her parents if this situation could be resolved amicably and to the satisfaction of all involved. The interview might start with an explanation that it is important for everyone to respect the other's views as far as it is possible. It would then be ideal if permission could be obtained from the daughter to discuss the case with her parents. This might be best achieved if the daughter stayed for the discussion and a promise was made that no discussions would take place 'behind her back'. If this agreement cannot be achieved then it might be wise to postpone any further discussion until you (and the parents if they wish) have sought legal advice. You will need the support of your hospital's solicitors and your defence union if you belong to one. If, however, agreement can be obtained then it would be wise in effect to go through the process of informed consent with the daughter once again with the parents listening in. It is possible that once the parents have heard a calm and reasoned explanation of what is planned they may withdraw their objections. If they are not prepared to move their ground then the judgment by Lord Scarman may need to be explained to them, so that they are aware that currently the law sides with their daughter being allowed to decide for herself. Nevertheless, it would be wise to take legal advice before proceeding with the surgery.

Scenario 3

- Introduction
- Explain that wishes of the patient are paramount
- Look for compromise
- Reassure that everything is being done to avoid the risks mentioned

It is clear that 'informed consent' is not possible. Your duty, therefore, is to act 'in the best interest' of the patient. Clearly from the figures that you have here, the best interest for this patient is to have surgery to fix the fracture. It is also in the best interest of your service as it will save money and bed space. The needs of your service should not take priority over the needs of the patient but the patient's daughter may feel that this is the reason why you are advising surgery over non-operative treatment. It is also possible, but very unlikely that the daughter has personal reasons why she wants non-operative treatment. For example, it may be that the fees for the nursing home are very high and that the daughter is paying these. While her mother is in hospital her daughter may be saving money, and this might be contributing to her insisting that her mother does not have surgery. Therefore the views of relatives and of next of kin should be sought **only** to find out as accurately as possible the wishes that the patient would have expressed if the had been able to. They do not 'own' the patient, and therefore their views about how they want the patient treated, or even how they would want themselves treated if they were in this situation, are not relevant, and should not be taken into account.

The options of treatment and the likely outcome of these possibilities should be discussed with the daughter, just as if it was she herself who was having the surgery. Then, it has to be explained to her, tactfully, that it is the views of her mother and the best interests of her mother which are paramount. If the daughter insists that her mother has always been terrified of surgery, and that if she was fully competent, that then she would refuse surgery, then that should be your decision. But if the daughter says that it is she herself who is against surgery, then once again you may need to explain that it is the wishes and best interests of her mother which are paramount, and that a decision based on these is the correct one.

Scenario 4

- Introduction
- List to their view
- Explain situations
- Emphasize that the patient's views are the most important

The situation needs to be explained to the parents just as if they were the patient. It needs to be emphasized that the chances of their son surviving without a blood transfusion of some sort is very low, and that surgery without transfusion is unlikely to be of any value. You then need to emphasize that it is the views of their son not them which are paramount, so you must emphasize that it is the actual views of their son (not the views they hope that he would express) that you need help with. If they are adamant that his views would be that, even if it will cost him his life, he would decline transfusion, then you must record all details of the conversation in contemporaneous notes and then respect the son's wishes as presented by his parents.

Scenario 5

- Explanation of situation
- Explanation of law
- Listen to their views
- Lay out options including ward of court

The situation has already been explained to the parents just as if they were the patient, and you just need to be sure that they have fully understood the choices and the consequences of their choice. It is clear that the child is too young to be able to make the decision for herself. The child is not 'Gillick competent', and so the child's views are not likely to help resolve this issue. The only option here is to apply for this child to be made a 'ward of court'. The court then takes on responsibility for the welfare of the child and will take over the rights of the parents to decide whether surgery should be undertaken or not.

Scenario 6

- Introduction
- Explain
- Explore trust
- Offer a second opinion

Your responsibilities are to act in the patient's best interests, but clearly you are in a dilemma because there is a significant chance that you will find yourself facing litigation however well you treat this patient. It might be best here to explain that firstly no guarantee can be made on the outcome of any treatment (especially one as difficult as this). So it will not necessarily be negligence if the outcome is not as good as he hopes or expects. Even more importantly, the successful results of treatment rely heavily on trust and respect between the patient and the treating doctor. If he, the patient, does not trust your opinion and your ability to perform competent surgery, then it is not in his best interests to proceed. He should either find a doctor whom he does trust, or should not consider further surgery. It will also be very important to record very clearly what has been said, as contemporary notes are very valuable in preventing any subsequent disputes about what was and was not said. What you cannot do is refuse to treat him unless he promises not to sue you. That deprives him of a fundamental right and will not be respected in law

Scenario 7

- Introduction
- Listen to patient
- Explain risks
- Negotiate

There is no point in going over the issues again. At the end of the day you cannot be forced to do an operation which in your heart of hearts you do not think is in your patient's best interests. However, it is also not ideal to deny a patient the opportunity to have something done which she has set her heart on. It is not our business to discuss her unreasonable expectations about resolution of her marriage difficulties, so the best solution may be to offer to refer her for a second opinion, preferably to a colleague who has special expertise in managing these kinds of problems. You should not be allowed to be talked into performing surgery, which you do not feel is in the patient's best interests.

Scenario 8

- Purpose
- Patient
- Problems
- Plan
- Purpose

'Good evening sir. I am so sorry to ring you at home, but I would like to let you know about one of our patients who is unwell, and to confirm with you that I am doing the right thing. The patient is Mr. Jones, the 70-year-old on whom you did a routine knee replacement first on the list yesterday morning. I have been asked to see him because he has a temperature of 38 degrees and is slightly confused. His pulse is up at 100 and blood pressure down from 170/90 to 120/60. He has also only passed 100ml of urine today. I have not exposed the wound but the distal neurovascular status of that limb is fine, and there is only 250ml of blood in the drain. His chest is clear. He is not short of breath and his oxygen saturation is 98%. There is no sign of heart failure, and his ECG and cardiac enzymes are normal. He has only passed 100ml of urine today, so we have left the catheter in. His blood results show a haemoglobin of 12 and a slightly raised creatinine. I don't think there is anything too serious going on but am worried that he might be going into septic shock. So, I have informed the ICU outreach team who will visit first thing in the morning. In the meantime I have sent blood cultures, started him on IV flucloxacillin and arranged for hourly observations. I was also going to give a further fluid challenge of 250ml of Hartmann's now. Are you happy with this plan, or is there anything else that you would like me to do?'

Scenario 9

- Basic data. Name of patient, date, etc.
- Position, incision, findings, procedure, closure, checks, post-operative instructions
  12th November 2009. 14.00 Day Case Theatre St Margaret's Hospital
  Name: Reginald Jones. DOB: 12/1/1947
  3cm sebaceous cyst posterior triangle left side of neck. Not infected
  Surgeon: James Harvey
  Preparation. Skin cleaned and 10ml 1% lignocaine with adrenaline infiltrated around the cyst. Draped
  Incision 4cm horizontal incision just avoiding the punctum of the cyst. Cyst wall identified as separated from surrounding tissues using blunt dissection only. Accessory nerve seen in floor of wound, protected. Cyst removed almost intact and sent for histology. Haemostasis obtained using swabs and pressure. Accessory nerve confirmed intact before closure. Fat layer closed using catgut. Skin closed interrupted 4/0 Nylon. Discharge home as soon as ready. To GP for removal of stitches in 5–10 days

Scenario 10

- SOAP

  10.30am 12 November 2009. Dr James Harvey (2447)

  Asked to see wound red and discharging

  S Patient feels a little hot and sweaty, and the knee is more painful than yesterday. 'Throbbing.' Feels that it is also stiffer. No cough. No pain passing urine. Bowels open OK this am

  O Patient looks well but a little flushed. Pulse 90 regular. Temp 37.8. Fluctuating between 37.2 and 37.9 for last 12 hours. Wound looks red and swollen. Erythema has crossed the line drawn around it by the nursing staff at 9.00am this morning. Some sero-sanguinous discharge. Feels hot. Range of movement not tested (too painful). Distal neurovascular status OK

  A May be discharging haematoma but could be superficial or deep infection

  P FBC, CRP, wound swab. Inform consultant, and patient to go nil by mouth for the time being in case consultant decides he wants to take him back to theatre for wash-out. Antibiotics not to be started until I have discussed with consultant

Scenario 11

- Basic details
- Legible
- Concise summary of diagnosis and treatment
- What if?
- Review when

  Date 15th April 2009. Dr Jamey Harvey (2447) for Mr Pradip Datta

  Discharge summary on James Paget. DOB: 31/8/1991

  Admitted 10 April 2009 following motorcycle accident. Only injury open fracture left shin. Wound closed primarily. Locking intramedullary nail. Slight post-op pyrexia so on flucloxacillin oral 250mg qds for 5 days (2 days to run)

  If wound becomes more red and painful or discharges please refer straight back to emergency department where we will see him

  Stitches out 10 days

  Review Monday trauma clinic 6 weeks. X-ray of tibia on arrival please

Scenario 12

- Simple language
- Multiple tests, repetition over time
- Explanation of pain tests, pupillary, cephalo-ocular and calorific tests
- Checks for understanding

'Hello, I am Dr X. I have come to talk to you about what we are planning to do next. Is that OK with you?' …

'As you know your son has shown no sign of recovery and as we explained to you we fear that his brain has now actually died although his physiology continues while we continue to support him here on the Intensive Care Unit. Obviously it is important that we are all certain what the situation is before we make any further plans. So, we are going to do a set of tests, and repeat all of them again after 24 hours so that if there is any sign of life we do not miss it. The tests that we do each test a different part of the most fundamental part of the brain called the brainstem. Without activity in the brainstem recovery is not possible. Is that quite clear?' …

'First we are going to make sure that he is neither cold nor has any drugs in his body which could mask our tests. Once we have checked that we are going to test whether his brain and especially the balance organs in his ears can detect movement or a stimulus of cold water which causes them to feel as if the head is moving. Then we are going to test whether he responds to pain in several places, and whether his eyes respond to light or to pain. Finally we are going to turn off the ventilator for a few minutes to allow the build up of gases in his blood which should make him want to breathe. Before we do that we will give him enough oxygen so that his body can come to no harm during this test. Is that quite clear?'…

'If all these tests point to his brainstem being dead, then we will repeat them at 24 hours just to make doubly sure. Do you have any questions?'

Scenario 13

- Introduction
- Check what she wants to hear
- Simple clear language
- Support
- Offer to stop there
- Simple discussion of donation
- Time to think about it

Doctor: 'Hello Mrs Jones. Thanks for allowing me to see you. I have come to give you the results of the tests we have just performed on your son. Do you remember what they were all about?'

Mrs Jones: 'They were to see if my son's brain has died. It has hasn't it?'

Doctor: 'I am so sorry but I am afraid that is right. There is no sign of activity so I am afraid that all hope has gone.'

Mrs Jones: Face in hands. 'Oh no! What am I going to do? I am alone now.'

Doctor: 'Is there anyone who can be with you to help you through this difficult time?'

Mrs Jones: 'My sister is coming from Canada and arrives tonight.'

Doctor: 'That's good. Now do you want to talk about things any further or would you rather hold it there while you come to terms with your loss?'

Mrs Jones: 'No If there are other things that need discussing then I would prefer to discuss them now.'

Doctor: 'Well, I am going to discuss this with you gently, but obviously your son was a strong and fit young person and it might be possible for some of his organs to be donated to give someone else a new chance at life. Have you any idea what your son would have wanted. Did he ever mention this possibility to you?'

Mrs Jones: 'Oh yes. One of the girls at his school had a kidney transplant and he told me that he thought that it was a wonderful thing. I am sure that he was strongly in favour. Oh dear! This is all so sad. Do I have to decide anything now?'

Doctor: 'No, absolutely not. Why don't we stop there and leave you to give this some thought as it is a big decision and you have a lot on your plate at the moment. It is something that you may want to talk over with your sister when she arrives.'

Mrs Jones: 'Yes I will do that.'

Scenario 14

- Introduction
- Explain the uncertainty
- Choice of entering or not
- Invite questions at the end

'I gather that you know what has happened to your Achilles tendon and that I am doing a trial comparing repair with nylon and with wire. The reason that we are doing this trial is that we genuinely don't know which material is better. In order to do the trial you will not know which treatment you are to receive. That decision will be made using a computer which will randomly allocate you to one of the treatment groups. When we review your progress after surgery, we will again make sure that neither you nor the surgeon reviewing your case knows which treatment you have received, so that there is no way that the results can be biased. I must emphasize that you do not have to enter the trial if you do not want to. It will make no difference to the way in which we treat you overall. The decision is yours, and you have plenty of time to think about it. Are there any questions that I can answer for you?'

Chapter 12 **Ethics**

Introduction

Ethics does not just define a minimum acceptable standard. It is also the study and implementation of a set of the highest values to which each of us individually aspires.

These values may include courtesy, consideration for others, and honesty, as well as a commitment to the highest technical standards.

Surgeons are rightly regarded as highly trained professionals who are also usually working as team leaders. Patients and staff may and do expect to be able to put their trust in them. With this respect comes responsibility and so the standards of behaviour expected of a surgeon are considerably higher than those expected of the rest of the population. Each new generation of surgeons will model their behaviour on their teachers (putting a heavy burden on those who do teach), but this alone is not enough. They should also continuously strive to raise standards, so that they end up standing on the shoulders of the last generation.

There have been many attempts to codify these codes of behaviours starting with the 'Hippocratic' oath. Some codes have focused on over-arching principles. They have been comprehensive but lacked guidance in specific cases. Others have been detailed but proved cumbersome, rigid, and impractical. The General Medical Council (GMC) has taken on the statutory duty of defining these standards and judging those doctors who have been charged with breaching those standards. This code is encapsulated in the GMC's *Good Medical Practice*. Those containing the word 'must' are minimum standards. Those with the word 'should' are more aspirational. They are common sense and could equally be applied to any professional whose skills and knowledge can do harm as well as good, and should provide a framework on which trust can be built.

Rules to guide one's actions

1 **Best interests** You should always act in your patient's best interests. This means that any advice or treatment which you offer a patient should be chosen to be the best possible option for the patient, and any other criteria (such as what 'you' want to do) should be secondary to this. This does not mean that you have to lay down your life for your patient, but when you offer treatment it must be in the patient's best interests

2 **Acting within limits of competence** As a professional you should make sure that you only take on responsibilities which you have received adequate training to carry out safely. You should also be up to date in current practice. Finally you need to be performing the task so regularly that your performance will not be compromised by lack of practice

3 **Probity** Honesty with patients and your colleagues is more than just socially advantageous—it is an absolute requirement in doctors. This higher requirement of standard of behaviour is necessary because of the privileges given to us as licensed professionals. If we are to be allowed such great powers then our behaviour when using them must be beyond reproach

4 **Respect** Medicine relies on trust. Trust is engendered by respect. If you respect your patients then they will in turn be likely to respect you. If you respect your colleagues then their jobs will be made easier and they too will hopefully reciprocate. This respect between colleagues is not a charter to close ranks and cover-up mistakes from patients. All of us, at one time or another, have felt that a colleague's work as a doctor has been substandard and has harmed a patient. When giving a second opinion it is tempting to try to gain credit with a patient by blaming the other doctor. Do not do this. Firstly, you may not know all the facts, and so may be falsely maligning a colleague. Secondly, you will cause the patient to lose trust in the medical profession and this may cause them untold misery if they require further complex and dangerous treatment. Thirdly, it does little to help put the situation right. If you believe that a colleague's actions *may* have harmed a patient then that information needs to be given to the appropriate authority for them to investigate and then decide on the most appropriate action. This will be discussed in Chapter 10 on clinical governance

5 **Up to date** It is your duty as a professional to make sure that you are completely up to date in your understanding of the conditions which you are treating, and with the current treatment options.

This will mean reading the literature and attending conferences where these topics are discussed. This is sometimes called Continuing Professional Development (CPD). It is equally your employer's responsibility to assist you in keeping up to date, and it is also their responsibility to make sure that they check regularly that you are, in fact, performing to an adequate standard. They are therefore quite right to ask you to provide evidence that your practice is adequate

6 **Review** Good professionals continuously gather material needed to demonstrate their competence to continue in practice. This evidence will now be needed for revalidation One important way to check that you are performing to an adequate standard is to audit your practice, continuously checking that your quality of work is within the same 'norms' as others doing the same work under equivalent conditions. If you identify areas of weakness then you need to take action to rectify these (courses, extra training, etc.) or stop offering that service. A key area here is to learn from mistakes. Your review will therefore need evidence that you recognize that you have made mistakes (we all do), and that you have analysed how they occurred and taken action to make sure that they do not happen again

Scenarios

Scenario 1

You have a patient, whom you think would benefit from a new type of hip replacement which you have pioneered and which you want to demonstrate to a group of visiting surgeons who are coming to your hospital next month. She is a perfect patient ideally suited to the procedure and you have no one else suitable on your waiting list at the moment. Your patient is very frightened of having any surgery on her hip and although her X-rays show advanced arthritis, she says that she can control the pain with pain killers (just) and can manage her own shopping. She says that she realizes that she needs a hip replacement and is very keen to have your new type, but just feels that she would like to wait a little longer before she has surgery. Carry out the conversation that you would have with her.

Scenario 2

A patient who is 19 years old and a Jehovah's Witness comes in following a road traffic accident. A CT scan confirms severe damage to the spleen and the liver, and he is sinking rapidly into deep shock. He was conscious on arrival and told the staff of his religion and that he must not receive blood. He has now lapsed into coma. His only near relative is his brother, who has arrived, and wants him to be given blood if this will save his life. You are quite clear that without blood you cannot safely open the abdomen, as the bleeding will not be controllable in the first instance, but that with a massive blood transfusion the chances of gaining control are good. You have blood ready and a team experienced in the management of liver trauma. The actor here is the patient's brother. Please carry out the conversation that you would have with the brother

Scenario 3

A patient wants you to do her surgery as she trusts you, but this is not an operation you have performed for the last 18 months since a new consultant arrived, and he has taken over the management of these cases. You really like this patient and have done a lot of surgery for her in the past. You also liked doing this operation. The actress here is going to take the part of the patient. Please carry out the conversation that you would have with her.

Scenario 4

A patient has inoperable cancer of the pancreas and is quite rapidly deteriorating. His wife and children are adamant that he must not be told his diagnosis. The patient asks to see you and asks you to tell him his diagnosis and whether it is fatal. This actor is the patient. Please carry out the conversation that you would have with him.

Scenario 5

A patient has inoperable cancer of the pancreas and is quite rapidly deteriorating. His wife and children are adamant that he must not be told his diagnosis. This actor is the patient's daughter. Please carry out the conversation that you would have with her.

Scenario 6

A patient has come to see you with recurrent dislocation of a total hip replacement done some 12 months ago. She has been referred by her GP for a second opinion as the original surgeon is not prepared to do anything further. You review the X-rays and the femoral component appears to be riding high in the cup. You go back and review the operation note which is short but reports no problems. However, when you check the labels of the implants used it is clear that a 28-mm head has been put into a 32-mm cup. This discrepancy is a major surgical error and is undoubtedly the cause of the multiple dislocations that she has experienced since the hip was put in. This actor here is the patient. Please carry out the conversation which you would have with this patient.

Scenario 7

You are having a problem with a colleague who wants you all to standardize on a new technique for repairing anterior cruciate ligaments which uses an expensive new synthetic implant placed through the arthroscope. You have always used part of the patella tendon harvested at an open operation. You have obtained consistently good results with this technique for over 15 years and see no reason to change. Your colleague has set up a meeting with you about this as he wants to spend a lot of money on new instruments and these implants. Describe how you would prepare for this meeting.

Scenario 8

Imagine that you are a consultant. Describe how you would prepare for your annual appraisal to demonstrate that you are practising to an adequate standard.

Answers

Scenario 1

You must explain to your patient that her wishes are paramount. You can certainly explain to her that there are a visiting group of distinguished surgeons coming to the hospital next month and that her operation would be a perfect one to show them, but you must qualify that with the comment that if she does not yet feel ready for the surgery, then she should not have it, and that at the end of the day the decision is hers and hers alone

Scenario 2

The relative is going to try to persuade you to give blood if this will save his brother's life. However, you must respect the patient's wishes which he has made quite clear while he was still conscious. The temptation will be to say (to yourself and indeed to the relative) that the situation is hopeless anyway, but this would not be strictly true. You will need to empathize with the brother, sharing in his frustration at the situation, but you need to stand fast and respect the patient's views.

Scenario 3

You may wish to review with her that you go back a long way, and that you are touched by her trust in you. You should also explain that there is now a very good surgeon who specializes in this work and that you pass all the work to him, because in this way better results will be obtained.

If she insists that she wants you to be the surgeon, a compromise might be to offer to see whether it is logistically possible to do the operation together.

Scenario 4

The patient's wishes are paramount and therefore, having checked that he wants to be told his diagnosis and prognosis, you need to go into the standard system for breaking bad news (see Chapter 13). First, you need to find out what he already knows and then what he hopes and fears about the current situation. Once you have this information you can plan what you need to say and how best to go about it. If a patient says 'I haven't got cancer, have I?', then he has made clear what he does and does not want to hear. At each stage you need to check whether he has any questions and what he has understood by what you are saying. If it is clear that he is in denial then it may be best not to try to break down a deliberate attempt by him *not* to understand what you are saying, but come back to it at a later stage. Each stage of bad news needs to be couched in reasonably optimistic terms and any support which can be given described and emphasized. For example, he may be very anxious about pain, and you may be able to reassure him that pain control should not be a problem.

If the relatives are adamant that he is not to be told then the patient's wishes are still paramount and he is to be told as much as he wants to know.

Scenario 5

The patient's wishes are paramount, and this will need explaining to the daughter, but in the first instance it may be helpful to explore with the daughter why the family does not want her father told. In many cases they will claim that it is to spare his feelings, when actually it is their own feelings which they are hoping to spare. However, you may wish choose to explain to them that once everyone knows what they are talking about, and there are no secrets, it may give the patient a last and much needed opportunity to discuss things that he wants to. Once again the discussion needs to be handled gently and with sympathy, but you must remain firm that although the patient does not have to be told his diagnosis, his wishes in the matter must be respected.

Scenario 6

This is a difficult case. There is a real temptation to show the patient what you think is wrong, and then to point out that this is a gross surgical error, which should never have happened, and that there is almost certainly compensation payable if she instructs a solicitor. However, you do not yet know the full facts of the matter. The labels in the notes may be incorrect, and you know nothing of the circumstances surrounding this error. If the facts turn out to be wrong, and there is a perfectly reasonable explanation for what has apparently happened, then you will have unfairly insulted your colleague, involved your Trust in a lot of unnecessary expense, and damaged the patient's trust in another doctor. Against that, your patient has a right to know what has happened and to decide for herself what she wants to do about it. The best path here is probably to explain that you think that there may be a mismatch between the components and that this is likely to explain the problems that she has experienced. You should decline to speculate how this might have happened, and focus on what can be done now to try to put things right. It is important that you document carefully everything that is said in this and future meetings. Also, you have a responsibility to report this as a possible serious untoward incident (SUI) so that it can be discussed in the next clinical audit meeting (see Chapter 10), and actions taken to ensure that it does not happen again.

Scenario 7

It looks possible that your well-proven technique which has worked well over the years has reached its sell-by date. However, this new synthetic ligament may be yet another expensive flash in the pan. There have been plenty of these 'here today, gone tomorrow' ideas before. The first thing that you need before any meeting is more information, so a literature search and/or a meeting with the company representative marketing the product might prove very helpful. On the basis of this you need to decide whether:

- There is overwhelming evidence that the new technique is better—if so you need to give in at the meeting and arrange to learn the new technique
- There is some evidence that the new technique might be better—in this case suggest at the meeting setting up some form of trial to determine what is best
- There is no evidence whatsoever—why not suggest at the meeting that your colleague performs a preliminary trial to determine what results are obtainable with this new technique before he adopts it unreservedly?

Scenario 8

Define appraisal as a mainly formative and constructive process aimed at identifying problems and finding solutions to these. Also note that there is a summative element aimed at determining fitness to practice, which feeds in to re-validation. The process of appraisal is in itself an integral part professional behaviour and therefore must be performed.

Actions

First, you need to find out from management/Internet/colleagues if there are standard forms for appraisal (there are). Second, you need to populate the required fields. These will include your job plan (does it fit national guidelines?). You also need to report your workload (number of cases managed) and compare this with national recommendations. Complications and complaints will need to be listed alongside comments on the action you have taken to reduce these in future. Any audits performed with their outcome should be described. CPD should be listed. A list of problems you are experiencing in doing your job should be accompanied by suggestions as to how these might be overcome. Goals from last year need reviewing with comments on whether they have or have not been achieved and why. New goals for the following year need to be set, which should be appropriate to address the problems experienced in the previous year. Minutes of the meeting need to be written and agreed and the documents signed off.

PART 2
HISTORY-TAKING AND COMMUNICATION SKILLS

Introduction

This part specifically deals with 'Communication' for which there are five stations in the examination. Hence this part has not been divided into sections and has been written as a whole. The following part deals with all the aspects of communication that you as a candidate will be tested upon. The examination in this part is a reflection of a day in your life as a CT1/2 or ST1/2.

Chapter 13 starts by instructing you in the nuances of good and **effective communication** as a doctor in your career as a surgeon. It should help you to become an effective communicator not only as a junior surgical trainee but should put you in good stead as you go up the professional ladder. Every aspect that you might come across has been discussed with appropriate examples which are all true episodes. This chapter will help you to prevent such mishaps in your professional dealings.

Chapter 14 deals with **history-taking**. It is said that the vast majority of diagnoses can be reached by a good history. The importance of taking a good history cannot be over-emphasized. In history-taking, listening is a very important part. If the patient realises that you are a good listener, he or she will open up to you and volunteer a good history. In the interest of consistency you will be asked to take a history from a pretend patient (actor).

Chapter 15 will give you practice on **dealing with difficult situations**. This will be in two forms. You will be asked to read a scenario and consult with a colleague on the phone. You will also be asked to read a scenario and explain a problem to the prospective patient or a family member (actors). There will be two examiners sitting in the bay who will mark you on your powers of communication. There will be no interaction between you and the examiners.

Chapter 16 will give you practice on **written communication**—writing a letter to a GP. This would usually be with regard to an unforeseen circumstance that has arisen with regard to patient management— for example, a postponed operation, a postoperative complication, or a death.

In each chapter 10 scenarios are discussed as examples. All the stations are for 9 minutes. If you finish your task well before the allocated time, then consider that your answer might be incomplete.

Chapter 13 **Effective communication**

Please note there are no Scenarios in this chapter; they are in the subsequent chapters in Part 2.

Introduction

The importance of communication cannot be overstated. Communication is the keystone upon which rests the art and practice of medicine. A poor communicator usually ends up as a poor doctor in the widest sense of the term. Nevertheless there are and have been excellent technical surgeons and good physicians who are very poor communicators; they leave their patients frustrated and unhappy. The majority of problems in the management of patients resulting in legal wrangles arise from ineffective communication—errors of commission, or, more often, errors of omission.

It is therefore apt that the present format of the MRCS OSCE examination lays stress upon and tests the skills on effective communication in the daily professional life of a young surgical trainee. It is gratifying to see that similar importance is being given to good communication in the undergraduate curriculum of most medical schools. Expertise in communication expected of a surgical trainee obviously will not be of the same magnitude as that of a consultant with whom the buck stops. Similarly a surgical trainee in the later years should be able to face more complicated communication problems than in the earlier years of training.

It is certain, however, that communication delayed is communication denied, particularly when it concerns a possible error in management. Often a complaint can be prevented by the person at the helm of the team pre-empting the problem and volunteering an explanation to the patient and/or relatives concerned before they ask any questions. The patient and relatives should be made to feel 'we were kept informed at all times'. The situation is not dissimilar to an airline flight not taking off as scheduled and the passengers being kept fully informed as to the cause of the delay and the impending solution.

This chapter is based on the author's observations and experiences over 38 years in the National Health Service as a junior doctor and a consultant. Some of the examples used are his own and others are taken from 'Personal View' columns in the British Medical Journal (BMJ) and appropriately acknowledged.

*In this chapter on communication when referring to a consultant, trainee, or the patient the word 'he' is used as a generic term; it is obvious that the person in question may be male or female.

The doctor as a communicator

This initial chapter of Part 2 of this book, 'History-taking and communication skills', deals with aspects of communication at the level expected of a junior doctor in the examinations. It also reflects the daily life of any hospital doctor, particularly a consultant, who should lead by example and the trainee should emulate (Fig. 13.1). The hospital consultant has to communicate with a large number of professionals—medical and non-medical. As this book deals with the MRCS examination to be taken by a basic surgical trainee (BST), the hospital consultant, for practical purposes will be depicted as a consultant surgeon and his daily life as a communicator.

It would be apparent that much of the communication aspects that are dealt with will pertain to consultants, sub-consultants, and trainees. It must never be forgotten that the one person who is of paramount importance for whom the entire medical profession exists is **'the patient'**. Therefore every aspect of communication should be geared solely towards providing the best possible service to this person—our patient.

The outpatient appointment—history-taking

The art of history-taking seems to have taken a back seat. In this day and age of advanced imaging techniques, not enough importance is given to taking a good history. At times an imaging technique is ordered on the strength of the referral letter; whilst such an approach does save time, it belittles the importance of history and clinical examination. After exchanging the usual pleasantries, the opening sentence should be, 'I have had a letter from your GP but tell me in your own words how it all started'. Having said that to the patient (who may be accompanied by a relative/carer), the clinician should show interest in the patient by maintaining eye contact and studying the patient's body language. While listening attentively, one should look for the patient's ill-fitting clothes, observe the belt for the 'belt-holes' going up two or three notches—tell-tale signs of weight loss—and nicotine staining of fingers.

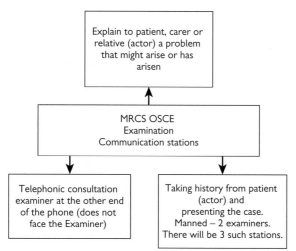

Figure 13.1 Communication stations in the examination.

Listening is a very important part of communication. The doctor by his body language should make that apparent. Within a few minutes the patient realizes that his consultant is a 'listening doctor' and will then open up and volunteer important aspects of history that are really worrying the patient. A good listener is automatically a good observer and would have elicited a few physical signs well before laying hands on the patient. 'While I was talking, he was all the time either looking at the computer or writing his notes', sadly is an oft-repeated comment from a patient. That is poor communication.

When one starts out, it is very tempting to 'write everything down' just in case you miss something. But, actually it may be much better to wait until the end before writing, as then you can give your full attention to the patient while he is talking and then produce a clear, relevant, and concise description in the notes. During this time the patient could be getting undressed.

The 'open-access endoscopy'—a boon or a curse to communication?

This, by and large, has taken communication out of the equation in patient management. The patient goes to the GP with upper GI symptoms of abdominal pain or lower GI symptoms of altered bowel habit. A brief history is taken and clinical examination carried out followed by the statement 'I'll send you to the specialist for a camera examination'. The patient is automatically put on the waiting list for an OGD or flexible sigmoidoscopy/colonoscopy as the case may be. The occasional patient may simultaneously be on the waiting list for an USS for gallstones. The patient returns home reasonably satisfied that he/she is going to see a specialist for camera examination and 'all will be sorted out' thereafter. The endoscopy might be done by a nurse specialist.

Come the day of endoscopy, the patient might have a brief history taken by a junior doctor in the day case unit just before being wheeled into the endoscopy suite. The briefest of history is elicited by the specialist while the sedative is about to be injected—a history probably only adequate to make sure that the correct endoscope is being inserted into the right orifice.

In bygone days when routine lower GI endoscopy had a long waiting list, I was asked to see patients in view of their unremitting symptoms. After a history and clinical examination pointed towards the possibility of a colonic carcinoma, an urgent barium enema was the routine (which had a much shorter wait than an endoscopy). On more than one occasion a large bowel carcinoma was diagnosed and surgically treated before the endoscopy appointment was due. On another occasion a patient on the open-access waiting list for an OGD came in with a perforated duodenal ulcer.

The moral of these episodes is obvious: there is no substitute for a good history and clinical examination. A good history starts you on the correct diagnostic path in the vast majority of patients. Perhaps an example might illustrate how modern-day technology and management can fail a patient badly.

A well-built man in his late fifties saw his GP with upper abdominal pain, vomiting, and weight loss. He was put on open-access OGD. This was carried out with gastric biopsies which showed curious gastritis (or words to that effect). He was treated with a course for *Helicobacter pylori*. He was no better; all his symptoms were worse. A US was therefore done which showed gall stones. The GP arranged a surgical referral and he was placed on the waiting list for a laparoscopic cholecystectomy which was duly carried out uneventfully.

Several weeks passed and he was much worse and had lost so much weight that he had problems keeping his trousers up. This was a patient who had been overweight. On his insistence he was referred back to the surgeon; before he was seen, this time a CT scan was arranged. This came back as showing an advanced gastric cancer. The patient died a year after the onset of his symptoms. At no stage in the chain of care did anybody bother to take a history and as far as the patient could remember nobody ever felt his abdomen. Every time he was seen in hospital, doctors only spoke to him when he was lying in a bed or on a couch just before his OGD which was done three times. The reader of this episode may feel that hindsight is a wonderful thing. It is not so: if only somebody in the chain of care had bothered to take a history and listened to him, the diagnosis was written all over the place. An example of failed communication: nobody followed-up the 'curiousness' of the histology report; nobody tried to find out the outcome of his cholecystectomy—did that cure his symptoms? This was an abject failure in communication. The final outcome might not have been much different. But that is not the point.

The written communication

The written communication in medical practice takes various forms. From the moment a patient is seen in the hospital, a detailed note should be made of the patient's history. It is useful to make a note of the patient's mood, manner, for example, if the patient is in pain, avoids eye contact, and makes analogies. It is useful to note down the patient's own words within quotes for the sake of accuracy. Often line drawings depicting physical findings are a great way to keep accurate notes.

The trainee should note down progress of the patient in the ward on a daily basis. Any contact with a patient should be recorded with the date and time. One cannot lay enough stress on the importance of good note-keeping, something that is reiterated time and again by the GMC and the Medical Defence Unions. It is a sad indictment of the medical profession that whenever there is a medico-legal problem and the team requires details of an episode, it is the nursing kardex that has far better information than the medical notes.

The letter to the GP should be succinct but contain all relevant information—provisional diagnosis, present medication, synopsis of the day's visit, plan of management, and follow-up. A good letter is a GP's dream. If the patient has been seen by another colleague in a different department in the past, it is imperative to copy the letter to that specialist as it may be relevant in future particularly in cases such as inflammatory bowel disease (IBD) or gastroesophageal reflux disease (GORD). In such instances the pathologist should be kept in the picture too with copies of correspondence; these patients may suffer from dysplastic changes of various grades in future when a meeting may be necessary between the surgeon, gastroenterologist, and pathologist to collectively review the slides of suspected high-grade dysplasia which may be regarded as carcinoma in situ requiring prompt surgical treatment.

Referral letters to other hospital colleagues should be copied to the patient's GP who should be the hub in the patient's overall management. Sometimes an inpatient is referred to another colleague by letter; a personal phone call is a better approach. In the 1970s a consultant surgeon wanted a medical opinion from his consultant physician colleague who shared the same Nightingale type ward with him. Having written a referral letter in the patient's notes, he left a message with the ward sister to inform the physician. After 3 days when the patient had not yet had a medical opinion, the surgeon sent a telegram to the physician!

The written communication which is often the source of irritation to the allied specialities such as radiology, pathology, biochemistry, haematology, and microbiology is the request form. The clinician—consultant and trainee—is guilty of inadequate information too frequently, a situation that creates quite a lot of angst between departments. Who suffers as a result? It is the hapless patient.

Finally, in this age of super high-speed technology, the patient is right to expect good coordinated communication between various departments when he or she is seen. Sadly it is not uncommon for the patient to be told that 'we cannot find your notes', 'I cannot see the reports of the tests', 'I cannot find the referral letter from the other consultant'. Even if the filing system is at fault, it still amounts to poor communication.

The dictation

The dictaphone, a great innovation that it is and which plays a major role in our lives, can be a secretary's nightmare on two counts—long, rambling letters and inability to understand what is being said. It is surprising how often the user has no idea about the benefit of brevity which is a sure way to have the letter read completely. Rudolph Virchow said 'Brevity in writing is the best insurance for its perusal'. There is a tendency to go on and on and the reader therefore loses the wood for the trees.

It requires practice to formulate a good letter. Carelessness is at the heart of a poor letter. Once a doctor has learnt the art of good letter-writing it becomes second nature and would put him in good stead for ever. Blaise Pascal is reputed to have said 'The present letter is a very long one, simply because I had no leisure to make it shorter'. Once when there was a medical secretaries' strike, doctors had to write letters by hand. Never were the recipients, particularly GPs, so happy as the missives were short and to the point.

The other problem that secretaries face is inability to understand what is being said. This is not a problem of just those whose first language is not English. The problem is universal—particularly swallowing one's words. When using the dictating machine, it is important not to talk as though you are having a conversation with somebody face-to-face. The contents of the letter may reflect a conversation but the delivery must be slow and deliberate mentioning the particular punctuation mark as and when it should be used. Difficult words need to be spelt out as should certain proper nouns. Medical secretaries quickly get to know whose letters are a pleasure to type. Those whose letters are short and pithy and where the language and diction are easily understood, have their tapes typed more promptly.

The telephone communication

Alexander Graham Bell's invention had been the greatest boon for communication until the Internet came along. Where would the doctor be without the telephone? For inter-hospital referral to a specialist unit in a tertiary centre, the referral ideally should be consultant to consultant irrespective of the time of day. It is surprising how often a consultant instructs the trainee to ring up a consultant at another hospital to refer the patient. This is extremely rude and should not happen.

Often when the consultant does talk to his counterpart, he asks his secretary to get the other consultant on the phone and connect the person to him. Is he really so busy that he cannot hang on the phone while he is being connected? This is the height of professional discourtesy. One appreciates that it can take a while to track down a colleague in another hospital. But the onus is on the consultant making the referral and hence they should find time to hang on to the phone. Whilst waiting on the phone for the other consultant to be tracked down, one can be on the computer getting other things done. The person making the referral, consultant or trainee, should be armed with every detail and have the notes on hand.

A good telephone manner is an art. It is well to remember that the person at the other end of the phone, who is to receive a patient, may not always understand what is being said—for a host of reasons. It is the telephone manner that gives a mental picture of the doctor at the end of the line and vice versa. Slow and deliberate conversation is the order of the day.

Consultants in the middle of the night when rung up by their trainee about a patient who might need an urgent referral, e.g. a head injury, who feel that the patient needs a neurosurgical referral, should never ask the trainee to make the telephone call to the consultant in the tertiary hospital. If the consultant neurosurgeon is woken up in the middle of the night, it is mandatory that he or she is woken up by the consultant and not a trainee from the referring hospital.

It is important to plan the conversation before making a phone call to one's consultant or to a doctor in another hospital. One should take some time over this before picking up the phone. The referring doctor should try to put oneself in the shoes of the person receiving the call who may have been asleep or busy with another patient. He should therefore lay out the problem slowly, clearly, and succinctly, perhaps starting with what he really wants—advice or the patient to be seen and taken over. The good consultant in the tertiary hospital will almost always take the patient over following a decent telephone presentation of a difficult case.

Communication between the consultant and the trainee

Mentoring of the trainee

For a consultant this is one of the thorniest aspects of one's job while at the same time it can be the most rewarding. Nowadays this task is made even more difficult because in most instances the consultant does not have a say in the appointment of his junior staff. That decision is made in an ivory tower far away from the hospital where the trainee is due to work. The working pattern is such, that during the tenure of appointment (4 or 6 months), the consultant may see the same person once or twice. The ethic of a team consisting of a consultant, registrar, and house officer is something in the distant past.

So under these circumstances there is hardly a rapport between the consultant and his trainee; there is no time to develop such a relationship. Communication with one's junior staff is essentially on two fronts—clinical training of which teaching is a part and trying to help the underperforming doctor. The former is quite simple: train your junior staff on the job and ring fence time for formal teaching. This function must be taken seriously by the consultant and not do it 'if I have time'. It would turn out to be the best investment for our national health service.

The second task is much more demanding. Underperformance is usually noticed by the nurse in charge who brings it to the attention of the consultant. The consultant should see the person concerned and allocate sufficient time to talk to the particular trainee in a sympathetic manner. This should be a one-to-one confidential conversation, one of the most challenging tasks confronting a consultant.

The consultant should try to elicit if there is anything personal or otherwise that is bothering the trainee; is there a cultural problem? In the interest of political correctness, the consultant should not shy away from raising the question, difficult though it might be; or is it purely lack of knowledge or motivation? It should be looked upon as an opportunity to help rather than admonish. The latter approach will be necessary in persistent underperformance whatever the reason.

In this two-way relationship the trainees should watch what they think their consultants do well, and what irks them. They should then make sure that when they are consultants they do not forget these lessons.

The trainee as a good communicator

It is obvious to assume that a trainee learns from his consultant and this should be true about communication too. However, that presumes the consultant is a good communicator himself. It is imperative to stress the importance of communication at the induction, a routine procedure at the start of any new job. This is usually done by all the departments, the common denominator being effective communication, the cornerstone of good patient management.

When seeing a patient for the first time, the junior doctor must introduce who he or she is and what the patient can expect from him or her during the hospital stay. Good history taking is essential as is note keeping. When going off or coming on a shift, thorough handover is only possible with effective communication. Filling forms, mundane though it is, must be thorough. It often pays to take a filled X-ray form to the department and talk to the radiographer or radiologist in an emergency or urgent patient. They may also have some really useful suggestions about extra imaging or tests which might help to clarify the situation. This approach makes the staff in the X-ray department feel as a part of the team, not just somebody at the end of a form. As a registrar or a consultant, whenever I have personally requested a radiologist for an unscheduled imaging, I have never been refused. It is amazing what a bit of personal contact can achieve—and the patient benefits as a result.

It is always good to be prepared to make time when talking to a patient who has cancer, or who has not progressed according to plan after an operation. One should be prepared for the possible questions. It is the same when talking to relatives, particularly outside the usual working hours, as relatives can only sometimes come during visiting hours when the consultant might not be in hospital. Never start by saying, 'I have just come on duty and don't know much about your mother, father…'. This creates an awful impression on the relative about the doctor, the unit, and the hospital. Find out everything about the patient in question from the nursing staff and colleagues before going to see the relatives. Nowadays with shift system in vogue, there is a lack of continuity of care; so before going to see the relatives one must be armed with all the information from the handover as the patient and relatives will want to know the outcome of investigations.

When it comes to investigations, it is good to let the patient know why he is being approached with a syringe and needle. Complicated investigations such as an angiogram would require more detailed explanation warranted by the need of a consent form. Often the first time the patient is told that he is going to have an X-ray is when the porter comes to take him to the radiology department because the doctor who wrote the form did not bother to tell the patient about it—poor communication.

Rarely the trainee may have to give bad news. This may be in the form of having to break the news of a diagnosis of cancer or an unexpected post-operative complication. I say 'rarely' because the harbinger of any bad or unexpected news must always be the person at the helm with whom the buck stops—the consultant. It is poor form if the junior doctor is thrust unsupported to do this most difficult task of breaking bad news.

Communication in a multidisciplinary team (MDT) meeting

In order to give the patient the best possible clinical outcome, the surgeon should liaise with several colleagues, medical and paramedical, within the hospital and in the community. Such a group is referred to as the MDT, which comes into its own in the overall management of cancer. The MDT management is also the way forward in patients with multiple trauma; certain situations in gastroenterology such as GORD and IBD also benefit from a team management.

In a chapter such as this the detailed role of every member in a MDT cannot be described. The principles of communication in a MDT would be outlined. At the outset it is important that one person should assume the role of team leader who should have a strategic overview of a difficult situation and liaise with other members and chair the meetings. Usually this would be the surgeon although the role of individual members of the team may change from time to time as the patient progresses in his/her journey through cancer.

The surgeon must not attempt always to have the last word or the 'maximum say' in a MDT meeting; such an approach would not bring the best out of the other team members. A weekly meeting, even if there are no new patients, should be held where as many of the team members should make an attempt to attend and assess the progress. It should be appreciated that at some meetings certain members of the team may have more to contribute than others.

The number in a team would vary according to the condition for which the patient is being treated. For instance, for a benign gastroenterological condition, the surgeon, the physician, and the pathologist would form the core of the team; the pathologist particularly may play a major role in helping to make a decision with regard to the best form of treatment as in the degree of dysplasia at the gastro-oesophageal junction or the large bowel.

In a polytrauma patient, the number of team members will depend according to the systems involved. A patient could easily be under the combined care of the neurosurgeon, cardiothoracic surgeon, orthopaedic surgeon, general surgeon, plastic surgeon, and the intensive care anaesthetist. A physiotherapist is an important member of the MDT with long-term rehabilitation in mind. However, in such a situation it is essential that the patient does not 'fall between several stools'.

Finally, the cancer patient may be under a MDT of many members depending upon the particular cancer and the stage. For instance, head and neck cancer may require a very large team—the head and neck surgeon, maxillofacial surgeon, plastic surgeon, clinical and radiation oncologist, radiologist, dentist, dietitian, speech therapist, social worker; the list can go on.

In summary, this section highlights the importance of every member of the MDT who should play an important role in the optimum recovery of the patient. It may sometimes give the impression of 'treatment by committee' bringing with it the problems in its wake that sometimes a committee may do. Problems should not occur when a patient is managed by a MDT as long as there is good and effective communication orchestrated by the team leader, a person to be so designated at the very outset.

Breaking bad news

'Bad news' is 'any information likely to alter drastically a patient's view of his or her future whether at the time of diagnosis or when facing the failure of curative intention' (R Buckman in 'Breaking bad news: why is it still so difficult?' *BMJ* 1984; 288:1587–99).

This can take various forms: telling the patient that he has cancer; the operation has had to be postponed as a bed in ITU is unavailable because the last bed was occupied by an emergency the night before; the patient has to go back to theatre for a post-operative complication. Examples of very poor communication when it comes to breaking bad news are legion in number throughout the health service.

A few examples should make the medical profession shudder in disbelief. Nowhere is the saying 'Example is better than precept' more true. Hence here are some examples of how not to communicate. After a US of his testis showed a solid lump, a young junior doctor was rung up by the consultant surgeon on a Friday evening and told, 'Yes it looked malignant. Come in on Monday, we will do a frozen section and chop the thing out for you. Bye.' The doctor wrote 'I was devastated… Fortunately one of the nurses sensed that something was seriously wrong. I was protected in the office until I had had the chance to dry my tears properly' (Graham Rich, 'Denial is dangerous', Personal view, *BMJ* 1990: 300:270).

A lady had a breast cancer diagnosed. The senior registrar said that she 'needed a mastectomy probably with axillary clearance'. When the patient saw the consultant he said 'a mastectomy was not necessary and that removal of the lump would be sufficient'. The patient 'was incredulous, baffled and angry' (Anonymous, 'An open letter to my surgeon', Personal view, *BMJ* 1992; 305:62).

What should be done so that such examples never occur again? Sadly, they still do, except some are much worse. For a start, bad news must always be given by the consultant in charge of the patient. What is the junior to do if this does not happen in his unit? He will have to learn as best as he can by being thrown in at the deep end. Ideally a comfortable room should be chosen for the meeting—congenial surroundings make a lot of difference. It is good principle to have such a meeting with the charge nurse in attendance and a trainee being present. This helps to prevent any future misunderstanding as the patient and the relatives will certainly have other follow-up questions. The patient should be encouraged to have the next of kin at the meeting.

The patient's permission should be sought for the presence of the nurse and the trainee who is primarily there to learn the art of communication in difficult situations. Although confidentiality is presumed, the patient is reassured about it. The team must be prepared for a longish conversation and allocate adequate time for the process. The consultant must desist from looking at the watch during the interview; nothing is more off-putting and rude.

At this meeting it is prudent to tell the next of kin that it is his/her responsibility to pass on the information to other interested members of the family. This is to prevent the same conversation having to be repeated to other family members later on. An exception to this can be made when a very close family member, e.g. offspring, has to travel from afar to visit the patient in view of the adverse news. The patient should never be given the impression that the consultant is in a hurry. After all, attentive listening is an essential part of good communication. Sir Thomas Holmes Sellors said 'In the NHS the patient listens to the doctor. In private practice, the doctor listens to the patient.' True though the statement is, it should really be: the doctor always listens to the patient.—NHS or private.

The patient with cancer

The acronym SPIKES is a useful protocol for delivering bad news about cancer.[1] The six steps are:

1 **Setting** up the interview
2 Assessing the patient's **perception**
3 Obtaining the patient's **invitation**
4 Giving **knowledge** and information
5 Addressing the patient's **emotions** and empathy
6 **Strategy** and **summary**

---

[1] Baile WF, Buckman R, Lenzi R, et al. SPIKES – A six step protocol for delivering bad news: application to the patient with cancer. *The Oncologist* 2000; 5:302–11.

Although waiting for the patient's INVITATION may be seen as a natural progression in the management, a good case can be made for not waiting for a call from the patient. A good consultant would take upon himself to break the news to the patient when all information is on hand by inviting the patient and next of kin for an interview. While breaking the news about cancer, it may be useful to use different words during the course of the same conversation.

Patient asks, 'Do I have cancer?'
Consultant, 'I am afraid you do'.
Then some patients are known to say, 'Does that mean it is malignant?'

The other way round is sometimes equally true—when the doctor says 'it is malignant' (a word better not used at the outset), the patient says 'thank goodness it is not cancer'. The moral of this lesson is that during a conversation with the cancer patient, words such as 'cancer' and 'malignant' should be used interchangeably, albeit in a considered manner. Once the initial breakthrough of informing the patient about cancer has been made, the subsequent supplementary questions (some of them would have been answered at the initial interview anyway) can be answered by the charge nurse or the trainee; hence the importance of the presence of the charge nurse and junior doctor at the first interview. At the end of the day one should be honest without sounding hopeless. In this regard the tone of the conversation and body language is just as important.

Cancer patients should be treated as fellow human beings who are in distress, not as cases to be managed. We should be ready to inform, be prepared to explain and answer questions with compassion—the principal ethic of our profession. We should not keep them in the dark thinking 'the patient may not be able to take it, it would be too devastating'. Devastating it may be at first, but we should not underestimate the resilience of the human body and mind. Ralph Waldo Emerson said 'Knowledge is the antidote to fear'. It is fear of the unknown that is much worse. Some patients with cancer may be in denial. They need to be seen repeatedly; this is best done in the presence of a near relative.

The ultimate communication—the dying patient

'We are there to cure sometimes, relieve often and comfort always' (Sir James Calnan). We will comfort our patients only if we are good communicators. How to talk to a patient that is dying is hardly taught and hence doctors tend to avoid a patient with terminal cancer on the ward. On a ward round such a patient should never be ignored (unless the patient is asleep). If the patient happens to be asleep during the formal ward round, the team or the consultant must make it a point to see and talk to the patient at a later time when the patient is awake.

Such a patient will almost certainly have disseminated cancer. Not all such patients will spend their last days at home or in a hospice. Some are looked after in a surgical ward. That patient will need the most reassurance. It is a challenging task. Everyone knows that death will come one day. What the cancer patient is concerned about is the manner and the extent of suffering that will precede the inevitable. Something on the lines 'I will be there whenever you need me to relieve pain and sickness. We are in it together and will travel the road as companions' may be a nice and comforting way of putting it.

The patient with a post-operative complication

The professional life of a surgeon, enjoyable and rewarding that it is, can be blighted by one problem— the post-operative complication. Such a situation does arise unfortunately, in spite of doing one's best and the consultant, as the team leader, has to face it and set it right. There is always a cause for a post-operative complication although it may be difficult at times to pinpoint one single reason because there may be many. Whatever the cause, the consultant shoulders the responsibility. Once this has happened, good and prompt communication can forestall a complaint or even litigation. This also goes towards softening the blow that the patient and relatives suffer from this setback.

On most occasions the team can guess that 'things are not right'. Some professionals do not like to admit that their work is ever less than perfect; so they are in a 'denial mode' oblivious to the fact that a complication may be developing. In this regard listening to the senior nurse on the ward would go a long way towards promptly identifying the problem. A sort of 'case conference' initiated by the consultant about a 'non-progressing' post-operative patient is a good start. As this would be an ill patient, it is presumed that the patient will be in a side room. The team led by the consultant should explain in detail the problem, the result of the investigations, why things are not progressing, and the next step of action—an operation or perhaps an interventional radiological procedure.

If the problem is to be set right by an interventional radiological procedure, the onus is on the clinical team to explain in detail the nature of the procedure; this should not be left to the radiologist although it is hoped that the radiologist would also explain what is going to be done. The clinical team should also take consent from the patient to offer to explain to the next of kin the course of action. It should never happen that when the next of kin come to visit, they are told that the patient has had another operation without them ever being informed about it in the first place. In the discussion, sometimes the patient may have to be warned about the possibility of a stoma (when one was not expected) and that he may end up in the ICU.

This should be the ideal approach. Such good communication where the patient and relatives are fully informed at every step will calm a distressing situation and defuse the anger and disappointment felt. Not saying anything much makes the patient and relatives suspicious and they may feel that bad news is being shrouded in a veil of secrecy and silence. There is a real temptation to avoid patients when things are not going well or a mistake has been made. They will not go away. Much as the period of plucking up courage to go to see the patient is miserable for the surgeon and often frightening for the patient, this unpleasant task should be done sooner rather than later. Only then both parties can get on with their lives again.

An example will testify how poor communication can add insult to intense grief. In the days of open cholecystectomy, a gentleman underwent 'a routine gall bladder operation. Three weeks later he was in an intensive care ward with extensive brain damage on a ventilator. Two weeks after that he was dead…. What was, and still is, indefensible is the appalling breakdown in communication that occurred once my father entered the hospital'(Gill Whalley Personal View, *BMJ* 1985; 291:671).

Communication regarding intra-operative problems

Sometimes during an operation, the procedure does not go according to plan. In spite of that, the post-operative outcome remains good as expected, albeit occasionally requiring a few extra days stay in hospital. Should the patient be told about such episodes? I think they should, as it may have a bearing just in case the patient may need another operation elsewhere in future.

A retired doctor underwent open heart surgery. After the essential part of the operation, there was a problem in getting his heart started. The team was so worried that his family was summoned to the hospital straightaway. They spent several agonizing hours in the hospital whilst the team got the patient's heart going again. He spent 7 hours in the theatre instead of the expected 3 or 4 and a longer than anticipated stay in the ICU. The ultimate outcome was fine. The patient wrote, 'I have wondered why I was told so little, both before and after the operation. Was it better for me not to know, or did the fact of my being a doctor lead all concerned to assume that I did not need to be told anything. The latter is not appropriate. The former is open to debate.' (FB Coates, 'Never too old' Personal View, *BMJ* 1992: 304:1449).

In the middle of an emergency appedicectomy for perforated appendicitis in a fit young man, the patient suddenly became very blue with intense coughing. There was a panic at the anaesthetic end of the table and I was asked to stop immediately. After intense activity at the head end of the table, things seemed to have returned to normal and I was asked to proceed. The operation finished without any further problems and the patient went home some 5 days later. The anaesthetist told me that the patient had an attack of status asthmaticus during the operation which was the cause of the problem. The anaesthetist was unaware of the history of asthma. Neither of us informed the patient about this although when asked, the patient said that he did suffer from asthma for which he occasionally used the inhaler. I said to him that in future if ever he needed an anaesthetic, he should inform the anaesthetist about his asthma. No questions were asked by the patient and I said nothing else. In retrospect that was very poor communication on our part. I should have known the dictum, 'The fact that a patient does not ask does not mean that he has no questions' (Dame Cecily Saunders).

Communication with relatives (carers)

This is an essential part of a doctor's job. This takes on an added significance when bad news has to be given. When the progress of the patient does not go as it should, the relatives may ask for an appointment to see the consultant or a doctor looking after the patient (a trainee). It may even be necessary to make an appointment to see them outside working hours because it may just not be possible for the next of kin to come during the daytime hours. This may mean that the consultant may have to come to the hospital specifically for this purpose. Good doctoring can at times be a 24-hour vocation like the clergy, old-fashioned though such an idea is. If the bad news entails a post-operative complication, going this extra mile will demonstrate not only good communication but also a caring attitude. It may also prevent a complaint leading on to litigation.

Communication with the nursing profession

The medical profession owes their nursing colleagues a debt of immeasurable gratitude. Whilst the consultant might get the overall credit for a patient's recovery, such an outcome would never be possible without the nursing care, something that is often taken for granted. In the present climate of restricted working hours for trainees, it is the consultant and nurse in charge who provide continuity of care. Good and effective communication between the nurses and surgical staff is essential for the patient's post-operative recovery. In this regard listening to the nurse is the mainstay of communication. It is the nurse who keeps a watchful eye on the patient over longer periods than any doctor and therefore quickly spots anything untoward. The good trainee therefore takes all the help he can get from the nursing staff by listening to them. Good communication engenders a rapport between the surgical and nursing teams. This is the hallmark of a successful working relationship and the winner is the patient.

Communication with hospital colleagues

Good rapport with one's colleagues makes professional life so much more enjoyable; the enjoyment is reflected in giving one's best which ultimately benefits the most important person—the patient. Effective communication is at the heart of good rapport.

Often it pays to discuss face-to-face with the radiologist the best imaging technique in a complicated case; one should not hesitate to ring up the consultant radiologist on call in an emergency for advice. Unfortunately the only time the radiologist is rung up as an emergency is when the duty radiographer refuses to do a particular X-ray as it is not in the guidelines of the Royal College of Radiologists. Similarly, referral for a medical opinion ideally should be 'consultant to consultant'. It is appreciated that that this may not always be possible. Referral between registrars may result in an equally good outcome.

It is always very instructive to have a dialogue with the pathologist in difficult cases, e.g. those with dysplasia in the GI or GU tract. A phone call to the microbiologist and pharmacist, haematologist, or biochemist can be very rewarding. If seeds of good communication between other departments are sown by the consultant into the minds of his trainees, it will bear good fruit as the trainee will grow up with such an attribute while ascending the professional ladder. Poor communication from the clinician towards non-clinical colleagues is a sign of rudeness, even arrogance which unfortunately still exists.

Communication with the GP

Whilst communication between GPs and hospital doctors, usually consultants, after the outpatient clinic visit of a patient is usually good, information of a patient who is a hospital inpatient is often lacking. When a patient does not progress satisfactorily during a stay in a hospital, the GP should be informed either by a phone call or an interim letter from a member of the team, usually the junior doctor. This is the ideal situation where the trainee can be taught to communicate well with colleagues in the community. Otherwise the GP might have to wait a while before the detailed discharge summary arrives. A brief telephone conversation about a patient's progress, or lack of it, fosters huge goodwill between the hospital team and the GP, thus engendering good rapport.

Communication with administrators and managers

In this day and age of increasing bureaucracy, good communication with the administration and managerial staff helps one's professional life to run smoothly. As a junior doctor the only time one meets the administrative staff is at the start and end of a job to sign papers or when something has gone wrong. In such rare situations it pays to talk to them face-to-face. A personal touch is infinitely better than a telephone conversation.

As consultants, it is a part of one's job to be a member of various committees. Some enjoy the work whilst others do not. It is essential for every consultant to share the responsibility of committee work in turn. In a large hospital this may come just once during a consultant's professional life. An even temperament helps. The 'us and them' attitude of some consultants and managers does not help. Both parties are on the same side with one goal in mind—efficient delivery of care. The differences, implacable sometimes though it seems, are to be bridged to achieve the common goal. Unfortunately often one hears of a 'difficult' colleague at meetings whose modus operandi is always confrontation instead of cooperation. An attitude of 'give and take' is effective communication in such circumstances.

Trainees who have a penchant for medical politics and are good at communication could get involved with various committee work. This makes such juniors good communicators, which bodes well for the rest of their careers when they become consultants.

Academic communication

Speaking at meetings

A significant aspect of a trainee's professional life is presentation at meetings. It should be looked upon as a privilege and a pleasure to be savoured, not a chore to be endured. Depending upon the forum and the audience, it can appear daunting too. But on the whole it should be an enjoyable experience on two counts, the preparation before and the presentation on the day. Moreover, this may also provide opportunities for travel abroad.

A huge amount has been written in books and journals on how to hone one's skills in this regard. The reader should refer to them. There are short 1-day courses on 'presentation skills'. These courses are not inexpensive and are meant for anyone wishing to improve skills as a speaker—business executives, managers, doctors. Early on in one's career, attending one of these courses is invaluable. This enables a junior doctor during the formative years to learn the 'tricks of the trade' which will be ingrained for ever.

The advent of PowerPoint has revolutionized presentation skills. Unfortunately on occasions the speaker is so enslaved by the computer that he is keener to show off how good he is with computer skills than concentrating his efforts on the material being presented. To some the medium seems to be more important than the message. It is important to keep under wraps one's addiction to animation schemes. In the pre-computer era, during the days of 35-mm slides, the very nature of the presentation meant more preparatory work. The work entailed typing out the material and sending them to the medical photography department. This subconsciously meant that the talk gets rehearsed during preparation. The downside of computer technology, which has simplified matters, is that the prospective speaker leaves preparation to the last minute and therefore a slip-shod nature creeps in. Certain rules are worth remembering:

1 An hour's preparation for every minute of presentation
2 For a slide, remember the rule of 7—no more than 7 lines (excluding the title) and no more than 7 words in each line
3 The title should be no more than 5 words
4 Eight slides for every 10 minutes of a talk
5 A table of statistics is an audio-visual death—avoid it
6 Aim for 8.5 minutes for a 10-minute talk, 25 minutes for a 30-minute talk
7 Talk at a relaxed pace with a well-projected voice
8 A strong start and an equally strong finish
9 Rehearse as often as you feel necessary
10 Never over-run—'Make sure you have finished speaking before the audience have finished listening' (Dorothy Sarnoff)

Medical writing

This aspect of communicating one's professional work is less intimidating than medical speaking. Once again a large amount of published material is available to help the inexperienced writer master this art. The junior doctor should look out for opportunities to publish. Here there will be no attempt to teach the nuances of good writing. To ensure acceptance, the quality of work presented and the method of presentation are both important. For this last point, conformity to the 'Instructions to authors' is mandatory.

The essence of good writing is to keep to the point, use short sentences, ensure good grammar and decent punctuation, and avoid wastage of words. However good a writer is, it is estimated that on average after the eighth or ninth draft the paper is finally sent to the editorial board. If the material is good and the presentation poor, the author would usually be asked to rewrite and submit. This usually means that the paper would be accepted after the presentation and language is improved—a much encouraging situation than outright rejection. Should the paper be rejected, disappointing though it is, there is no need to despair; try again, perhaps in another journal. This author has had more rejections than he would care to recollect.

Chapter 14 **History-taking stations**

Introduction

There will be two history-taking stations. Both stations last for 9 minutes each. The stations are manned by two examiners. There will be a 'patient' who is an actor.

Before entering each station you will have 1 minute to read the Scenario. It would normally take you about 30 seconds so that you will have another 30 seconds to gather your thoughts regarding the Scenario.

In one station you are supposed to be in an outpatient clinic where you are eliciting a history from a 'patient'. You are allocated 6 minutes when you will hear a bell. But in some instances, depending upon the Scenario, you may finish early.

Then you briefly present the relevant points and you will be asked by one of the examiners the differential diagnosis, investigations, and management. Although the examiners take it in turn to ask the questions, both will mark your performance.

The other station will be the ward where you have been asked by the nurse in charge to see a postoperative patient. Once again you have 6 minutes to ask relevant questions. You then present to the examiners and answer questions from one of the examiners (who take turns) with regard to the possible diagnoses, investigations, and management.

What the examiners are specifically looking for in this station

In taking a history, there are certain generic questions that you must ask while gathering information. You must also follow a routine pattern so that you do not miss out any vital information. The following is a useful 10-point check list:

- Introduce yourself, shake hands unless there is any cultural reason for not doing so
- Commence by asking 'Tell me in your own words how it all started. What are your concerns and what do *you* think might be wrong with you?'
- Past history
- History of medication
- Family history
- Systemic history
- Summarize your history to the patient
- Close interview by explaining what is to be done
- Be a good listener; do not reel off leading questions
- Make sure you have created a rapport with your patient

The history-taking Scenarios in this chapter will be divided into two parts—scenarios in the outpatient clinic and those on the ward. The lists of Scenarios will be given first. Then the salient points for the sample answers will follow for each section.

In all these Scenarios in Part A, assume you are CT or ST 1 or 2 to Mr Gardner, a consultant general surgeon or Mr Mackenzie, a consultant orthopaedic surgeon, and you are seeing the patient on his behalf.

Part A: Scenarios in the outpatient clinic

Scenario 1

Dear Mr Gardner

Mrs Angela Mackay 37 years

The above lady who is a solicitor complains of central abdominal pain on and off for 4 months. This is associated with nausea. On at least three occasions the pain has been so bad that she has had to take time off work. I cannot find any abnormality. Kindly see and advise.

Yours sincerely

Dr Neil Wilson

Scenario 2

Dear Mr Gardner

Mr John Smith 58 years

The above patient who is a postman complains of pain in both his calves for the past 6 months. This has been gradually getting worse so much so that it is affecting his work. Although he has not been off work, according to him it is taking longer for him to complete his daily round. He is a smoker. Thank you for seeing him

Yours sincerely

Dr Neil Wilson

Scenario 3

Dear Mr Gardner

Mr James O'Brien 68 years

This patient complains of throbbing backache for almost 3 months. He feels that the pain starts in the epigastrium and radiates to the back and is there all the time. On examination I think I can feel a mass in the epigastrium which seems to be pulsatile. He has angina for which he is on propranolol. Thank you for seeing him.

Yours sincerely

Dr Neil Wilson

Scenario 4

Dear Mr Gardner

Mr Colin Gunn 48 years

The above patient has a lump in his right groin which he noticed 6 weeks ago. This gives him some discomfort. He has been a type 1 diabetic since he was 22 years old. Thank you for seeing him.

Yours sincerely

Dr Neil Wilson

Scenario 5

Dear Mr Gardner

Mr Peter Harrison 72 years

This patient complains of increasing constipation for the past 4 months. Occasionally his motions are accompanied by blood. He has some abdominal discomfort. There is no change in his weight. I am concerned that he may have an obstruction in his large bowel. Thank you for seeing him.

Yours sincerely

Dr Neil Wilson

Scenario 6

Dear Mr Gardner

Miss Rebecca Jackson 32 years

The above primary schoolteacher complains of loose motions for the past 6 weeks. This is associated with blood and mucus. She also has some tenesmus and has lost almost a stone (6kg) in weight during this period. I feel she needs to be investigated. Thank you for seeing her.

Yours sincerely

Dr Neil Wilson

Scenario 7

Mr John Mackenzie

Consultant Orthopaedic Surgeon

Dear Mr Mackenzie

Mr Alan Miller 44 years

The above patient who works as a builder's mate has developed severe pain in his right buttock radiating to the back of the thigh and leg for the past 2 weeks. He is limping and has sleepless nights. I have prescribed for him voltarol which gives him transitory relief. Thank you for seeing him urgently.

Yours sincerely

Dr Neil Wilson

Scenario 8

Mr John Mackenzie

Consultant Orthopaedic Surgeon

Dear Mr Mackenzie

Mr David Manson 33 years

During a game of football 3 weeks ago, the above patient twisted his right knee. To start with his pain was quite severe and he was treated with crutches and analgesics. His knee is still swollen and he limps although he has been able to dispense with his crutches. He has been off work as a telephone engineer. Thank you for seeing him.

Yours sincerely

Dr Neil Wilson

Scenario 9

Dear Mr Gardner

Mrs Elizabeth Marshall 58 years

This lady noticed a lump in her left breast 3 weeks ago accidentally in the bath. I fear that she may have a sinister lesion. Thank you for seeing her urgently.

Yours sincerely

Dr Neil Wilson

Scenario 10

Dear Mr Gardner

Miss Jean Grant 26 years

This primary school teacher complains of weight loss for the past couple of months or so. She has been perspiring unusually. She has diarrhoea occasionally and has noticed some irregularity of her periods. On examination the only abnormality I could find was tachycardia. Thank you for seeing her.

Yours sincerely

Dr Neil Wilson

The history to be taken for the above Scenarios is now given below. Routine generic history—past history, drug history, family history, personal history, systemic history—will not be mentioned. The salient points with regard to the relevant history for each patient will be mentioned.

In the examination situation, you will be given a sheet of paper to write down some points if you so wish. However, this will take up valuable time. You must be able to remember salient points of the history without needing to write them down; moreover, you should not be reading out the history even if you write some facts down.

Part B: Scenarios on the ward

In the following Scenarios, the action takes place on the ward or Accident and Emergency Department. You are a CT2 or ST2 surgical trainee called by the nurse in charge to come and see the patient. You will have about 5 minutes to take a history from the patient. As the situation may be an emergency in the middle of the night and the 'patient' is post-operative and very ill, some part of the history may be supplemented by the nurse (the examiner) as would happen in a real situation.

When you enter the station you will be faced with two examiners and one 'patient'—an actor. Once you feel that you have come to a conclusion and in your mind have formulated a plan for management, the patient will leave the station and one of the two examiners, who will ask you to present and ask questions.

What are the examiners looking for in this station?

- Brief summary and good presentation
- Come to a correct conclusion; if the examiner does not agree, he/she may ask you to reconsider. Do not feel downhearted if you feel that your conclusion was not the one that the examiner expected. Your subsequent discussion may still be sufficient for you to pass that station
- Outline your management

Scenario 1

Surgical ward: 13.00

A 60-year-old woman has been admitted as an emergency with a 4-day history of severe right upper quadrant pain, vomiting, jaundice, and intense pruritus and is very toxic—high temperature with rigors and hyperdynamic circulation. What do you suspect? Outline your management.

Scenario 2

Surgical ward: 02.30

A 70-year-old patient, ASA anaesthetic category 3, underwent an emergency closure of a perforated duodenal ulcer. The anaesthetic and operation were uneventful. On the 1st post-operative day he complained of feeling very unwell with a systolic BP of 80mmHg with no unusual signs in his abdomen; there was impaired conscious level and peripheral vasoconstriction. What will go through your mind? Outline your management.

Scenario 3

Accident and Emergency Department: 10.00

A fit 25-year-old man fell from a height of 40 feet at a building site. He has been brought in unconscious with a GCS score of 13 and flaccid limbs. What would he be suffering from and outline your initial A&E management.

Scenario 4

Surgical ward: 09.00. Post-operative ward round

A 60-year-old man had a right hemicolectomy. On the 1st postoperative day he has developed a temperature of 39°C, is very short of breath and looks slightly cyanosed; his oxygen saturation is 92%. What will you suspect and how will you manage the condition?

Scenario 5

Orthopaedic ward: 11.00

A 65-year-old lady had a hip replacement 10 days ago. She is ready to be discharged. She went to the toilet just prior to leaving the ward for home. She collapsed in the toilet. What is your diagnosis and management?

Scenario 6

Surgical ward: 10.00

A 50-year-old man underwent a laparoscopic closure of a perforated duodenal ulcer. His post-operative period during the first 4–5 days was uneventful. However, thereafter he did not progress satisfactorily, had swinging pyrexia, hiccoughs, was tachypnoeic, toxic, and complained of pain in the right upper quadrant and right shoulder tip. What would you suspect and outline the management.

Scenario 7

High Dependency Unit: 12.00

A 60-year-old man underwent a Whipple's operation for periampullary carcinoma. On the 2nd postoperative day, while still in the HDU, his urinary output has reduced to 300ml in the previous 12 hours. The catheter is not blocked. What will you suspect and how will you manage?

Scenario 8

Surgical ward: 01.00

A 65-year-old man with atrial fibrillation underwent a successful lower limb embolectomy under local anaesthetic. A couple of days later in the same limb he developed severe throbbing pain over a period of 4 hours; the limb looked pink. What will you suspect and how will you manage?

Scenario 9

Orthopaedic ward: 18.00

A fit 28-year-old motorcyclist had a fracture shaft of femur and fracture-dislocation of his elbow treated by internal fixation. On the 2nd post-operative day he is confused and agitated and later in the day has a fit. What will you suspect and how will you manage the condition?

Scenario 10

Urology ward: 10.00

A 77-year-old man underwent a TURP. On the 2nd post-operative day he is confused, restless, and has some visual disturbance. What will you suspect and how will you manage?

Part A: Answers to history-taking Scenarios

Scenario 1

Clinical suspicion: gallstone or peptic ulcer disease

In this 37-year-old lady find out everything about the pain—total duration, duration of each bout, radiation, relationship with food, associated nausea (it is in the letter) and vomiting, and how the pain is relieved. Is there any heartburn?

There will probably be no physical findings. Summarize by saying that she could be suffering from gallstone or peptic ulcer disease. Besides routine blood tests she would require an upper abdominal US and oesophagogastroduodenoscopy (OGD). Take her menstrual history and if she is on the contraceptive pill.

Scenario 2

Clinical suspicion: intermittent claudication

Find out his approximate claudication distance. Is the claudication distance less when he walks uphill, or walks fast, or against a head wind, or when his postman's bag is unduly heavy; smoking history. Family history, history of angina, details of smoking history, and drug history are particularly relevant.

Explain to him that he will have routine blood tests, particularly serum lipids, non-invasive tests such as treadmill test to accurately assess his claudication distance, and ankle–brachial pressure index (ABPI). Explain details of initial conservative management and that an angiogram, which is a road map for the vascular surgeon, would only be carried out if and when intervention, surgical or radiological, is contemplated. This would only be done once he has given up smoking.

Scenario 3

Clinical suspicion: abdominal aortic aneurysm (AAA)

Elicit all details of the abdominal pain and its radiation to the back. Can he sleep at night? Has he found any particular position that lessens the pain, such as leaning forward? Does he feel any pulsations in his abdomen? Get details of his general health. What is the extent of his exact disability from his angina should he be considered for an operation. Is there any family history of atherosclerosis?

Explain what an AAA is. He would need an abdominal US to measure the size. If it is >5.5cm in diameter then he would need an operation fairly soon. In such a case he would need some more specialized tests to assess his suitability for operation. Finally mention to him that as he has symptoms, even if the size is <5.5cm, he would be better advised to have an operation provided his general assessment is satisfactory.

Scenario 4

Clinical suspicion: inguinal hernia

The history with regard to his hernia will be straightforward. Is there any history of irreducibility or pain? Get details of his insulin medication. Ask him if he has any other effects of his diabetes—vision, any problems with his cardiovascular system.

Explain the approaches—open and laparoscopic. He will need to come in the day before his operation and stay overnight as he is an insulin dependent diabetic. These procedures are usually performed under general anaesthetic but open operations in patients unfit for GA can be done under spinal anaesthetic or local anaesthetic.

Scenario 5

Clinical suspicion: carcinoma of left side of colon

Concentrate on alteration in bowel habit in the form of constipation. How often do the bowels open? What was 'normal' bowel frequency for the patient? Does he take laxatives for a satisfactory motion? Is he left with a feeling of insufficient evacuation after a motion? Ask about weight loss.

Is the rectal bleeding bright or dark red? Bright red bleeding usually would be from coincidental piles which bleed from straining at stools. Dark red bleeding is more sinister and may be from the growth itself or incidental diverticular disease. Ask about family history—parents and siblings so as to exclude familial non-polyposis colon cancer (HNPCC).

Explain what investigations will need to be done: besides routine blood tests including carcino-embryonic antigen (CEA), barium enema, and colonoscopy. 'Patient' will ask if he has cancer. You will have to give an honest answer while at the same time you should not alarm him. You should say something on these lines: 'We have to do tests such as a camera examination to see if there is a blockage from cancer. If there is a block we will take a small piece from the site to be examined under a microscope. Only then we will be sure of the diagnosis. We would then assess spread by doing a CT scan, CXR, and US. We would then be able to give you a detailed plan of treatment. Let us take one step at a time'.

Scenario 6

Clinical suspicion: ulcerative colitis

Take a detailed history regarding alteration of bowel habit. Diarrhoea may mean different things to different people. Some may interpret diarrhoea as frequency, whilst others may mean loose motions but not frequent visits to the toilet. So you need to find out specifically in the case of this school teacher if it is frequency or loose motions or both. Is there just mucus or blood also?

Ask if there is any specific event in her life that has triggered this episode. Is there any weight loss?

The patient may ask if she could have cancer. You need to explain with tact and empathy that it probably is not cancer, but you are going to get various tests carried out. You would do blood tests, put her on urgent waiting list for colonoscopy and biopsy, and barium enema. You will also be doing a rigid sigmoidoscopy and biopsy at this visit itself which will give you an idea of the diagnosis.

Scenario 7

Clinical suspicion: lumbar disc prolapse

Ask specifically about exact daily disability—in particular sphincter disturbances, bladder and rectal. Is the pain increased by coughing and sneezing? Is there any sensory and motor disturbances?

This man, who earns his living by hard physical labour, will be worried about his job and earning potential. You need to explain that in the vast majority of people this problem settles down. However, if he has sphincter, sensory or motor disturbances, you will arrange a MRI which is the gold standard for investigations. You should explain that plain X-rays of the lumbar spine do not help greatly.

Scenario 8

Clinical suspicion: ligamentous damage of the knee—cruciate ligament, collateral ligament, or meniscal tear

Ask if he is back to work. Does his work as a telephone engineer entail going up and down ladders? Then almost certainly he would be off work. Does his knee lock or give way?

He would want to know how long he would be off work and what is going to be done. Explain to him the complex nature of the anatomy of the knee joint. He could have damage to the collateral ligaments, cruciate ligaments, or menisci (cartilages). You will examine him at this visit and first get an X-ray done. This would be followed by MRI. Meanwhile he would be referred for physiotherapy.

Scenario 9

Clinical suspicion: breast cancer

Ask specifically how she noticed this lump although the GP's letter says 'accidentally'. Ask about nipple discharge, menarche, menopause, and detailed family history.

The lady would be distraught. Reassure her and explain what is going to be done—the components of triple assessment: after clinical examination, a bilateral mammogram followed by Tru-Cut biopsy. FNAC is the other alternative but this is not as successful as Tru-Cut biopsy. This would be a one-stop breast clinic and she would have all tests completed at this visit itself. The histology may take a few days to come back. Also finally explain that her case would be discussed in a MDT meeting so as to give her the benefit of the best possible outcome.

Scenario 10

Clinical suspicion: primary thyrotoxicosis

This patient will have symptoms pertaining to most systems—GI, metabolic, gynaecological, cardiovascular, and ophthalmological. Has she noticed any fullness of her neck? You need to ask questions with regard to all the systems. Find out if there was any precipitating factor.

She would be quite agitated and fidgety. Try to calm her down and explain the nature of the illness. Say to her that this is an eminently treatable and even curable illness. She would need blood tests and her condition can easily be treated with some tablets. She would be under surveillance for a few months if not a year.

Part B: Answers to Scenarios on the ward

Scenario 1

Diagnosis

Septic shock from acute cholecystitis + stone in CBD ± acute pancreatitis; may also be Mirrizzi's syndrome.

Outline of management

- Resuscitate: analgesia, blood tests for culture, full biochemical profile including serum amylase, FBC, prothrombin time, IV fluids,' best-guess' antibiotics
- USS of gall bladder and CBD
- If CBD diameter is > 7mm, do magnetic resonance cholangiopancreatography (MRCP). If stones are seen in the CBD, patient should have vitamin K, ERCP, and endoscopic papillotomy. Once the jaundice is better, within the next few days should undergo laparoscopic cholecystectomy

Scenario 2

Diagnosis

Post-operative cardiogenic shock.

Outline of management

- Patient already has a drip
- ECG:
  - ◆ ST elevation in precordial leads
  - ◆ Development of new Q waves—wide and/or deep
  - ◆ T-wave inversion
- Pulse oximeter
- Blood for:
  - ◆ CK-MB (creatine kinase, membrane bound)
  - ◆ ALT (alanine aminotransferase)
  - ◆ AST (aspartate aminotransferase)

- ◆ LDH (lactic dehydrogenase)
- ◆ Troponin T assay
- Transfer to CCU
- CVP
- Consider a pulmonary artery floatation catheter (PAFC)
- Oxygen therapy
- Aspirin
- Nitrates, angiotensin-converting enzyme (ACE) inhibitors and opiates
- IV beta blockers
- Consider reperfusion strategy

Scenario 3

Diagnosis
Neurogenic and spinal shock from head injury and C-spinal injury.

Outline of management
- C-spine should already have been stabilized
- Urgent CT scan of head and spine for extradural haemorrhage and C1 and or C2 fracture
  - ◆ Identify and control life-threatening problems
  - ◆ Immobilization—part of pre-hospital care; this is maintained until C-spine injury is excluded
  - ◆ X-rays
  - ◆ IV fluids—be careful; over-zealous administration of fluids may cause pulmonary oedema because hypotension is due to vasodilatation; in uncertain cases a Swan–Ganz catheter may be useful. Hypovolaemic shock causes tachycardia and neurogenic shock causes bradycardia. Vasopressors may be indicated.
  - ◆ Urinary catheter
  - ◆ NG tube to prevent aspiration
  - ◆ Medication: methylprednisolone 30mg/kg immediately followed by 5.4mg/kg per hour for the next 23 hours
  - ◆ Transfer to neurosurgical centre for definitive management
  - ◆ Rehabilitation—long term

Scenario 4

Diagnosis
Post-operative atelectasis.

Outline of management
- Vigorous physiotherapy ± IV doxapram
- Antibiotic—amoxycillin
- Oxygen therapy with inspired oxygen concentration of 30–40% with humidification
- Urgent fibreoptic bronchoscopy
- Minitracheostomy
- Continue with physiotherapy and monitor with blood gases and pulse oximetry—aim for oxygen tension to be no less than 10kPa

Scenario 5

Diagnosis
Pulmonary embolism.

Outline of management
Resuscitation
- Patient may need intubation and ventilation

Investigations
- Echocardiogram
- Pulmonary angiogram ECG and CXR; blood gases
- VQ scan
- Duplex Doppler US of leg veins
- Pulmonary angiogram

- Contrast venography and plethysmography
- Spiral CT—very sensitive

Treatment

- Anticoagulation
- Emergency embolectomy
- IVC filters
- Thrombolysis—in haemodynamically unstable patient with refractory shock; IV or pulse spray directly into embolus

Scenario 6

Diagnosis

Post-operative pyrexia—subphrenic abscess.

Outline of management

Resuscitation

- Oxygen
- Analgesia
- IV fluids
- Antibiotics after blood has been sent for culture

Confirmation of diagnosis

- Blood: culture, FBC, CRP
- CXR
- US
- ?CT

Definitive treatment

- US- or CT-guided needle drainage. This may require more than one attempt because there may be several loculi of the abscess
- Open operation—extra-peritoneal approach; anterior or posterior depending upon the site

Scenario 7

Diagnosis

Pre-renal failure from hepatorenal syndrome.

Outline of management

Prevent by:

- Adequate hydration and pre-operative induction of diuresis
- For 12–24 hours pre-operative 5% dextrose saline IV
- Mannitol (osmotic diuretic) or frusemide (loop diuretic) IV at anaesthetic induction
- Catheterize—hourly urine output
- Further diuretics if urine output <40ml/h in peri-operative and post-operative period
- Pre-operative oral chenodeoxycholate and oral lactulose for a few days—controversial

Treat hyperkalaemia by:

- 10–20ml of 10% clacium gluconate or chloride IV: stabilizes the myocardial membrane
- 50ml of 50% dextrose + 10 units of soluble insulin: drives potassium into cells
- 200–300ml of 1.4% sodium bicarbonate IV: drives potassium into cells and corrects acidosis; beware of fluid overload in acute renal failure
- Calcium resonium 15g tds orally or rectally: binds potassium and releases calcium in exchange

Definitive treatment

- Treat hyperkalaemia
- Peritoneal dialysis
- Haemofiltration
- Haemodialysis

Scenario 8

Diagnosis

Limb compartment syndrome.

Outline of management

Clinical features
- Pain—severe and out of proportion to the apparent injury
- Pain on passive movement
- Swollen and tense compartment
- Progression of the above over a short time period
- Paraesthesia—especially loss of two-point discrimination
- Pallor and pulselessness—usually with a vascular injury
- Paralysis—late symptom

Clinical diagnosis
- Normal resting pressure: 0–8mmHg
- Pain and paraesthesia: 20–30mmHg
- Fasciotomy: >30mmHg
- If pressure of >30mmHg is present for 6–8 hours irreversible damage occurs

Aetiology
- Orthopaedic
- Iatrogenic
- Soft tissue injury
- Part A
  - ◆ Scenario 5 – constipation vs loose stools
  - ◆ Scenario 9 – accidentally vs incidentally
- Part B
  - ◆ Scenario 4 & 5 – management
  - ◆ Scenario 7

Treatment
- Urgent fasciotomy
- Two or three long incisions—over posterior compartment and anterior or lateral compartments if necessary

Scenario 9

Diagnosis

Fat embolism.

Outline of management

Diagnosis
- Mental confusion
- Decreased conscious level
- Seizures
- Respiratory failure
- Petechial skin haemorrhages (3rd day)

Treatment
- Ventilation
- Systemic antibiotics
- Diuretics

Aetiology
- Major orthopaedic trauma
- Head injury

- Acute pancreatitis
- Cardiac massage
- Parenteral nutrition
- Liposuction
- Bone marrow transplantation

Scenario 10

Diagnosis

TURP syndrome.

- Restlessness, muscle twitching, disorientation, visual disturbances, seizures, and collapse
- Hypertension, severe hyponatraemia

Outline of management

Cause

- Occurs following prolonged prostatic resection of large glands and likely when >9L of glycine (1.5%) irrigation is used. Large volume of irrigating fluid enters the vascular space causing dilutional hyponatraemia resulting in disturbance of muscle and nerve function

Treatment

- Needs ITU monitoring—CVP, serum osmolality, serum Na
- Supportive
- Furosemide
- Hypertonic saline through CVP line (250–500ml of 3–5%) when there are seizures

Prevention

- Keep level of irrigating fluid below 20cm above the operating table
- Stop resection if large veins are opened
- Use irrigating resectoscope
- IV normal saline postoperatively for 12 hours

Chapter 15 **Dealing with difficult situations**

Introduction

You will have 9 minutes:

- You read the Scenario with biochemical data
- Make a diagnosis
- Gather your thoughts and write them down if necessary
- Lift up the phone
- There will be an examiner at the other end
- You present your case to take the patient over/or ask for advice

Allocate 5 minutes to read the Scenario, gather your thoughts, make a diagnosis, and rehearse in your mind what you are going to say. You should then present your case succinctly within the next 4 minutes. You must be prepared for occasional interruption. The better prepared you are with your thoughts the less you are likely to be interrupted by the examiner at the other end of the phone.

Part A: Scenarios on telephone communication

Scenario 1

A 60-year-old man had a right hemicolectomy. On the evening of the operation he has developed a temperature of 39°C, is very short of breath, and looks slightly cyanosed; his investigations are as follows:

- Oxygen saturation is 92%
- Arterial blood shows P_aO_2 of 8kPa.
- pCO_2: 7.5kPa
- pH: 7.3
- HCO_3: 18mmol/L

Ring the ITU registrar for help and possible transfer to the ITU.

Scenario 2

You are in A&E and faced with a 4-week-old male neonate who has developed incessant vomiting which is not bile-stained. His biochemistry is as follows:

- Arterial pH: 7.48
- Cl: 90mmol/L
- HCO_3: 38mmol/L
- K: 2.8mmol/L
- Na: 128mmol/L

Ring the paediatrician for help and transfer.

Scenario 3

A 30-year-old male patient has been brought to the A&E department having been extracted from a house on fire. You have resuscitated the patient according the ATLS protocol. Ring the regional burns unit for transfer. His blood results are as follows:

- pO_2: 10kPa
- pCO_2: 7kPa
- pH: 7.38
- HCO_3: 20mmol/L
- Hb: 17g/L

Scenario 4

A 65-year-old patient underwent repair of a leaking AAA 2 days ago. In the ITU he has now developed:

- Gross abdominal distension
- Type 2 respiratory failure
- Urinary output of 0.5ml/min (30ml/h)

- BP = 80mmHg
- CVP = 12cm

Ring the vascular surgeon as you are worried.

Scenario 5

A 25-year-old male patient in the neurosurgical ITU is brainstem dead. Ring the regional transplant unit for organ harvesting.

You must be prepared for questions on criteria of brainstem death.

Scenario 6

A 70-year-old patient underwent an abdominoperineal resection 2 days ago. He has now become oliguric. His blood results are as follows:

- Urinary output in the last 24 hours: 700ml
- Ph: 7.30
- HCO_3: 18mmol/L
- K: 6.2mmol/L
- Cr: 260mmol/L
- U: 20mmol/L

Ultrasound of kidneys show normal size and shape of both kidneys.

Ring the renal physician as you are worried.

Scenario 7

A 40-year-old male patient was involved in a RTA. He has a fractured pelvis. He has been resuscitated but a urethral catheter has not been inserted for fear of urethral damage. The orthopaedic department would like you to decide on what should be done next. You are not sure whether to insert a catheter or not. Ring your consultant for advice.

Scenario 8

A 30-year-old patient underwent internal fixation for fracture of tibia and fibula. On the 1st post-operative day he complains of severe throbbing pain with numbness in the foot. The temperature is normal and dorsiflexion of toes produces severe pain. You are worried because you are unable to control his pain. Ring your consultant.

Scenario 9

A 25-year-old footballer was injured while heading a ball. He was unconscious for less than a minute and then continued to play. At the end of the game he felt drowsy and has been brought to the A&E department. As SHO in the A&E department you are worried. Ring the neurosurgical registrar on call who is in another hospital.

Scenario 10

A 70-year-old man has been brought to the A&E with incessant upper and lower GI haemorrhage which is dark red from the rectum and bright red from above. He is almost exsanguinating in spite of blood transfusion with two wide-bore cannulae. He has a scar from the xiphisternum to the pubic symphysis of an operation. He wife said that the operation was for a ballooning of his abdominal blood vessel about 2 years ago. Ring your consultant about this problem as you don't know what is happening. His recordings are:

- BP: 70 mm systolic, diastolic not recordable
- Pulse: 130/min, thready
- He is not responding very well: GCS score 14

Part B: Scenarios on ethical dilemmas

Here you will be examined by two examiners—one surgeon and a lay person. You will have 1 minute to read the Scenario. When you go in you will face three people in the bay, including an actor who may be acting as a patient or a relative (carer). The actor will have questions for you pertaining to ethical problems. The examiners mark you after listening to how you tackle the problem and answer the person's questions.

You must start off by introducing yourself. The Scenarios will tell you who you are supposed to be, for example, SHO to Mr.... or SHO on call: 'I am Dr Smith, Surgical House Officer to Mr Jones or surgical junior doctor on call. I gather that you have some questions for me, I'll try my best to answer them.'

Once you feel you have finished, you must end by saying 'Is there anything else I can help you with?' If you find that the bell has not yet gone, then do not leave early. Summarize what you have said to the patient/actor/carer.

Scenario 1

A 45-year-old lady, Mrs Mackay, is due to have a mastectomy for carcinoma and breast reconstruction. She is a Jehovah's Witness and does not wish to have a blood transfusion under any circumstances. Discuss the problems with her.

You need to know about blood substitutes and auto-transfusion.

Scenario 2

A 25-year-old male, Mr Johnson, has been brought in with a stab injury to his chest. He is in the operating theatre undergoing surgery. Sergeant Jones from the local police wants to have his details as the person might be a suspect in a murder enquiry. You do not wish to divulge any details as it infringes on the patient's confidentiality. Explain to the police what your line of action is going to be.

Scenario 3

A 75-year-old patient, Mr Macdonald, has an obstructing annular carcinoma in the middle one-third of the rectum. This has been proven by an emergency gastrograffin enema. He does not wish to have an operation particularly because it will entail a permanent colostomy. You need to talk to him about the consequences and explain the future.

Scenario 4

A 60-year-old patient, Mr Mackenzie, had a thoracotomy for a lung cancer with a view to pneumonectomy. At operation it was found to be inoperable. At a routine postoperative CXR on the first postoperative day, he was found to have a retained swab. Talk to the patient about it.

Scenario 5

A 70-year-old patient, Mr Campbell, underwent a palliative left hemicolectomy for cancer of the descending colon. He has multiple liver secondaries. His son and daughter wish to see you with regard to the diagnosis. You have asked the patient's permission to talk to the family and he has agreed.

At the interview the offspring are very adamant that their father should not be told the diagnosis as 'he would be devastated'.

Answer their concern.

Scenario 6

A 10-year-old girl, Mary Calder, fell off a swing in the school playground and injured the left side of her chest. Her mother, a single parent, could not be contacted. Mary was brought to the hospital and was taken to theatre for a ruptured spleen. When she went to school to collect her daughter she heard about the incident. She came to the hospital and was incandescent with fury as her daughter had an operation without her consent. Explain the situation to the mother.

Scenario 7

It is 10pm. You have requested your consultant who is on call to come in to see a patient. Your consultant smells very strongly of whisky. He is conversing quite normally. The patient had a FAST (focused abdominal sonography in trauma) following abdominal trauma and requires an urgent laparotomy for a suspected intra-abdominal bleed. You are unhappy with the situation. What do you do?

Scenario 8

You are arranging a vascular operating list for your consultant who is on holiday. This is his first list on his return. Before he went on holiday he asked you to put three vascular cases in his all-day list—a AAA, a femoro-distal bypass, and a carotid endarterectomy.

The clinical manager, Mr Wheeler, has asked you to alter the list as the hospital is behind targets. Instead of doing the three cases listed above, he wants you put on four varicose vein operations and two A-V shunts for dialysis. The hospital is hoping for foundation status. You cannot contact your consultant who is sailing in the Bahamas.

Scenario 9

An 82-year-old patient, Mr Miller, has an inoperable bronchogenic carcinoma. He has uncontrollable pain all over his hemithorax and has skeletal secondaries. His son has approached you with a request to increase his analgesics to a lethal level to hasten his end. Talk to him about it.

Scenario 10

A 75-year-old female patient, Mrs Sutherland, with severe Alzheimer's disease has had a fracture neck of femur treated with hemi-arthroplasty. Talk to the patient's son/daughter about the futility of cardiopulmonary resuscitation (CPR) should she develop a cardiac arrest while in hospital.

Part A: Answers to telephone communication Scenarios

Scenario1

Answer: postoperative atelectasis.

ITU Registrar (ITU R): 'What do you think is the problem?'
Candidate (C): 'I think he has postoperative atelectasis.'
ITU R: 'Why do you think so?'
C: 'He has got tachypnoea, cyanosis, bronchial breathing at the left base, the left side of chest is not moving very well. The blood results show respiratory acidosis.'
ITU R: 'What have you done so far?'
C: 'I have put him on 100% oxygen sat him up, given him a saline nebuliser and have asked the physiotherapist to come in as an emergency. As his oxygen saturation is down to 90% on high-flow oxygen I am worried that he may tire and go into respiratory failure. I am therefore ringing you before things get any worse just in case these measures do not work.'
ITU R: 'What do you expect me to do then?'
C: I would be grateful if you could review him with a view to transferring him to ITU as I suspect he will benefit from some ventilator support .
ITU R: 'I'll come and see him.'

Scenario 2

Answer: congenital hypertrophic pyloric stenosis.

Paediatrician (P): 'What do you think is the problem?'
Candidate (C): 'The baby has probably congenital hypertrophic pyloric stenosis.'
P: 'Why do you think so?'
C: 'The baby has non-bilious vomiting and is the right age, 4 weeks, for that condition. Oh, he is the first born male child. He seems to have hypchloraemic, hpokalaemic metabolic alkalosis.'
P: 'Have you put up a drip?'
C: 'No, I haven't yet as I have very little experience cannulating babies. However, if you prefer, I don't mind performing this under your supervision.'
P: 'Have you done a test feed or an ultrasound?'
C: 'No, I have ordered the ultrasound but the radiologist preferred that you saw the patient first. I would be grateful if you could review the patient and arrange transfer to the paediatric ward. Thank you'

Scenario 3

Answer: management of a burns patient.

Candidate (C): 'I am ringing you about a 30-year-old male patient who was extricated from a burning building about 2 hours ago. I have resuscitated him according to the ATLS protocol and at present he is stable. I would like to transfer him please.'
Regional burns unit (RBU): 'What actually have you done so far?'

C:

- 'We have given him 20mg of morphine intravenously
- I have inserted two wide-bore cannulae into both hands through which I am giving him dextrose saline and normal saline
- I have inserted an indwelling catheter
- His Hb shows haemoconcentration at 17g/L
- His blood gases show respiratory acidosis
- His CXR looks normal
- He has an estimated burnt area of about 18% mainly in his lower limbs and part of trunk
- His has some singeing of his nasal hair
- He is on 100% oxygen
- The nurses have dressed the burns with flamazine unless you wish something different
- Tetanus prophylaxis has been given'

RBU: 'You seemed to have coped well. Why do wish to transfer him? We have no beds at present.'

C: 'He is stable. But his lower limb burns are partly circumferential and I am worried about impending compartment syndrome and he might need escharotomies. Moreover he might be a candidate for early skin grafting.'

RBU: 'Very well, thank you. Give me the details and we will take him over as soon as we can within the next day or two. Meanwhile keep a close eye on his respiratory system.'

Scenario 4

Answer: abdominal compartment syndrome.

Candidate (C): 'Your patient in the ITU who had repair of a leaking AAA 2 days ago has not been too well over the past 6 hours or so. He is oliguric, he seems to have type 2 respiratory failure with gross abdominal distension. His systolic is 80mmHg and CVP 12cm of water.'

Vascular surgeon (VS): 'What do you think he has got?'

C: 'I feel he might have abdominal compartment syndrome needing immediate abdominal decompression.'

VS: 'Arrange theatre and the anaesthetist. I'll be in straightaway.'

Scenario 5

Answer: brainstem death.

Regional transplant consultant (RTC): 'Can I help you?'

Candidate (C): 'We have a 25-year-old motorcyclist who unfortunately had a bad RTA and is regarded as brainstem dead. I wonder if you could send a team please for organ harvesting?'

RTC: 'Give me more details before I can send a team.'

C:

- 'The patient is apnoeic and on a ventilator and in deep coma
- The cause of brain damage is traumatic brain injury
- There is no history of drug ingestion
- His oculocephalic reflex was not done because of possible C-spine injury
- His vestibulo-ocular reflex, gag reflex, cough reflex jaw jerk, cilio-spinal reflex and oculo-cardiac reflex are all absent
- He has no EEG activity
- Two independent consultants, one of them a neurologist have seen him and carried out the tests twice 24 hours apart and have confirmed brain death
- We have spoken to the relatives and the patient himself was carrying an organ donor card'
  'The family have generously agreed to organ donation.'

RTC: 'Very well. Thank you. We are sending a team.'

Scenario 6

Answer: postoperative pre-renal renal failure.

Candidate(C): 'I am contacting you as the duty renal physician because I am worried about a 70-year-old patient who had an abdomino-perineal excision 2 days ago. He is not putting out enough urine.'

Renal physician (RP): 'The surgeon must have tied off the ureters, have you excluded that?'

C: 'Yes. In the immediate postoperative period he had 1.5L and on the 2nd day he had 1.2L of urine. Moreover, the ultrasound of kidneys shows normal anatomy. He is not hypotensive. There was minimal response with a fluid challenge.'

RP: 'What is his biochemistry?'

C: 'He has metabolic acidosis the blood results being [repeat the results from the Scenario).'

RP: 'What would you want me to do?'

C: 'I wonder if he might be a candidate for a short session of haemodialysis should his potassium go much higher?'

RP: 'I'll come and see him.'

Scenario 7

Answer: possible urethral injury.

Candidate (C): 'I have been asked to see a patient in the orthopaedic department with a nasty fracture of his pelvis following a RTA. He has been resuscitated according to the ATLS protocol. They asked me to consider putting in a catheter. I did not think it might be the best thing to do.'

Consultant Surgeon on call (CS): 'You are right. You should never put a catheter because you might convert a partial rupture into a complete one. Ring the duty radiologist to consider doing an ascending urethrogram. Have you done a rectal examination?'

C: 'Yes I have. The prostate is in its normal place and is not high riding or floating. So if the urethra is damaged it must be a partial tear.'

CS: 'Once the urethrogram is done let me know, I'll come and see the patient. He will probably need a suprapubic cystostomy.'

Scenario 8

Answer: acute limb compartment syndrome.

Candidate (C): 'This patient who underwent internal fixation of a fracture of his tibia and fibula last night complains of very severe pain in his entire lower limb. I have given him 20mg of IV morphine to no effect. I am worried.'

Consultant Orthopaedic Surgeon (COS): 'Has he got sensation in his toes? Can he feel you touching them?'

C: 'He has diminished sensation and he seems to have lost two-point discrimination. I am worried that he might have compartment syndrome and needs urgent fasciotomy.'

COS: 'Arrange theatre and anaesthetist. I'll see the patient in theatre straightaway.'

Scenario 9

Answer: extradural haemorrhage.

Candidate(C): 'Am I speaking to the neurosurgical registrar on call?'

Consultant Neurosurgeon (CNS): 'No I am the consultant on call. Registrars do not carry a pager these days after midnight.'

C: 'Good evening, Sir. I have a 25-year-old patient who seems to have all the features of an extradural haemorrhage. I would like you to take him over please.'

CNS: 'Give me some more details.'

C: 'He was playing football when, while heading a ball, he was knocked unconscious for a few minutes. However, he regained his consciousness to continue playing. He was then brought to the A&E department being drowsy with a Glasgow Coma Score of 13 to 14. His pulse is 60 per minute and his blood pressure is 120/80 mm hg. He has a linear fracture of his right temporo-parietal area and we are arranging a CT scan very shortly.'

CNS: 'What have you done for him so far?'

C: 'He has an IV cannula, an indwelling catheter with his C-spine immobilized. The anaesthetist is considering ventilating him with a view to transferring him to your care. Can we give him some mannitol?'

CNS: 'Yes. Transfer him with all his notes, X-rays, and send the CT scan pictures by teleradiology as soon as you have them.'

Scenario 10

Answer: arterio-enteric fistula.

Candidate (C): 'I have this 70-year-old man who is in extremis from severe upper and lower gastrointestinal haemorrhage. It is bright red blood from the top and dark red blood from the rectum. In spite of two large-bore cannulae and vigorous blood transfusion, we cannot bring his blood pressure up. There is no history of indigestion. He has no abdominal tenderness but a long scar from his xiphisternum down to his umbilicus. I don't know what is happening. I need your help.'

Consultant Surgeon (CS): 'Do you know what the scar is for?'

C: 'His wife says that 2 years ago he underwent an operation for ballooning of his tummy blood vessel and he had some sort of a graft put in. I presume it was for an AAA.'

CS: 'He has an aorto-enteric fistula. Inform the anaesthetist, take him to theatre and I'll see you all in theatre. He needs to be opened up immediately. I'll see his wife before I scrub up.'

Part B: Answers to Scenarios on ethical dilemmas

This is as usual a 9-minute session. As you go in, introduce yourself to the patient or carer or family (actor) as the case may be. The sheet pinned to the partition will tell you all about the Scenario and who you are. Start off by: 'Good morning/afternoon' shake hands with the actor 'I am Dr… I have come to see you to explain about the situation and answer your questions'.

Scenario 1

Patient (P Mrs Mackay): 'Doctor, I am due to have my breast removed for cancer. I have opted to have my breast reconstructed at the same time. The surgeon has explained to me what the operation entails. It sounds like a big operation that may take several hours. My religious beliefs prevent me from having any blood transfusion. I should not be transfused under any circumstances.'

Candidate (C): 'Mrs Mackay, we would not do anything to contravene your wishes and beliefs. I would like to give a few options that may help us together to make a decision as to best way forward.'

'As you wish to have the reconstruction carried out at the same time, it is a major procedure where there might be considerable blood loss. And usually blood transfusion may be necessary. But as you do not wish to have any blood transfusion, one alternative would be to consider having removal of the breast carried out at the first operation and then at a later date having the reconstruction.'

'If you still wish to have both parts carried out as one operation, we have many varieties of blood substitutes which are synthetically manufactured which can be used. Would you have any objection to that?'

P: 'No as long as the material is not from another living creature.'

C: 'No, it will not be. Gelofusine and Haemaccel are two infusions which we can use. There is of course another alternative called autologous blood transfusion. This can be done in two ways.'

'Provided your haemoglobin is over 11g/dl we can take blood from you once weekly and use it during your operation. This would mean your operation would be delayed by a couple of weeks but you would be having your own blood put back.'

'The other alternative is to remove blood from you after you have been anaesthetized. The blood would be replaced by electrolyte containing fluids (crystalloids). At the end of the operation your own blood would be replaced back. We would involve the haematologist in you operation.'

P: 'Thank you, doctor. I'll have a think and get back to you.'

Scenario 2

Candidate (C): 'Hello Sergeant Jones. I am Dr Smith who admitted the victim of a stab injury an hour ago. What is it you wanted to see me about?'

Policeman (P Sergeant Jones SJ): 'We would like to know some details of the injury suffered by the young man.'

C: 'Sorry Sergeant Jones, I cannot divulge any details as medical confidentiality prevents me from doing so. I need his permission to do so and that I can only obtain once he recovers from the anaesthetic.'

SJ: 'The patient, we think, was involved in a violent assault and robbery and we might charge him for attempted murder. This is an extreme situation doctor.'

C: 'I understand. I can see that there is no desperate urgency about this as the patient will be with us for quite a few days while he recovers. When I get the opportunity I will get in touch with my Medical Defence Union to take their advice. I will then get in touch with you.'

SJ: 'Thank you, doctor.'

Scenario 3

Candidate (C): 'Good morning/afternoon Mr Macdonald. I am Dr… I have come to explain about the problem that you have. Could you please tell me what you know about your condition so far?'

Patient (P): 'Doctor, I have not been told much except that I have a block in my bowel and I need an operation for this. After the operation I'll be left with a bag on my tummy. I don't fancy that at all. I really don't want that.'

C: 'Mr Macdonald, I do understand your concerns. You do have a block very far down in your large bowel. This is blocking the passage of your motions. The X-rays show that you have a complete block. Without an operation you will have very severe trouble.'

P: 'What sort of trouble?'

C: 'Your bowel, which is like a hollow tube, before the block has already started distending and at one point will burst causing severe peritonitis which will result in death. We want to do the operation before such a catastrophe happens.'

'I know you do not wish to have the operation because of the need to bring out your bowel outside and your motions will be passed without your control into a bag. This procedure is done as a last resort.'

'At your operation the block will be removed and the unblocked bowel will be brought out over your lower left tummy as a colostomy. The part of the bowel past the block will be closed off. This will give a hope, although remote, for the bowel ends to be joined up at a later operation which will then get rid of your colostomy and bag. We will also have a special stoma therapy nurse to see you to get you used to the workings of a colostomy.'

P: 'So, that means I need a second operation?'

C: 'No, not always. If you are happy to continue with the colostomy and we find that most people are, then you do not need another operation.'

P: 'I'll have a think about it and a chat with my family and get back to you.'

C: 'This is an emergency Mr Macdonald. Can I come and see you again within the hour?'

P: 'Yes. Thank you.'

Scenario 4

Candidate (C): 'Mr Mackenzie, I have come to talk to you about your chest X-ray carried out today. Last night my consultant talked to you about the outcome of the operation. Can you remember that?'

Patient (P): 'Yes, he told me that nothing was possible because the cancer was too far spread.'

C: 'Your chest X-ray I am sorry to say shows that we have left a swab inside.'

P: 'Is this a mistake?'

C: 'I am sorry to say that it is.'

P: 'Firstly I have an operation where nothing could be done. It was an open and shut job as they say. And now you say that a swab has been left inside. That is adding insult to injury. What does that mean now?'

C: 'Another operation to take it out now. We would do that right away once you have given us your consent.'

P: 'I want to see the consultant about it.'

C: 'Of course, I'll arrange that, Mr Mackenzie. I cannot apologize enough on behalf of the team for this.'

Scenario 5

Candidate (C): 'Good evening. I am Dr… You are Mr Campbell's son and daughter. What can I address you as?'

Patient's family (John and Linda): 'Call us John and Linda (J&L). We are Mr Smith's son and daughter.'

C: 'You wanted to see me with regard to your father's diagnosis. You father has given me permission to speak to you about his illness. How much do you know at present?'

J&L: 'We know that he had a cancer of the bowel that has been cut out. We would like to know more details, as much as you know, doctor.'

C: 'Mr Campbell had a block of the bowel almost certainly from a cancer. I say "almost certainly" because we need to wait for the final report which can take up to 10 days or so. The operation went off very well and he should recover as expected. Unfortunately, as we suspected from the scans before his operation, his cancer has spread to the liver.'

J&L: 'How long has he got, doctor? Does he know about this?'

C: 'This is a very difficult question to answer. Cancer can be a very unpredictable disease and no doctor could ever put a time span to one's life with this disease. Your father has not yet been told about the details as he only had the operation yesterday and is still very tired. However, we are planning to inform him as soon as he starts improving.'

J&L: 'Doctor, we would request you not to disclose to him the diagnosis as the very word "cancer" would devastate him, let alone the spread to the liver.'

C: 'I can appreciate your concern. But if any patient were to ask us about the diagnosis and details of the operation we are duty bound to tell him about it. It is within his rights to know. You are putting me in a very difficult situation.'

J&L: 'Will he have any chemotherapy doctor?'

C: 'This was discussed in a multidisciplinary team meeting and it was decided not to give chemotherapy as the side effects might be worse that than the benefits that would accrue. Going back to your first question, could we come to a compromise? Once your father gets better, we should all have an open chat so that you and your father know what has been said. In this way there will be no air of suspicion or mystery and we are all open about it. You will be surprised how well most patients take the news about their illness although it may not always be good news. It is the fear of the unknown that worries patients most.'

J&L: 'Thank you, doctor.'

C: 'I am available for any further questions that you might have.'

Scenario 6

Candidate (C): 'Good afternoon Mrs Calder.'

Mother (M): 'Miss Calder, thank you. Can you tell me what is happening?'

C: 'Your daughter, Mary, was brought into the Accident and Emergency department having fallen off a swing and hurt her tummy. We were told that the school tried to contact you but were not successful.'

M: 'I was available on my mobile all the time. They obviously did not try hard enough.'

C: 'I appreciate you are angry about the situation. But if you can bear with me for a few minutes, I can explain to you in detail what actually happened. We are the surgical unit on call for emergencies. I was called down to see Mary after her playground injury. I was very concerned that she might have ruptured her spleen. I asked my consultant to see her. He asked for a scan which showed that she was bleeding severely from a ruptured spleen.'

'After resuscitation we took her to theatre straightaway. While we were making arrangements we tried several times to contact you including through the police. But we were unsuccessful. As this was a desperate emergency we had to take her to theatre to remove her spleen. If we had to wait for you to come and give us consent then her life might have been in danger and we might have been guilty of negligence.'

M: 'Are you not guilty of negligence now that you have operated upon a child without her guardian's consent?'

C: 'Miss Calder, I must say that we are not legally guilty of negligence as events will show. Mary has got through the operation and is well on her way to the recovery room as we speak.'

M: 'So, what happens now?'

C: 'Mary will be given a vaccine against infections in future. She will go home on an oral antibiotic which she needs to take for 2 years to prevent infections. We will also give you a card to that effect that she has had her spleen removed.'

M: 'I still think the authorities both at the school and hospital did not try hard enough to contact me.'

C: 'Please accept my reassurance that we certainly tried every avenue to contact you possible. We always do when dealing with children, unless it is an emergency, as was the case with Mary.'

'Would you like me to show you to the recovery room now? Mary may still be quite drowsy from the anaesthetic but you can stay with her until she is transferred to the ward. If there is anything else I can be of assistance with, please feel free to contact me.'

Scenario 7

This is a very difficult issue that you may actually come across. This could well be a clinical governance problem. In this Scenario there is no correct or wrong answer to the problem. How you discuss the situation with your two examiners will decide the outcome. In such a tricky situation it is unlikely that you will fail. The conversation in the station will probably go like this:

Examiners (E): 'Doctor, you have read the Scenario. What do you propose to do?'

Candidate (C): 'I have read the Scenario. This is a difficult dilemma and I am acutely aware of the importance of maintaining confidentiality when dealing with this delicate matter. I am torn asunder between the welfare of the patient and loyalty towards my consultant. However, I feel that the former, i.e. welfare of the patient takes precedence in this tricky situation. Although my consultant is conversing normally, I do not feel he is fit to perform an emergency laparotomy in his current state.'

'What do I do? I am not in a position to confront my consultant. There is no middle-grade doctor for me to discuss this with. I feel in my position I need to do something otherwise I'll not be able to live with my conscience should anything go wrong. I feel I have two choices. Firstly to ring up the clinical manager on call and the second choice is to talk to the consultant anaesthetist on call.'

'The patient has an intra-abdominal bleed. I have very little time. I would choose to speak to the consultant anaesthetist face-to-face and request him to come to the hospital.'

Scenario 8

Clinical manager (CM), Mr Wheeler: 'Doctor, as you know we have applied for foundation status for our hospital. Obtaining that status would make a huge difference to the standing of our hospital in future. We are short of surgical targets in a very small way. A few extra operations here and there within the next 6 weeks will make all the difference.'

'Can I ask you to put on four varicose vein operations and two A-V shunts for dialysis instead of the list that you have arranged? This would mean that six operations would be done instead of three.

Candidate (C): 'Mr Wheeler, I appreciate your concerns regarding our foundation status. Achieving that would be a tremendous feather in our cap. However, I have huge misgivings in altering the list. The reasons are:

1 The list has been made entirely on clinical needs and indications

2 The patient with AAA has a 6-cm aneurysm which, because of its size, has a high chance of rupture. If that happens that carries a very high mortality unlike an elective repair. Moreover, you may not be aware that he has already been postponed once at the last minute because of lack of an ITU bed

3 The patient for femoro-popliteal bypass has critical ischaemia and rest pain. He has given up smoking. He could lose his limb any day. Should he lose his limb while waiting any longer, he will end up with an amputation. He would then become a huge burden to his family, NHS, and society, not to mention the devastating consequences to his morale

4 The patient for carotid endarterectomy has already had a small stroke from which he has fully recovered. If we do not do his operation as soon as possible, he may develop a complete stroke with catastrophic consequences to him, his family, not to mention the social services and the NHS

5 All three patients have given up smoking and thus have kept their side of the bargain. If we now postpone their operation on non-clinical grounds, it would be betraying their trust. I am sorry, Mr Wheeler, I cannot alter the list for the reasons explained in detail'

Scenario 9

Candidate (C): 'Mr Miller, you wanted to see me with regard to your father. How can I help? How much do you know about your father?'

Mr Miller (M): 'I know that my father has got lung cancer for which no surgical treatment is possible. He had some radiotherapy which made him much more ill and so it has been stopped. I also know that the cancer has spread to his bones. He seems to be in agony. I would like you to consider giving him a strong dose of pain killer to relieve him of the miserable time that he is having. Can you not put an end to his misery please?'

C: 'I know what you are asking me to do Mr Miller. You wish me to give your father a lethal dose of pain killer. Am I right in thinking that?'

M: 'Yes, Doctor.'

C: 'Mr Miller, I am afraid I cannot do that. I understand that you are concerned as bony metastases can be very painful. However, we are doing our best to keep him as pain-free as possible using a morphine pump which he controls. We are also giving him morphine patches and extra pain-killers to help with this.

When you or other family members visit we try not to make him completely dozy so that he can have some conversation with you. As far as I am aware, his pain is fairly well-controlled. However, we can add a different pain medication through another pump which will also help to relax him. This may mean that he is slightly sleepy when you visit.'

'However, if you wish that he should be sleepy when you visit him, we can increase the pain killer to which we can add what is called an anxiolytic. But you do appreciate that we cannot give him a lethal dose of pain killer. I very much regret that nature has to take its course. I assure you we will keep him pain free and we will make this unfortunate journey together with your father keeping him as comfortable as possible all the way.'

Scenario 10

Patient's son, Mr John Sutherland (JS): 'Doctor, you wanted to see me about my mother. What was it about?'

Candidate (C): 'As you know your mother Mrs Sutherland had her hip replaced because of a break in the upper part of her thigh bone. The operation went off fine and from that point of view she is recovering well. I wanted to ask you about her Alzheimer's – how bad is it? Does she recognize you and other family members?'

JS: 'Why do you ask?'

C: 'Unfortunately it is my unpleasant task to talk to you about cardiopulmonary resuscitation should your mother's heart stop while she is in hospital. When making such a decision, we usually consider each patient's overall status in terms of general health and quality of life.'

JS: 'Are you saying that because of her age you do not wish to resuscitate her. After all you did her operation didn't you?'

C: 'You are right, we did her operation as we felt it would improve her quality of life as she was completely mobile prior to this. However, the reason for this conversation is to do with her Alzheimer's disease and her general frailty and not related to her age. From a medical point of view, we do not feel CPR is in her best interest were her heart or breathing to stop. Even if she were to survive CPR, it is unlikely she will recover to her previous quality of life. What are your thoughts about this? What would your mother have liked us to do?'

JS: 'Do I have to make that decision now and give you an answer straightaway?'

C: 'Not at all. This is actually a medical decision. However, before we make any firm decisions we felt it was important to hear your thoughts around this matter and also to find out if your mother had voiced her feelings about this before. I would ask you to take your time and have a family meeting and let me know how you feel about this. Please contact me once you have had time to think and talk this over.'

JS: 'Thank you.'

Chapter 16 **Written communication**

Introduction

At this station your written communication will be assessed. The examiner will provide you with a scenario and you will be provided information of the patient's details. You may also be provided supplementary information such as investigation results.

This would normally take 30 seconds to a minute. You will then have 8 minutes to think and write a letter to the GP regarding the scenario. You will need to write the patient's details as they are in the scenario. Then you write the letter. Allocate your 9 minutes as follows:

- Digesting all the material provided you: 1 minute
- Thinking about what to write: 3 minutes
- Writing the letter: 4 minutes
- Revising your letter: 1 minute

Although you are allowed to finish early, you will still have to remain seated in the station until the bell rings. If you have finished very early consider that you probably have not written enough. Your letter should have the following points:

- The name of the patient, obviously
- Give the reason for your letter
- If a complication has occurred, then what is being done to rectify it
- What is the future plan for the patient?
- Finish off every letter with 'If I can be of any further help please do not hesitate to contact me'

Please make sure that your handwriting is legible. The examiner will not take trouble over deciphering illegible writing.

The following Scenarios are in regard to letters to the GP.

Scenarios

Scenario 1

A 60-year-old patient who was to come in for an oesophagectomy for carcinoma of the oesophagus has had his operation postponed for lack of an ITU, bed the last of which was taken during the night with a bad road traffic accident.

Scenario 2

A patient has been admitted for laparoscopic cholecystectomy. The patient is an insulin-dependent diabetic. On admission her blood glucose is 17mmol/L and her HbA1c last week was 15 (normal = <7). Her operation is therefore postponed.

Scenario 3

Write a letter regarding a 55-year-old man who has been admitted for laparoscopic fundoplication. He is on warfarin and his INR is 7. Therefore his operation is postponed.

Scenario 4

A 60-year-old patient had a routine anterior resection for a low rectal carcinoma. On the 6th post-operative day he became unwell and an anastomotic leak was demonstrated. He underwent an emergency Hartmann's procedure.

Scenario 5

A 30-year-old female underwent a laparoscopic cholecystectomy. She became jaundiced the first day post-operatively. Investigations showed a damaged common bile duct. She is being transferred to a tertiary hepatobiliary unit. Write a letter to the GP informing him/her of this mishap.

Scenario 6

A 60-year-old man has been admitted with a right ureteric colic. He has a solitary kidney because the contralateral kidney was removed as a result of trauma 25 years ago. He is being transferred to a urological unit in a hospital where there are facilities for dialysis. Write a letter informing the GP.

Scenario 7

A 65-year-old male patient was admitted with severe acute pancreatitis a week ago. Unfortunately the patient died of systemic inflammatory response syndrome. Write a letter to inform the GP with the possible sequence of events that led to this outcome.

Scenario 8

A 50-year-old patient was admitted with a perforated duodenal ulcer. He underwent a laparoscopic closure. On the 5th post-operative day he developed swinging pyrexia. Write to the GP informing this outcome and what is being done as a result.

Scenario 9

A 35-year-old professional singer underwent a subtotal thyroidectomy for medically controlled Graves' disease. She has developed hoarseness of voice post-operatively. Inform the GP and explain what is going to happen.

Scenario 10

A 60-year-old patient underwent a superficial parotidectomy for a pleomorphic adenoma. Post-operatively he developed a facial palsy. Write to the GP informing him/her of the situation.

Answers

Please note that the following letters are a guideline to formulating the letter. In planning your letter to the GP the following points should be borne in mind:

- Your ability to write a polite and professional letter
- Explain why the difficult situation might have arisen
- Explain the future if you are describing a complication that has occurred. The examiner would like to see if you have a basic knowledge of the solution to the complication

Scenario 1

Date: 12/2/10

Name of patient: Mr James Smith

Dear Doctor

The above patient was admitted from the list for an oesophagectomy for carcinoma. Unfortunately in the early hours of the morning the last bed in the surgical ITU was taken by a bad road traffic accident patient who is on a ventilator. Although there are beds in the HDU, we would like Mr Smith to be allocated an ITU bed as post-operatively he might need to be ventilated.

Understandably he is disappointed and his family is irate and asked if the delay might make the cancer inoperable. While I could not answer the question definitely, I have assured him that we would allocate the next available bed to him and that we would telephone him.

I have apologized to the patient and his family for these unfortunate circumstances beyond our control. Please do not hesitate to contact me if I can be of any further help.

Yours sincerely

Scenario 2

Date: 12/2/10

Name of patient: Mrs Jean Mackay

Dear Doctor

The above patient who is an insulin-dependent diabetic was admitted from the list for a laparoscopic cholecystectomy. On admission her random blood glucose was 17mmol/L and according to her records her HbA1c last week was 15 (normal = <7). Under the circumstances the anaesthetist rightly decided not to proceed with the operation.

We did give her a choice of being referred to our local consultant physician but she preferred to have it seen to by you as you have been looking after her type 1 diabetes for many years now. Please contact us when you feel that her diabetes is under control. Meanwhile please do not hesitate to contact me if I can be of any further help.

Yours sincerely

Scenario 3

Date: 12/2/10

Name of patient: Mr James Smith

Dear Doctor

The above patient was admitted from the waiting list for a laparoscopic fundoplication for his GORD (gastro-oesophageal reflux disease). He has been on warfarin for almost 2 years for atrial fibrillation. As is our usual practice for patients on warfarin for AF, we advised Mr Smith to stop his warfarin 5 days prior to surgery. Unfortunately, Mr Smith forgot and today his INR is 7. Therefore his operation has had to be postponed.

At present he is on 5mg of warfarin a day. We have advised him to stop this and we have given him Vitamin K to reverse it. We also arranged for him to have repeat blood tests and I would be grateful if you would follow this up and adjust his warfarin dose accordingly, aiming for an INR of 2.5.

Once it is stable please let me know so that we can offer him the next available date for his operation. We have also provided Mr Smith with written instructions about stopping his warfarin 5 days prior to his operation. Meanwhile please do not hesitate to contact me if I can be of any further help.

Yours sincerely

Scenario 4

Date: 12/2/10

Name of patient: Mr James Smith

Dear Doctor

The above patient underwent a low anterior resection for cancer rectum a week ago. Unfortunately on the 6th post-operative day it transpired that he developed a leak from his anastomosis. He had to be taken to theatre as an emergency and the operation had to be converted to a Hartmann's procedure where the anastomosis was resected and the lower descending colon was brought out as an end colostomy and the rectum was closed off. He is now recovering in the HDU.

Understandably the patient and his family are upset at the stoma. I have explained the situation to them and have said that perhaps in a few months down the line we will be able to restore bowel continuity and the stoma could be dispensed with. Please do not hesitate to contact me if I can be of any further help.

Yours sincerely

Scenario 5

Date: 12/2/10

Name of patient: Ms Jean Mackenzie

Dear Doctor

The above lady underwent a laparoscopic cholecystectomy 2 days ago. On the 1st post-operative day she became jaundiced with itching. Blood investigations showed an obstructive pattern. Our worst fears were realized when imaging by MRCP (magnetic resonance cholangiopancreatography) showed the possibility of damage to the common bile duct. She has been transferred to the regional tertiary hepatobiliary centre.

The patient and her family have been kept fully informed and are understandably upset at the whole episode. Please do not hesitate to contact me if I can be of any further help.

Yours sincerely

Scenario 6

Date: 12/2/10

Name of patient: Mr James Smith

Dear Doctor

The above patient of yours was admitted last night with a right ureteric colic. His left kidney was removed 25 years ago for trauma. He is at present free of pain. A contrast spiral CT scan confirms the presence of a 5-mm stone in his lower right ureter.

To be on the safe side this patient is best managed in a hospital with facilities for renal replacement therapy which our hospital cannot provide. He is therefore being transferred to the care of the urologists in our neighbouring hospital. It is envisaged that he will be under the combined care of the urologists and nephrologists.

The patient and his family have been informed and they fully understand the situation. Please do not hesitate to contact me if I can be of any further help.

Yours sincerely

Scenario 7

Date: 12/2/10

Name of patient: Mr James Smith

Dear Doctor

I am sorry to inform you that the above patient died last night from the complications of severe acute pancreatitis. He was admitted a week ago as an emergency with acute pancreatitis which was stratified as severe. He was transferred to the ITU. He had contrast enhanced spiral CT scan (CECT) which showed infected pancreatic necrosis. This was treated by necrosectomy. In spite of vigorous treatment he succumbed to systemic inflammatory response syndrome (SIRS) going on to multiple organ dysfunction syndrome (MODS).

His family, although upset, fully understand the serious nature of the illness and are appreciative of the fact that everything possible has been done. Please do not hesitate to contact me if I can be of any further help.

Yours sincerely

Scenario 8

Date: 12/2/10

Name of patient: Mr James Smith

Dear Doctor

The above 50-year-old patient of yours was admitted as an emergency with perforated duodenal ulcer 5 days ago. Shortly after admission he underwent a laparoscopic closure of his perforation. He progressed satisfactorily until the 5th post-operative day when he became unwell with rigors and swinging pyrexia. Imaging with ultrasound and CT scan showed a subphrenic abscess. This has been drained under CT guidance and he is progressing and is apyrexial at present.

I have warned the patient and the family that sometimes the procedure may have to be repeated because of the loculated nature of the abscess. Please do not hesitate to contact me if I can be of any further help.

Yours sincerely

Scenario 9

Date: 12/2/10

Name of patient: Mrs Jane Smith

Dear Doctor

This patient underwent a subtotal thyroidectomy for medically controlled Graves' disease. In the post-operative period she has developed hoarseness of voice. Immediately after the operation the vocal cords were checked and they were moving normally. She was informed about this possibility during informed consent.

Today, on the 3rd post-operative day, the hoarseness continues albeit slightly better. It is envisaged that the problem might be one of neurapraxia. We hope she should recover fully. She and her family have been kept informed fully although they are understandably upset as this problem may affect her profession. Please do not hesitate to contact me if I can be of any further help.

Yours sincerely

Scenario 10

Date: 12/2/10

Name of patient: Mr John Smith

Dear Doctor

The above patient underwent a superficial parotidectomy for a pleomorphic adenoma. Although during the operation branches of the facial nerve were identified with a nerve stimulator, she has developed post-operatively incomplete facial palsy. Usually this is due to neurapraxia from post-operative oedema or sometimes from nerve ischaemia.

Having explained this to the patient and his family, they are rightly concerned and asked various questions about the future. I said that we hope this will recover and we should wait up to a maximum period of 6 months to assess recovery. If after that there is still residual palsy, then we would consider referral to a plastic surgeon for sling operations. Meanwhile please do not hesitate to contact me if I can be of any further help.

Yours sincerely

PART 3
APPLIED SURGICAL SCIENCES AND CRITICAL CARE

Section 1 **Applied surgical pathology**

Introduction

This section is directed towards helping the reader to be proficient in several stations. For instance, in the oral examination dealing with physiology and critical care (manned and unmanned), pathology, pre-operative assessment of a patient with comorbid conditions, and questions relating to patient discussion on the phone. There will be clinical examination of patients with skin lesions and practical discussion outlining the diagnosis and management. The common conditions are illustrated.

Chapter 17 **Microbiology**

Introduction

Infections are, regrettably, a ubiquitous part of surgical practice and are a significant cause of surgical morbidity and mortality. Patients may be admitted with infections with surgical relevance or develop infections while in hospital or during the post-operative period.

Hence, it is vital that all surgical trainees are familiar with the basic principles of microbiology and infection control. The examiner will be looking for evidence of knowledge in the following areas:

- Principles of infection control in surgery
- Surgically relevant microorganisms
- Antibiotic use in surgery—prophylaxis, treatment, and resistance
- Recognizing the septic patient (see Chapter 25)

Principles of infection control in surgery

Infection control is of paramount importance in surgical practice. In most hospitals, national and local guidelines are implemented by infection control teams to ameliorate the morbidity and mortality associated with infections and sepsis.

Pathogenic or potentially pathogenic microorganisms may originate from a variety of sources to cause infection. These include:

- Infected patients
- Apparently healthy staff or clinically non-infective patients
- Hospital environment
- Biological samples, e.g. blood, sputum, surgical specimen

Transmission of these microbes may occur by:

- Direct contact
- Parenteral inoculation
- Aerosol inhalation
- Faecal–oral route

In addition, in surgical patients, patients' own normal flora can enter the bloodstream and tissues and result in infection as the body's usual defences are breached (e.g. skin).

Hospital admission increases the risk of patients developing infections. Nosocomial infections or hospital acquired infections (HAI) are defined as infections that develop 48 hours or more after admission to hospital or 30 days after discharge from hospital.

Patients may also be more susceptible to infection in certain circumstances.

General factors:

- Extremes of age
- Poor nutrition—obesity and malnutrition
- Smoking
- Length of hospital stay
- Metabolic disease—diabetes mellitus especially if poor glycaemic control, renal failure
- Tissue ischaemia—poor perfusion, poor oxygenation, anaemia
- Hypothermia
- Coexisting infection at another site
- Malignancy and cancer treatment—chemotherapy, radiotherapy
- Immunosuppression:
  - ◆ Long-term steroid use
  - ◆ Previous splenectomy—susceptible to infection by encapsulated organisms
  - ◆ Transplant recipients—on immunosuppressive therapy
  - ◆ Disease-modifying antirheumatoid drugs
  - ◆ Treatment for immune-mediated conditions such as Crohn's disease

- ◆ Haematological diseases
- ◆ Immune deficiency (e.g. HIV, SCID)

Procedural factors:

- Emergency surgery
- Invasive procedures
- Necrotic tissue
- Presence of a foreign body including the use of prosthesis—joint implants, mesh
- Indwelling tubes/devices
- Trauma/burns
- Recent surgery, especially if long duration of surgery
- Poor surgical technique—tissue trauma, tension, haemostasis, poor blood supply
- Haematoma formation
- Inadequate sterilization/disinfection—surgical scrub, instruments, skin antisepsis

Microbiological factors:

- Bacterial colonization, e.g. MRSA in nares
- Inadequate or inappropriate antibiotic prophylaxis
- Antibiotic resistance, e.g. after protracted use of broad-spectrum agents
- Virulence of organism
- Size of bacteriological load

Basic principles

Recognizing this, a few standard precautions are necessary to help control infection when dealing with surgical patients.

On the ward:

- Conscientious hygiene—especially hand washing before and after patient contact. **Hand washing is the single most effective procedure for preventing nosocomial infections.** Alternatively alcoholic chlorhexidine preparations can be used on visibly clean hands. Cuts and abrasions should be covered with water-resistant occlusive dressing
- Screening for specific infections (e.g. MRSA) in all patients admitted to hospital and treating/ eradicating as appropriate
- In high-risk patients, testing for blood-borne infections should be carried out with the patient's informed consent. Discretion and patient confidentiality must be maintained at all times
- Isolation of infective patients
- Barrier nursing/use of personal protective equipment (PPE)—e.g. disposable gloves, aprons, masks, visors:
  - ◆ Dealing with infective patients
  - ◆ Performing exposure-prone procedures
  - ◆ Dealing with patients with susceptible patients (e.g. neutropenic)
- Blood and other body substance of all patient should be treated as potentially infective
- In patients clinically suspected to have an infection:
  - ◆ Where possible, obtain samples for culture prior to commencing antimicrobial therapy
  - ◆ Appropriate use of antimicrobial treatment—short, focused treatment with narrow-spectrum agents
- Vaccination of all staff against high-risk infections. **All healthcare workers must be immunized against hepatitis B and should be aware of their HIV and hepatitis C status**
- Regular cleaning of ward areas
- Patient should have a shower (preferably with an antiseptic agent) the night before or the morning of surgery

Throughout the **perioperative period**, certain measures help to reduce the incidence of infection:

- Appropriate antibiotic prophylaxis (detailed below)
- Normothermia—aim to keep the patient's temperature above 36°C
- Normoglycaemia—maintain blood glucose level <11mmol/L
- Good tissue oxygenation—aim to keep saturation >96%
- Good tissue perfusion—maintain a normotensive blood pressure and treat shock early
- Improve nutrition pre-operatively. If possible, delay surgery until optimal nutritional status achieved. Commence nutrition as soon after surgery as possible, ideally via the enteral route.
- Remove all indwelling tubes/devices as soon after surgery as practicable

In the **operating theatre**, standard theatre etiquette and the principles of asepsis should be adhered to minimize contamination and maintain a sterile operating field:

- Surgical site:
  - Hair removal itself does contribute to infection control and should only be carried out if hair mechanically interferes with the surgical wound or dressing. Pre-operative hair removal should be carried out immediately prior to surgery—preferably with electric clippers with a sterile disposable head. Razors are not recommended as it may cause nicks or skin abrasions which bacteria can colonize.
  - Pre-operative skin preparation of clean skin with a no-touch technique using an antiseptic solution and radiating from inside out—pay extra attention to high-risk areas such as the groin, perineum, and axilla. This should be repeated 2–3 times using a fresh sponge each time. The antiseptic solution should be applied for 2–5 minutes before starting surgical procedure. (Detailed further below.)
  - Sterile drapes—do not decrease infection rates in itself but helps to augment the surgical field for the scrub team
- Theatre environment:
  - Optimum temperature (18–25°C) and optimum humidity (40–60%)
  - Positive pressure ventilation or laminar flow theatres (orthopaedic or implant surgery)
  - Regular air changes—20–23 cycles per hour
  - Minimal fittings and furnishings, all made of easily disinfected material
  - Only necessary personal in theatres and traffic flow from clean to dirty
  - All personnel should be attired in surgical scrubs
- Scrub team:
  - Scrubbing-up of hands to elbows with antiseptic solution e.g. povidone-iodine 2% or chlorhexidine gluconate 1.5% solution. Use a stiff brush to clean fingernails at the beginning of the list
  - Use sterile, water-proof, bacteria-impermeable gowns and sterile well-fitted gloves
  - The scrub team should also use theatre caps, masks, closed footwear, and beard protectors (if required). These PPEs are not sterile and there should be no contact with these equipment once sterile
  - Masks have no effect on infection rates but will help deflect coughs and sneezes. Masks also provide protection for the scrub team from splashes as does the use of a visor
  - Double gloving is recommended to protect the scrub team from needlestick injury
  - Scrub team should remain sterile throughout the procedure and must only handle sterile objects. In the event of contamination, gloves or gown must be changed as needed
  - Gloves, gowns, and masks should be removed before leaving the operating theatre
- Sterile equipment—detailed below
- Handling of sharps:
  - Sharps must not be passed by hand—blades and needles should be passed in a kidney dish and sutures should be passed mounted on a needle-holder to decrease the risk of needlestick injury
  - Suture needles should only be handled with instruments—needle holder or forceps

- ◆ When tying a knot, the needle should first be placed in the needle-holder so the sharp point is facing in.
- ◆ Blunt tip needles should be used for mass closure of the abdomen
- ◆ If bent or mis-shaped, a needle should be discarded
- ◆ Disposed in yellow puncture-resistant biohazard container as soon as possible after use
- At the end:
  - ◆ The patient's skin should be cleaned of any blood or contaminant
  - ◆ The wound should be cleaned and dressed with an impervious dressing
  - ◆ Surgical specimens should be labelled, placed in secure containers, and sent off for analysis
  - ◆ Clinical waste and should be disposed of appropriately in yellow/orange biohazard bags

Skin antisepsis

A potential source of pathogens causing surgical site infections (SSI) is believed to originate from the patient's own skin flora. Skin preparation with an antimicrobial solution is critical in reducing SSIs. The ideal skin antiseptic agent has:

- A broad spectrum of activity
- Rapid antimicrobial activity
- Prolonged duration of action
- Effective in the presence of organic material, e.g. pus, blood
- Non-irritating or low allergic potential

The most commonly used skin preparation agents used today include iodophor or chlorhexidine containing products, which may be either aqueous- or alcohol-based solutions.

Alcohol-based agents (usually 70% isopropyl alcohol):

- Broad spectrum of activity—effective against bacteria, mycobacteria, viruses, and some fungi but not spores
- Rapid activity. Acts by denaturing protein and subsequently causing cell lysis
- **Flammable**. Caution with diathermy. Ensure solution has dried thoroughly before draping to avoid pools of potentially flammable alcohol-based solution

Chlorhexidine-based products (e.g. chlorhexidine gluconate 2% and isopropyl alcohol 70%):

- Broad spectrum of activity—effective against bacteria, viruses, and fungi but not spores or mycobacteria. (However, its effect is augmented in alcohol-based preparations.)
- Moderately rapid and sustained activity. Acts by disrupting cell membranes
- Non-toxic to skin or mucous membranes
- Inactivated by some organic material, e.g. pus

Iodopho-based solutions (e.g. povidone-iodine):

- Broad spectrum of activity—effective against bacteria, virus, mycobacteria, fungi, and spores
- Moderately rapid but has a shorter duration of action than chlorhexidine. Releases 'free' iodine which causes oxidation and cell damage
- Easily inactivated by organic material, e.g. blood, pus, faeces
- Irritant to skin, may cause hypersensitivity or allergic reactions
- Stains skin—area covered by solution can be verified

The choice of antiseptic should be made after patient assessment but recent data suggests that chlorhexidine 2% with alcohol is superior to povidone-iodine at decreasing SSIs.

Sterilization and disinfection of surgical equipment

This is unlikely to feature as a major part of an OSCE station but it is useful to understand the principles behind these processes

Some definitions:

- **Sterilization**—process of completely eliminating all viable microorganisms including spores and viruses from inanimate objects. It utilizes extreme temperatures, chemicals, and irradiation and hence is not suitable for use on skin or viable tissue
- **Disinfection**—process of reducing the number of viable microorganisms present on an inanimate object using physical or chemical agents. Not suitable for use on living tissue
- **Antiseptics**—chemical agent used to destroy microorganisms on living tissue

All surgical equipment which penetrate skin or mucous membrane or used for invasive procedures must be sterile. Instruments may be:

- Pre-sterilized single-use disposable items—these items should be opened just before use in an aseptic manner and disposed off as soon as practicable after use
- Reusable items which are sterilized before each use—a number of different methods can be employed to sterilize these objects

In most hospitals, sterilizations, disinfection, packaging, and storage of surgical equipment is carried out by a sterile services department.

Decontamination

Irrespective of the method of sterilization, thorough physical cleaning of instruments with warm water and soap to remove blood or other material is essential for disinfection or sterilization to be effective.

Sterilization

There are a number of methods of sterilization of surgical instruments and the three most commonly used methods are briefly described below:

- Autoclave/steam under pressure:
  - ◆ This is the most efficient and reliable method of sterilization
  - ◆ Usually at 134°C, 30 psi for 3 minutes or 121°C, 15 psi for 15 minutes
  - ◆ Only suitable for heat-resistant, non-moisture sensitive instruments—e.g. metal, glass, or some plastic instruments
- Ethylene oxide:
  - ◆ Highly penetrative gas, usually requires 12 hours (including time for aeration to rid the article of residual toxic ethylene oxide)
  - ◆ Suitable for instruments which cannot withstand temperatures above 60°C—e.g. electrical, electronic, fibreoptics, and heat sensitive plastics
  - ◆ Often used for single-use items
- Dry heat:
  - ◆ Dry heat at 160°C for at least 2 hours
  - ◆ Glass ware, oils and fats (e.g. petroleum jelly), carbon steel instruments

Disinfection

There are a number of different methods of disinfection of inanimate objects which include

- Low-pressure steam
- Boiling water
- Glutaraldehyde 2%:
  - ◆ Twenty-minute immersion will disinfect the instrument (rid it off most microorganisms but not spores)
  - ◆ For disinfection of heat-sensitive instruments—used for flexible fibreoptics, e.g. endoscopes
  - ◆ Toxic and an extreme irritant to skin—must be washed off before use

Infection control in high-risk patients

All patients should be treated as potentially infective and all routine precautions should be used with no exception. When dealing with patients known to have blood-borne infections (e.g. HIV, hepatitis B, hepatitis C) these precautions are even more important as potential breaches may have greater consequence. Certain additional measures may need to be taken and these include:

- Avoid invasive procedures in these patients if possible
- Confidentiality and discretion should be practised throughout but healthcare personnel involved in the patient's care should be informed of the patient's infectious status
- Using disposable instruments and equipment
- Use blunt suture needles where possible
- Use staples rather than sutures
- Invasive procedures should be performed by experience surgeons
- Only necessary theatre staff and equipment in the operating theatre
- Terminal cleaning of theatre after the procedure and appropriate disposal of contaminated waste

Surgically important microorganisms

Disease causing organisms include:

- Bacteria:
  - Gram-positive (stains blue with Gram stain) or Gram-negative (stains pink)
  - Cocci (circular) or bacilli (rod-shaped)
  - Aerobic, anaerobic, or facultatively anaerobic
  - May release toxins—endotoxins or exotoxins
- Viruses:
  - DNA viruses or RNA viruses with reverse transcriptase can integrate themselves into host DNA to replicate
  - Other RNA virus replicates within the cell
  - Host cell lysis to release virions into the bloodstream to infect more cells
  - May also stimulate cell proliferation—may result in neoplasia (e.g. EBV, HPV)
- Eukaryotes:
  - Fungi:
  - Yeasts—e.g. *Candida*
  - Moulds—e.g. *Aspergilus*
  - Dimorphic funghi—e.g. *Histoplasma*
- Protozoa:
  - Luminal—e.g. amoebiasis, giardiasis
  - Blood-borne—e.g. malaria
  - Intracellular—e.g. toxoplasmosis
- Parasitic worms:
  - Platyhelminths
  - Cestodes
  - Trematodes
  - Nematodes

Bacterial

Gram-positive cocci

Staphylococci

- Arranged in clusters.
- May be coagulase positive (*Staphylococcus aureus*) or coagulase negative (*Staphylococcus epidermidis*)

Staph. aureus

- 30% adults carry *Staph. aureus* in their anterior nares. Carriers transfer the organism to skin allowing a portal of entry
- Clinically it produces skin and soft tissue infections including:
  - Impetigo
  - Folliculitis
  - Cellulitis
- Deeper infections may occur after trauma or surgery:
  - Endocarditis
  - Pericarditis
  - Osteomyelitis
  - Lung abscesses/pneumonia

Staph. epidermides

- Form part of normal skin flora, are of low pathogenicity, and rarely cause infections in healthy individuals
- May cause nosocomial infections especially those related to an in-dwelling foreign body, e.g. catheters or prosthetic material
- In these circumstances, may cause septicaemia or prosthetic valve endocarditis

Streptococci

- Arranged in pairs or chains
- Classified by ability to lyse erythrocytes (α-haemolytic, e.g. *Strep. pneumoniae*—partial lysis, β-haemolytic, e.g. *Strep. pyogenes*—complete lysis, γ-haemolytic, e.g. *Strep. bovis*—non-haemolytic)
- May also be divided into Lancefield groups based on the number of polysaccharide antigens present on its surface
- β-haemolytic strains (Lancefield Group A, B, C, and G) are often responsible for systemic infections

Strep. pyogenes (Lancefield group A)

- Causes various cutaneous and systemic infections including:
  - Upper respiratory tract infections—pharyngitis, tonsillitis, quinsy
  - Ear infections—otitis media, mastoiditis
  - Soft tissue infections—erysipelas, wound infections, necrotizing fasciitis

Strep. pneumoniae

- Common diplococcus pathogen
- Found in the nasopharynx of 20% of adults
- Common cause of localized and systemic infections including:
  - Sinusitis
  - Meningitis
  - Pneumonia
  - Endocarditis
  - Osteomyelitis
- Infection can be prevented by the pneumococcal vaccine

Viridans group streptococci (α-haemolytic)

- These are respiratory, GI, and oral cavity commensals—low pathogenicity
- Infection usually occurs in immunocompromised hosts
- Principal virulence trait is to adhere to cardiac valves and cause endocarditis
- Account for 30–40% of cases of endocarditis
- Most occur in patients with valvular heart disease

- Other risk factors include:
  - Prosthetic heart valves
  - IV drug abuse

Enterococci

- Common commensal of the GI tract
- Significant cause of nosocomial infection including:
  - Urinary tract infections
  - Endocarditis
  - Intra-abdominal infection
- Risk factors for infection include
  - Severe underlying disease
  - Previous surgery
  - Previous antibiotic therapy
  - Renal failure
  - The presence of vascular or urinary catheters

Gram-positive bacilli

Surgically important Gram-positive bacilli are the anaerobes:

- *Clostridium* species (spore-forming):
  - *C. botulinum*—botulism
  - *C. perfringens*—gas gangrene/ myonecrosis. *C. perfringens,* found in soil and faeces, proliferates in necrotic tissue. It releases a powerful exotoxin (alpha toxin) which destroys nearby tissue, including muscle, generating gas. It can cause widespread muscle destruction (myonecrosis) resulting in renal failure, septic shock, and even death. Management includes resuscitation, aggressive debridement (including amputation if needed), and antibiotics (penicillin and metronidazole)
  - *C. tetani*—tetanus. *C. tetani* is found in soil and faeces, and produces a neurotoxic exotoxin, tetanospasmin. Patients develop painful skeletal muscle spasm resulting in 'lockjaw', risus sardonicus (sardonic grin), opisthotonus (arching of the back muscles), neck stiffness, dysphagia, and diaphragmatic spasm causing respiratory complications. Often requires ITU-level management. Although rare in the UK, tetanus has a high mortality rate in excess of 40%. However, it is a preventable disease with primary immunization, prompt attention to wounds, and the use of human tetanus immunoglobulin in non-immune individuals with 'dirty' wounds
  - *C. difficile*—pseudomembranous colitis
- *Actinomyces israelii* (non-spore forming):
  - Actinomycosis

Gram-negative cocci

- *Neisseria*:
  - *Neisseria meningitides*—meningitis, septicaemia
  - *Neisseria gonorrhoea*—gonorrhoea
- *Moraxella catarrhalis*—atypical pneumonia

Gram-negative bacilli

Many organisms in this group are of surgical relevance. They can be divided into aerobes and anaerobes.

Aerobic Gram-negative bacilli—**Pseudomonas aeroginosa:**

- Serious pathogen especially in:
  - Immunocompromised patients
  - Patients with burns, malignancy
  - Patients with indwelling tubes—e.g. catheter, endotracheal tubes

- Can survive in antiseptics and other fluids
- Important cause of nosocomial infections
- Causes:
  - ◆ Pneumonia
  - ◆ Septicaemia
  - ◆ Urinary tract infections
  - ◆ Wound infections

Anaerobic Gram-negative bacilli:

- *Escherichia coli*:
  - ◆ Urinary tract infections
  - ◆ Biliary tract infections
  - ◆ Wound infections—especially after lower GI surgery
  - ◆ Diarrhoeal illnesses
- *Klebsiella* spp.:
  - ◆ Urinary tract infections
  - ◆ Endocarditis
  - ◆ Septicaemia

Other Gram-negative bacilli include:
- *Proteus*—UTI, wound infections
- *Salmonella*—typhoid, enteric fever
- *Shigella*—dysentery
- *Yersinia*—food poisoning

*Necrotizing fasciitis

Necrotizing fasciitis is an uncommon but potentially fatal condition characterized by a synergistic, rapidly spreading infection along deep fascial planes with necrosis of subcutaneous tissue. It is commonly a polymicrobial infection involving streptococci, staphylococci, anaerobes, Gram-negative bacilli and *Bacteriodes*.

Necrotizing fasciitis is usually seen in patients with a recent history of trauma or surgery and most commonly affects the trunk, extremities, and perineum (involvement of the male perineum is termed Fournier's gangrene). Initially, patients present with erythema, pain, and swelling of the overlying skin. Due to its uncommon nature and non-specific signs, diagnosis is often delayed. However, it quickly progresses to affect a more widespread area with purplish discoloration, crepitus, putrid discharge, bullae, and necrosis. Necrotizing fasciitis is often associated systemic complications including disseminated intravascular coagulation, multiorgan failure, and septic shock.

Management includes resuscitation (usually on intensive care), broad-spectrum antibiotics, and aggressive surgical debridement. Repeated excisions are often necessary until the infection is adequately controlled. The role of hyperbaric oxygen in the treatment of necrotizing fasciitis remains contentious.

Surgical site infection

SSIs are infections at the surgical site which develops within 30 days of a surgical procedure (or within 1 year if an implant is in place). SSIs are defined by certain criteria which include:

- Evidence of inflammation—tenderness, heat, swelling, redness AND/OR loss of function
- Purulent discharge or evidence of an abscess
- Positive culture of aseptically obtained specimen (e.g. purulent discharge or wound swab)

SSIs can be divided into:

- Superficial incisional SSIs—only involves skin and subcutaneous tissue
- Deep incisional SSIs—involves deep soft tissue (muscle and fascial layers)
- Organ/space SSIs—involves any organ or spaces manipulated during the operation

Classification of operations

Operations can be classified into four different categories with increasing bacterial contamination and incidence of SSIs from Class 1 to 4:

1 **Clean** (e.g. hernia repair)—<2% of cases are complicated by SSIs:
   • No inflammation encountered
   • The respiratory, alimentary, and genitourinary tracts are not entered
   • No break in aseptic technique
2 **Clean-contaminated** (e.g. simple cholecystectomy)—<10%:
   • The respiratory, alimentary, or genitourinary tracts are entered without significant spillage (not the colon)
3 **Contaminated** (e.g. simple appendicectomy)—15–20%:
   • Acute inflammation encountered, without pus
   • Visible contamination of the wound
   • Spillage from a hollow viscus
   • Compound/open injuries operated on within 4 hours
4 **Dirty** (e.g. diverticular perforation)—>40%:
   • Perforated hollow viscus, necrotic tissue or pus
   • Compound/open injuries >4 hours old

Antibiotic use in surgery

Antibiotics are molecules that kill (bactericidal) or stop the growth (bacteriostatic) of microorganisms, particularly bacteria.
   Different classes have different mechanisms of action to achieve this which include

• Inhibition of cell wall synthesis
• Inhibition of protein synthesis
• Inhibition of nucleic acid synthesis
• Alteration of cell membrane function

Antibiotic treatment

Specific antimicrobial treatment for all infectious diseases is outside the scope of this book. We will discuss good practice when prescribing antibiotics and a few surgically relevant antibiotics.

Good practice recommendations for antimicrobial prescribing

Antimicrobial management is a key component of infection prevention, control, and treatment. Prudent antimicrobial prescribing is essential in reducing the prevalence of or *C. difficile* diarrhoea and antibiotic resistance. Factors that should be considered when prescribing antibiotics are:

Decision to prescribe

• Take microbiology samples before commencing antibiotics but do not delay treatment in a severely ill patient
• Should be clinically justified
• Ideally based on positive culture (but remember, treat the patient not the result—a positive result in a well patient may represent contamination or colonization, no necessarily infection)
• If empirical treatment—review early in light of microbial results and change or discontinue as soon as reasonable
• Consider non-antibiotic options—e.g. wound debridement, removal of foreign body
• Always consider:
   ◆ Sensitivity of organism involved (or likely organism, if empirical treatment)
   ◆ Previous antimicrobial history
   ◆ Previous infection with multiresistant organisms

◆ Allergies—document nature of reaction as well (e.g. anaphylaxis, rash)
◆ Toxicity—e.g. in renal failure, hepatic failure

Route—IV or oral

- Generally, oral is the preferred route
- Use IV in patients with:
  ◆ Severe infections—high tissue concentrations vital
  ◆ Oral route unavailable
  ◆ Antibiotic not available in oral form
- If using IV, change to oral as soon as practicable (review after 48 hours)

Review prescription regularly

- The need and choice of antibiotic treatment should be reviewed regularly:
  ◆ Duration of therapy—as short as possible for effective treatment
  ◆ Write stop/review date on prescription
  ◆ Route of delivery—ideally oral
- Review available microbiology results and rationalize antimicrobial treatment accordingly
- Advice from microbiology team

Minimize use of broad-spectrum antimicrobials (especially certain classes, e.g. quinolones, cephalosporins, broad-spectrum penicillins)

Use broad-spectrum antibiotics only if:

- Offending organism unknown, change accordingly once microbiology results back
- Other effective agents unavailable

Classes of commonly used antibiotics in surgery

1 **Aminoglycosides**
   - Interfere with protein synthesis vital for bacterial growth
   - Effective against aerobic bacteria especially Gram-negative bacteria—*E.coli, Klebsiella, Pseudomonas aeroginosa*
   - Dose-related side-effects—nephrotoxicity, ototoxicity
   - Require IV administration
   - E.g. Gentamicin, amikacin, neomycin, streptomycin
2 **Beta-lactams**
   - Act by interfering with peptidoglycan cross-links in the bacterial cell wall
   - Penicillins:
     ◆ Effective against Gram-positive organisms, some Gram-negative cocci and spirochaetes (e.g. syphilis, Lyme disease)
     ◆ Some subtypes such as ampicillin, piperacillin/tazobactam are also effective against some Gram-negative bacilli (e.g. *Pseudomonas aeroginosa, Enterobacter*)
     ◆ Penicillin combinations (e.g. co-amoxiclav—amoxicillin/clavulanate) the added part prevents bacterial resistance of the first component and widens the spectrum of its effect
     ◆ Good tissue penetrance, inexpensive
     ◆ Can cause antibiotic related diarrhoea
     ◆ Hypersensitivity and allergic reactions which range from a rash (in 10%) to anaphylaxis (in <0.1%)
   - Cephalosporins:
     ◆ Many generations—generally wider-spectrum of activity (especially to Gram-negative organism) and lower resistance from generation to generation
     ◆ Broad-spectrum—effective against both Gram-positive and Gram-negative organisms
     ◆ Good tissue penetrance
     ◆ 10% of patients with penicillin allergy will have an allergic/hypersensitivity reaction with cephalosporins

- ◆ Nausea (with alcohol), diarrhoea
- ◆ E.g. cefalexin (1st gen), cefuroxime (2nd gen), ceftriaxone (3rd gen), cefepime (4th gen), and ceftobiprole (5th gen)
- Other beta-lactams include monobactam (e.g. aztreonam) and carbapenem (e.g. meropenem, imipenem)

3 **Glycopeptides**
- Inhibit peptidoglycan sysnthesis in the bacterial cell wall
- Used to treat MRSA, *C.diff* diarrhoea, serious Gram-positive infections
- Side effects include nephrotoxicity, ototoxicity, 'red man syndrome'
- E.g. vancomycin, teicoplanin

4 **Macrolides**
- Irreversibly bind to ribosomes to inhibit protein synthesis
- Useful for streptococcal infections, upper respiratory tract infections, atypical pneumonia, *H. pylori* eradication (triple therapy), spirochaetes infections, leprosy, TB
- Used in patients with penicillin allergy
- Side effects include hepatotoxicity, vomiting, diarrhoea
- Drug interactions—antihistamines, warfarin, carbamazepine
- E.g. erythromycin, clarithromycin, azithromycin

5 **Quinolones**
- Inhibits bacterial DNA replication
- Useful for biliary infections, urinary tract infections, prostatitis, community acquired pneumonia, bacterial diarrhoea
- Same bioavailability orally and IV
- Side effects include arrhythmias, tendinitis, central nervous system disturbances
- E.g. ciprofloxacin, norfloxacin

6 **Sulfonamides**
- Inhibits folic acid production which is necessary for cell growth
- Used for urinary tract infections, enterocolitis, PCP in immunocompromised patients
- Side effects include Stevens–Johnson syndrome, toxic epidermal necrolysis, hepatic necrosis, blood dyscrasias, vomiting, diarrhoea
- E.g. co-trimoxazole, trimethoprim

7 **Tetracyclines**
- Inhibits bacterial protein synthesis
- Used for acne, Chlamydia, mycoplasma infections (TB, leprosy), brucellosis, syphilis
- Side effects include photosensitivity, diarrhoea, vomiting, browning of enamel, slow bone growth
- Avoid in pregnancy and in children <12 years
- E.g. tetracycline, oxytetracycline, doxycycline

8 **Other antibiotics**
- Clindamycin:
  - ◆ Effective against Gram-positive cocci and anaerobes
  - ◆ Used in bone and joint infections
  - ◆ Can cause *C. diff* pseudomembranous colitis
- Metronidazole:
  - ◆ Effective against anaerobes, *Entamoeba*, *Giardia*, *C. diff* diarrhoea
  - ◆ Metallic taste, nausea, alcohol is contraindicated
- Nitrofurantoin:
  - ◆ Used in urinary tract infections

Antibiotic prophylaxis (Box 17.1)

Antibiotic prophylaxis is recommended for:

- Procedures with a high-risk of post-op infection
- Procedures in which a post-op infection may have severe consequences (e.g. joint prosthesis)

Box 17.1 Example of prophylaxis for adults undergoing selected surgical procedures

Upper GI surgery

- Oesophageal, gastric, or duodenal surgery—IV cefuroxime 1.5g

Biliary surgery

- High-risk laparoscopic cholecystectomy or open HPB surgery—IV cefuroxime 1.5g + IV metronidazole 500mg
  (High risk—on-table cholangiogram, conversion to open, acute cholecystitis, jaundice, CBD stones, immunosuppression)
- ERCP in high risk patients—IV gentamicin 5mg /kg or oral ciprofloxacin 750mg
- (High-risk—pseudocyst, jaundice, incomplete biliary drainage, immunosuppression)

Lower GI surgery

- Small bowel, large bowel, appendicectomy—IV cefuroxime 1.5g + IV metronidazole 500mg
- Hernia repair with mesh—IV cefuroxime 1.5g

Breast surgery

- Breast surgery including reconstructive and implants—IV co-amoiclav 1.2g

Orthopaedic surgery

- Joint replacement with prosthetic device, closed fracture fixation/repair—IV ceftriaxone 2g

Vascular surgery

- Abdominal or lower-limb vascular surgery involving grafts or lower-limb amputation—IV co-amoxiclav 1.2g

---

The aim of antibiotic prophylaxis is to reduce the incidence of SSIs. Patients undergoing elective Class 1–3 procedures should receive prophylaxis, if indicated. Class 4 procedures involve operating on infected tissue; hence these patients need antibiotic treatment rather than prophylaxis.

Prophylaxis with antibacterial drugs works by reducing intra-operative microbial contamination to a level that will not overwhelm host defences. Administration must achieve a tissue concentration sufficient to prevent growth of organisms that enter the surgical site between the first incision to skin closure. Antibiotic choice is usually determined by local policy and local antibiotic resistance patterns. It should be narrow-spectrum and cover the expected pathogen for that operative site and type.

This is usually provided by a single standard therapeutic IV dose of an antimicrobial agent given at induction of anaesthesia and within 0–30 minutes prior to incision. Wound infection is more likely if prophylaxis is given >2 hours prior to the start of the procedure.

In some circumstances, additional doses will be required. This is usually only given for the 1st 24 hours after surgery.

- Prolonged duration of surgery (>4 hours)
- Increased blood loss (>1.5L in an adult or >25ml/kg in a child)
- Arthroplasty

In general, further post-operative doses do not confer any added benefit and increase the likelihood of unwanted effects

- Toxicity—e.g. gentamicin
- *Clostridium difficile* diarrhoea
- Antimicrobial resistance—e.g. MRSA
- Side effects
- Allergies

Antibiotic choice will need to be altered in patients with (refer to local hospital guidelines)

- With penicillin allergy
- MRSA

Splenectomized patients

Splenectomized patients are at increased risk of infection, particularly by encapsulated organisms (i.e. *S. pneumonia, H. influenza, N. menigitidis*). Hence these patients should be:

- Immunized—pneumococcal vaccine (every 5 years), HiB vaccine, meningococcal C vaccine and annual influenza vaccine
- Elective surgery—immunized 2 weeks pre-operatively
- Emergency surgery—as soon as possible post-operatively
- Commenced on life-long prophylactic antibiotics with penicillin (or erythromycin if penicillin allergic)

Antibiotic resistance

Antibiotic resistance is rising and occurs as a result of selective survival pressure on bacteria. There are different mechanisms by which bacteria can attain resistance (plasmid transfer, conjugation, transduction) and this is then passed to subsequent bacterial progeny.

Risk factors that may contribute to increased resistance include:

- Inappropriate prescription
- Partial completion of antibiotic course
- Extensive use of antibiotics in a sick patient with multiple bacterial infections.
- Natural evolution

Some specific resistant bacteria include:

Methicillin resistant *Staphylococcus aureus* (MRSA)

Beta-lactam antibiotics usually inhibit bacterial cell wall synthesis by inactivating penicillin-binding proteins. However, MRSA strains produce an alternative protein that allows continued cell wall synthesis, rendering beta-lactams ineffective against it.

Vancomycin is currently the 1st-line antibiotic when treating MRSA infections. However, some strains are developing intermediate and complete vancomycin resistant genes.

MRSA can be either hospital- or community-acquired and can cause serious systemic infections. These patients should receive antibiotic treatment based on local hospital guidelines.

MRSA is also easily transmissible and certain precautions should be practised to decrease/prevent MRSA transmission:

- Hand washing
- Patient screening—patients known to carry MRSA should have a course of eradication therapy prior to high risk surgery.
- Isolation of carriers/infected
- Removal of colonized catheters
- Timely treatment of infection

Vancomycin resistant enterococci (VRE)

Enterococci reside in the GI tract and female genitalia as a normal commensal. It has properties which help it evade several antibiotics including vancomycin but it does not usually cause disease in healthy populations. However, it can cause infections in immunocompromised patients, ITU patients, elderly patients, and patients with chronic diseases or those who have previously received vancomycin.

Antibiotic resistance in *Enterococcus* can either be:

- Intrinsic—low level of resistance, limited clinical significance
- Acquired—from transfer of genes from other bacteria, more likely to cause disease, e.g. *E. faecalis*

Patients with VRE infections should be treated with antibiotics based on sensitivity results and this may include aminoglycosides, cephalosporins, and clindamycin.

Similar prevention strategies (as employed for MRSA) should be in place.

Scenarios

Scenario 1

You are an ST2 doctor on the breast firm. Your consultant is about to start performing a mastectomy and you are assisting him in this operation. This is the first case on the list. Please demonstrate how you 'scrub' up, gown, and glove for this procedure. Please presume that you are in theatre scrubs and clogs.

Scenario 2

You are the on-call ST1 surgeon on nights. You are in theatre and have just finished closing up after an open appendicectomy, when your scrub nurse (actress) accidentally stabs her index finger with a contaminated needle. She is very worried and asks you for advice. Please demonstrate how you would proceed.

Scenario 3

You are the ST1 plastic surgery doctor on call. You have just received a call from A&E about a 6-year-old girl who has sustained a dog bite to her face. She has attended with her mum. She is currently clinically stable and is awaiting further review. The A&E ST1 doctor has taken a brief history from the patient as detailed below. Please detail how you would assess the wound and outline your initial management plan.

Mandy Palmer, a 6-year-old girl was bitten by her family pet (adult German Shepherd dog) on the right cheek 3 hours ago. She was playing with the dog at home when attacked. No other injuries sustained. Patient is up-to-date with immunization and has no past medical history of significance. She has no known allergies. The dog is healthy and has been vaccinated for rabies. The pet has been taken to the veterinarian.

(Actors play the parent and child. You are provided a photograph of a child with a dog-bite to her face.)

Scenario 4

You are presented a card with a history as below.

A 22-year old university student, Ciara Brown, has been brought in by ambulance with a 2-hour history of a severe left-sided loin-to-groin pain with a point of maximum tenderness in her left flank. She describes the pain as a constant, severe pain and finds that the pain does not improve in any position. She has been writhing around in bed trying to get comfortable to no avail. She also gives a history of nausea, vomiting, and two episodes of rigors since the onset of pain.

Systemic enquiry reveals increased urinary frequency and dysuria 24 hours preceding the onset of pain. Over the past 2 weeks she has been trekking in Peru and returned from her holiday the day before. She has no past medical history of note and is not on any regular medications.

Her vital signs are: Sats 97% on room air, RR 26/min, HR 108 /min, BP 107/92, Temp 38.3°C.

What is the most likely cause of this patient's condition?

1 Please detail your initial management of this patient. She is currently still in A&E. It is 7pm on a Friday evening.
2 The results of the patient's investigations are as follows:
   • Urine dipstick:
     ◆ Blood +++, nitrites++, leucocytes++
   • Blood tests:
     ◆ WCC 16.8 × 10⁹/L, CRP 208,
     ◆ Urea 9.2mmol/L, creatinine 158μmol/L
   • CT KUB:
     ◆ A 7-mm calculi in her right ureter
     ◆ Hydronephrosis, dilated pelvis and ureter
     How would you proceed from here?
3 It is now 10pm on a Friday night—the on-call radiologist suggests that it may be safer to arrange this for Monday morning and manage the patient conservatively over the weekend.

Scenario 5

Mrs Matilda Cooper is an obese 65-year-old patient who has been admitted to hospital with a 2-day history of upper abdominal pain, pyrexia, vomiting, and clinical jaundice. On examination, she is hypotensive, tachycardic, and drowsy. She is tender across her upper abdomen and is Murphy's sign positive. She is known to have gallstones and is awaiting a laparoscopic cholecystectomy. Her other past medical history of note is a pacemaker for heart block, ischaemic heart disease and osteoarthritis.

1 You are the ST2 surgeon on-call. From this brief history, what do you think the diagnosis is? How do you proceed?
2 The patient is transferred to HDU and the results of the investigations you organized are back.
   You are provided with three cards are shown below:

Abnormal blood tests			
Hb	12.2g/dl	Bilirubin	75µmol/L
WCC	18.2 × 10⁹/L	ALT	72 IU/L
Platelets	96 × 10⁹/L	Alk phos	230U/L
CRP	176	GGT	202IU/L
Urea	9.6mmol/L	Amylase	197U/Dl

Abdominal USS report:
There are multiple subcentimetre calculi within a thick-walled gallbladder. There is a small amount of pericholecystic fluid present. The CBD is dilated at 9mm proximally. However, due to patient's body habitus and overlying bowel gas and I am unable to follow the CBD more distally. There is a suggestion of an acoustic shadow at the distal end of the CBD ?stone. Clinical correlation or further imaging is advised.

Excerpt from HDU chart			
Time	0200	0600	1000
Temperature	38.2	38.4	38.7
Blood pressure (MAP)	104/82 (88)	98/64 (74)	88 /52 (63)
HR	104	112	124
Noradrenaline (mcg/kg/min)		0.01	0.02

Which diagnosis is more likely now and how do you proceed?

Scenario 6

A 54-year-old diabetic man was referred by his GP the day before with a 7cm × 5cm abscess on his back. The night team have clerked him in, consented him, and listed him for an incision and drainage procedure. The patient refused to have the procedure done under local anaesthetic and is currently anaesthetized and ready in theatre.

(You are presented with a model with the abscess prepped and draped. There is a scrub nurse and all the necessary equipment available.)

Please demonstrate how you would proceed.

Scenario 7

A 37-year-old builder, Mr Shane McKinnon, presents to A&E 10 days after an open mesh repair of a right-sided inguinal hernia. He complains of a 3-day history of a hot, tender, erythematous area overlying his wound repair site. He has been started on flucloxacillin by his GP 48 hours prior to his presentation to A&E but feel his symptoms have continued to progress. He is apyrexial and clinically stable.

1 What is the likely diagnosis? What else are you concerned about? How are you going to manage this patient?
2 If the USS suggested a fluid collection with a density consistent with pus around the mesh site—how would your management differ?

3 Mr McKinnon's USS does not show any evidence of a deeper infection, hence he is discharged home from A&E with a course of oral antibiotics. Two days later, you receive a telephone call from the Microbiology Registrar informing you that Mr McKinnon's wound swab has yielded MRSA. Her advice is to change the antibiotic to doxycycline, if he is still symptomatic. She also recommends he receive eradication therapy. You telephone Mr McKinnon to explain this. Please demonstrate how you would proceed

Scenario 8

You are the Surgical ST2 in orthopaedic clinic.

Mr John Bernard, a 73-year-old obese retired policeman underwent an elective right total hip replacement for osteoarthritis. His in-hospital recovery was unremarkable barring a mild wound infection he developed 10 days post-operatively. He was commenced on antibiotics for this and discharged with community nurse and physiotherapy follow-up. He lives on his own and was previously independent with a frame. He has COPD and type 2 diabetes.

You are seeing him in the outpatient department 3 weeks post-operatively. This is his first review since discharge.
You: 'Hello Mr Bernard. How are you? And how is that new hip of yours?'
Mr Bernard: 'Well Doctor, I feel fine but this wound infection isn't going away. My doctor gave me another course of antibiotics after I left hospital but the wound is still tender and its now getting difficult for me to walk on this hip. In fact, even getting out of bed is getting difficult.'

He shows you his right hip. You notice that standing up to loosen his trousers causes him a significant amount of pain. The wound is clearly inflamed and tender. There is a small amount of purulent-looking discharge at the medial aspect of the wound.

1 From inspecting this wound and from the history you have been provided, what is your concern and why?
2 How do you plan to manage Mr Bernard?
3 Which organisms commonly cause prosthetic joint organisms?
4 What are the management principles in this situation?
5 Clearly, the consequences of a prosthetic joint infection are very serious. Do you know of any preventative strategies that are employed to help minimize the risk of these infections?

Answers

Scenario 1

1 Preparation:
  - Ensure your nails are short and clean.
  - Remove any jewellery from your hands or forearms—you should be 'bare below the elbow'. Any cuts or abrasions should be covered with a plaster.
  - (The above two statements apply to the entire examination)
  - Put on your theatre cap, visor and mask
  - Lay out your gown and gloves—these should be opened with a no-touch technique
  - (For procedures with potential contamination (e.g. laparotomy) use an apron)
2 Scrubbing (should take around 3 minutes):
  - Set the taps running and set the flow and temperature as comfortable. If you need to, spend a few extra seconds to get this right at the start—do not adjust the taps with your hands once you've started scrubbing
  - Wet your hands and forearms up to your elbows—keep your hands above elbow level for the rest of the scrub
  - For the first scrub of the day, use a sterile nail brush to clean under your fingernails using the bactericidal soap solution provided—usually iodophor-based (e.g. Betadine) or chlorhexidine-based (e.g. Hibiscrub). Do not use the brush on skin. Discard the brush and wash off the soap
  - Using your elbow, pump a few millilitres of bactericidal wash into the palm of your other hand and begin by washing your hands carefully and thoroughly. Take particular care to clean the palmar and dorsal surfaces of your hands, the web between your fingers, around your thumb, and around your wrist. Repeat these motions between 5–8 times
  - Then rub the soap along your forearm, moving from hand to elbow. Repeat for the other side. Your hand get progressively dirtier as it moves down from hand to elbow

- Wash off the soap under running water, starting with your hands and moving along your forearm to your elbow. Ensure you keep your hands above the level of your elbows so the dirty effluent runs down your elbows and not your hands
- Repeat this wash-and-rinse routine a further two times
- Finally, wash only your hands thoroughly and ensure that you rinse off the soap in a hands to elbows direction
- Turn the taps off using your elbows. Stand at the sink with your hands raised for a few seconds to allow any excess water to drip off your elbows

3 Gowning:
- Using the sterile towel provided in your gown pack, dry your hands, moving from hand to elbow, and discard the towel into the foot-operated bin. Remember to dry between your fingers. Repeat with a fresh towel for the other side
- Pick up your gown carefully with both hands—ensuring that you only touch the inner side of the gown. Step back from the table and while holding the gown near the neckline with the inner side facing you, allow it to unfold in front of you.
- Put your arms into the arm holes but not out past the cuff

The circulating nurse (one of the examiners) will assist you by fastening the gown behind you

4 Gloving:
- Using the cuff of your gown as a mitten, pick up the left glove with your right hand and place it on your left hand with the thumbs aligned and the finger facing your elbow
- Stretch the glove cuff over the gown cuff and slide you fingers in. Pull back on your gown cuff
- Repeat for the other side
- Offer the paper tag of the wrap-around tie to the circulating nurse, do a 180° turn, pull back on your tie and fasten the gown at the side
- Keep your hands elevated and close to your body

Scenario 2

1 First aid

You:
- 'Julia, the first thing you need to do is to unscrub. One of the other scrub nurses will scrub in and take over the remaining tasks
- You need to gently encourage bleeding of the wound by putting some pressure around the puncture site. Do not suck the wound
- Then, wash the puncture site thoroughly with soap and running water. Be careful not to scrub the area to avoid causing further breaks in the skin
- Pat it dry and cover it with a waterproof dressing'

Julia: 'Mr Conway, I have cleaned and dressed the puncture site. What should I do next?'

2 Risk assessment

You:
- 'Once that is done, you need to go down to A&E where you will be asked to fill out a needlestick injury form.
- You will be asked about the circumstances of the exposure including details such as:
  ◆ Were you wearing gloves at that time?
  ◆ Type of needle involved—this was a solid needle which has a lower risk of transmission than a hollow needle.
  ◆ Was there skin puncture? How deep was the injury?
  ◆ Was it fresh/stale blood on the needle?
- They will also ask you about:
  ◆ Your personal details
  ◆ Your hepatitis B status
- In addition, they will also need to know details of the source:
  ◆ Patient's name, hospital number, date of birth
  ◆ Source HIV/hepatitis B/hepatitis C status
  ◆ Is the source in a high-risk group for blood borne viruses?
- Once, they have all the relevant information they will perform a preliminary risk assessment to decide if you need any post-exposure-prophylaxis (PEP)
- They will also take some blood from you to test and for storage. In addition they will also check your pregnancy status'

Julia: 'I don't know the source infective status or if he is in a high-risk group. Can I take some blood from him now to check his status, while he is still under anaesthetic?'

You:

- 'No, we cannot take blood from him without his consent. Also, you will not be allowed to contact him directly about this and will need to do this through a third person.
- Once, he is more awake I will discuss the incident with him and find out the relevant information from him to determine if he is known or at high-risk of a blood borne viral infection. If he consents, I will arrange to take blood from him for testing and for storage.
- However, looking at his past medical history and social history from his admission notes, everything suggests that he is at low risk of a blood borne viral infection'

Julia: 'If he is HIV, hepatitis B or C positive, what is the risk of me contracting it from him?'

3 Transmission risk

You:

- 'The average risk of transmission of blood borne viral infections after a needlestick injury is estimated to be
  - ◆ 33% for hepatitis B (1 in 3) but the risk is significantly lower in individuals who have been immunized.
  - ◆ 3.3% for hepatitis C (1 in 30)
  - ◆ 0.33% for HIV (1 in 300)
- If he consents for a blood test, his blood will be tested for these infections. Both his and your samples will also be stored for further testing at 3 and 6 months, if required'

Julia: 'OK, will I still be allowed to work?'

4 Occupational Health

You:

- 'Once you have been to A&E, ring Occupational Health and leave them a message with your contact details and a brief description of the incident so they can contact you tomorrow
- They will be able to advise you about taking sick leave. However, in cases where the risk of any disease transmission is low, this should not have an effect on your job
- They will also be able to provide you with further information and advice and follow you up for further testing'

Julia: Is there anything else I need to do?

5 Incident reporting

You: 'Yes, you need to fill in an incident form/DATIX form to report the incident and inform your manager in the morning.'

Julia: 'Thank you, Dr. Conway.'

You: 'You're welcome. Let me know if there is anything else I can do to help.'

Scenario 3

** There are 2 parts to this question:

- Part 1—assessment of the wound (5 minutes)
- Part 2—outline of management (2 minutes)

**Important points to note from the history:

- Time of injury: delayed presentation >6 hours—higher risk of infection, may benefit from delayed closure
- General health: immunosuppression—higher risk of infection
- Immunization status: incomplete immunization—needs tetanus booster
  (Tetanus vaccination schedule: 3 doses in infancy, 1 booster in pre-school, 1 booster as a teenager—provides good immunity.)
- Details about the animal: unprovoked attack, wild animal—consider rabies

Part 1—assessment of the wound

- Reassurance—examining children can be challenging. It is vital to gain the child's trust from the start and to talk them through each step of the examination using language they would understand. Parental presence goes a long way when assessing children—have the child sat on a parent's lap if possible
- Inspection of the wound (describe what you see in the photograph):
  - ◆ Site of wound
  - ◆ Size, depth, number, and classification of wounds—puncture, lacerations, crush injury, avulsion
  - ◆ Evidence of devitalized tissue
  - ◆ Evidence of foreign body

- 'Feel and move' (perform the relevant steps on the child):
  - Examine wound through a range of motion
  - Sensory and motor function of nearby nerves
  - Vascular injury—feel for pulses, warmth, bleeding, visible vessels

'This photo demonstrates a dog bite to the right cheek of a girl. I see two lacerations of approximately 5cm each on her cheek and some surrounding superficial abrasions. The superior of these lacerations is along her zygomatic bone and the inferior along her mandible. There are also two superficial puncture marks of approximately 1cm diameter. The superior of these is located 2cm lateral to the external canthus of her right eye and the inferior puncture mark is lateral to her right naso-labial fold. There is some devitalized skin around the wounds but the underlying soft tissue looks healthy. There are no foreign bodies seen within these wounds.'

'During the examination, Mandy was talking, laughing and crying and I notice that she had good, symmetrical use of her facial muscles, in particular her buccinators, masseter, and zygomaticus. This was also confirmed on formal examination. Her cranial nerve function, in particular CN V and CN VII are also preserved. There are a few clots but no evidence of bleeding from any of the wounds and none of them lie in the path of major facial vessels.'

** In some injuries (e.g. hand injury), wounds should also be assessed for

- Tendon or tendon sheath involvement
- Bony injury
- Joint space violation

Part 2—outline of management
- Examination under anaesthetic:
  - To allow a more thorough pain-free inspection of the wound (in adults you may consider examining the wound under local anaesthetic)
  - Take a wound swab
- Wound debridement:
  - Remove necrotic/devitalized tissue, clots and particulate matter, if any
  - Aim to reach clean edges but avoid excessive resection on the face as this may make closure/reconstruction difficult
  - Scrub abrasions thoroughly to avoid tattooing
- Copious irrigation of the wound with 0.9% NaCl
- Primary closure: 'As this patient presented early and has an adequately cleaned facial wound, I think primary closure would be appropriate. However, I would discuss this with my consultant before proceeding'
- (In non-facial wounds, especially wounds on the hand, wounds with extensive crush injury or delayed presentation >6 hours from injury—higher risk of infection and hence, delayed closure may be more appropriate)
- Prophylactic antibiotics—5–7-day course of co-amoxiclav is usually sufficient.
- Tetanus vaccine:
  - As she would have only received one booster as part of the vaccination schedule, it is prudent to give her a booster shot of tetanus vaccine
- Arrange for the wound to be reviewed again in 48 hours. If healing well, suture removal 5 days post-closure
- Warn parent about the possibility of infection and to return to hospital if any concerns especially if pyrexial, septic, cellulitic, swelling, or if she has difficulty talking, chewing, laughing

Scenario 4

From the above history, I suspect this patient may have an infected ureteric calculus. This requires urgent intervention.

1 I would proceed by:
- Taking a full history and examination, paying particular attention to:
  - Any previous episodes of pain
  - Family history
  - Dehydration—trekking in hot climate, long-haul flight
  - Previous episodes of UTIs
  - Sexual history
- Arranging basic investigations:
  - Urine dipstick
  - Send urine for microbiology and culture

- ◆ Blood test—FBC, U&Es, CRP, Ca^{++}, PO$_4^{2-}$, urate, INR
- ◆ Blood culture
- ◆ CT KUB (if not available consider X-ray KUB + abdominal USS)
- Initiating resuscitation and symptom control
  - ◆ Prompt analgesia—e.g. diclofenac IM or PR (if not contraindicated)
  - ◆ Anti-emetics
  - ◆ Judicious IV and oral fluid. Start a fluid balance chart to monitor input /output
  - ◆ Broad spectrum antibiotics with Gram-negative cover—e.g. amoxicillin, metronidazole and gentamicin (check renal function 1st). Change antibiotics accordingly once culture results back
  - ◆ Regular monitoring of vital signs
2 This patient has an obstructed infected urinary system and needs urgent decompression. After discussing the patient with the Urology Consultant, I will contact the on-call radiologist with regard to inserting a percutaneous nephrostomy under US guidance urgently. I will ensure that the patient's coagulation is within normal limits and that she has received the antibiotics that were prescribed for her before she proceeds for drainage.
3 This is an urgent intervention and should not be delayed. If the collecting system is not decompressed urgently, the patient may develop ipsilateral renal dysfunction, Gram-negative sepsis and SIRS.

Scenario 5

1 I think the main differential here is gallstone pancreatitis or cholangitis.
  I will proceed by:
  - Taking a history and performing an examination:
    - ◆ Only covering pertinent points as this patient is clearly unwell
  - Arranging basic investigations:
    - ◆ Blood tests—FBC, U&Es, LFTs, amylase/lipase, CRP, coagulation profile
    - ◆ Arterial blood gas
    - ◆ Blood culture
    - ◆ Urine dipstick ± MC&S
    - ◆ Urgent abdominal US—to investigate for ductal stones
  - Initiate resuscitation and symptom control:
    - ◆ Analgesia
    - ◆ Anti-emetic ± NG tube
    - ◆ IV fluids
    - ◆ Catheter and hourly fluid balance chart
    - ◆ Broad-spectrum antibiotics with anaerobe and Gram-negative cover—e.g. amoxicillin, metronidazole and gentamicin (check renal function first). Change antibiotics accordingly once culture results back
    - ◆ Regular monitoring of vital signs
    - ◆ Transfer to higher level care—HDU
2 This patient presents with Charcot's triad of right upper quadrant pain, fever, and jaundice suggesting cholangitis. This is further supported by her raised inflammatory markers, biochemical jaundice, and deranged LFTs with an obstructive picture. In addition her amylase is only minimally raised, making acute pancreatitis unlikely.

(In fact, she demonstrates Raynaud's pentad—Charcot's triad +hypotension + altered mental state).

On reviewing her HDU charts, she is clearly deteriorating despite active resuscitation and antibiotics. This patient has acute severe cholangitis with an infected, obstructed biliary system. She needs urgent decompression. Although the USS report is somewhat equivocal, I do not feel further imaging is required. Furthermore, this patient has a pacemaker, hence an MRCP is contraindicated.

After discussing this patient with my consultant and ensuring she is optimally resuscitated, I will contact the on-call Consultant Gastroenterologist to request an urgent ERCP for decompression 9 stone retrieval 9 sphincterotomy. I will ensure her coagulation profile is within normal limits and that she has appropriate antibiotic cover.

Scenario 6

Procedure:

- Hold the scalpel between your thumb and forefinger:
  - ◆ Make a stab incision over the most fluctuant point of the abscess along its long axis.

◆ Maintain steady firm pressure as you extend the incision to enter the subcutaneous tissue. The incision should be large enough to ensure adequate drainage.

- Deroof the overlying skin, especially if necrotic. This prevents premature closure of the overlying skin allowing the abscess cavity to drain adequately during healing. You can form either:
  ◆ An elliptical incision for small abscess cavities
  ◆ A cruciate incision for larger abscess cavities.
  (Where possible, make your incision parallel to Langer's lines to improve cosmesis)
- Purulent contents will start draining as you make the incision—insert a swab into the abscess cavity to take a sample of pus for MC&S.
- Allow the rest of the pus to drain either spontaneously or with gentle pressure.
- Using your finger or a curette, bluntly dissect within the abscess cavity to break loculations:
  ◆ Ensure that you explore the entire abscess cavity including any deep tracks that may be present
- Gently irrigate the wound with copious amounts of sterile normal saline until the effluent is clear
- Apply direct pressure on bleeding points for 1–2 minutes to ensure haemostasis. Alternatively, you can use diathermy if available
- Loosely pack the abscess cavity with packing material (e.g. proflavin soaked ribbon gauze), starting at one end and working around the entire cavity:
  ◆ Ensure the cavity is adequately packed to keep the abscess cavity 'open'—this allows further drainage of infected debris and permits the wound to heal from the base upward.
  ◆ However, it is essential to ensure the cavity is not packed too tightly as this may cause ischaemia of the surrounding tissue, interfere with wound drainage, and add to patient discomfort.
- Apply a sterile non-adherent gauze dressing over the wound and secure this with an adhesive dressing tape

Document the procedure in patient notes.

Post-operative instructions:

- Routine post- operative observation
- Home later today/tomorrow
- Leave dressings in place for 48 hours—then regular dressings by practice/district nurse
- Does not need antibiotics unless evidence of cellulitis. Patient advised to seek medical advice if any concerns

Scenario 7

1 This patient has developed a post-op wound infection at the site of his hernia repair. My concern is of mesh infection.

After taking a history and examining the patient, I will arrange basic investigations which include

- Wound swab for MC&S
- Urine dipstick and MC&S
- Blood tests for FBC, U&Es and CRP

I will remove the skin stitches to allow any pus/fluid to drain. This fluid should also be swabbed and sent for MC&S.

If there is a large area of inflammation or the patient is systemically unwell, I will arrange for the patient to have a groin USS to visualize the mesh and to assess for a deeper collection. If there is no suggestion of a deeper infection, I will commence the patient on antibiotics (penicillin and flucloxacillin) and analgesia. This is usually an oral course with advice to return if there is no improvement in 48 hours. However, if there is a large area of inflammation or the patient is systemically unwell, he should be commenced on IV antibiotics for a 48-hour period. Once there is clinical improvement, the patient can be discharged to complete the rest of the course with oral antibiotics.

2 In this case, I would admit the patient and commence them on IV antibiotics. I will discuss the patient with my consultant, arrange further imaging with a CT scan and arrange for the patient to have the mesh removed

3 I will telephone Mr. Mckinnon to explain the result to him
  You: 'Hello, is that Mr McKinnon?'
  Patient: 'Yes, this is he.'
  You: 'My name is Dr Nielson. I met you on Wednesday in A&E when you came in with an infected wound.'
  Patient: 'Ay. I am glad you rang, Doc. That wound is no better. It is still red, hot, and tender. I don't think the antibiotics are working too well, Doc.'

You: 'Well, that is the reason I rang. While you were in hospital 2 days ago, I swabbed the wound to look for the specific bug that is causing the infection. And the swab results have come back showing a certain bug called MRSA for which we need special antibiotics to treat.'

Patient (sounds worried): 'MRSA? I have MRSA? My nan died of MRSA. Is this serious Doc? How did this happen?'

You: 'Let me explain what this means. MRSA is the short form for methicillin resistant *Staphylococcus aureus*. The last two words, *Staphylococcus aureus*, is a type of bug which is very common and many people have it growing as part of the normal bugs on their skin. These bugs are found both in hospitals and also in the community, There are broadly two groups of these bugs—those that are sensitive to common antibiotics and those that are resistant to common antibiotics and for which we need stronger antibiotics to treat. This second group is MRSA. Although it can cause serious infections if it gets into the bloodstream, wound infections are usually less serious and respond well to appropriate antibiotic treatment.'

Patient: 'OK, so you can treat it? What do you need me to do, Doc?'

You: 'Yes, there are specific antibiotics that we use to treat MRSA. As you are still having symptoms of infection we need to give you the antibiotic that fights MRSA. You will need to take this antibiotic for 7 days. Discard the antibiotics that we gave you on Wednesday. You will also need to use a special soap (chlorhexidine 2%—Hibiscrub) for handwashing, bathing, or showering for 7 days. I have faxed a letter to your GP practice and they will be able to give you a prescription for this. I have also faxed an information leaflet about MRSA infections, which you can pick up from your practice.'

Patient: 'Ok, so if I do all that, I won't have MRSA anymore?'

You: 'Once you complete the treatment, you should attend your practice nurse who will repeat the swabs to ensure that you are clear. However, if you are admitted to hospital over the next 6 months it is important that you let your doctors know that you have had treatment for MRSA recently.'

Patient: 'What should I do if the infection doesn't get better?'

You: 'If you do not see any improvement in 48 hours, you should either see your GP or come back via A&E.'

Patient: 'OK, thank you for ringing Doc.'

Scenario 8

1 Thank you Mr Bernard.
  - Mr Bernard has a post-operative wound infection and my main concern is of a prosthetic joint infection. Apart from the overlying skin infection he is also complaining of pain on mobilizing and I noticed that he only used a limited range of motion when getting undressed and dressed.
  - Although, this is an uncommon complication affecting <2% of all hip prosthesis, Mr Bernard is at higher risk of infective complications in view of his raised BMI and diabetes. In addition, I am unsure if he has been on steroids for his COPD which is a further risk factor for prosthetic joint infections

2 My management plan for Mr Bernard is:
  - Admit to hospital
  - Blood tests—FBC, CRP, ESR, U&Es, LFTs, coagulation
  - Blood culture
  - Wound swab
  - Hip X-ray—often non-specific, can be used to monitor serial changes
  - USS—to assess for joint effusion
  - If the patient has raised inflammatory markers and /or a joint effusion seen at US, perform a joint aspiration under sterile condition and radiological guidance. Take multiple samples and send aspirate for MC&S

3 Prosthetic joint infections are commonly caused by Gram-positive cocci—*Staphylococcus aureus* including MRSA and coagulase-negative staphylococci. Less commonly, it may be caused by streptococci, Gram-negative bacteria, anaerobes or fungi
  - Early infection (<3 months) is usually acquired at the time of surgery or as a consequence of a wound infection, while delayed (3–12 months) or late infections (>12 months) occur as a result of haematogenous spread from bacteraemia from any cause

4 Basic principles and management of prosthesis
  - Identify the offending organism and commence on sensitive antibiotics. (Start empirical treatment while awaiting results—microbiology advice.)
  - Formal debridement of necrotic tissue, drainage of abscess
  - Obtain further soft tissue samples to confirm the diagnosis
  - Well-fixed prosthesis and healthy soft tissue—retention of prosthesis + prolonged course of antibiotics (6 weeks IV or 6 months oral)

- Loose prosthesis and healthy soft tissue—one-stage revision + 6 weeks oral antibiotics
- Loose prosthesis and damaged soft tissue—two-stage revision + 6 weeks of oral antibiotics
- Surgery contraindicated or patient refuses—consider prosthesis removal or arthrodesis
- Amputation is used as a last resort in joint infections that are not responding to antibiotics or in joints with severe soft tissue damage not amenable to reconstruction

5 Preventative strategies include:
- Hand washing—**single most important precaution**
- Screen and eradicate MRSA—pre-operatively
- Pre-operative preparation—optimize comobidities and treat any infections pre-operatively
- Ring-fencing of elective orthopaedic beds—decreases MRSA infection rate
- Ultra-clean laminar flow theatres
- Standard theatre etiquette
- Prophylactic antibiotics
- Meticulous, aseptic technique—minimize trauma, remove devitalized tissue
- Wound care
- Some surgeons advocate the use of prophylactic antibiotics in patients undergoing invasive dental procedures

Chapter 18 **Carcinogenesis and neoplasia**

Introduction

Cancer can be defined as a disease in which cells display uncontrolled growth, invasion, and sometimes metastasis. These features distinguish benign from malignant tumours. Normal tissues within the body divide and reproduce under the control of signalling systems, in order to replace damaged or dying cells. In contrast to this, malignant tissues lose their ability to respond to such growth controls. The resulting replication, out of proportion to tissue requirements, leads to tumour growth. As well as an increase in cell number, malignancies can develop the ability to invade surrounding tissues, breaking through basement membranes to invade tissues directly or to gain access to blood vessels or lymphatic channels enabling metastasis. Having invaded a new site, and started to replicate, the malignant cells continue to replicate and destroy the invaded organs.

Cancer is the second most common cause of death in the developed world after cardiovascular disease. A surgeon's role in the management of cancer involves diagnosis, staging, and treatment. Knowledge of the principles underlying cancer development and progression is an important step in understanding the natural history of this set of diseases. Only by knowing the fundamentals can a surgeon develop effective methods to investigate, counsel, and manage patients with cancer.

Definitions

Before starting, there are certain terms which will be used and with which the student should be familiar (Table 18.1). Understanding these basic terms will allow more complex themes to be developed later in the chapter.

Tumour biology

In the normal cell, a strict control is maintained over growth and proliferation. Cancer cells become unresponsive to the normal controls exerted over growth and proliferation. This loss of control results in abnormal behaviour, manifesting as enhanced growth potential, abnormal appearance, immortality, and loss of adherence to other cells.

Normal cells develop into cancer cells over a number of steps. The initial transformation involves a genetic event or mutation, resulting in either gaining the function of an oncogene or losing the function of a tumour-suppressor gene. Subsequent genetic events lead to progressive change of the genome as the cell develops a more aggressive genetic profile.

In keeping with this idea of genetic steps in tumourigenesis, most human cancers are thought to develop in a progressive fashion. The model of colon cancer (Fig. 18.1), which develops from the normal

Table 18.1 Basic definitions

Term	Definition
Carcinoma	Cancers derived from epithelial cells
Sarcoma	Cancer derived from connective tissue (mesenchymal cells)
Lymphoma/leukaemia	Cancers developed from blood-forming (haematopoetic) cells
Germ cell tumour	Cancers derived from totipotent cells
Blastoma	A tumour resembling embryonic tissues
Metastasis	Spread of a cancer from one part of the body to another
Oncogene	A gene that contributes to creating a cancer
Proto-oncogene	A gene that when mutated can become an oncogene
Tumour suppressor gene	A gene that protects against cancer
Apoptosis	Genetically programmed cell death
Incidence	The number of new cases within a specified time frame
Prevalence	The number of patients in a population with the disease

epithelium through adenoma to malignancy, is one example. Progression of breast tissue through atypical ductal hyperplasia to carcinoma in situ and ultimately carcinoma is another.

Expression of genes involves transcription to mRNA, translation into protein, and function of that protein. Each step involved is controlled by complex factors, any one of which can be affected to alter cell behaviour.

DNA contains many genes relating to the control of cell growth and proliferation. When the mutation of one of these genes results in code that contributes to cancer, the new gene is called an oncogene, and the original is described as a proto-oncogene. Oncogenes can code for growth factors, growth factor receptors, intracellular signalling molecules, or nuclear transcription factors.

From the above description, many distinct mechanisms for the development of cancers have been described, but they can largely be broken down in to six groups (Fig. 18.2).

Limitless cell replication

Normal cells are limited in their potential to replicate. The ends of chromosomes are composed of thousands of repeats of base pairs, or telomeres. Telomeres prevent the ends of chromosomes from fusing which would result in cell death. Each cell replication results in the loss of telomeres, and when a critical level is reached, the chromosomes fuse and the cell dies.

Telomerase is an enzyme that promotes the addition of telomeres to DNA, so protecting the chromosome from fusion and increasing the ability to duplicate. Many tumour cells exhibit raised telomerase activity, providing the cells with unlimited proliferation potential.

Increased sensitivity to growth signals

Cells respond to signals that can be local (paracrine), systemic (endocrine), or even produced themselves (autocrine). This is true of both normal and cancer cells. Cancer cells behave abnormally and may

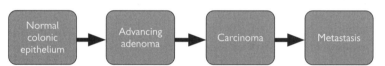

Figure 18.1 Simplified model of colon cancer development.

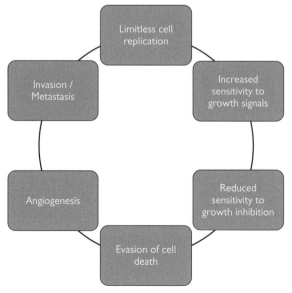

Figure 18.2 Features of the biology of malignant cells.

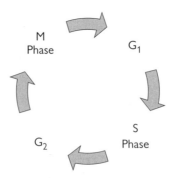

Figure 18.3 The cell cycle.

produce growth factors to stimulate their own proliferation, or factors that stimulate the surrounding microenvironment to become more suitable for their development.

Factors secreted by the tumour cells themselves, cells within the surrounding stroma or cells which infiltrate the tissues such as lymphocytes can all affect tumour growth. The abnormality can result from changes in the growth signals themselves, the membrane bound receptors for such signals, or the intracellular mechanisms triggered by the signal–receptor interactions.

Reduced sensitivity to growth inhibition

Normal cell division is under the control of both growth stimulation and inhibition. In order to escape this regulation, cancer cells must also overcome the inhibition exerted upon them.

The cell cycle which results in duplication of single cells is split into four separate steps (Fig. 18.3). During the S phase, DNA synthesis occurs, and the cell generates a copy of its genetic material. During the M phase, this genetic material is divided between two separate daughter cells. Between these two phases are the G1 and G2 checkpoints, which are periods the cell uses to prepare for the upcoming S and M phases. When a cell leaves the cell cycle, and no longer proliferates, it is said to be in the G0 or quiescent phase.

Progression around the cell cycle is tightly controlled by both stimulatory and inhibitory factors which are coded for by oncogenes and tumour-suppressor genes. Factors that inhibit growth can lead to the cell passing out of the cell cycle at the M stage, and into either G0 or a state of terminal differentiation, from where no further replication is possible.

Cells monitor their external environment when in the M phase, and are guided either back in to the cycle or in to a state where further growth is prevented. The retinoblastoma protein is crucial to this step as a negative regulator. Genetic events that result in changes in this protein or its action can promote cell division resulting in tumour growth.

The path out of the cell cycle to terminal differentiation can also be blocked classically by overexpression of the oncogene *c-myc*, which in turn maintains the cell in the cell cycle leading to further replication.

Evasion of cell death

The rate of growth in cell number is dependent not only on the rate of cell division, but also on the rate of cell death. Apoptosis, or programmed cell death, leads to a characteristic set of events including cell membrane disruption and chromosomal degeneration. The process is used by normal tissues particularly in the embryonic state and by the functioning immune system. p53 is a key regulator in apoptosis, sensing irreparable DNA damage and stimulating the events of programmed cell death. Functional inactivation of p53 is seen in more than half of human cancers.

Abnormalities in tumour cells make them potential targets for the immune system, and increased rates of malignancies are seen in the immune-suppressed population. Highly immunogenic cells are targeted by the immune system, whilst those with a reduced immunogenicity are tolerated. Over time this survival advantage for one set of cells results in their selection for growth. It is thought that early-stage tumours are more likely to be immunogenic, and so targeted for destruction. The genetic instability of the surviving cells results in production of colonies of cells less susceptible to immune destruction. It is these cells which escape the immune response and form viable tumours.

Other mechanisms of cell death include necrosis, autophagy (the catabolic destruction of a cell's own contents), and mitotic catastrophe (where damaged DNA replicates leading to cell death). These mechanisms and their interaction with the evolution of cancer are less well defined.

Angiogenesis

As a tumour grows, it requires energy which in turn requires blood flow. Tumours may be present but lack the potential to recruit the blood they require which maintains them in a dormant state.

Again the system of angiogenesis relies on both stimulatory and inhibitory pressures. Growth factors, such as vascular endothelial growth factor (VEGF) promote angiogenesis whilst interferon alpha is amongst the angiogenesis inhibitors. The anti-VEGF antibody, bevacizumab (Avastin), has been shown to prolong survival in patients with advanced colon cancer.

Control of angiogenesis then is dependent on multiple factors which can be altered by genetic mutations. Increased functional activators of angiogenesis, or decreased functional inhibitors result in disruption of normal homeostasis and allow tumours to develop new blood vessels, which is integral to both growth and metastasis.

Invasion and metastasis

Over 90% of human deaths due to cancer are caused by distant metastases. Development of a metastasis involves detachment of cells from the primary tumour, invasion of blood or lymphatic vessels (intravasation), transport to the target organ, extravasation of the tumour cells, and proliferation in the new environment.

Both intravasation and extravasation are a result of tumour cells interaction with the extracellular matrix. Cadherin proteins are responsible for normal tissue organization, and in tumours, loss of epithelial cadherin may be a prerequisite for tissue invasion and subsequent metastasis.

Cells not only have to escape their environment and invade a distant organ, but on arrival they must be able to adapt to their new surroundings. Integrins are the receptors on a cell's membrane which allow it to attach to the tissues surrounding it. Shifting their expression of integrin molecules allows cancer cells to interact with different extracellular matrices, and so to survive in multiple environments.

Increased production of proteases or reduced production of protease inhibitors allows cancer cells to destroy the surrounding extracellular matrix, so allowing for tissue invasion. The protein destruction may allow cells to invade through epithelial layers, across stroma and into blood vessels.

In 1889 Paget observed breast cancer metastasizing preferentially to the liver, lung, adrenal, and brain. From this pattern he hypothesized that specific cancer cells would only grow in suitable environments, the so-called seed and soil hypothesis. The explanation for this phenomenon is unclear. It may be that cells with the potential to invade and metastasize do so at an equal rate in all tissues, but only when they find a suitable environment are they able to proliferate and regenerate a tumour. Alternatively it may be the specific endothelial cells within target organs that express specific adhesion molecules which attract the metastatic cells, promoting their extravasation and subsequent growth. A third explanation is that chemokines from target organs attract metastatic cells with appropriate receptors.

Carcinogens

A carcinogen is any agent that contributes to tumour formation. They can be classified as chemical, physical, or biological.

Chemical carcinogens

A wide range of both natural and synthetic chemicals have proven carcinogenic potential (Table 18.2). Some can act directly and are described as direct, other indirect carcinogens require some form of transformation for their action. The active forms of these chemicals interact with DNA within cells.

Most carcinogens are indirect, and so production of the active chemical depends on the balance of metabolic activation and inactivation. The cytochrome P450 system is responsible for many chemical

Table 18.2 Chemical carcinogens

Chemical carcinogen	Related cancers
Asbestos	Lung cancer, mesothelioma
Tobacco smoke	Lung, upper airway, oesophageal
Vinyl chloride	Hepatocellular carcinoma

carcinogen activation pathways and heterogeneity in the genes that code for these enzymes results in different levels of individual risk. Ten per cent of Caucasians have a form of enzyme that renders them high risk from cigarette smoke.

Radiation carcinogenesis

Cancer caused by radiation develops many years after exposure. Ultraviolet (UV) light and ionizing radiation are the two most important forms of radiation inducing cancers in humans.

UV light is associated with skin cancers (squamous cell carcinoma, basal cell carcinoma, and possible malignant melanoma). The level of risk depends on the amount of exposure, the type of rays (UVB being most important), and the quantity of melanin in an individual's skin. Widespread DNA damage caused by UV radiation exposure may overwhelm the body's ability to repair leading to mutations which can lead to cancer.

Ionizing radiation includes particles such as alpha and beta particles, protons and neutrons, and also electromagnetic X-rays and gamma rays. High doses of radiation can of course prevent the growth of tumours, but low-dose exposure can increase the risk of malignancy. Sub-lethal exposure leads to genomic instability that can result in malignant transformation. In survivors of the atomic bombs dropped on Hiroshima and Nagasaki an increased risk of tumours has been described. Different tissues display different vulnerabilities with haematopoietic cell lines being most vulnerable. Thyroid, breast, and lung are intermediate in vulnerability with skin, bone, and the GI tract being most radioresistant.

Infectious carcinogens

Infections can induce malignancy by direct cellular transformation, alteration of the expression of onco-genes, interference with DNA repair, or damage of the immune system.

An estimated 15% of human cancers worldwide are caused by viruses (Table 18.3). *Helicobacter pylori* has been linked to gastric cancer. The exact cause is unclear but may be linked to the body's immune response to infection.

Chronic inflammation is known to lead to the development of cancers. The classic example being Marjolin's ulcers, areas of squamous cell carcinoma which develop in areas of chronic ulceration. Another example is the colonic carcinoma linked with long-term ulcerative colitis.

Epidemiology and screening of cancer

Epidemiology

Population-based cancer statistics tend to be reported in a number of standard ways. Both incidence and mortality rates are of interest, as not all patients who develop cancer go on to die of the disease. Incidence tends to be reported on a 1-year basis within a population of 100,000.

Cancer is a disease that disproportionately affects older patients, with around 80% of cancers affecting patients aged 55 years or older. As the overall population ages, the burden of cancer is going to be far greater in the coming century than the last. Coupled with increasing healthcare costs, the financial impact of treating the aging population is a problem facing all countries. The most common cancer diagnoses and causes of cancer death are shown in Table 18.4.

Screening

Screening a population for cancer has become commonplace in the UK. Primary prevention refers to an intervention that is applied to a normal population whereas in secondary prevention the intervention is

Table 18.3 Examples of virally induced cancers

Virus	Associated cancer
Human papilloma viruses	Cervical and anal cancers
Hepatitis B + C	Hepatocellular carcinoma
Epstein-Barr virus	Burkitt's lymphoma, Hodgkin's disease, Nasopharyngeal carcinoma
Human immunodeficiency virus	Kaposi's sarcoma

Table 18.4 UK Figures for leading cancers in 2008 for men and women (excluding skin cancers)

Men		Women	
Percentage of new cancer diagnoses per year			
Prostate	24%	Breast	31%
Lung	15%	Lung	12%
Colorectal	14%	Colorectal	12%
Percentage of cancer deaths per year			
Lung	24%	Lung	21%
Prostate	12%	Breast	16%
Colorectal	11%	Colorectal	10%

Table 18.5 Two by two table

	Disease present?		Totals
Test result	Yes	No	
Positive	A	B	A+B
Negative	C	D	C+D
Totals	A+C	B+D	

aimed at patients who are known to be at risk. There are four criteria that must be met for a screening programme to be appropriate:

1 The disease must represent an important health problem
2 The disease must have a detectable pre-clinical phase
3 Treatment of pre-clinical stage disease must have better outcomes
4 An appropriate screening test must be available

Screening programmes tend to be aimed at diseases which result in major morbidity and/or mortality. They should have a high prevalence within the population being screened. Having identified such a disease, the characteristics of the disease are important. Ideally the disease will have a long pre-clinical latency period during which treatment will result in cure.

Having decided on a disease, there must be a test which is suitable for the disease in question. It must be of reasonable cost, and acceptable to both the healthcare provider and the patient group to whom it is applied.

Assuming a screening test is designed to give a positive or negative result, its effectiveness is measured in a standard fashion based around the classic two by two table (Table 18.5).

Within this table one can see that patients may get the correct result—a true positive (A) or a true negative (D). In this situation the test correctly identifies the disease state of the patient. If the test is incorrect, however, the patient will be called a false positive (B) or a false negative (C). There is no way for an individual patient to know whether their test is correct or not, but by measuring the test result against a 'gold standard', the overall results can be interpreted.

The statistics used to describe this kind of test are the sensitivity, specificity, the positive predictive power, and the negative predictive power.

- Sensitivity is the proportion of patients with the disease (A+C) that are correctly identified using the test (A). The formula then is A/(A+C)
- Specificity is the proportion of patients who do not have disease (B+D) that are correctly identified (D). The formula is D/(B+D)
- The positive predictive power is the proportion of positive test results (A+B) that have the disease (A). The formula is A/(A+B)
- The negative predictive power is the proportion of negative test results (C+D) that do not have the disease (D). The formula is D/(C+D)

Even a highly sensitive and specific test will be unsuccessful if compliance rates are low. Populations should be educated about the risks of the disease, the benefits of screening, the details of the screening, and ways to access the service. Healthcare providers are pivotal to ensuring high compliance and should advise their patients about appropriate screening programmes available to them.

The introduction of an effective screening programme should lead to a reduction in morbidity or mortality within a group. There are, however, some features of the disease's clinical characteristics that will change on introduction of screening that must be considered.

Diseases will be detected earlier by screening than they normally would have. This early detection gives rise to 'lead-time bias'. Survival times will now be measured from detection at screening rather than clinical presentation, so making outcomes in the screened group seem more favourable.

Within cancers, there is variation in presentation. Some will have long pre-clinical phases which are likely to be detected by screening. Others may progress more rapidly through the pre-clinical phase and are more likely to represent aggressive disease. The fact that screening programmes are likely to detect the more indolent group is described as 'length-bias' and should be accounted for when comparing screened and non-screened populations.

Patients will select themselves for screening. This tends to favour more health conscious patient groups with differing smoking and alcohol habits. This form of bias is difficult to avoid, and providing care to those most at risk can be challenging.

Examples of UK screening programmes

Breast cancer screening

Breast cancer accounts for around one in three new cancer diagnoses in women in the UK. X-ray examination is used to detect pre-clinical breast masses which can then be targeted for biopsy and treatment. Screening mammography is uncomfortable but not painful and has acceptable sensitivity and specificity in the over 50-years age group. The breast screening programme in the UK started in 1988 and now 1.5 million women between the ages of 50–70 years are screened each year. The introduction of breast screening has been shown to result in a reduction in deaths from breast cancer.

Colorectal cancer screening

Colorectal cancer is the third most common cancer in men and women. Most colorectal cancers develop from adenomatous polyps and have a long pre-clinical phase. In the UK, individuals aged 60–69 will be invited to be screened then sent a kit to test for faecal occult blood. Those testing positive will be assessed for colonoscopy. This programme which started in 2009 is based on evidence suggesting a 16% reduction in disease specific mortality.

Tumour markers

The ideal tumour marker should be expressed exclusively by the tumour, be easy to collect, and there should be a cheap and reliable test available. They may help distinguish benign from malignant disease, represent tumour burden, assist in staging disease, or guide therapy.

Tumour markers may be proteins or genetic mutations. Tumour markers which can be detected in blood or urine have gained most widespread use due to ease of access and testing (Table 18.6).

Table 18.6 Examples of tumour markers

Protein	Abbreviation	Diseases	Uses
Carcinoembryonic antigen	CEA	Colorectal cancer	Prognosis and monitoring for recurrence
α-fetoprotein	AFP	Hepatocellular cancer	Prognosis and monitoring (screening with USS)
α-fetoprotein/human chorionic gonadotrophin	AFP/hCG	Germ cell tumours	Diagnosis, prognosis, and monitoring
Prostate specific antigen	PSA	Prostate cancer	Screening and monitoring
Carbohydrate antigen 125	CA 125	Ovarian cancer	Monitoring for recurrence

Specific changes in DNA such as in the *ret* proto-oncogene in multiple endocrine neoplasia syndrome 2, can act as biomarkers for diseases. They can be used to identify patients at risk of disease before even developing the cancer. Treatment such as prophylactic total thyroidectomy for medullary thyroid cancer can prevent the malignancy before it exists.

Management of cancers

The role of the surgeon in the management of cancer has changed over the past decades. Few patients are managed in isolation, with the modern standard of care requiring discussion within local MDTs, linked to regional cancer networks.

Within these teams, surgeons work hand-in-hand with oncologists, but also with clinicians from pathology, radiology, anaesthesia, and critical care. Aside from doctors, these teams also consist of nurse specialists, dieticians, physiotherapists, occupational therapists, and speech therapists. Together this group of individuals can provide a broad range of support services which meet the complex needs of their patients. These needs will change as the patient progresses from diagnosis to treatment and beyond.

Surgical oncology

Surgery is still the mainstay of treatment for most solid tumours. Used as a single modality, surgery offers the highest rate of cure compared with other treatment modalities. Almost all patients with a solid tumour will be at least considered for surgical intervention. Despite the move towards team-oriented management of cancers, the surgeon maintains a unique role.

For most patients with solid tumours, the surgeon remains the first point of contact. It is the surgeon who will be required to obtain tissue for biopsy. Surgeons often arrange imaging to provide staging information and ultimately it is commonly a surgeon that presents the case to the MDT. This position requires surgeons to understand the biology of the diseases that they treat, to be familiar with the treatment options, their likely consequences, and outcomes. The surgeon may have to offer counselling to patients receiving the diagnosis of cancer for the first time, and be the one to introduce them to other individuals within the MDT.

The biopsy

A biopsy will be used to determine the histology of the tumour in question, which is essential prior to definitive treatment. Decisions made without histological evidence lead to significant errors, and should be avoided whenever possible.

Superficial lesions can be biopsied directly or with the use of suitable endoscopes. Deeper lesions may require image-guided biopsies or even surgical procedures in order to obtain tissues.

Fine-needle aspiration (FNA) using a hollow needle removes cells from the tumour mass. The tissue architecture is not normally represented, so diagnosis must be made on the cellular features alone. This may prevent the diagnosis of invasive malignancy, as in follicular lesions of the thyroid. Despite this drawback, FNA is cheap, fast, and relatively painless and is the first-line investigation in many situations.

The technique of core biopsy involves removing a core of tissue from the tumour, using a large-bore needle. Tissue architecture is maintained and more tissue is obtained, both of which can aid the pathologist in making a diagnosis.

Incisional biopsy describes the open removal of a piece of tumour for analysis. Since there is a risk of tumour seeding at the wound site, incisions should be made in such a way as to facilitate their excision as part of the definitive surgical procedure. This option is used when needle biopsies have failed to reveal a diagnosis and when a tumour is sufficiently large to make complete excision impractical without a diagnosis.

Excisional biopsy removes the tumour completely. Although it should encompass the entire macroscopic tumour mass, it should not prevent later wide field local excision to achieve oncological control. Whereas excision biopsy is accepted for small skin cancers, follicular thyroid lesions, and breast nodules, it should be avoided in cervical lymph node metastases as the outcome of squamous cell carcinoma is adversely affected by excisional biopsy. A full head and neck examination followed by FNA is more appropriate.

Staging

Cancers can be described by their local, regional, and distant extents. These descriptions can then be translated in to international staging systems, which offer prognostic information and guide treatment choices. Specific staging systems exist for many cancers and are often based around the TNM system based on features primary tumour extent (T_{1-4}), nodal disease (N_{0-1+}), and metastases (M_{0-1}).

Surgery

Once a recommendation to proceed with surgery has been made, the nature of the operation and potential for complications, as well as alternative therapies should be discussed with the patient. When planning surgery it should be remembered that the first attempt at surgical cure has the highest rate of success. Once tissue planes and lymphatic channels have been disrupted, further surgery will be more challenging and patterns of spread will be abnormal.

The primary disease should be excised with a surrounding cuff of normal tissue. As malignancies grow they develop a pseudo-capsule. This normal tissue, compressed by the enlarging tumour, makes an attractive target as a margin, but cancers tend to infiltrate this pseudo-capsule, and such enucleation can lead to malignant cells being left behind. The margin required to ensure that all malignant cells are excised varies between cancers and generally the more aggressive the tumour, the wider the margin required.

Cancers often spread from the primary site to the regional lymphatics. For this reason, the regional nodal basin may be dissected out or assessed for disease. Clinically obvious disease may be resected, but in cases where there is no palpable disease, a number of choices exist.

These nodes may simply be observed, and treated should clinically positive disease develop in the future.

Resection of these nodes will detect micrometastases (clinically negative but histologically positive lymph nodes). This information can be used to re-stage the disease, and may affect prognosis and treatment plans. The additional information gained must be weighed against the potential risks of more invasive surgery (such as lymphoedema following axillary clearance).

A recent concept has been the sentinel node biopsy. This involves injection of a dye or radiolabelled tracer to the site of primary disease, and subsequent identification of the first lymph node to which it drains. This node can be excised and submitted for careful analysis. If this is shown to be positive for disease, further surgery can be scheduled to excise the remaining nodes, if negative the nodal basin is assumed to be free of disease. This approach has been adopted for some diseases including breast cancer and malignant melanoma.

Once a cancer has metastasized to distant structures, surgical resection at the primary site will not cure disease. Despite that, surgery has a role in selected patients. An example is colonic cancer with an isolated liver metastasis. These patients can be considered for surgery with metastectomy, and 25% can expect to survive at 5 years. Patients with disseminated thyroid cancer may live for long periods following diagnosis, and surgery to remove the thyroid as a debulking procedure improves concentration of radioiodine in the systemic metastases, so improving prognosis.

Following surgical resection of cancer, reconstruction must be considered. Options include simple primary closure of skin or viscera, local or regional reconstructive techniques, or procedures involving free tissue transfer. The adequacy of oncological resection must not be compromised to achieve reconstruction. Breast reconstruction following mastectomy is an example of how this range of techniques can be applied to provide superior outcomes for these patients.

The surgeon's role in palliative treatment should not be overlooked. Procedures may be indicated to relieve pain, haemorrhage, or obstruction. These operations are designed to improve quality of life rather than to extend longevity. The risks of surgery must be weighed against the benefits and such decisions rely on an understanding of the biology of the disease and the likely sequelae of both action and inaction.

Radiation oncology

Radiation can be used to cure cancer either alone, or in combination with chemotherapy, surgery, or both. It can also be used in palliation of advanced cancers and even in benign disease.

Radiation is delivered to human tissue with high energy photons (X-rays or gamma rays) or charged particles (protons or electrons). The intracellular target for this radiation is the DNA. The energy results in breaks and abnormal cross links within the DNA molecule. In most cells this damage will not manifest immediately, but instead when the cell tries to divide it dies. Some cells undergo apoptosis following exposure to radiation. The fact that radiation effects may not present immediately means that slowly growing tumours will retain histologically normal cells for long periods following therapy. Although biopsy of these tissues following radiotherapy may show viable cells under the microscope, the DNA damage which is undetectable, will render these cells non-viable.

Medical radiation is measured by 'absorbed dose' which is the energy absorbed per unit mass. The unit of absorbed dose is the Gray (Gy). The extent of DNA damage following radiotherapy varies dependent on a number of factors, the most important of which is the level of tissue oxygenation. Hypoxic cells are relatively radioresistant, as oxygen prolongs the life of free radicals which mediate the indirect effects of treatment.

Chemotherapeutic agents can act as radiosensitizers by promoting cellular oxygen levels and hindering DNA repair mechanisms.

External beam radiotherapy uses beams of uniform intensity to treat the target, whilst attempting to minimize the dose to surrounding structures. Pre treatment planning is used to design treatment fields which optimize delivery of energy to the tumour whilst sparing the normal tissues.

Intensity-modulated radiation uses beams of varying intensity which can conform to the shape of the tumour. This adaptation of external beam radiotherapy allows high levels of energy to be delivered to the tumour volume whilst sparing the surrounding tissue. In turn this opens the possibility of delivering higher doses to improve cure rates. The technique has found application in prostatic cancer, where the rectum can be spared and in head and neck cancers where damage to salivary tissue can be reduced.

Stereotactic radiosurgery delivers a single high dose of radiotherapy, with high levels of accuracy, to a small intracranial volume. If multiple fractions are delivered, the technique is called stereotactic radiotherapy. The patient must be positioned correctly to allow energy delivery with a precision of millimetres. To effect this, a stereotactic frame is attached to the skull to improve targeting. This technique has been used for primary and metastatic brain tumours in conjunction with external beam treatment, and for benign lesions including arteriovenous malformations and acoustic neuromas.

Delivering radiation from a close proximity to the tumour is a technique called brachytherapy. Radioactive sources are placed either in body cavities near the tumour (intracavitary), or within the tumour itself (interstitial).

Fractionation describes the delivery of a total dose of radiation over a series of smaller dose fractions. This spares normal tissues by allowing them time to repair. Generally once a day dosing schedules are employed for 5 days per week, over 3–7 weeks.

Hyperfractionation involves smaller doses given more frequently resulting in a higher total dose but the same treatment time. Accelerated fractionation involves a shorter treatment time with multiple daily doses. Hypofractionation delivers a lower number of doses in larger fractions and is often employed in palliative treatments.

The acute side effects of radiation therapy include skin desquamation, mucositis, and diarrhoea, as rapidly proliferating tissues are affected soon after initiation of treatment. Controlling these acute symptoms will prevent treatment breaks which can affect the outcomes following therapy.

Chronic side effects are related to slowly proliferating cell lines. Damage to the vasculature in the area treated may also contribute to these effects. The nature of these side effects will depend on the treatment area and volume. Introduction of techniques such as intensity-modulated radiation therapy and stereotactic radiotherapy may lead to a reduction in these undesirable outcomes.

Medical oncology

Medical oncologists are involved in all aspects of the management of cancer including prevention, curative treatment, palliative care, and clinical research. We will focus on the use of chemotherapy.

Chemotherapy is the use of drugs against disease, or in the field of oncology, drug therapy for cancer. Our understanding of cancer cell growth has evolved over the past century. Initial experiments suggested that all cancer cells within a tumour are proliferating at the same rate. This results in the cancer cell number doubling at a predictable, exponential rate. Chemotherapeutic drugs follow first-order kinetics, which is to say that the percentage of tumour cells killed by a given dose is a constant, regardless of the number of viable cells. From these two principles, experimental models can predict rates growth and tumour control.

In vivo systems are more complex, and most solid tumours do not consist of homogeneously dividing cell populations. The growth factor or percentage of cells that are proliferating varies between and within tumour types. This is influenced by factors such as relative hypoxia at the centre of a tumour mass, resulting in high growth factors in small tumours such as micrometastases and lower growth factors in the primary tumour.

Chemotherapeutics must target cancer cells preferentially. Unlike viruses and bacteria, cancer cells use the same 'self' proteins that are present on normal cells. They do, however, respond differently to growth control, a mechanism which gives them a survival advantage over normal cells. Drugs can target this difference to affect cancer cells more than normal cells. It appears that the final pathway in cell death for many cancers is apoptosis.

A second method of targeting chemotherapy is related to the expression of specific proteins that are produced either by infective viruses such as Epstein–Barr, or by genetic mutations such as *RAS* mutations. By targeting therapy against such proteins, drugs can be delivered selectively to cancerous cells.

In order to achieve high kill and low resistance rates, combination chemotherapy is in routine use. The drugs chosen should have different effects on the cancer cells, so using separate mechanisms to achieve cell death. The dose limiting toxic effects should be different to allow full dose treatments to be given. Drugs with different resistance patterns should also be chosen where possible.

Most drugs are used intravenously, either through temporary or surgically placed venous catheters. Intraperitoneal delivery has been used for ovarian and GI malignancies. It allows high concentrations to be achieved but requires an adhesion free abdomen to be successful. Intrathecal delivery bypasses the blood–brain barrier, and is used for treatment of disease in the central nervous system (CNS) and for prophylaxis in cancers with high rates of CNS disease such as Burkitt's lymphoma. Intra-arterial delivery can be used if a tumour has a well-defined arterial supply. It has found most application in tumours of the liver.

Having decided what drug or combination to use and the route of delivery, timing is the next issue. Adjuvant treatment is used in combination when surgery or radiation has removed macroscopic evidence of cancer. This is ideal for treatment of micrometastases which should be rapidly proliferating and have high sensitivity to chemotherapy.

Neoadjuvant therapy describes the use of chemotherapy prior to surgery or radiation. It results in immediate exposure of cancer cells to treatment effects, removing any pre-surgical or radiation delay. It provides an assessment of the responsiveness of the primary tumour, which may act as a surrogate in assessing the response of micrometastases. There may also be a reduction in the bulk of primary tumour. Such 'downstaging' of primary disease may allow less destructive procedures to be considered as definitive therapy.

Chemotherapy may be used during the same time period as radiation, as concurrent therapy. In this setting chemotherapy may both destroy cells and act as a radiation sensitizer.

The evolving field of medical oncology has changed over the past few decades with improvements in drug design. Targeting against specific cancers allows for tailored treatments with more effect and fewer side effects. Improved supportive treatment of the unwanted effects of treatment such as myelosuppression has led to reduction in morbidity and the potential for increased dosing. These developments have resulted in medical oncologists becoming an indispensable member of all cancer MDTs.

Scenarios

Scenario 1

A 66-year-old man with altered bowel habit is found to have an adenomatous polyp in the sigmoid colon. Why should this lesion be removed?

Scenario 2

A 50-year-old non-smoker with asbestos exposure develops shortness of breath and an abnormal CXR. What is the most likely malignancy in this setting?

Scenario 3

Results of a recently introduced screening tests show improved survival in the screened population. What factors would you consider when analysing these results?

Scenario 4

When planning an excisional biopsy of a mass, what must the surgeon consider in relation to the scar?

Scenario 5

A patient asks his surgeon what immediate effects he should expect from upcoming radiotherapy. What is the appropriate response?

Scenario 6

Following definitive surgery to remove cancer, a patient is recommended a course of chemotherapy. What is the appropriate term for this treatment and what is the intended target?

Scenario 7

A 68-year-old female with an enlarging mass in the neck is investigated with CT scanning. The results suggest that the mass is unresectable, as it invades the base of skull. What must be done to determine the most appropriate treatment plan?

Scenario 8

What are the potential advantages of image-modulated radiotherapy?

Scenario 9

Following surgical excision of a malignant melanoma, with sentinel lymph node sampling, the node is found to harbour malignant cells. The remaining nodes were felt to be clinically normal during the procedure. What steps should the surgical team now take?

Scenario 10

In terms of mucosal malignancies, which two categories of metastases exist and how do they impact on patient management?

Scenario 11

Give examples of the members of staff encountered within a MDT dealing with cancers in the UK.

Scenario 12

What is the sensitivity and specificity of the test described below?

Excerpt from HDU chart		
Test A	**Disease present?**	
Test result	**Yes**	**No**
Positive	80	40
Negative	20	60

Answers

Scenario 1

Colonic cancer has been shown to develop from normal mucosa to adenomatous polyps, then overt malignancy and metastasis. The polyp should be removed to prevent this sequence of events.

Scenario 2

Both of these chemicals have a carcinogenic effect. Exposure to asbestos is related to the development of the rare pleural malignancy, mesothelioma. Exposure is also linked with bronchogenic carcinoma which is in fact more common amongst those exposed to asbestos than mesothelioma

Scenario 3

A number of biases, including lead time bias, length bias, and the fact that a population that presents for screening is self-selected can all affect the results of a screening programme, and are likely to produce favourable results.

Scenario 4

The risk of tumour seeding in to the incision means that it should be placed and orientated in a manner which allows incorporation into the incision required for definitive surgery.

Scenario 5

Patients are likely to be anxious about upcoming treatment and it is important that a surgeon understands some of the expected side effects of treatments their patients will receive. Immediate effects are seen from cells that are rapidly proliferating. Desquamation, mucositis, and diarrhoea are the most common, but the site of treatment will affect the side-effect profile.

Scenario 6

The goal of definitive surgery is to remove macroscopic tumour cells. Chemotherapy may be recommended following surgery to destroy microscopic cells, and in particular micrometastases. These small tumour deposits may be rapidly proliferating and so are highly sensitive to this form of chemotherapy, known as adjuvant therapy.

Scenario 7

Although the mass may not be amenable to surgical resection, without a histological diagnosis, appropriate plans cannot be made. The most likely diagnosis is squamous cell carcinoma, but lymphoma and tuberculosis are within the differential diagnosis, which makes diagnostic biopsy essential. The options available include FNA, core biopsy, and incisional biopsy, as the CT scan has shown that excisional biopsy is impossible.

Scenario 8

By using image guidance, often in the form of CT or MRI scanning, radiation oncologists can design the radiation fields with great precision. This improved targeting can in turn result in lower levels of collateral damage to surrounding structures. Examples of this include sparing the spinal cord for tumours close to the spinal column, and sparing the eye in tumours of the midface.

Scenario 9

Sentinel node biopsy is a procedure used in the absence of clinically positive metastatic nodes within the draining nodal basin. If nodes are felt to be likely to harbour metastases, a therapeutic surgical strategy should be considered from the outset.

The presence of metastatic cells within the clinically normal excised node suggest that other, non-dissected nodes within the nodal basin may also harbour malignant cells. Following discussion within the MDT and the patient, plans should be made to excise the remaining nodes in order to surgically stage the disease and remove malignant cells.

Scenario 10

Mucosal malignancies give rise to regional and distant metastases. Regional metastases involve the draining lymphatic basin. Distant metastases involve structures beyond the primary site or regional lymphatics. Whilst regional metastasis is a poor prognostic sign, many lesions can still be cured with appropriate treatment. By the time malignancies have given rise to distant metastases, the chance of cure is far lower. There are some exceptions to this rule, and experience with surgery for isolated distant metastasis is growing in certain specialties.

Scenario 11

Modern cancer management in the UK is coordinated by an MDT. These teams will vary according to specialty but generally will include surgeons (who may have varying surgical backgrounds), oncologists with an interest in radiotherapy and chemotherapy, pathologists and radiologists. Other clinical members of the team may include cancer nurse specialists, physiotherapists, occupational therapists, and speech therapists. Non-clinical members may include administrators, secretaries, and data managers.

Scenario 12

Sensitivity describes the percentage of patients with the disease who test positive, which here is 80/80 + 20 = 0.8, or 80%.

Specificity describes the number of patients without the disease who test negative, 60/60+40 = 0.6, or 60%.

Chapter 19 **Oedema and thromboprophylaxis**

Oedema

Thromboprophylaxis

Oedema

Introduction

Oedema is abnormal swelling caused by accumulation of fluids in the tissues. If there is a high concentration of protein in the fluid then the oedema does not 'pit'. If the oedema has been present constantly for many years fibrous tissue is laid down and the oedema becomes indurated. Lymphoedema is a subset of oedema and is a result of pathology in the lymphatic system.

The causes of oedema can be simply subdivided into local and systemic. The causes of lymphoedema can then be divided into congenital and acquired.

Physiology

Blood coming to the tissues through the arteries is at high pressure. This is to enable it to transport oxygen rapidly from the lungs to the tissues. As the blood passes through the arterioles to the capillaries, the pressure is reduced to much lower levels, which can be tolerated by the capillary bed. There are smooth muscle pre-capillary sphincters at the entry to the capillary bed which ensure that the appropriate pressure reduction is achieved. These sphincters are under adrenergic control but appear also to be very sensitive to accumulation of metabolites in the tissues which their capillaries supply. They are therefore able to open up if the tissues start metabolizing rapidly.

The walls of the capillaries themselves are normally highly permeable to water and small molecules, but relatively impermeable to large molecules such as albumin. As the blood enters the capillary bed through the pre-capillary sphincter, the hydrostatic pressure inside the capillaries is higher than the pressure in the interstitial tissue. Therefore, water, glucose, and salts leak out of the capillaries into the interstitial tissues. By the time the blood reaches the far end of the capillaries, its pressure has fallen (though friction with the capillary walls) but its oncotic pressure has risen because it has lost water but not the larger protein molecules. These create an osmotic pressure gradient in the opposite direction to the hydrostatic pressure gradient which eventually (as the protein concentration rises) exceeds it. Water therefore re-enters the capillaries flowing down the osmotic gradient. Not all the fluid, electrolytes and small molecules re-enter the capillary system and the surplus enters the lymphatic system and is drained back into the venous system via the lymphatic duct.

Causes

The causes of oedema can be related to the physiology of fluid movement in and out of the capillary bed and so this makes a popular question in the MRCS exam:

- Local
- Systemic
- Venous
- Lymphatic

Local causes

- **Reperfusion injury** Relaxation of the pre-capillary sphincters in response to accumulation of metabolites will lead to a rise in hydrostatic pressure in the capillary bed and so an increase in fluid accumulation in the interstitial tissues. This is a normal and appropriate physiological response. However, this is also in large part responsible for the oedema, which develops in a limb suffering from a reperfusion injury.
- **Inflammation** The amount of fluid escaping from the capillaries depends to a degree on the permeability of the capillary walls. This is measured in units denoted by the Greek figure sigma and varies from zero (full permeability) to 1 for totally impermeable. Under normal conditions the capillary wall is fairly permeable to water, sugar and salts (σ = close to 0) and almost totally impermeable to proteins like albumin (σ = close to 1.0). However, if the capillary is inflamed or damaged then the permeability rises. Water leaves even more rapidly but protein leaves too.

If protein has escaped into the interstitial tissues there is no longer such a high oncotic pressure gradient to reverse the effect of the hydrostatic pressure gradient. This is a second reason why water (with protein) accumulates in the interstitial tissues in inflammation.

- **Infection** This is doubly important as it is both a cause of oedema, and tissues with chronic lymphoedema are also more susceptible to becoming infected. Staphylococci and streptococci can spread by the lymphatics and will produce rapidly extending red streaks which are also swollen. Antibiotics need to be started as soon as possible (once swabs have been taken for M,C&S. If the condition does not respond rapidly then the infection may be resistant to that antibiotic and a change should be considered. Limbs with chronic oedema need constant skin care to ensure that cracks which form in the skin do not act as an entry point for bacterial or fungal infection. Filariasis is a mosquito-borne nematode worm infection (*Wucheri bancroftii*) associated with poverty and poor hygiene which affects over 100 million people in parts of Africa, India, and South America. The worms invade and block the lymphatics causing severe lymphoedema. Massive oedema caused by filaria is called elephantiasiasis

Systemic causes

- **Low albumin** If the protein concentration (mainly albumin) in the blood is abnormally low, as occurs and liver failure, malnutrition and renal failure, then the oncotic pressure gradient which draws fluid back into the capillary no longer works so well and fluid remains in the interstitial tissues, and oedema forms
- **Fluid overload** Renal failure and overhydration will increase the blood volume, and so increase venous back pressure. It will also dilute the plasma and so reduce the oncotic pressure gradient
- **Gravity** If there is anything which raises the pressure at the venous end of the capillary then the oncotic pressure gradient created by the proteins will not exceed the hydrostatic pressure gradient working in the opposite direction. The result will be that fluid will not be drawn back into the capillaries and oedema will form. Gravity can provide this excess pressure so a dependant limb which is not moved will accumulate venous blood and so the venous pressure will rise and oedema will develop. If the limb is moved regularly the muscles moving the limb squeeze the venous blood out of the veins and reduce the static venous pressure. Gravity induced oedema tends to improve overnight when the patient is lying flat. The patient also notices that they have to get up frequently at night to pass urine, as the fluid comes back out of the tissues
- **Drugs** Drugs may cause or reduce oedema by either affecting the total body fluid balance (diuretics), cardiac output (inotropic drugs), or capillary permeability (anti-inflammatory agents)

Venous causes

- **Incompetent valves in veins** However, if the veins which prevent reflux of venous blood are incompetent then the muscle pumps will not be able to move the venous blood away and venous pressure will remain high
- **Obstruction to venous return** Similarly, if there is any obstruction to venous return either because of external pressure (e.g. a bandage which is too tight), or because of occlusion of the lumen of the vein (thrombosis) venous pressure will rise and oedema will result. An important fact to remember is that pain and swelling in a leg is often attributed to venous insufficiency. The diagnosis may appear to be confirmed by a finding of superficial reflux on duplex ultrasound. However, care needs to be taken. Studies of 'normal' legs show superficial reflux in up to 25% of cases so this finding is not necessarily explanatory. If the real cause is some form of lymphatic insufficiency, then ligation of the sapheno-femoral junction will inevitably further damage the lymphatics which travel with these veins and make the situation worse
- **Heart failure** If there is right heart failure then there will be raised venous pressure which may raise the hydrostatic pressure in the capillary bed

Lymphatic causes

Not all the fluid which leaves the blood as it flows through the capillary bed returns into the vascular system. That which is left behind is scavenged by the lymphatic system which returns this relatively protein-rich fluid to the venous system via the lymph nodes and then the lymphatic duct into the junction of the jugular with the left subclavian vein. The lymphatics have non-return valves and contractile walls which help to move fluid up the system. Although the lymph ducts are relatively thin-walled and are collapsed in their rest state, accumulation of interstitial fluid actually opens their lumen by creating tension on the walls through microfibrils If the lymphatic system is absent or obstructed this scavenging system will fail and fluid will accumulate in the tissues. Maldevelopment of the lymphatics can be congenital, or acquired. Acquired causes will include fibrosis secondary to radiotherapy, trauma damaging the soft tissues, and parasitic infection occluding the lumen (such as filariasis). Simply cutting or removing lymphatic channels does not usually cause lymphoedema as new channels grow and collateral channels open up. However, if there is extensive scarring from trauma or radiotherapy this will not be possible.

History

The history needs to systematically check for possible causes of lymphoedema checking for any evidence of heart, liver, or kidney failure. A check also needs to be made for any surgery especially for malignant disease, and of any courses of radiotherapy. A drug history is also valuable.

Examination

The distribution of oedema may give a clue to its likely cause. Bilateral oedema is more likely to be produced by a systemic cause than unilateral. Local oedema is more likely to have an inflammatory cause. Pitting oedema is the result of the accumulation of mainly fluid and not protein so is more likely to be systemic in origin (heart, liver, and renal). A full cardiovascular examination will be needed to exclude heart failure. An abdominal examination will be needed to check for an enlarged liver or kidneys, a caput medusae, and the shifting dullness of ascites. A peripheral vascular examination will be needed to exclude varicose veins arising from valve incompetence and/or deep vein occlusion. If the lymphoedema is only in one limb then a check for lymphadenopathy will also be needed as well as well as for signs proximally of surgery, trauma, and radiotherapy.

Investigations

The urine will need testing for protein to exclude hypoproteinuria secondary to nephrotic syndrome. A check of the creatinine, urea and electrolytes, will exclude fluid overload, while liver function tests will exclude oedema secondary to hypoproteinaemia.

Imaging might include a duplex ultrasound examination of the venous system to check for patency of the deep vein system and competence of the perforator veins. Lymphangiograms are painful and difficult to perform and can damage tissues in their own right. They have therefore been replaced by isotope lymphoscintigraphy, and now by CT scan and MRI. Malignancy (lymphangiosarcoma) may be diagnosed by skin biopsy or fine needle aspiration.

Prevention

When planning block dissection of lymph nodes and radiotherapy to the axilla in the treatment of carcinoma of the breast, great care needs to be taken to ensure that no more extreme measures are taken than are necessary.

In major surgery, care needs to be taken to avoid a patient developing a significant deep vein thrombosis (DVT) which may not recannulate and may damage the perforator veins leading to venous hypertension.

Treatment

Treatment can be divided into non-operative and operative. Non-operative measures include optimization of heart, renal, and liver function. If the patient is leaving the lower limbs dependant for long periods then help and advice on keeping them elevated and regular mobility will improve matters. Well-fitting graduated pressure stockings will increase the hydrostatic pressure in the interstitial tissues and so improve both venous and lymphatic drainage. Pain may be a major element and is helped by reduction of swelling.

Careful graduated and regular massage over an oedematous limb milking fluid up the lymphatics can also reduce oedema. This is called manual lymphatic drainage (MLD). After an initial intensive phase lasting several months, the maintenance phase can be continued by the patient themselves. At the same time they are educated in the importance of regular and meticulous skin care.

Bandaging is probably best done with non-elastic bandages in the acute phase (they are safer), and the pressure applied needs to be graduated (reducing as the bandage is applied higher up the limb). Compression garments need to be made to measure if they are to apply the optimum pressure gradient and must be put on before the patient gets out of bed in the morning. Pneumatic (inflatable pressure garments) are of questionable benefit.

Exercise is beneficial and indeed should be the only time when the limb is dependant. Otherwise wherever possible it should be kept elevated.

Acute inflammatory episodes are common and each one causes further damage to the lymphatics. It is therefore important for the patient to learn to recognize and start antibiotics as soon as possible to abort the attack and minimize damage.

Surgery is rarely valuable in the treatment of lymphoedema. It can be divided into procedures for diversion, and those which involve excision. Diversion surgery now involves super-microsurgery and this requires special equipment and expertise. Reduction surgery either involves removal of wedges of tissue with primary closure (Sistrunk), or subcutaneous fat excision (Homans). A modification of this (Thompsons) is to de-fat the skin then tuck it under the opposite fascia in the hope that it will act as a conduit for new lymph channels to form. All these operations have a high complication rate and a poor cosmetic result. In the Charles operation (specifically for severe filariasis) the skin and fat is all excised and split skin applied to the underlying muscle fascia. This is primarily a debulking operation.

Scenarios on oedema

Scenario 1
Please take a history from this lady to try to determine the cause(s) of her bilateral ankle oedema.

Scenario 2
Perform a brief examination to determine why this patient has oedema in her left arm.

Scenario 3
Perform a brief examination to determine why this patient has oedema in both legs.

Scenario 4
This lady has had swollen ankles for many years. Explain to her how you propose to help her manage this problem.

Scenario 5
This patient is a chronic alcoholic with ascites and oedema. He is a scientist and wants an explanation of why fluid is accumulating in his ankles. He does not understand medical terminology.

Answers for scenarios on oedema

Scenario 1
Introduction.

How long has she had it? Was there anything that started it? E.g. a pregnancy, thrombosis, an injury. Is it congenital or did it come on when living in the tropics?

Ask whether the oedema improves overnight and about nocturia (suggests gravitational effect).

Take a rapid cardiovascular history checking for evidence of cardiac insufficiency, e.g. dyspnoea, orthopnoea, angina, and palpitations.

Check for any history of liver problems (jaundice) or renal problems (stones, repeated infections, investigations, and surgery).

Take a brief vascular history asking about deep vein thrombosis and varicose veins.

Ask about medication especially inotropic drugs and diuretics.

Thank and close.

Scenario 2

Introduction.

Obtain adequate exposure. Look at skin for scars, redness, or atrophy, soft tissues for swelling and/or wasting, bone for deformity. There will be a mastectomy scar and the breast may or may not have been reconstructed. The incision should be checked for extension into the axilla for lymph node clearance. If radiotherapy has been used there may be the atrophic skin and soft tissue changes characteristic of this. Describe the oedema in relation to the other side. Size and extent. Check distal neurovascular status, and range of movement of the joints of the arm especially the shoulder. Thank the patient and help cover her up again. The reason is going to be a mastectomy with or without axillary clearance and radiotherapy.

Thank and close.

Scenario 3

Introduction.

Obtain adequate exposure. Look at skin for scars, redness, or atrophy and signs of old or current leg ulceration. Check soft tissues for varicose veins swelling and/or wasting. Describe the severity and extent of the oedema and whether it is equal in both legs. Check for pitting around the ankle. Now lay the patient down and check her hands for general stigmata, (palmar erythema, clubbing and spider naevae). Check the eyes and mouth for jaundice and anaemia. Check the pulse for rate and rhythm. Check the neck for raised jugular venous pressure. Feel the heart for displaced apex and listen for murmurs. Check the abdomen for hepatosplenomegaly. Balotte the kidney and check for shifting dullness. Check the groins for masses or lymphadenopathy which might be obstructing drainage from the legs.

Thank and close.

Scenario 4

Introduction.

Wash your hands. Introduce yourself. Explain what you want to do, and ask permission. Find out first from her what treatments have been tried before. If these have not been covered, explain about keeping legs elevated whenever possible and about how walking and moving the feet help pump fluid away. Discuss massage, and the use of graduated stockings, and avoiding constricting clothing in the groin such as corsets. Discuss the advantages and disadvantages of diuretics.

Thank and close.

Scenario 5

Introduction.

Blood travels around your body in blood vessels. When blood reaches the tissues it is destined to serve it enters a mesh of tiny thin-walled vessels called capillaries. Their walls are leaky to oxygen, carbon dioxide, sugars, water, and waste products, so this capillary bed is the point where the requirements of life are provided to the tissues and waste products are removed. The process of transfer is a delicate balance of pressure exerted by the blood pressure and by osmosis. When the blood first enters the capillary bed it is at higher pressure than the tissues around it and so fluid and nutrients leak out. By the time the blood reaches the far end of the capillary bed ready to connect to the venous system, the pressure has dropped. However, proteins dissolved in the blood have not been able to escape so they draw water back into the capillaries by osmotic pressure. Because of your illness your liver is not able to manufacture as much protein as is needed to run this system. Your blood is low on protein so does not draw this fluid back as well as a healthy person. The result is that fluid accumulates in your tissues.

Thank and close.

Thromboprophylaxis

Introduction

Blood clotting is a normal process vital to the survival of all mammals. The biochemical system for bringing about thrombosis (clotting) and clot clearance (fibrinolysis) is a complex one which is in a continuous state of dynamic equilibrium (see Fig. 19.1). Normally the enzymes which prevent the formation of thrombus (clot) inhibit those which are ready to produce a thrombus, and blood flows freely through arteries, capillaries, and veins. If that equilibrium is disturbed then a cascade of enzymes are activated so that blood loss from a damaged vessel is stopped as soon as possible. The damaged vessel is then repaired, and finally the clot is cleared away so that normal circulation can resume.

However, the clotting process can also be initiated inappropriately or over-exuberantly, and at other times the thrombus which forms is not adequate to control the bleeding and the patient continues to lose blood (and clotting factors). This section will look at those pathological states.

Thrombosis (appropriate and inappropriate) is usually initiated by one of three events:

1 Damage to a blood vessel wall (this is a normal healthy physiological response
2 An imbalance of the enzymes which control clotting (this is pathological)
3 Stagnation or turbulence of blood flow (this too is abnormal)

These three factors are commonly but incorrectly attributed to Virchow and so are called Virchow's triad (Box 19.1).

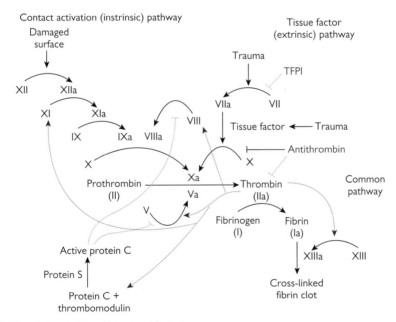

Figure 19.1 Cascade for clotting of blood and for lysis.

Box 19.1 **Virchow's triad**
• Vessel wall damage
• Hypercoagulability
• Stasis or turbulence in blood flow

Physiologically appropriate initiation of thrombus formation

Arteries have smooth muscles in the wall and when damaged can go into spasm and limit the rate of blood loss. In both arteries and veins the exposure of collagen in a damaged vessel wall, and the release of cytokines from the damaged areas are the initiating factors which transforms thin non-sticky platelets flowing freely in the bloodstream, into fat sticky structures which glue themselves to the damaged vessel wall and to each other. This aggregation of platelets and red cells, which are also caught in the net, creates a plug or clot which stops the bleeding (primary haemostasis). At the same time proteins which are precursors of coagulation factors in the plasma are activated and start the process of laying down fibrin, (secondary haemostasis). Once healing has occurred fibrinolysis (the removal of thrombi and emboli) is activated. This is controlled by plasmin, a fibrinolytic enzyme. If the thrombus which forms grows too large or is not removed quickly then a permanent blockage of the veins will occur. Post-phlebitic syndrome (also called post-thrombotic syndrome, PTS) is the consequence of permanent blockage of veins and loss of competency of valves. This leads to swollen legs and can be the underlying cause of chronic leg ulceration. If during any stage of thrombosis formation and then fibrinolysis, a thrombus breaks away from the vessel wall to which it was attached, it will float away through the bloodstream as an embolus, until it enters a vessel too narrow to allow it to pass, where it will block that vessel. Thrombi forming in the venous system, which then embolize tend to pass through the right side of the heart and end up lodging in the lungs (pulmonary emboli, PEs). Small ones are of no clinical significance and probably occur all the time, but large ones cause pulmonary hypertension and prevent blood being oxygenated properly in the lungs. Large PEs can cause sudden death. If the patient has a patent foramen ovale, the venous emboli may pass from the right side of the heart to the left and then proceed to the brain causing cerebral emboli (infarcting stroke). The lung has a large capacity to absorb small emboli without the patient having any symptoms. Equally thrombi can form (especially in the deep veins of the calf) without the patient noticing anything. It is therefore likely that the majority of deep vein thromboses and indeed small PEs occur all the time without any of us being aware of them.

Humans who are confined to bed for any reason are believed to be more susceptible to developing deep vein thrombosis (DVT) than those who are active. It is believed that the stasis of the blood in the deep veins of the calf when lying in bed or even sitting in a chair for long periods (as in long aeroplane journeys) creates an environment when inappropriate clotting becomes more likely. Thrombi which form in the deep veins below the knee are not thought to be associated with life-threatening PEs, but those which extend into the femoral vessels are. Thrombi in the pelvic veins tend to be large and especially dangerous if they break off.

Patients undergoing surgery usually lie still for a period of time on the operating table and may then be confined to bed during the recovery period. Therefore all patients undergoing surgical operations probably carry an increased risk of significant DVT and of PE directly proportional to the length of the operation and of the recovery period. However, patients receiving epidural, spinal, and regional blocks appear to have a reduced risk of DVT compared with general anaesthesia although the reason for this is not known.

Some patients who have malignant disease appear to have an alteration in the enzymes in the blood leading to hypercoagulability. So they are at even higher risk when they undergo surgery for their malignant disease. Obese patients and those who are pregnant, on the contraceptive pill, and hormone replacement therapy (HRT) are also at increased risk, but the reason for this is not known. It has also been suggested that the twisting of the hip joint in total hip replacement may damage the intima of the femoral and pelvic veins making thrombus formation more likely, but the epidemiological evidence for this is lacking. Similarly the use of the tourniquet in total knee replacement is thought by some to raise the risk of DVT because of venous stasis below the cuff and possible intimal damage from the cuff itself. Once again there is no epidemiological evidence to support this. However patients with polytrauma undoubtedly do have an increased risk of DVT and PE for a multitude of possible reasons. Patients with polytrauma may lie still for long periods (if unconscious or not yet found). Polytrauma itself leads to a hypercoagulable state. Soft tissue trauma damages vessel walls, and both dehydration as well as infusion of crystalloids to rehydrate the patient alters coagulability of blood. It is becoming increasingly clear that some patients are much more susceptible to developing DVT than others, for example, the G20210A mutation of the prothrombin gene increases the risk of developing a DVT by at least eight times, but as

---

Box 19.2 Minimizing risk of DVT and PE

- Stasis—operating table, bed rest, sitting for long periods
- Malignant disease—hypercoagulability
- Obesity
- Pregnancy, the contraceptive pill, and HRT—?cause
- Damage to vessels by trauma or surgery
- Dehydration and infusion of crystalloids
- General anaesthetic compared with spinal or regional block
- Patient susceptibility as revealed by previous events

Box 19.3 Causes of increased risk of DVT

- Early mobilization
- Mechanical (static and dynamic) to avoid calf vein stasis
- Use regional rather than general anaesthesia

---

yet there are no tests available for determining increased susceptibility. A list of the causes of increased susceptibility to DVT is summarized in Box 19.2.

Minimizing patient risk

The best approach to the danger of DVT and PE in surgery is a) to try to minimize patient risk (Box 19.3) and then b) to consider thromboprophylaxis for those most at risk.

- **Early mobilization** It is now generally accepted that it is good for patients psychologically as well as physiologically to mobilize as soon as possible provided that adequate pain relief is given. The risk of hypostatic pneumonia, urinary tract infection, bed sores, and DVT are probably all reduced by early mobilization. It can also reduce the cost of care of the patient if this results in early discharge from hospital
- **Avoiding stasis** There are both static and dynamic mechanical systems designed to prevent stasis of blood in the deep veins of the calf. Static methods such as graded compression stocking are designed to keep the calf veins empty by compression although if they do not fit properly they can actually cause obstruction and distension. Dynamic methods such as foot and calf pumps or electrical stimulators of the calf muscles replicate the pumping action on the venous plexus of the foot and the deep calf veins normally produced by walking and reduce the risk of venous thromboembolism (VTE) by over 70%. They do this either by electrodes applied to the calf muscles or by intermittently compressing the foot and/or lower leg with a pneumatic inflatable cuff.
- **Avoiding general anaesthetic** Where possible, spinal, epidural, and regional blocks offer substantial advantages in terms of pain relief (especially post-operatively) compared with general anaesthetic. They usually require more time and more skill by the anaesthetist, but to the advantages of regional anaesthesia have to be added the reduced risk of VTE by around 30%. However, it should be noted that if chemical thromboprophylaxis is used, then most anaesthetists will decline to perform spinal or epidural anaesthesia because there may be an increased risk of uncontrolled epidural bleeding leading to cord or root compression

All the above methods of prevention should be considered in every patient undergoing surgery, as the risk of doing harm with these techniques is low. Therefore the risk/benefit balance is always likely to be tilted towards benefit.

Chemical thromboprophylaxis (Box 19.4)

Patients at higher risk of developing DVT and PE must be considered for additional chemical thromboprophylaxis. Here a careful risk/benefit analysis needs to be performed because any anticoagulant which

---

Box 19.4 Chemical thromboprophylaxis

- Aspirin—cheap, oral, safe, not very effective
- Heparin—cheap, injected, fairly effective
- LMWH—cheap, injected, very effective
- Warfarin—cheap, oral, effective, risky to use
- Pentasaccharides—safe, effective
- Factor Xa and thrombin inhibitors— expensive, oral, safe,

---

actually works will inevitably increase the risk of bleeding both during surgery and afterwards. Bleeding is a risk to patients and haematomas are a classic site for the start of infection, so the benefits must outweigh the potential risks. Some chemical thromboprophylactic agents such as aspirin are weak in preventing thromboembolic disease and as a general rule have mild complications. Others like warfarin are very powerful but also carry significant risks of complications.

There is good evidence that if thromboprophylaxis is given before any traumatic event (such as surgery) the agent is much more potent in preventing VTE than if it is given afterwards. Obviously surgeons would prefer to operate first, then give VTE afterwards, once haemostasis has been obtained, but there is a penalty in that this weakens the VTE effect of the agent. In the case of trauma it is only possible to give VTE after the event so it may be prudent to give a stronger thromboprophylactic agent or a higher dose than in a patient undergoing elective surgery. As mentioned before, most anaesthetists will not give an epidural or spinal anaesthetic if chemical thromboprophylaxis has been started, so this too is a contraindication to pre-operative thromboprophylaxis.

- **Aspirin** Aspirin is cheap, and can be taken orally once a day. Its action is to reduce platelet stickiness. It is not primarily an antithrombotic agent. The risk reduction of VTE is less than can be achieved with heparin or other new antithrombotic agents. It carries a risk of causing GI inflammation and even bleeding
- **Heparin** This is well-tried and proven but must be given by injection. Its use has now been superseded by newer safer drugs
- **Low-molecular-weight heparin (LMWH)** This class of drugs are safe and do not need careful monitoring like warfarin. They are cheap and can be given by subcutaneous injection once or twice a day. They are more effective than heparin and as effective as warfarin. There is no evidence that they cause increased bleeding but must be given with care in patients with renal disease
- **Warfarin** This drug is taken orally and requires a loading dose to bring its plasma levels up to therapeutic range (this takes up to 48 hours). It affects the extrinsic pathway of clotting and requires very careful monitoring of the prothrombin time, using the prothrombin ratio or the international normalized ratio (INR). This should be kept between 2.0 and 3.0 for the warfarin to be safe and effective. The body's ability to metabolize warfarin in the liver is affected by many drugs and alcohol so considerable care needs to be taken when changing the patient's medication. Near patient testing of the INR is now available so patients can test their own blood and then phone in for advice on the appropriate dose to take next. The effects of warfarin overdose can be reversed by giving the patient vitamin K
- **Pentasaccharides** Fondaparinux is the first and commonest of this group of synthetic agents which inhibit Factor Xa. It is given once a day by injection and is more effective than LMWH in preventing VTE, but may also have a higher complication risk in terms of increased risk of post-operative bleeding
- **Direct Factor Xa and thrombin inhibitors** This new class of drugs may revolutionize thromboprophylaxis as they can be given orally and have a broad safe therapeutic range
- **Combination therapy** There are good grounds for believing that a combination of mechanical and chemical methods of thromboprophylaxis offers the safest option for the patients who are most at risk of VTE. Mechanical methods can be safely used during surgery itself, then after surgery chemical methods can also be introduced once the dangers of bleeding are less immediate

---

Box 19.5 **The Wells score of predicting the likelihood of PE**

The Wells score

- Clinically suspected DVT: 3.0 points
- Alternative diagnosis (such as asthma) is less likely than PE: 3.0 points
- Tachycardia: 1.5 points
- Immobilization/surgery in previous 4 weeks: 1.5 points
- History of DVT or PE: 1.5 points
- Hemoptysis: 1.0 points
- Malignancy (treatment for within 6 months, palliative): 1.0 points

Score >4: PE likely. Consider diagnostic imaging.

Score 4 or less: PE unlikely. Consider D-dimer to rule out PE.

Diagnosing deep vein thrombosis and pulmonary embolism

The diagnosis of DVT and of PE is notoriously difficult on clinical grounds alone. Calf sensitivity is only present in 50% of patients with a DVT. In PE, shortness of breath, cyanosis, wheezing, and a pleural rub are all late signs. The Wells score (Box 19.5) is the most commonly used to determine thresholds for further action.

The ECG may show characteristics or cor pulmonale (right heart strain) with an S wave in lead 1, a Q wave in lead 3, and an inverted T wave in lead 3 (S1Q3T3). Neither this nor the CXR is particularly sensitive. In a patient where VTE is suspected, a D-dimer combined with clinical findings improves the sensitivity and specificity so that a decision can be made whether to ask for Doppler ultrasound examination of the leg veins and/or a CT or MRI scan of the lung fields. Arterial blood gases will also be helpful. The arterial pressure of oxygen will usually fall as will the partial pressure of carbon dioxide (as a result of hyper-ventilation).

Treating deep vein thrombosis and pulmonary embolism

As soon as significant DVT or PE is diagnosed, the patient should be given oxygen, started on a loading dose of IV heparin, and started on warfarin. Blood gases will give an indication of the severity of the PE. If serious it may be considered appropriate to give thrombolysis (streptokinase or one of the other thrombolytic drugs).

Inferior vena cava filters

In patients with known DVT and a high risk of PE it may be decided that very high-risk strategies such as an inferior vena cava filter should be used to prevent massive PE. This may be especially useful where a patient is having repeated PEs or where for whatever reason anticoagulation cannot be used.

Summary

VTE can lead to DVT, PE, and post-phlebitic syndrome. All surgical patients need to be assessed for their risk of VTE, and then appropriate measures taken to minimize that risk. Some measures (such as minimizing bed rest) and mechanical methods are appropriate to most patients. Chemical thromboprophylaxis should be reserved for high-risk cases and may then be combined with mechanical methods such as stockings and calf pumps. The diagnosis of DVT and PE is difficult to make reliably but a high index of suspicion allows you to reliably identify those patients who need further investigation to exclude VTE. The treatment of proven cases should not be delayed and involves anticoagulation, combined with thrombolysis in life-threatening cases.

Scenarios for thromboprophylaxis

Scenario 1

One of your 70-year-old patients has become suddenly short of breath, 2 days after falling and sustaining a fractured neck of femur. She had a dynamic hip screw on the day of the fall and was mobilized for the first time today. On the round this morning you noticed that one of her calves was swollen. Before the fall she was fit and well with no medical problems. You have been called by your house-officer to see her this evening and have written up a care plan on the assumption that she may have had a pulmonary embolus. She has asked you to explain to her brother (the actor here), who is a retired lawyer, what this is.

Scenario 2

You are going to perform a high tibial osteotomy on a 40-year-old lady who has early arthritis of the knee and is on the contraceptive pill. You are seeing her in the clinic some 6 weeks before surgery. Explain your plan of action to this patient (actor) with regard to thromboprophylaxis, what is happening, and what you are doing.

Scenario 3

You have been asked by one of the nurses who works on your ward to explain to her quickly how clotting works. You have only 5 minutes to do this. This actor is your physiotherapist.

Answers to scenarios on thromboprophylaxis

Scenario 1

Candidate: 'Hello. My name is Dr James and I believe that your sister would like me to explain to you what I think is going on. … OK, and how much do you know already?'

Brother: 'Only that she has fallen and broken her hip.'

Candidate: 'As you know she unfortunately slipped and fell, breaking her hip. We fixed the fracture that evening and everything went well. However, I did notice this morning that she had a swollen calf. That could be bruising but it could also be a clot forming in her calf: what we call a deep vein thrombosis or DVT. Most patients get a swollen calf after this kind of surgery but she has now become a little short of breath so we are now busy trying to find out what is wrong and what needs to be done.'

Brother: 'So what is wrong?'

Candidate: 'I think that the most likely diagnosis at the moment is that she has got a DVT, and that a piece of that clot has broken off and travelled up into her lung. This is making her short of breath as not all of her lung is working properly. So, what we are going to do is work on three fronts simultaneously as we obviously don't want to delay things unnecessarily. On the first front we are doing tests to try to find out if the diagnosis I am working on is correct. At the same time we are starting treatment to stop any more clots breaking off, and finally we are giving her body all the support that we can to cope with the problem she is having at the moment. To deal with the last issue first, we are going to give her oxygen by a mask to make it as easy as possible for her lungs to get oxygen into her body. We have also put up a drip so that we can give drugs and fluids quickly if she needs them. Now to the second part. We are starting now to give her heparin through the drip. This thins her blood and should prevent any more clots from forming. Finally, we are taking blood tests to check how well her lungs are working. These tests are called blood gases. We are also taking blood to tell us whether there is likely to have been a clot in her bloodstream. This test is called a D-dimer. We have already carried out a test of her heart to make sure that she has not had a heart attack, and we will be getting a chest X-ray just to be sure that she has not got a pneumothorax or a chest infection. The team from the Intensive Care Unit (called the Outreach Team) will visit in a moment to make sure that they are happy with what we are doing. They will be ready to take her onto the Intensive Care Unit if her condition gets any worse. However, if all goes well, and I am sure that it will, then we will replace the blood thinning drug heparin with a tablet called warfarin over the next few days, and then she will remain on that for some months just to make sure that she has no further problems. I hope I have explained that clearly. Have you got any questions?'

Scenario 2

Candidate: Hello. My name is Dr James and I want to talk to you about one of the risks of your surgery which we need to discuss and plan so that we can keep any chances of anything going wrong to an absolute minimum. I understand that you are currently on the contraceptive pill, and as you know this has a small risk of you developing a clot in your circulation. The operation that we are planning to do also has the same risk so we need to work out how we can deal with this double small risk. Is it possible for you to stop the contraceptive pill say 4 weeks before the surgery? … It is? That is good. Even so I think we need to take a belt and braces approach to this, and I would like to propose that we give you a low dose of a blood-thinning drug over the period of your surgery, and continue that at least until you are out of plaster, as that is the highest risk time. We will also use pressure boots on your other leg during the surgery to keep the circulation going all the time that you are lying quiet on the table. I will also discuss your case with the anaesthetists, because if we can do your surgery under spinal anaesthetic then that will also reduce the risk of a clot forming. If you are happy with that then I will plan to start the blood-thinning drug straight after surgery as the anaesthetists prefer us not to use these while they are giving a spinal anaesthetic. I hope I have explained that clearly. Have you got any questions?'

Scenario 3

Candidate: 'Hello. I gather that you want a quick talk on how clotting works. How much do you know already?'

Actor: 'Not much. That is why I want you to explain things.'

Candidate: 'OK well here goes. When you get a cut the blood vessels which are damaged start to bleed. If they are arteries they have muscle bands in their walls which contract or go into spasm. That reduces but does not stop the bleeding. However, the damaged blood vessel walls also release signal chemicals that tell the blood nearby that the vessel has been damaged. In the blood there are tiny cells called platelets, which are normally thin and spiky. When they detect these chemical signals they swell up and become very sticky, trapping other platelets and even red cells. This is the start of a clot which serves to block up the damaged vessel and stop bleeding. These chemical signals also activate other enzymes in the body so that there is a rapid chain reaction resulting in the production of fibrin (a sort of scar tissue). This fibrin is the scaffolding of the clot and, given time, strengthens it so that it cannot be knocked off and the bleeding starts again. Some patients are born without all the correct enzymes which enable them to form a proper clot, so they do not stop bleeding when injured. They are called haemophiliacs, and the condition runs in families. Other patients seem to have a blood system which is a little too trigger happy and they clot too easily. Those patients are at risk of developing very large clots if they have an operation. If they develop a large clot it can block the vessels in their legs giving them a deep vein thrombosis and this later can go on to create a chronically swollen leg with leg ulcers. If the clot in the leg breaks away it can be carried up into the lung and cause a pulmonary embolus. We use TED stockings and blood thinning drugs like low-molecular-weight heparin to try to prevent patients from developing abnormal clots, while still allowing them to form normal clots so that they stop bleeding after surgery. The other things that we do to try to prevent patients from getting clots are to use spinal anaesthetics and to get patients up as early as possible after surgery. I hope I have explained that clearly. Have you got any questions?'

Chapter 20 **Trauma**

This chapter on trauma contains material that can be asked in the stations in 'Anatomy and surgical pathology' and 'Applied surgical science and critical care'—all of these stations being in the generic context or specialty context. Concentrate on the scenarios which are common everyday problems.

Introduction

Trauma is the leading cause of death in the world for young adults. Most of that mortality and morbidity is avoidable. Much more can be done to relieve the human suffering caused by trauma using simple prevention measures than anything that a surgeon can do for an individual patient.

Pre-hospital care

Surgeons are expected to have good skills in the management of trauma and will therefore hopefully always volunteer to manage injured patients if they come upon them at the roadside or in the workplace.

Safety

It is the first responsibility of anyone handling the case and situation to make sure that both the patient and anyone involved in helping them is safe (Fig. 20.1).

In the case of accidents where there are many casualties, the most valuable task you can perform as a surgeon may be initially to stand back, assess the severity of the injuries, and organize the help that you have available to manage the cases.

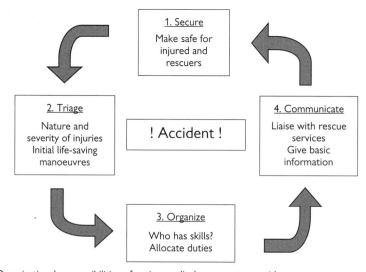

Figure 20.1 Organizational responsibilities of senior medical person at an accident.

Triage

Triage is the process of deciding the priority for managing patient so that the best use can be made of limited resources. The simplest system divides cases into three types (Box 20.1).

Obviously there are simple measures, which can and should be taken as you assess a casualty for triage status (such as moving them into the recovery position to maintain airway) but the essence of good triage is speed (see Fig. 20.1).

Communication

The more information that the rescue services can be given about the nature of the incident the more likely they will be to arrive with the correct number of people and equipment needed to handle the situation quickly and efficiently (Box 20.2).

> Box 20.1 **Principles of triage**
>
> **1** Beyond hope in the current situation
> **2** Can be saved if immediate and simple treatment is undertaken
> **3** Not suffering from any life threatening condition so can wait until other more urgent cases have been treated

> Box 20.2 **Basic information for rescue services**
>
> **1** Time of the incident, e.g. 09.50 or 20 minutes ago
> **2** Nature of the incident, e.g. lorry rolled over into ditch
> **3** Estimated number of casualties, e.g. two
> **4** Severity of injuries, e.g. both are conscious but are trapped in the cab
> **5** Any special features about the site or accident, e.g. there is water in the bottom of the ditch which makes access difficult

Handover

When patients arrive at a definitive care centre such as an Emergency Department, it is always valuable for the whole team to listen carefully to the handover from the rescue services, who are delivering the patient (Box 20.3).

In patients where extrication has been difficult and attendance at hospital has been delayed, it is actually less likely that there will be anything catastrophically wrong, as the patient has already survived some time without full resuscitation. However, those patients whose presentation is delayed suffer other problems. They may have become hypothermic, and an unnoticed trickle of blood loss may have continued long enough to produce hypovolaemic shock.

> Box 20.3 **Critical information at handover of a patient to emergency department staff**
>
> **1** Time since the accident
> **2** Amount of energy involved in the accident
> **3** Any treatment given during transport especially analgesia, and
> **4** Any changes in the conscious state or other vital signs of the patient

Initial assessment and primary resuscitation

The system used for this is based on the Advanced Trauma Life Support (ATLS®) courses which have provided a common language as well as a logical system for individual resuscitation (Box 20.4)

> Box 20.4 **<C>ABC**
>
> • <C> = Catastrophic haemorrhage
> • A = Airway with cervical spine control
> • B = Breathing with oxygen
> • C = Circulation

Catastrophic haemorrhage

In major disasters involving such things as terrorist activity '<C>' has been added before the 'A' for Airway, because if there is catastrophic (<C>) external haemorrhage from blast or gunshot wound, control of this bleeding may need to take priority over everything else.

Airway, breathing, and circulation (ABC)

Airway, breathing, circulation, and mental state can be assessed quickly by greeting the patient and asking their name. If the patient is able to reply then the airway is clear (because the patient can speak). Breathing is under control for the same reason. Finally, circulation is adequate because the brain is well enough perfused for the patient to answer a question. An added bonus is that an initial measurement of mental state has also been performed and can be recorded using the AVPU system (Box 20.5).

If the patient cannot or does not respond to being asked their name, then a quick check needs to be made of whether the patient is cyanosed. If they are, then the first problem is likely to be in the airway or breathing.

Box 20.5 The APVU system

- A = Alert and orientated
- V = responding to Verbal commands
- P = responding only to Painful stimuli
- U = Unresponsive

Airway

The mouth is opened and cleared of debris with a finger sweep or better still using a Yankauer sucker. At the same time, you are listening for any sound that air is passing down into the lungs, and if so, whether it is passing freely or the airway is partially obstructed. If the tongue is falling back and occluding the pharynx then a chin lift or jaw thrust will give temporary relief. Guedel oropharyngeal airway can be slipped in over the tongue or a nasopharyngeal airway passed via the nose to release you for other work. If an oxygen mask is already in place then misting of the mask will indicate that the air is passing in and out of the lungs. If it is not possible to clear the airway then endotracheal intubation is needed immediately (a crash induction). If that is not immediately successful then a needle cricothyroidotomy will be needed to buy time before a tracheostomy is performed.

Breathing

The patient should now be given 100% oxygen at 15L per minute via a 100% mask, while a check of breathing is carried out. During the transition from airway to breathing, a quick check of the neck should be performed to make sure that there is no sinister pathology there (Box 20.6).

If the patient is not breathing at all, and making no effort to do so either, then the patient needs to be ventilated manually with an Ambu bag and will need endotracheal intubation as soon as this is feasible. This will make ventilation much easier. In all patients, a pulse oximeter should be applied as soon as possible.

Box 20.6 Check of the neck for sinister pathology

- Deviation of the trachea (may be caused by tension pneumothorax)
- Surgical emphysema (broken ribs with leakage of air into tissues)
- Penetrating wounds damaging critical structures
- Distended neck veins (raised intrathoracic pressure)

Ventilation rate

The whole chest should now be exposed at this stage. The respiratory rate should be measured and recorded. An abnormal respiratory rate (too fast or too slow) is a sensitive indicator of underlying serious problems, and a change in respiratory rate an important indicator as to whether the condition of the patient is improving or deteriorating.

Chest symmetry

Next a check needs to be made whether both sides of the chest are expanding equally. A cyanosed patient with respiratory distress raises the possibility of a tension pneumothorax. If one side of the chest is not moving and is overinflated then the diagnosis is confirmed. A CXR should not be taken as there is no time. This is a surgical emergency. A large-bore needle should be introduced into the 2nd intercostal space midaxillary line to reduce the tension immediately. If the patient improves then the diagnosis was correct, and a chest drain can be introduced later when there is time available.

If several ribs are broken in more than one place there may be a flail segment in the chest wall, which collapses each time the patient tries to draw a breath. This will hinder proper oxygenation of the lungs and may be an indication for endotracheal intubation. The other indications for early intubation are listed in Box 20.7.

Finally a quick, but full examination of the chest needs to be performed checking for penetrating (and bubbling wounds). Breath sounds and percussion note also needs to be checked looking for signs of a pneumo- or a haemothorax. Beware—the back of the chest can be difficult to examine at this stage but is a common site for stab wounds.

Box 20.7 **Indications for endotracheal intubation in trauma**
• Severe facial injuries making it impossible to keep the pharynx open
• Head injury with GCS score <9
• Patient not breathing for themselves
• Flail chest
• Patient violent and cannot be restrained and treated
• Patient going into the scanner at high risk of losing airway

Circulation

Oxygen can only reach the tissues if there is a viable circulation. The patient's pulse and blood pressure should be recorded as soon as possible and then monitored regularly. It is a rise in the pulse accompanied by a fall in blood pressure which warns of deepening shock, although in young fit people the blood pressure does not always drop until shock is well advanced. If a patient has a low blood pressure but is fully conscious then the brain is perfusing adequately. Current thinking is that we should no longer 'chase the numbers' and try to raise the blood pressure with large volumes of intravenous fluids, as this can affect the concentration and activity of clotting factors in the blood. If, however, the blood pressure is so low that perfusion is compromised, mental state will deteriorate and urine output will fall, so both of these should be monitored carefully. Two wide-bore cannulae, one in each antecubital fossa, is optimal. In children intraosseous infusion may be easiest. Blood samples should be taken at the time of cannulation and sent immediately to the laboratory (Box 20.8).

Box 20.8 **Blood samples to be sent to the laboratory in acute trauma**
• Blood for cross-match (amount and type depends on severity of injury)
• Full blood count (provides base line)
• Creatinine and electrolytes (provides base line)
• Liver function tests (provides base line)
• Amylase (to exclude pancreatic damage)
• Glucose (to exclude hypoglycaemia)
• Sample for drug screen (for later analysis if needed)
• Cardiac enzymes (if a pre-existing medical condition is suspected

If the patient's tissue perfusion is compromised (as shown by low urine output or reduced mental state), then 250ml of crystalloid (saline or Hartmann's solution) should be given and the response of the patient monitored. This is called a 'fluid challenge'. If the patient's blood pressure rises and pulse falls and this improvement is sustained then the patient is a 'full responder' and further fluids do not need to be given at this stage. If however the patient improves and then starts to deteriorate again (a transient responder), it is likely that there is continuing haemorrhage and that the source needs to be found (Box 20.9). Blood will need to be given while the search proceeds. If the patient does not respond to the

---

Box 20.9 Sites of severe blood loss

- The chest (haemothorax)
- The abdomen
- The pelvis (associated with pelvic fracture)
- The floor (external bleeding)
- 1L of spilt blood produces a puddle nearly 1 metre in diameter

---

fluid challenge at all (a non-responder) then there is likely to be ongoing catastrophic haemorrhage and immediate preparations need to be made to perform a laparotomy and if necessary a thoracotomy to find and control the source of haemorrhage. In the meantime group O negative blood will be needed to sustain a circulating volume.

As soon as the first ABC has been performed there needs to be a careful review of what has been found and what action needs to be taken. If the situation is highly unstable, then it may be appropriate to repeat the ABC forthwith to assess the direction of any trends, as these may be much more important in guiding treatment than any absolute values (Box 20.10).

Box 20.10 Review of initial assessment

- Re-check ABC
- Review findings and determine patient's trend
- Formulate a plan of initial treatment and further investigation
- Record this in the notes and inform the team

D = Disability

After ABC it is usual to assess mental state as once again. It is changes which may be more informative than an absolute level. The Glasgow Coma Scale (GCS) is the usual scale used (Table 20.1) but most neurosurgeons will now insist that each part of the score is given separately rather than the old system of relying on an aggregate score.

Table 20.1 The Glasgow Coma Scale

	1	2	3	4	5	6
Eyes open	Do not	To pain	To voice	Spontaneous		
Verbalization	None	Incomprehensible	Inappropriate words	Confused	Orientated	
Movements to pain	None	Extension	Flexion	Withdrawal	Localizes	Obeys commands

Minimum score = 3.
Maximum score = 15.
Patients with a GCS <9 may need endotracheal intubation to protect their airway.

E = Exposure

All the patient's clothes must be removed and a careful head-to-toe examination needs performing to locate and document all injuries. This will include log-rolling the patient to check the spine, and a rectal (and vaginal) examination. Patients should not receive a urinary catheter until a check has been made that there is no damage to the integrity of the urethra (by inspection and rectal examination) as otherwise catheterization may make the damage worse. The urinary catheter will allow accurate measurement of urine output. This will be very useful in monitoring tissue perfusion. Be careful at this stage to make sure that the patient stays warm and that their dignity is preserved as much as possible.

Initial imaging

Initial imaging may be introduced at any stage after the initial ABC assessment. The three sets of films required are cervical spine, chest, and pelvis.

A **FAST scan** (focused assessment with sonography for trauma) in units with the equipment and the expertise may be valuable in trying to exclude intra-peritoneal bleeding. A check can be made for fluid in the Rutherford–Morison pouch (between the liver and the right kidney), the pouch of Douglas in females and the rectovesical pouch in males. The spleen can also be checked for haemorrhage, and finally the heart can be viewed to exclude pericardial tamponade. The FAST scan is not especially sensitive (it sometimes misses pathology) but is highly specific (reliable if positive).

High-speed multislice **CT scanners** are revolutionizing the early assessment of polytraumatized patients. Intracranial and cervical spine injury can be rapidly excluded, while scans of the thorax, abdomen, and pelvis are also highly sensitive and specific.

Secondary survey

The secondary survey must not be rushed as any injury missed at this time may not be discovered until it is too late to repair the damage done.

The head (see Box 20.11)

> Box 20.11 **Secondary survey of the head**
>
> - Inspect the scalp, ears, and nose for blood
> - Palpate the scalp for boggy swelling or indentations
> - Check the eyes for subconjunctival haemorrhage and its posterior border
> - Check facial bones and mandible for stability

The neck

If the cervical spine is tender to palpation or the patient has any neurological deficit in the upper limbs, then a CT scan is the only way to reliably exclude an unstable fracture or dislocation. The same applies if the patient's conscious state is so poor that they cannot cooperate in a full physical and neurological examination.

The back

At the time of the log-roll a careful visual inspection is made of the back of the chest, the loins, and the pelvis to check for bruising and penetrating wounds. The spine is palpated for tenderness. This is also the appropriate time to perform a rectal examination. A urinary catheter should only be inserted after a rectal exam has excluded urethral damage.

The abdomen

The healthy abdomen moves freely with respiration. If the patient is conscious a check needs to be made for tenderness in all four quadrants as well as in the loins. The absence of bowel sounds may indicate free fluid (blood or bowel contents) in the peritoneum.

The pelvis

A fractured pelvis is a potent cause of bleeding. Blood at the urethral meatus suggests damage to the urethra.

The limbs

The limbs and digits should be palpated from end to end and each joint carefully put through a full range of movement, checking for penetrating wounds, fractures, and dislocations. Finally a check needs to be made that there is adequate circulation (pulses and capillary filling) and that nerves are intact, testing sensation and motor power.

Record findings

The time and actions in the primary and secondary survey should be laid out with any further actions taken. A preliminary care plan should now be drawn up, listing injuries and prioritizing their treatment. Where possible all events should have a time written against them (Box 20.12).

Box 20.12 Secondary survey

- Clear the cervical spine using CT if necessary
- Log-roll to check the back for wounds and fractures
- Repeat examination of the chest
- Check the abdomen and pelvis including rectal and vaginal examination
- Closely inspect all joints checking distal neurovascular status
- Review all imaging
- Record in notes

The management of wounds

The principles of the management of wounds revolves around the questions:

1 What anatomical structures are in the vicinity which might be affected?
2 How much energy was involved?
3 Is there any possibility of contamination?

The energy involved determines how wide the track of damage is likely to be. High-velocity injuries create a spindle-shaped area of damage around their path which greatly extends the damage which they can cause (Box 20.13).

Contamination is a critical factor in the treatment and outcome of a wound. If a wound is potentially contaminated then it must be cleaned as soon as possible if contamination is not to develop into infection. Antibiotics may be an adjunct but are **never** a substitute for good wound cleaning. This is especially important with fractures. Once infection has become established in bone (osteomyelitis), it is well-nigh impossible to eradicate. Chronic osteomyelitis will be the likely result. Wounds that may be contaminated must not be closed as otherwise the presence of contaminated haematoma and even dead tissue creates the perfect environment for the growth and then spread of infection. This is especially true of the deadly infection *Clostridium perfringens* (gas gangrene). Patients with wounds must also have their tetanus prophylaxis status checked. If it is not certain that a wound is clean after vigorous initial cleaning then it should be left open, packed, and reviewed after 24–48 hours. If it is then found to be clean it can be closed, but if there is still doubt after further cleaning then it should be packed and reviewed again. This is called delayed primary closure (DPC).

Box 20.13 Management of wounds

- Assess wounds by site, energy, and contamination
- Check for nerve, vessel, tendon, and bone injury
- Take a photograph to avoid repeated exposure
- Explore and clean contaminated wounds within hours
- Antibiotics are no substitute for proper debridement
- Do not close contaminated wounds
- Wounds must be covered

Cover

Photographs should be taken as soon as possible to avoid the risk of contamination from repeated inspections, then the wound needs to be kept covered.

Pain

Pain relief should be strong enough to relieve the pain, and repeated frequently enough to prevent the pain from returning. It is much best to start with a small dose of a strong analgesic, such as morphine, and quickly titrate the dose until the pain is removed.

Prophylactic antibiotics and thromboprophylaxis

If wounds are contaminated then prophylactic antibiotics may help during the cleaning of the wounds by delaying the conversion of contamination to infection. Polytrauma cases are at risk of thrombosis and so thromboprophylaxis should be considered, certainly after the initial trauma has settled, and the risk of further bleeding has reduced (Box 20.14).

Box 20.14 Initial management of patients with wounds

- Provide adequate pain relief
- Give prophylactic antibiotics
- Consider thromboprophylaxis

Fractures

The energy of the injury, the direction of the forces applied, and the frailty of the patient all give a clue to the likelihood of fracture even before the examination begins and tenderness with or without deformity are found.

The main types of fracture as derived from the history are:

- Traumatic—normal bone, excessive force
- Pathological—weak bone, normal force
- Stress—normal bone, excess repetitions of normal force

Classification by position, shape, and stability

The position of a fracture can then be described in simple terms, see Table 20.2.

Table 20.2 Fracture description according to position

Site	Shape	Situation	Special
Diaphyseal (shaft)	Transverse	Displaced	Intra-articular
Metaphyseal	Oblique/spiral	Undisplaced	Open/closed
Epiphyseal	Comminuted	Impacted	Involving the epiphyseal plate

Management of fractures

The principles of the management of a fracture are:

- Clean and cover
- Reduce
- Hold

All wounds near to a fracture must be explored as soon as possible to determine whether the wound extends down to the fracture site. If it does then the track and fracture must be laid open, dead tissue removed, and the wound washed out vigorously.

Fractures which are displaced usually need reduction. This is especially true of fractures which extend into a joint, as failure to obtain a good reduction will lead to post-traumatic arthritis in a joint. If there is a step of >2mm. then this is felt to be inevitable.

Once reduction has been achieved then the fracture needs to be prevented from re-displacing. If the fixation is absolutely rigid then normal bone healing is delayed as there is no stimulus for callus formation, but the patient may be able to mobilize normally, provided that the fixation is strong enough. The advantages to soft tissue healing of early mobilization (reducing stiffness and swelling) and psychologically (the patient is able to return to a normal life) usually far outweigh the problem of delayed bone healing, especially if the fixation is strong enough to allow near full activity. Nevertheless, fracture healing will inevitably become a race against time, as repetitive loading on the fixation device starts weakening it through fatigue. If the bone healing is excessively delayed then that fixation will break, and need replacing (Box 20.15).

Box 20.15 **Management of fractures**

- Explore and clean open fractures
- Reduce displaced fractures especially if intra-articular
- Hold the fracture with appropriate fixation
- Provide pain relief

Checking distal neurovascular status

Before starting reduction of a fracture, a final check should be made of the distal neurovascular status, and this should then be recorded in the notes.

Reduction of fracture—closed

Closed reduction is most easily performed if careful thought is given to the direction and nature of the deforming force that caused the fracture in the first place. If the fracture is impacted (they usually are) then this impaction will need to be released by distraction before any correction of position can be obtained (Fig 20.2A)

Anatomical reduction of a closed fracture can be obtained by making use of the periosteum, which is likely still to be intact on the concave side of the fracture. It is important not to damage this intact area as it is providing some of the blood supply to the fracture and will act as a guide to obtaining good reduction. Therefore, as soon as the fracture is felt to have disimpacted, the fracture is angulated sharply in the direction, which *increases* the deformity (Fig. 20.2B). This hinges the fracture on the intact periosteum and allows the jagged ends of the fracture to be opened enough to move across each other to correct

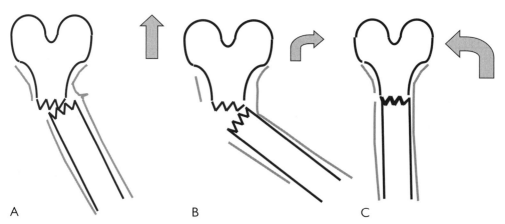

A   B   C

Figure 20.2 A) Fracture reduction. Impacted angulated fracture. Periosteum buckled on concave side, torn on convex side. B) Fracture disimpacted by overangulation and distraction until the cortices on the concave side can be hooked back into position. C) Correction of distortion using intact periosteum to act as a fulcrum, and as a 'stop' to over-reduction.

any displacement. The intact periosteum should prevent any overcorrection, and so once displacement has been corrected the fracture angulation can be returned to normal and then overcorrected in the opposite direction (Fig. 20.2C). The fracture ends should now engage with each other hinging down on the intact periosteum (Box 20.16). So long as the limb is now held with the fracture slightly overcorrected it should not be possible for the fracture to slip out of position again, as the intact periosteum is holding the fragments tight together.

A fracture does not have to be held to heal. Indeed some slight movement at the fracture site stimulates callus formation and rapid healing. Broken ribs are not held. They move with respiration, and yet they heal very quickly. However, they are very painful while they do so. Nevertheless fractures which are unstable will fall back out of position if they are not held once they have been reduced.

Box 20.16 Stages in the closed reduction of a fracture

- Consider the direction of the forces which caused the fracture
- Disimpact the fragment ends
- Overcorrect the deformity to allow reduction
- Hinge the fracture into reduced position using the intact periosteum as a guide

---

Methods of holding a fracture

Balanced traction

This is a traditional method for holding fractures and once again relies on intact periosteum and soft tissues to align the bone fragments. It is safe but requires a long stay in hospital.

Plaster of Paris

Plaster of Paris (or fibreglass castes) is a simple and cheap way of holding a fracture. However, there are some major dangers which need to be borne in mind. The first is that for the first 24 hours after a fracture a completely circumferential closed plaster should not be used, because if the limb swells inside it, then it will create what is in effect a compartment syndrome. Therefore it is good practice to apply a heavily padded back-slab until the swelling has peaked and then to change this for a closer-fitting complete plaster once the swelling is settling.

External fixators

This system is designed to combine the advantages of 'no major surgery' with the benefits of getting a strong and secure hold on the limb so that a patient can even walk on an unstable fracture. External fixators are especially valuable where there is such extensive soft tissue damage over a fracture that internal fixation cannot be used.

The AO system of plates and screws

The AO system provides a large range of plates and screws designed to hold reduced the vast majority of the most common fractures. It is especially useful for achieving anatomical reduction of intra-articular fractures (such as the ankle), and bones where fixation requires careful contouring of the plates (pelvic fractures). The strength of the fixation allows early mobilization. Its disadvantage is that however careful the surgeon there will inevitably be some disconnection of soft tissue from bone even if periosteal stripping is avoided. This loss of blood supply may compromise bone healing, and if great care is not taken may also introduce infection.

Intra-medullary nails

These nails are very useful for long-bone fractures as they fit inside the bone and provide good strong fixation, which allows early pain-free mobilization. When combined with interlocking screws, they can also control rotation and compression.

Joint replacement

Some fractures unfortunately also cut end arteries and may lead to devascularization of the bone supplied by those arteries. In this case reducing and holding the fracture is unlikely to be of any use, and a
better strategy may be to replace the compromised bone end altogether.

Fusion

Joints which are so badly destroyed by a fracture that they cannot be reconstructed may be best treated
by removing the joint altogether and fusing the two bones together (an arthrodesis). This will at least give
the patient a strong and pain-free limb even if mobility is reduced (Box 20.17).

Box 20.17 Methods of holding a fracture

- Simple sling and analgesia, e.g. midshaft of humerus
- Plaster of Paris, e.g. distal radius fracture in an elderly patient
- Balanced traction, e.g. fractured femur in an infant
- K-wires, e.g. supracondylar fracture of elbow
- AO plates, e.g. intra-articular ankle fracture
- Intramedullary nail, e.g. fracture midshaft femur in an adult
- External fixator, e.g. open fracture of the tibia with soft tissue loss
- Partial or complete joint replacement, e.g. subcapital fractured neck of femur
- Fusion, e.g. intra-articular complex fracture of the wrist

Compartment syndrome

This is a specific and very dangerous soft tissue injury which may accompany a bone fracture but can
occur without fracture following a soft tissue crush injury. It is a surgical emergency. Compartment syndrome occurs because some muscles in the body are contained within fascial sheaths, a compartment
which is effectively unable to expand in response to a rise in pressure. If one of these compartments fills
with haematoma or with fluid, veins which drain the compartment are forced shut by a rise in the pressure
in the compartment around them. From that moment on, blood can enter the muscle compartment
through the high-pressure thick-walled arteries but cannot easily leave because the veins have collapsed.
The pressure therefore continues to rise to mean arterial pressure when all circulation in that compartment ceases. There is intense pain and if something is not done within hours the muscle will become
ischaemic and then necrose. It is important to note that the distal pulses may still be present, as the thick-
walled artery continues to pump blood through the compartment even when the perfusion of the muscles around has effectively ceased. The commonly affected muscle compartments are the calf, the forearm
and the intrinsic muscles of the hand and foot. Diagnosis is on clinical suspicion (a crush injury or a fracture haematoma draining into a compartment) and is confirmed by the presence of intense pain on passive stretching of the muscles in the affected compartment. Compartment pressure studies are difficult to
perform and do not give reliable results, but may need to be performed in the unconscious patient.

The treatment is to remove any dressing or plaster which might be constricting circulation and if there
is not an immediate improvement in the patient's condition, a fasciotomy must be performed. This
operation involves laying open the fascia of all the potentially affected compartments from end to end,
and then leaving the wound open until the swelling has started to go down.

Nerve injuries

Nerves can be damaged in acute trauma or be subject to chronic compression where they travel through
bony or ligament walled tunnels, e.g. carpal tunnel syndrome. Many fractures and dislocation are classically associated with nerve injuries (Table 20.3).

Classification

- **Neuropraxia** is the most minor injury. The nerve is stretched or crushed but remains in continuity.
  Recovery of full function can be expected within hours or days

Table 20.3 Nerve injuries associated with common fractures and dislocations

Injury	Associated nerve damage
Cervical and thoracic spine fracture/dislocation	Spinal cord
Scapulothoracic dissociation	Brachial plexus injury
Anterior dislocation of the shoulder	Axillary nerve neuropraxia
Spiral fracture of the humerus	Radial nerve
Elbow fractures	Ulnar nerve
Distal radius	Median nerve in carpal tunnel
Posterior dislocation of the hip	Sciatic nerve
Fracture of the upper fibula	Common peroneal nerve

- **Axonotmesis** is a more severe injury. The myelin nerve sheath remains intact but a proportion of the axons are disrupted. In this case the axons distal to the damage will die (Wallerian degeneration) and then new axons will sprout from the damaged proximal ends. These axons will travel down the old sheaths left by the Schwann cells at about 1–2mm/day. Recovery should be good but may take many weeks depending on the site of the injury and the age of the patient
- **Neurotmesis**—in this case the nerve internal structure is disrupted and in the worst case the actual nerve is transacted. If the disrupted ends are not brought together (or a graft used to bridge a defect) then there will be no recovery. Even in the best circumstances recovery may only be partial as axons enter the wrong myelin sheath and so do not make the correct connection (Box 20.18)

Box 20.18 Classification of nerve injuries

- Neuropraxia: structure intact—recovery in hours or days
- Axonotmesis: myelin sheath intact—recovery slow but good
- Neurotmesis: complete transection of nerve—needs surgical repair for good recovery

---

Head injuries

The initial assessment of head injuries is described in the initial management of trauma earlier in this chapter. A limb can recover after a period of ischaemia lasting over an hour, but only a few minutes of ischaemia will permanently damage the brain. The situation is further complicated by the fact that the brain is enclosed in the skull, a rigid box. Any significant swelling of the brain following injury will result in a disproportionate rise in intracranial pressure. This can both compromise the blood supply to the brain tissue and force the brain stem down into the narrowing funnel of space in the upper cervical spine, fatally compressing it. This is called 'coning'. The key to the optimal management of a brain injury is to maintain circulation and oxygenation to the brain. This will best be achieved by ensuring that

- Ventilation (airway and breathing) is adequate to maintain normal blood gases
- Blood pressure (circulation) is adequate for good tissue perfusion
- Intracranial pressure remains within physiological limits

The patient's state of consciousness is an important monitor of progress so the measurement of the GCS score needs to be repeated at regular intervals. A deterioration in the score is more important than any individual reading, and should trigger an immediate review for reversible causes.

Any intracranial bleed is much commoner in patients who are on anticoagulants, so this must be checked when obtaining a history (Box 20.19).

Extra-dural haemorrhage

The rare but highly treatable cause of brain compression is the extra-dural haemorrhage. The initial injury may be relatively trivial but if the blow is to a thin part of the skull such as the temporal bone

---

Box 20.19 Basic principles for management of head injuries

- Good oxygenation
- Adequate perfusion
- Maintain intracranial pressure at physiological levels
- Monitor for change in conscious state

---

where the middle meningeal artery runs across its inner surface, a fracture may damage the artery causing intracranial bleeding. The initial period of unconsciousness (concussion) may be short and followed by a period of recovery (the lucid interval). As the volume of blood leaking into the extra-dural space increases, the intracranial pressure starts to rise, the patient's conscious level will now deteriorate. The initial signs of brain compression may be one-sided with dilatation of the ipsilateral pupil combined with contralateral spastic weakness, but later signs become bilateral and then death commonly results from coning.

The key to treatment is early recognition of the possibility of an extra-dural. A CT or better still MRI scan will localize the haemorrhage and guide the surgeon to the best site for burr holes. These need to be performed as quickly as possible. Once the pressure has been released a cranial flap can be raised to identify and control the bleeding vessel.

Spinal injuries

Spinal injuries are uncommon but important both because the consequences are severe and because there is much which can be done to minimize permanent damage. If there is evidence of neurological damage immediately after the accident this may be temporary (spinal shock) or permanent, or a mixture of the two. At first it may be very difficult to distinguish the two types of damage, but any sign of sacral sparing (preservation of sensation and motor power in the perineal area) suggests that there may be an element of spinal shock and that further improvement can be expected as the effects of the shock wear off over the next few days. If the neurological damage is permanent then after some days the spinal shock wears off (flaccid paralysis) and is replaced by spasticity of the affected muscles. This change from flaccid to spastic paralysis may raise false hopes that control is returning when actually the opposite is the case.

The patient will need early catheterization under as sterile conditions as possible (to reduce the chance of introducing infection). Arrangements will also need to be made to arrange safe and regular turning of the patient to prevent pressure sores from developing. Spinal shock with loss of sympathetic tone will mean that fluid resuscitation will need to be performed with great care to avoid fluid overloading (Box 20.20).

Box 20.20 Management of spinal injuries

- Assess stability of fracture pattern
- Plot neurological level checking for sacral sparing
- Turn regularly to avoid bed sores
- Catheterize under sterile conditions
- Beware fluid overload

Chest trauma

Chest trauma can be divided into sharp or blunt.

Sharp or penetrating injuries

These may cause a pneumo- or haemothorax, injure the spinal cord, the heart or major vessels, or damage the mediastinum including the oesophagus. All these structures need considering when planning imaging.

Blunt trauma

This may break ribs, and damage the lungs either by creating a pneumothorax or damaging lung function by creating large volumes of contused lung, which is useless for gas exchange. If the patient is not able to maintain their blood gases, then a flail chest may need stabilizing, painful broken ribs may need a nerve block, and the patient may need ventilating.

Abdominal trauma

Abdominal trauma can also be divided into blunt and sharp. As a general rule sharp injuries need exploration, as perforation of bowel will lead to peritonitis. It is much easier to clean out contamination early than manage full-blown peritonitis later. A full laparotomy will be needed through an extensile incision and the bowel should be inspected from end to end searching for holes and necrotic segments.

Blunt trauma may rupture the liver, spleen, or diaphragm, or tear bowel from its mesentery (especially at the duodeno-jejunal junction). If staff skilled in the use of FAST scan are not available then a CT scan is very valuable in diagnosing free fluid in the peritoneum. Oral contrast or rectal contrast may help in the diagnosis of torn bowel. Splenectomy and even partial hepatectomy may be indicated if repair of these organs is impossible. Diaphragmatic rupture will need repair while avascular bowel may need resection. The decision whether to bring out a defunctioning colostomy should be based on a) the level of the repair, b) the damage done to bowel and blood supply by the original injury, c) the delay between injury and repair, and d) the experience of the surgical team.

Abdominal compartment syndrome (ACS) occurs when the contents of the bowel expand so much that the elasticity of the abdominal wall is no longer able to accommodate the bowel without a rise in pressure. If this occurs, the blood supply to the bowel may be compromised. If a patient is at risk of developing ACS, the bowel should be left open at the end of the laparotomy and covered with sterile drapes until such time as closure without compression can be achieved (Box 20.21).

Box 20.21 Management of abdominal trauma

- FAST scans help determine the presence of fluid/blood in the peritoneal cavity
- CT scans have even better sensitivity
- The whole of the bowel needs careful checking for leaks and vascular damage
- Abdominal compartment syndrome is treated by leaving the abdomen open

---

Imaging in trauma

If a fracture or dislocation is suspected in extremity trauma, then it is normal to ask for X-rays of the affected area. A minimum of two films are needed taken at as near to a right angle to each other as possible. In polytrauma a basic set of films is always taken of a) the cervical spine, b) the chest, and c) the pelvis as these are critical areas where injury needs to be identified early.

CT scanning is becoming faster and safer and more accurate in defining the severity of a fracture. It also allows three-dimensional reconstructions to be performed. This will help in planning surgery, in terms of surgical approach and placement of fixation. This is especially valuable in intra-articular, pelvic, and spinal fractures, but is also crucial in identifying intracranial, thoracic abdominal injuries

---

Box 20.22 Imaging in trauma

- Two-plane X-rays remain the bedrock of trauma imaging
- CT scanning is becoming increasingly central to the assessment of a polytraumatized patient
- MRI carries risks because of access to the patient during scanning
- US is valuable for initial assessment of the abdomen and for checking for vascular integrity

---

MRI is valuable in diagnosis of soft tissue injuries especially if they are not accessible to US. This is especially the case for spinal cord and intracranial lesions. However, the acquisition time makes this investigation risky for a patient who is anaesthetically unstable so should be used with care.

US is becoming increasingly useful for both diagnosing intra-abdominal bleeding (see above) and in diagnosing soft tissue injuries such as rupture of tendons or tearing of ligaments. It is also valuable for checking whether the circulation to a limb is intact using Doppler (Box 20.22).

Scenarios

Scenario 1

Written scenario outside the OSCE station.

You are driving along a motorway when a large lorry ahead of you is hit by a gust of wind and tips over the central reservation and collides with a fully loaded coach on the other carriageway. You manage to stop on the hard shoulder without collision.

Question Describe what you would do initially.

Scenario 2

Written scenario outside the OSCE station.

A rugby player is brought into the Emergency Department by his colleagues having suffered a knock-out during a game that afternoon. He apparently recovered, but then collapsed in the bar of the club-house some hours later. His colleagues bundled him into a car and have carried him into the Emergency Department.

Question Demonstrate your management.

Scenario 3

Written scenario outside the OSCE station.

A patient of around 40 years is brought into the resuscitation room having been found by the police collapsed in the street. As the police arrived two men were seen running away. He was brought in by ambulance. His cervical spine is protected and he is on oxygen. His airway is now fine since a Guedel airway was put in. There are no wounds visible on his neck or his chest. His respiration rate is 40, and he looks blue despite receiving 100% oxygen at 15L per minute. The pulse oximeter records a saturation of 90%. He has wide-bore cannulae in both antecubital fossa and has Hartmann's solution running slowly. A full set of bloods have been sent. His blood pressure is 110/70 and pulse 120. He is grunting incomprehensible words between breaths.

Question What is the likely diagnosis? Demonstrate your examination and management.

Scenario 4

Written scenario outside the OSCE station.

A 16-year-old has fallen 3 metres off a wall. He has come into the emergency department conscious but in shock. His blood pressure is 100/60, pulse 120, and he complains of abdominal pain. The airway and breathing are OK and the cervical spine is stabilized. Two wide-bore cannulae have been inserted, and bloods sent. He weighs approximately 60kg, and so in view of his shocked state, you decide to give a fluid challenge of 1200ml of Hartmann's. His blood pressure rises to 120/60 and pulse falls to 90, but within 10 minutes the situation of low blood pressure and raised pulse has returned.

Question What is the likely diagnosis? Demonstrate your examination to confirm this.

Scenario 5

Written scenario outside the OSCE station.

A 16-year-old girl is brought in after a fall from a horse. She was wearing a helmet but appears to have struck the side of her head on a fence post as she fell. Initially she was unconscious and unrousable but after 10 minutes recovered consciousness and was able to walk back to the stables with assistance. However, an hour later she lapsed back into coma, and has been brought in by ambulance. Her cervical spine has been immobilized and her airway is protected with a Guedel tube. Her breathing rate is 25, and she is not cyanosed. Chest examination is grossly normal. She has had bloods taken and two wide-bore cannulae inserted. Fluids are not being run in. Pulse is 50 and blood pressure 160/100. She responds to pain but not to verbal commands.

Question What is the likely diagnosis? Demonstrate your examination to confirm this and describe your management plan

Scenario 6

Written scenario outside the OSCE station.

A 20-year-old motorcyclist is brought in following a high-speed crash. He has had initial resuscitation and you have completed your primary survey. He is fully alert. He has had his initial X-rays.

Question Demonstrate your secondary survey on this model please.

Scenario 7

Written scenario outside the OSCE station.

A patient has been brought in to the resuscitation room following a bee sting on his lip. He is known to be allergic to bee-stings and has been brought in by ambulance with increasing difficulty breathing. The patient is on oxygen and has been given adrenaline to no avail. He has two wide-bore cannulae in place. The anaesthetist has attempted endotracheal intubation and failed. The patient's airway is now effectively completely obstructed, although he is still making a respiratory effort.

Question Demonstrate your next actions on the simulation model.

Scenario 8

Written scenario outside the OSCE station.

A joy rider is brought in following a car chase having rolled over and been ejected from the car. He is stable on ABC and after the secondary survey but has some fractured ribs, a closed mid-shaft fracture of the left femur, a degloving with an exposed oblique fracture of the right tibia. He also has a crush fracture of L5 with no neurological deficit, displaced transverse fractures of the midshafts of the radius and ulna on the right, three metatarsals on the left foot.

Question Describe and justify your management plan.

Scenario 9

Written scenario outside the OSCE station.

The actor in this station has a Colles' fracture of the right wrist, as shown on this X-ray. It is anaesthetized.

Question Please could you show me how you would reduce that fracture and apply a plaster?

Scenario 10

Written scenario outside the OSCE station.

This young male actor has fallen on his outstretched hand. You have taken a history and performed a quick examination which reveals tenderness at the base of his right dominant thumb. There are no wounds and distal neurovascular status is normal.

Question Please explain your care plan to the actor.

Answers

Scenario 1

NOTIFICATION. Your first responsibility is the same as any member of the public. That is to inform the Emergency Services as quickly as possible of the time, location, and nature of the incident, with any possible extra advice (such as that the motorway looks as if it is going to be blocked in both directions).

SAFETY. Your next responsibility is as a professional, who should expect to take a lead in organizing the situation on the ground until the Emergency Service staff arrive. The priority is safety, so once the Emergency Services have been informed, volunteers need to be found to reverse back up the hard shoulder with their hazard lights on, to give vehicles approaching the accident site warning that they need to stop.

LEADERSHIP. Until the Emergency Services arrive, it will be a real help if someone at the site of the accident takes a leadership role, identifying volunteers, and allocating them to tasks appropriate to their skills. This applies in particular to medical assistance, and you should be ready and able to take this role.

TRIAGE. If you find yourself as the senior doctor on site, your next role is to perform triage, **not** to start treatment. This seems to be a paradox, but at this stage an expert doctor is more valuable 'triaging' all the patients rather than locking on to treating the first casualty that they come across. Obviously as you go from patient to patient performing triage, quick and simple actions, which might save the patient (such as moving them into the recovery position to open the airway) should be undertaken. If no other facilities are available (and that is usually the case) then simply writing the triage code in biro on the patient's forehead will be adequate. Category 1 is patients who are beyond hope in current circumstance. These would be patients who have no pulse, nor any signs of breathing, or who have catastrophic injuries. Category 2 are those in whom simple measures will make a significant difference. These might be patients whose airway needs clearing and protecting, or severe haemorrhage which can be controlled with local pressure or a simple tourniquet. Category 3 are patients whose life is not immediately threatened. These will be those with simple fractures, and the walking wounded. Category 1 patients should be left for the moment, as should category 3. All your resources should be focused on category 2 patients.

TEAM PLAYING. By this time Emergency Services will have arrived, and will take over control of the incident. Your role will be to give them all the information that you have already gathered, and then, if you wish, to offer your services as a doctor on site.

Scenario 2

The key to this case is that ABC has not yet been performed. This case may look like an extra-dural haemorrhage but simple causes of deterioration have not yet been excluded.

This patient should be managed according to the principles of ABC.

A is airway with cervical spine control. The patient's cervical spine should be stabilized with manual in-line immobilization until a cervical collar, sandbags, and tape can be applied. At the same time the mouth should be opened and a finger and/or a Yankauer sucker used to clear any loose teeth, vomitus, blood, or mucus from the oropharynx. Then your cheek should be laid close to the patient's mouth and nose while looking down at the chest. Your cheek will tell you if any air is moving in and out. Your ear will tell you whether the air is moving freely. Your eyes will tell you whether the patient is attempting to breathe. If the airway is compromised, a chin lift or jaw thrust is needed and then replaced by a Guedel airway. The size of the airway needs to be measured against the distance between the front of the incisors and the angle of the jaw. It should be inserted upside down, then rotated into position. If the patient is so deeply comatose that they are apparently not able to protect their airway, then endotracheal intubation will be needed to protect them from inhalation.

B is breathing and oxygen. The patient needs to be given 100% oxygen through a rebreathing bag at 15L per minute. If, however, the patient is not attempting to breath then they will need ventilating through an Ambu bag and face mask, until an endotracheal tube is in place. At this stage the neck needs to be checked for wounds, dilated veins suggestive of raised intrathoracic pressure, or deviation of the trachea. Now the chest needs to be checked. The key life-threatening condition is tension pneumothorax. So, the first thing to do is to go to the bottom of the bed and measure the respiration rate while noting whether the chest expansion is equal on both sides. If one side of the chest appears over expanded and is not moving with respiration then a tension pneumothorax should be suspected. A visual check needs to be made for wounds over the chest especially those which are bubbling or sucking. Then check with a stethoscope for air entry in both apices and bases. A pneumo- or a haemothorax will have reduced breath sounds. Percussion note will be bright over a pneumothorax and dull over a haemothorax or collapsed lung. By this time a pulse oximeter should be in place and the patient can be checked for signs of cyanosis as well as checking the reading on the pulse oximeter. Before moving on to circulation go back and check the airway quickly. Is the mask fogging up on exhalation, and are the breath sounds quiet not raucous?

C is for circulation. The patient's pulse and blood pressure should already have been taken. Now, a check needs to be made for any signs of external bleeding. One wide-bore cannula needs to be placed in each antecubital fossa, and bloods taken for Full blood count, cross-match, urea and electrolytes, liver function tests, glucose, and drug screen. If the blood pressure is falling and the pulse is rising, then the patient is going into hypovolaemic shock. The source of the bleeding needs to be sought (it is likely to be the chest, the abdomen, the pelvis, or the floor) and brought under control if possible. Meanwhile fluid needs to be given to stabilize the shock and to determine the degree of shock. Current teaching is to give 20ml/kg of crystalloid so that is around 1.5L for a 70-kg man. If the shock stabilizes (blood pressure rises to normal and pulse falls) then no more fluid needs to be given.

A patient in whom this occurs is called a 'responder'. If the blood pressure and pulse improve but then deteriorate, then blood is continuing to be lost, so blood now needs to be given while a search is made for the source of the bleeding. This patient is a 'transient responder'. If the blood pressure and pulse do not improve, the patient is a 'non-responder'. Blood needs to be given at once (O negative or type specific) and the patient needs to be moved immediately to the operating room, ready to attempt to control bleeding with a laparotomy, or thoracotomy as appropriate.

Scenario 3

The key to this question is that tension pneumothorax is likely to be the diagnosis.

Candidate: 'This patient has had ABC performed and there appears to be an acute problem with breathing. The most urgent cause of this will be tension pneumothorax so this needs to be excluded first. However, first I will quickly re-check airway. I am laying my cheek near to his mouth and nose and watching his chest. What do I feel, hear and see?'

Examiner: 'Air is moving and there are no sounds of airway obstruction. The chest is moving but more on the left than the right'

Candidate: 'Airway appears to be OK at the moment so I am moving to the end of the bed to observe the chest. I am looking for over expansion and inequality of movement.'

Examiner: 'The right side of the chest appears over-expanded compared with the left, and as I said before it is moving less.'

Candidate: 'I am now percussing the chest first the apices, and then lower.'

Examiner: 'The right side is hyper-resonant.'

Candidate: 'I am listening for breath sounds first at the apices and then at the bases.'

Examiner 'Breath sounds are fainter on the right.'

Candidate: 'I am now checking the neck, looking for distended veins and for a trachea deviated to the left.'

Examiner: 'The veins do appear distended and the trachea is deviated to the left.'

Candidate: 'I have a probable diagnosis of tension pneumothorax on the right and I am going to decompress this with a wide-bore cannula inserted into the 2nd intercostal space at the midclavicuar line. My fingers are locating the manubriosternal joint (the angle of Louis) and tracing laterally from there. I would now insert the needle into this space aiming to glance over the top of the 3rd rib and angled slightly upwards. What do I hear and what happens to the patient's condition?'

Examiner: 'There is a hiss of air. The patient's condition is improving. Respiration rate is down to 20 and the cyanosis has improved. Saturation is now 98%.'

Candidate: 'I need to tape in the cannula, and note that this patient will need a chest drain once I have completed my primary and secondary surveys. I now need to check the airway again as before.'

Examiner: 'It is OK.'

Candidate: 'Breathing. Expansion, percussion note, air entry and pulse oximeter reading.'

Examiner: 'All normal.'

Candidate: 'Circulation. What is the blood pressure and pulse please?'

Examiner: 'All normal.'

Candidate: 'I now need to go on to Disability and in the first instance I will use the Glasgow Coma Scale. If I ask him, will he speak to me?'

Examiner: 'He is now articulating words but not responding to you appropriately.'

Candidate: 'Will he open his eyes?'

Examiner: 'Yes. When you ask him.'

Candidate: 'I am now squeezing his finger nail. What is his motor response?'

Examiner: 'He is flexor but not coordinated.'

Candidate: 'He scores 3 for eyes. 4 for verbal and 3 for motor, so overall he scores 10. I now need to move to E (exposure), but before I do this I need to check ABC once again.'

Examiner: 'Quite right, but please take that as done and your findings are OK. Now proceed.'

Candidate: 'I want to remove all clothing and start a top of head to tip of toes inspection checking for wounds, bruises, distortion of bone and joints, tenderness and distal circulation. I would then log-roll the patient, check the back for injuries and the spine for tenderness, then perform a rectal examination to check for injuries, anal tone and the position of the prostate.'

Examiner: 'OK. We will stop there thank you.'

Scenario 4

The key to this case is a probable diagnosis of intra-abdominal bleed from either a ruptured spleen or liver.

Examiner: 'This dummy is your patient. Please continue from where the scenario leaves off.'

Candidate: 'First I would check ABC…'

Examiner: 'I quite agree, but please take that as read, and proceed to the next stage, explaining the reasons for your actions'

Candidate: 'This patient is in significant hypovolaemic shock. He has responded to a fluid challenge of 20ml per kg but has quite quickly started to slip back again. He is therefore a 'transient responder'. This suggests that he has lost and is continuing to lose blood from somewhere. Crystalloid is not going to sustain his circulation, so we now need blood, and if it has not already been ordered I would ask for 6 units of blood to be made available as soon as possible. If 'O-neg' blood is not available then I would ask for type specific as we do not have time to wait for a full cross-match. While waiting for that to arrive I would put up 2L of Hartmann's to run over 30 minutes or if there was going to be a significant delay I would give two bags of colloid. I would then start searching for the source of the bleeding. This is likely to be in one of four sites—the chest, the abdomen, the pelvis, or the floor (external). A careful physical examination of the chest (for a haemothorax), the abdomen (for peritonism and dullness), and the pelvis (for instability) should be performed. If a chest X-ray has not already been performed (it is part of the initial assessment) then it should be performed now. If a FAST scanner is available it should be used to check for blood in the pelvis, around the liver and the spleen and in the paracolic gutter. An alternative would be a CT of the trunk to exclude haemothorax, ruptured diaphragm, damage to the liver and or spleen, and bleeding from fracture disrupting the pelvic veins. Finally we need to check that the patient is not bleeding out from a hidden wound or into long-bone fractures. Throughout this stage of investigation, we need to be monitoring the vital signs carefully, titrating the amount of blood given against the conscious state of the patient, blood pressure, pulse, central venous line pressure, and urine output. Once the source of the bleeding has been found it needs to be brought under control. The methods at our disposal are a) pressure and tamponade—this may be the best way to control bleeding from pelvic veins in an open book pelvic fracture, b) interventional radiology to close off bleeding vessels, or c) open surgery to repair or remove bleeding organs (splenectomy), repair or ligate bleeding vessels, or suture up tears in viscera (such as the liver).'

Scenario 5

The key to this case is extra-dural haemorrhage.

Examiner: 'This dummy is your patient. Please continue from where the scenario leaves off.'

Candidate: 'First I would check ABC…'

Examiner: 'I quite agree, but please take that as read, and proceed to the next stage, explaining the reasons for your actions.'

Candidate: 'This patient may have an extra-dural haemorrhage. She has suffered a blow to the head which rendered her unconscious. After a short 'lucid' period she has lapsed back into coma. There appears to be no cause for this in the airway, breathing, and circulation but I have not yet checked the blood sugar, as hypoglycaemia could be a cause for this.'

Examiner: 'I quite agree, but her blood sugar has come back as normal.'

Candidate: 'My first priority is to ensure that the patient is well perfused and well oxygenated. Her blood pressure appears, if anything, to be high. Do we have a pulse oximeter on the patient?'

Examiner: 'Her oxygen saturation is 98%.'

Candidate: 'I now need to examine the head for signs of trauma and to perform a neurological examination to get a base-line Glasgow Coma Scale score and to check the cranial nerves. If I look in the ears and nose, and feel over the skull do I see any signs of bleeding or CSF, and is there any bruising anywhere?'

Examiner: 'There is a soft bruise in the left temporal region.'

Candidate: 'I now need to perform the tests to calculate the Glasgow Coma Scale score. Will she open her eyes to order or to painful stimulus?'

Examiner: 'She opens her eyes to pain.'

Candidate: Right. Well that scores 2. Will she answer questions, or if not is she saying anything?'

Examiner: 'Only incomprehensible sounds.'

Candidate: 'Right. Well that scores 2 too. What movements does she show in response to pain?'

Examiner: 'Withdrawal.'

Candidate: 'Right. Well that scores 4 so her total score is 8. I now need to check her pupils and response to bright light.'

Examiner: 'The left pupil is dilated and responds only minimally to light. The right pupil is normal.'

Candidate: 'That fits with an extra-dural haemorrhage on the left compressing the right oculomotor nerve over the edge of the tentorium. I now need assistance and my actions will depend on the facilities which I have available, as this is a surgical emergency. I need to contact the nearest neurosurgical service, and discuss with them whether they want a CT scan and whether they want the patient transferred to them or whether they will come to the patient. I need to discuss with the anaesthetic team the advisability of endotracheal intubation to allow more careful control of the intracranial pressure with hyperventilation and even mannitol. I need to inform theatres that I may need to perform burr-holes and ask them to make a theatre ready. I also need to arrange for regular neurological observations to determine whether the patient's condition is stable or currently deteriorating as this will decide whether it is safe or wise to perform a CT scan before decompression surgery or not.'

Scenario 6

The key to this scenario is a systematic secondary survey with log-roll.

Candidate: 'First I would check ABC…'

Examiner: 'I quite agree, but please take that as read, and proceed to the next stage, explaining the reasons for your actions'

Candidate: 'I am going to explain to the patient what I am doing and ask him to tell me if he feels any discomfort or pain. I am going to start at the top of the head and look and feel over the scalp for cuts bruises or depressions in the skull. I am going to check in the ears for blood suggesting fractured base of skull. I am looking in the nose for blood and clear fluid which may be CSF. I am checking the sclera of the eyes for haemorrhage especially that which has no posterior margin and which may indicate a fractured base of skull. I am going to look down from above the patient's face to look for any asymmetry suggestive of a zygomatic arch fracture. I am touching the cheek testing for signs of inferior orbital nerve palsy and feeling for tenderness over the zygomatic arch both of which are associated with the same fracture. I am feeling over the mandible from the temporomandibular joint forward checking for steps or tenderness. I am asking the patient to clench his jaw and asking whether he feels that his teeth meet together normally and whether there is pain over the neck of the mandible as either of these suggest a mandible fracture. I now feel with one finger inside the mouth checking for pain or steps and look for loose teeth. I now hold the front incisors and with my other fingers on the bridge of the nose I test for instability of maxilla and signs of a Le Fort fracture 1, 2, or 3. I then take my fingers out of the mouth and check for stability of the nasal bones. To complete my head examination I perform a rapid check of the cranial nerves one by one. Would you like me to do that now?'

Examiner: 'No. Let us take that as read and proceed to the next part.'

Candidate: 'If the cervical spine has not yet been cleared I check for any wounds on the neck then palpate carefully down the spinous processes of the cervical vertebrae asking the patient if any are tender. If not I perform a quick neurological examination of the hands asking the patient to grip my fingers then to spread their fingers wide apart. I am checking for equal and normal power. If this too is normal, then I ask the patient to gently put their neck through a full range of flexion rotation and lateral deviation but to stop at once if they feel pain. I have now completed my neck examination and proceed to the upper limbs. First I test distal neurovascular status checking pulse and sensation to soft touch over the distribution of the radial, median and ulna nerves asking the patient if the two sides feel the same or different. I then check over each limb for signs of bruising or of wounds, then look for swelling and finally for deformity. I then palpate over the soft tissues and bones for tenderness, steps and crepitus. This examination starts at the sternoclavicular joint and works on out to the finger tips. I now repeat the examination of the chest performed during the primary survey but this time I also spring the chest to check for fractured ribs. This completes my chest examination.'

'For the abdomen I first stand at the end of the bed and watch whether the abdomen moves easily with respiration. I then check the skin for wounds and bruising. I check the external genitalia for injuries especially making sure that there is no blood in the external meatus. I then palpate the four quadrants of the abdomen and check for tenderness in the loins balloting the kidneys. I check for bowel sounds and if I am performing a log-roll at this stage for the first time palpate down the spine for tenderness and perform a rectal examination checking visually for injuries and checking anal tone. The pelvis needs to be palpated carefully for steps and tenderness indicative of a fracture.'

'Finally the lower limbs need to be inspected for wounds, bruises and deformity, then palpated for tenderness once the distal neurovascular status has been checked. A careful examination of the knee should be performed checking for effusion, patella dislocation and ligament instability. Any abnormalities need to be recorded and the appropriate investigations to clarify the diagnosis performed.'

Scenario 7

The key to this case is the performance of a needle cricothyroidotomy.

Examiner: 'This dummy is your patient. Please continue from where the scenario leaves off.'

Candidate: 'This patient has a critically obstructed airway, and therefore needs a needle cricothyroidotomy. However he will almost certainly need a tracheostomy after that as this is only a temporary holding procedure so the ENT surgeons need to be called urgently.'

'In the meantime I would like to have a wide-bore cannula, or better still a needle cricothyroidotomy set if available. I am going to extend the patient's neck, and locate the thyroid cartilage (the Adam's apple). I am now going to identify the space between this cartilage and the cricoid cartilage immediately below it, and fixing the thyroid cartilage between my left finger and thumb insert the cannula into the cricothyroid membrane aiming slightly upwards initially then angling downwards once I have entered the trachea. I am then going to remove the steel cannula and connect the cannula directly to a high pressure oxygen line blowing oxygen in for 5 seconds then leaving air to run back out for 10 seconds. I am then going to repeat the injection of oxygen.'

Scenario 8

The key to this case is the open fracture which should now take priority over the other injuries.

Examiner: 'I have here a spare copy of the scenario so that you can remind yourself of the injuries. Would you like to discuss with me your care plan here with your reasons?'

Candidate: 'You have told me that the patient is stable with respect to airway, breathing, and circulation. However, I would like to know the distal neurovascular status of all four limbs please. I would also like to know if the patient is in pain.'

Examiner: 'Good. The sensation and pulses to all four limbs are present and grossly normal. Analgesia has been given and the patient is comfortable.'

Candidate: 'My next priority is therefore the open fracture of the tibia. This needs to be photographed then covered as quickly as possible with sterile saline gauze to minimize the chance of further contamination. This patient needs to go to theatre as soon as feasible to clean this tibial wound before contamination becomes infection. Internal fixation is unlikely to be safe here, so an external fixator might be the best option once I have discussed the case with the plastic surgeons. It may be that in the first instance the wound needs to be packed and left open only undertaking delayed primary closure once the wound is completely clean and all dead tissue has been removed.'

'At this time it would be appropriate to consider a locked intramedullary nail for the femoral fracture. This will enable early weight bearing on this limb. We also need to bear in mind the possibility of a compartment syndrome developing so the limb needs careful observation.'

'The undisplaced metatarsal fractures in the left foot will be most comfortable in a plaster, but this should just be a back-slab initially until the swelling has peaked. Then a below-knee plaster can be applied.'

'The rib fractures require no active treatment. They will heal rapidly, but intercostal nerve blocks will enable the patient to breathe deeply and cough and so reduce the risk of a post-operative chest infection.'

'The crush fracture of L5 is a stable fracture with no neurological deficit. It can therefore simply be managed with analgesia.'

'The forearm fractures are closed and unstable and will be best treated with plates and screws. This will enable anatomical reduction to be obtained and offer the best chance of getting back full pronation and supination.'

'I think that has covered all the fractures.'

Examiner: 'Good. Is there anything else that you need to consider?'

Candidate: 'This patient has had a set of severe injuries and is therefore at risk of pulmonary embolus. Thromboprophylaxis would be advisable. He also has an open fracture so prophylactic antibiotics should be used to cover the initial surgery. He is also at risk of developing SIRS, so he needs careful monitoring and his hydration state and oxygen needs to be monitored carefully.'

Scenario 9

Candidate: 'I would first like to take consent.'

Examiner: 'Good, but please could you assume that this has been done, and that you have introduced yourself to the patient.'

Candidate: 'I would make sure that all my plaster equipment is ready. I need a stockinette bandage, some padding wool, six folds of plaster shaped for a back-slab, a crepe bandage, and some warm water.

Examiner: 'We have all these here ready for you'

'I would then take the arm, and if you (the examiner) could provide counter-traction on the upper arm, pull straight out on the hand until I feel disimpaction of the fragments. When that happens I bend the wrist into 90 degrees of dorsiflexion (i.e. into the direction of the deformity) to unhook the fragments, and then distract while rolling the distal fragment into palmar flexion. I can feel with my finger tips whether the fracture feels reduced, and if it does, I put on the stockinette bandage then wrap the lower arm up to the base of the fingers in padding wool. I then soak my plaster slab in the water and lay it onto the back of the patient's forearm, fixing it in place with a wet crepe bandage. When the plaster has set, I tidy up the patient's arm, take a check X-ray, arrange for analgesia, and an advice sheet about checking circulation and returning if they are worried. Finally I make an appointment for the patient to attend the next fracture clinic so that the plaster can be changed to a complete light-weight fibreglass plaster.'

Scenario 10

Candidate: 'I understand that you are tender at the base of your thumb. One of the possibilities here is that you may have fractured your scaphoid bone. This is a small bone here at the bottom of your thumb. I am going to get some x-rays now but I am afraid that, even if there is a fracture, this does not always show up on X-ray. So, we are going to treat it as if it is fractured whatever the X-ray shows, and put your wrist into a plaster from just below your elbow to the middle joint of the thumb. This will protect the wrist and this bone for the time being. In about 1 week we are going to remove that plaster. If the tenderness has gone we are going to assume that the injury was only a sprain and discharge you from the clinic, but if the scaphoid bone is still tender then we will do some more X-rays. If that confirms a fracture of the scaphoid, then I am afraid that you will be in plaster for 6 weeks while we wait for it to heal. The reason that we are being so cautious is that the scaphoid bone has an odd blood supply which comes into the bone in only one place right here at the distal end. If the scaphoid bone has a break across its middle (the waist), then the blood supply to the fragment at the wrist end is at risk, and that part of the bone may die if we do not look after it carefully. So we keep it carefully guarded while we wait for it to heal and for the blood supply to grow back into the proximal fragment.'

Actor: 'What happens if it does not heal up?'

Candidate: 'There are other options then. One of the things which can be done is to fix the fracture together with a tiny screw, and to put a little bone graft there to stimulate the body to heal it up. But I would emphasize that this is not a common complication, so we just need to cross our bridges as we get to them.'

Chapter 21 Surgical disorders of the skin and subcutaneous tissue

Introduction

The skin is regarded as the largest organ in the human body. In this chapter the basic anatomy and physiology will be described followed by the common surgical skin conditions that surgeons encounter in clinical practice. Finally a description will be given of how to examine and present a skin lesion in the examination.

Basic sciences

Skin anatomy

Human skin is:
- One of the largest organs in the body—1.8m² surface area and consists of approximately 16% of body weight
- Composed of three layers—epidermis, dermis, and hypodermis (subcutaneous layer) (see Fig. 21.1)

Epidermis
- Acts as a protective barrier
- Composed of keratinized stratified squamous epithelium
- Consists of four layers:
  - Basal layer
  - Prickle cell layer
  - Granular cell layer
  - Horny layer
- The functional unit of the epidermis are keratinocytes. Keratinocytes produce keratin which progressively mature through each layer
- The epidermis also contains melanocytes and antigen-presenting Langerhans cells
- The epidermis varies in thickness at different sites, being thickest on the palms and soles

Dermis
- Consists of a dense, highly vascular fibroelastic connective tissue matrix with numerous sensory receptors
- Contains fibroblasts; which synthesize collagen, elastin, and glycosaminoglycans; as well as dendritic cells and other immunocompetent cells
- Epidermal appendages, hair follicles, sweat glands, sebaceous glands, and nails are epithelial structures which extend into the dermis and hypodermis

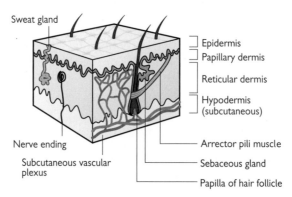

*S. lucidum only present in thick skin of the palm and soles of the feet

Figure 21.1 Skin layers. From *Training in Surgery*, Gardiner and Borley (2009), with permission from Oxford University Press.

Hypodermis

- Hypodermis or subcutaneous layer consists of loose connective tissue and adipose tissue

Langer's lines or cleavage lines are:

- Lines of minimum tension
- Correspond to the alignment of collagen fibres within the dermis and define the direction in which skin is least flexible.
- It differs in different parts of the body but can be identified by manipulating skin to find the natural crease.
- Generally lies perpendicular to the direction of pull of the underlying muscle.
- It was first given detailed attention by the Austrian anatomist Karl Langer in 1861
- Incisions made parallel to Langer's lines tend to heal with a narrower scar producing better cosmesis

Skin physiology

Skin is a metabolically active organ with a number of different functions as listed below:

1 Protection:
  - Physical barrier from entry of microorganisms and particulate matter
  - Against mechanical/chemical or thermal insults
  - Reduces penetration of UV radiation
  - Waterproof
2 Prevents loss of body fluid
3 Sensory organ—for touch, temperature, pain, and pressure
4 Immune surveillance
5 Metabolism:
  - Vitamin D synthesis in the epidermis
  - Energy store in the form of triglycerides in the subcutaneous layer
6 Thermoregulation (discussed in Chapter 5)

Scars—hypertrophic and keloidal

- Scars form as part of normal skin healing when there is damage to the dermis
- Skin is replaced with fibrous tissue and the wound usually regains its strength quickly in the first 7–10 days. This is when non-absorbable sutures would normally be removed
- Over the subsequent months or even years, the scar continues to undergo remodelling before gaining its final strength
- As fibrous tissue and collagen is laid down, it is also continually being digested and these two processes are usually in balance to produce the final shape and size of the scar

Poor healing

- If inadequate scar tissue is laid down or excessive amounts are removed, the wound will not heal well and this can lead to wound dehiscence or incisional hernia formation
- Conversely, if excessive scar tissue or collagen is laid down, the wound may heal with an abnormal scar—hypertrophic or keloid
- Abnormal scars occur more frequently in wounds with increased tension across the edges and consequent misalignment of the collagen fibres.
- Hypertrophic and keloid scars contain collagen nodules and a high density of fibroblasts. Keloid scars also demonstrate increased proliferating fibroblasts and random orientation of collagen fibres which in hypertrophic scars, are orientated parallel to the epidermal surface
- Both types of scars are completely benign

Examine this lesion/scar

Describe scar in terms of site, size, shape and area of tissue loss. If abnormal, state reasons you think it is either a hypertrophic or keloidal scar as below.

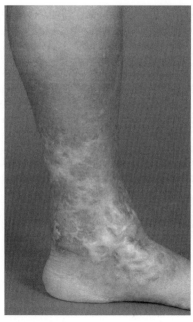

Figure 21.2 Hypertrophic scar after thermal injury (courtesy of Dr. Richard Weller, Royal Infirmary Edinburgh). See also Colour Plate 14.

After examining the lesion—ask patient

- Do they have any other abnormal scars?
- What caused the wound? Were they any problems with healing?
- Is it symptomatic? Have they sought treatment?

Hypertrophic scars (see Fig. 21.2)

- Red, raised fibrous lump and often pruritic in the early phase
- Within the boundaries of the original wound
- Often as a result of large areas of dermal damage—thermal injuries, deep abrasions
- Often arise within 4 weeks and grows intensely for several weeks
- Usually undergoes spontaneous resolution with time (within the first 12 months the appearance of the scar starts to improve)
- Usually asymptomatic—most people seek medical intervention due to cosmetic concerns
- Can occur anywhere on the body and affects all skin types
- More common in patients <30 years, uncommon at the extremes of age

Keloid (see Fig. 21.3)

- Firm, protrubent, smooth skin-covered growths. Usually devoid of hair follicles and skin adnexa
- Extends beyond the boundaries of the original wound
- Often as a result of trauma to skin—surgery, injury, acne, piercings
- May arise immediately following trauma or have a delayed onset
- Grows indefinitely, does not usually regress spontaneously—tends to recurs after excision (>50%)
- Usually asymptomatic—mainly a cosmetic problem, if large may catch on clothing, occasionally pruritic, rarely painful
- Tends to occur on earlobes, face, neck, chest, and shoulders but can occur anywhere
- More common in dark-skinned races, e.g. Afro-Caribbean.
- Familial—possibly a polygenetic inheritance. Often seen in people aged <30 years, rare at the extremes of age

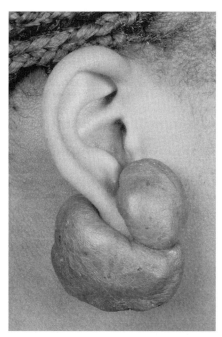

Figure 21.3 Keloid scar. From *Training in Surgery*, Gardiner and Borley (2009), with permission from Oxford University Press.

Treatment of hypertrophic and keloid scars

Currently, no scar can be completely removed. Hypertrophic scars usually regress after 12–24 months and treatment should ideally be considered after this period. Keloid scars rarely regress and are often resistant to treatment. A number of treatment options to minimize these scars are available which include:

- Excision—associated with a high recurrence rate. Outcome better when combined with another treatment, e.g. radiotherapy
- Pressure garments—need to be worn for 18–24 hours for at least 6–12 months. Works best on recent scars
- Intralesional steroid injections—every 4–6 weeks. Needs long-term use
- Silicone sheets and gel
- Laser therapy
- Radiotherapy (typically post-excision surgery)—superficial, low-dose, single use only

Minimization of scar formation

- Use Langer's lines
- 'Hide' along hair lines or in natural skin creases
- Minimal tissue handling—meticulous technique
- Accurate apposition of edges
- Tension free apposition—undermine skin to bring edges together without tension
- Asepsis, if contaminated clean wound well—prevents infection, improves healing
- Use smallest diameter of suture and remove non-absorbable sutures as early as possible—minimizes inflammatory reaction to foreign material, avoids tattooing
- Avoid UV exposure—causes pigmentation in new scars

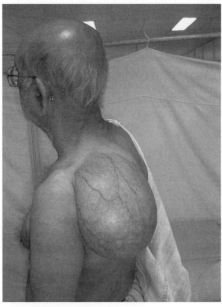

Figure 21.4 Giant lipoma. See also Colour Plate 15.

Benign skin lesions

Lipoma (lipomatous hamartoma) (see Fig. 21.4)

- Affects 1% of the population—commonest soft tissue tumour (hence, commonly seen in exams)
- Composed of mature fat cells which are distended with fat
- Occurs in areas where fat normally occurs—i.e. hamartoma (a focal malformation of disorganized tissue normally found at that site)
- Found anywhere in the body where fat can expand (hence rarely seen on the scalp, palms, or soles of feet). Commonly seen on the trunk, shoulder, thigh, and forearm
- Patients of any age—most commonly adults of 30–60 years. Rare in children
- Typically benign—malignant transformation has not been convincingly demonstrated. (Liposarcomas are a separate entity and do not arise from pre-existing subcutaneous lipomas. Suspect malignant process if rapid growth, firm/scirrhous lump with neovascularization.)

Presentation

Patients usually present with a:

- Smooth, lobulated painless lump. No punctum
- Diffuse margins
- Soft with some fluctuance (due to low density of fat)
- Typically mobile:
  - ◆ Skin moves over it ('slip sign')—lies in the subcutaneous layer
  - ◆ Not attached to deeper structures—becomes more prominent when underlying muscle is contracted (exception would be an intramuscular lipoma which would become less prominent when the specified muscle is contracted and is tethered to the muscle)
- Usually painless and asymptomatic. Occasionally, patients complain of discomfort associated with pressure symptoms, repeated friction with clothes/brastrap, or catching on things. Large lipomas near joints can result in restricted range of movement
- Overlying skin is normal (look for scars—may be recurrent)

- Not pulsatile, not reducible, not compressible, not transilluminable, no fluid thrill
- Often >1 in a patient

Any size—usually 1–3cm in size. However, can grow into large masses of 10–20cm in size and weigh up to 5kg (giant lipomas).

Treatment

- Not necessary—unless painful or restricts movement. Often removed for cosmetic reasons or if there is doubt on the nature of lump (to exclude malignant lumps).
- Usually simple excision—usually linear incision and pressure as lipoma 'pops' out whole and its freed from surrounding tissue
- Liposuction—less scarring. However, it may not remove the entire lipoma, which can lead to re-growth
- Newer methods—no scarring:
  - Injection of compounds which trigger lipolysis
  - Ultrasound waves (similar to lithotripsy for renal calculi)

Recurrence: 1–2%. Especially with deep lipomas as complete excision is not always possible.

Multiple lipoma

- Lipomatosis—hereditary condition, multiple lipoma
- Dercum's disease (adiposis dolorosa)—rare. Generally in obese, postmenopausal women who present with painful lipomas, swelling, weakness, and fatigue

Sebaceous cyst (epidermoid cyst/epidermal cyst/pilar cyst/trichilemmal cyst)

True sebaceous cysts are cysts which:

- Arise from sebaceous glands
- Contain sebum
- Are relatively rare

However, in practice, the term 'sebaceous cyst' is often used to describe:

- Epidermoid cysts—arise from epidermal tissue (common)
- Trichilemmal/pilar cysts—arise from hair follicles (common)

These cysts contain keratinous debris:

- Whitish-yellow cheesy material
- Similar appearance to sebum

Seen on hair-bearing skin:

- Usually scalp, face, neck, trunk, scrotum (not palms/soles of feet)
- 90% of pilar cysts occur on the head and neck

Benign, slow growing—malignant change has been reported but very rare.
All age groups—rare in children.
Sporadic usually (pilar cysts also have an autosomal dominant inheritance pattern).
May be solitary but often multiple.
Usually asymptomatic—may catch on clothes, get caught when combing hair if on scalp.

Presentation

- Smooth, raised dome-shaped lump
- Variable size—from a few millimetres to a few centimetres
- Not tender (unless infected)
- Well-defined edges
- May vary in consistency from soft to firm

- Intradermal—fixed to skin but mobile over underlying structures
- Overlying skin may be normal or may have a punctum—blocked outflow, seen in 50% of epidermal cysts (punctum not seen on pilar cysts)

No specific treatment required. Treat conservatively if patient asymptomatic. May resolve spontaneously. If infected—ask about diabetes, will usually require incision and drainage of pus.
If symptomatic/recurrent infection/cosmetic concerns—excise, usually under local anaesthetic:

- If cyst small, warn patients that scar may be larger than cyst
- Make an elliptical skin incision around cyst, excise entire cyst (preferably intact) with lining
- Recurrence to be expected if lining not completely removed

*Scalp lesions—shave area before starting. Prone to bleeding—use local anaesthetic with adrenaline, have diathermy handy, use mattress suture for haemostasis (as cosmesis usually less important on scalp).
*Gardener's syndrome—variant of familial adenomatosis polposis (FAP). Autosomal dominant condition. Patients have multiple colonic polyps, osteomas and soft tissue tumours (epidermoid cysts, fibromas, desmoids tumours).
*Cock's peculiar tumour—proliferating trichilemmal cysts which are clinically and histologically similar to squamous cell carcinomas (SCCs).

Dermoid cyst (see Fig. 21.5)

Dermoid cysts are cysts lined by skin (stratified squamous epithelium) and contain skin adnexa but are found in the subcutaneous tissue deep to skin. Dermoid cysts are true hamartomas.
They may be congenital or acquired:

- Congenital dermoid cysts are developmental inclusion cysts usually found along embryonic lines of fusion of dermatomes. Often found on the head and neck—medial and lateral edge of eye, floor of the mouth, and midline of forehead, nose, or neck. Less commonly found on the trunk, typically in the midline
  - ◆ Midline cysts may have a deep extension which penetrates through bone and the meninges to communicate with cerebrospinal fluid. Hence, appropriate assessment and imaging of midline cysts may be required
- Acquired dermoid cysts are forced implantation cysts of skin into the subcutaneous tissue as a result of trauma. There may be an overlying scar. Often seen in areas subject to repeated trauma, e.g. fingers

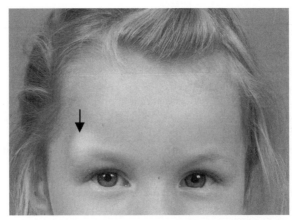

Figure 21.5 Dermoid cyst. From *Training in Surgery*, Gardiner and Borley (2009), with permission from Oxford University Press.

Presentation

- Usually asymptomatic. Rarely gets infected
- Smooth, spherical swelling usually around 1–4cm in size
- Soft, non-tender, may be fluctuant or rubbery
- Almost always benign. Carcinomatous change rare

Treatment

- May be left alone or excised if troublesome. Midline cysts should be appropriately imaged pre-operatively to establish deeper extension
- Cysts may recur if not completely excised

Dermatofibroma/fibrous histiocytoma

Benign neoplasm of dermal fibroblasts—probably secondary to an abortive immunoreactive process (previously thought to be secondary to minor trauma, e.g. insect bites but this theory has now fallen out of favour).

Cutaneous lesions (rarely, may involve deep soft tissue)—may occur anywhere, most commonly on the lower limbs of young and middle-aged females.

Arises within skin and hence is inseparable from skin and freely mobile over deeper structures.

Presentation

Patients usually present with:

- Non-tender pink to brown pigmented nodule, usually solitary
- Well-circumscribed, smooth hemispherical lesion
- Characteristically woody (firm) to palpate
- Usually asymptomatic, does not usually progress nor resolve spontaneously

Treatment

Treatment is not necessary. If cosmetic concern or diagnostic ambiguity, offer excision and histology.

Neurofibromatosis (NF)

Skin and subcutaneous manifestations (see Fig. 21.6)

NF is an inherited disorder (autosomal dominant or primary mutation, variable expression) which results in tumours of neural and fibrous elements. There are two distinct forms of NF:

- NF1 (von Recklinghausen's disease)—gene defect on chromosome 17
- NF2—gene defect on chromosome 22, rarer form, bilateral vestibular schwannomas, benign central neural tumours, fewer cutaneous manifestations than NF1

Associated cutaneous manifestations

- **Neurofibroma**—cutaneous (within the skin layer or pedunculated on skin) or subcutaneous neurofibroma are non-tender, usually multiple, fleshy, well-circumscribed, nodules of varying size. If attached to a nerve trunk, these lesions may be tender and cause paraesthesiae in the distribution of the relevant nerve. Neurofibromas are benign but have malignant potential with sarcomatous change (5% of NF1)
- **Plexiform neurofibroma**—rare (only seen in NF1), diffuse enlargement of neural tissue within the subcutaneous tissue resulting in severe deformity, often involves overlying skin
- **Café-au-lait patches**—light brown macules (≥6 lesions of at least 1.5cm in an adult—among the diagnostic criteria for NF1). If you see one, ask patient to point out others
- **Axillary/inguinal freckling**

Other associations—acoustic neuroma (deafness), gliomas, meningiomas, Lisch nodules, hypertension, learning difficulties, osseous lesions, GI lesions which may bleed or obstruct.

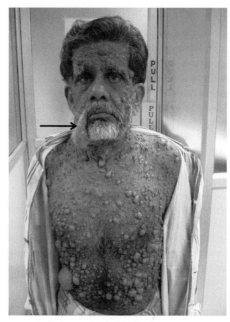

Figure 21.6 Cutaneous, subcutaneous, and plexiform (as marked with arrow) neurofibromata. See also Colour Plate 16.

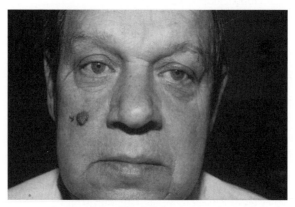

Figure 21.7 Seborrhoeic keratosis. See also Colour Plate 17.

Management is largely conservative. Excision should be considered if lesions restrict movement, have pressure effects on adjacent structures or malignant change is suspected.

Seborrhoeic keratosis (basal cell papilloma) (see Fig. 21.7)

Benign tumour of the basal cells of the epidermis characterized by hyperkeratosis, hyperpigmentation, and acanthosis (proliferation of the prickle cell layer). It is a very common lesion, usually seen in individuals >40 years and its frequency increases with age (very common in over-70s especially in areas which are inaccessible and rarely firmly washed).

Presentation

- Crusty, skin coloured, brown or black lesion—stuck-on appearance
- Variable shape and size, well-defined edges
- Velvety or warty surface (no relation to warts)

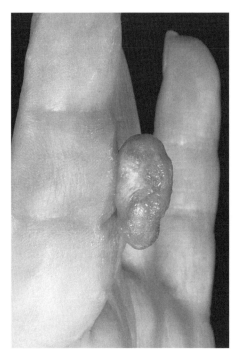

Figure 21.8 Pyogenic granuloma. From *Training in Surgery*, Gardiner and Borley (2009), with permission from Oxford University Press.

- Often multiple—can be found anywhere, commonly on the trunk
- Asymptomatic but may be an annoyance (catch on clothes, cosmetic concerns)
- Can be picked off leaving a pink patch which may bleed slightly (characteristic)

*Sudden onset of multiple lesions may signal visceral malignancy—Leser-Trelat sign.
*Pigmented lesions may resemble malignant melanoma.

Treament

No specific treatment is needed unless patient wishes for treatment or there is diagnostic uncertainty. Options include excision, cryotherapy, curettage, and cautery or shave biopsy.

Skin tag/benign papilloma/fibroepithelial polyp/acrocordons

- Harmless overgrowth of skin with a fibrovascular core. Very common—especially in obese, diabetic, pregnant, and elderly people
- Usually a small (<5mm) pedunculated swelling. Can occur anywhere on the body but often seen in areas where skin creases—eyelid, neck, axilla, groin
- Asymptomatic but may catch on clothes
- Treatment is unnecessary unless cosmetic concern or frequently catching on clothes and irritating patient. Excision with a sharp pair of scissors is usually all that is required. Haemostasis with diathermy or a single suture may be required

Pyogenic granuloma (see Fig. 21.8)

- Capillary haemangioma—common, benign lesion, grows rapidly over a few weeks
- Misnomer—not pyogenic, nor a granuloma
- Commonly seen in children and young adults, female preponderance, common in pregnancy
- Can occur anywhere on skin—most commonly seen on the head and neck, upper trunk, hands, and feet. Typically an oral condition in pregnancy

- Cause unknown—weak association with minor trauma, hormonal influence, drugs
- Arises from skin, not attached to deeper structures

Presentation

Patients usually present with:

- A solitary bright red/pink, fleshy hemispherical or pedunculated nodule, usually <1cm on a base of about 0.5cm
- May bleed on contact (palpate carefully), ulcerate, or crust
- Epithelialization present if long-standing
- Well-defined edges, usually not tender, not pulsatile

Treatment

- Not required for lesions which arise during pregnancy as regression common in post-partum period, otherwise regression uncommon
- Excision with diathermy to base, curettage and cauterization, cryotherapy, silver nitrate, laser

Recurrence common if incompletely removed as feeding blood vessel may extend into dermis. Differential diagnosis—amelanotic melanoma, especially if recurrent.

Pyoderma gangrenosum (see Fig. 21.9)

- Uncommon (1 in 100,000), ulcerative condition of uncertain aetiology, likely immune-related
- 50% of patients have an associated disease (inflammatory bowel disease, arthritides, haematological dyscrasias)
- Can occur anywhere but most commonly on the legs. Can occur at any age but most commonly in the 5th and 6th decade
- Sudden onset, often after minor trauma. The resultant papule or pustule breaks down and forms a painful ulcer with a necrotic base which enlarges rapidly. Several ulcers may develop simultaneously. Edges of the ulcers are purple and undermined

Treatment is non-surgical. Usually consists of immunosuppressive treatment such as systemic steroids, cyclosporine, and tacrolimus. Topical steroids may be considered for mild disease.

Differential diagnosis—vasculitic (Behçet's disease, Wegener's granulomatosis), infectious (tertiary syphilis, herpetic ulcers), trauma (insect bites), drug reactions, SCC.

Radiotherapy marks

Radiotherapy uses high-energy X-rays to ionize and damage DNA structure in tumour cells. Normal tissue will also be affected by these rays, particularly tissues with rapid turnover such as the epidermal layer in skin, but these tissues have a greater ability to recover than tumour cells.

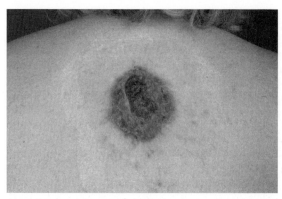

Figure 21.9 Pyoderma gangrenosum in a patient with inflammatory bowel disease (Courtesy of Dr. Richard Weller, Royal Infirmary Edinburgh). See also Colour Plate 18.

It is helpful to be able to recognize the changes associated with radiotherapy as, although it is unlikely to be seen as a case on its own, you may see a patient with radiotherapy marks in conjunction with other changes. (e.g. a female patient with a mastectomy scar and history of radiotherapy).

Ongoing/recent radiotherapy

- Erythema (sun-burnt appearance)
- Desquamation
- Dryness
- Itchy/sore—be gentle when examining
- Tattoos

After radiotherapy

- Usually completely reverse over a period of weeks to months
- Telangiectasia, permanent dilatation of capillaries, usually develops
- Tattoo marks are permanent

Premalignant and low-grade skin tumours

Keratoacanthoma, KA (molluscum sebaceum, cutaneous sebaceous neoplasm, verrugoma)

A fairly common epidermal tumour derived from hair follicles and characterized by rapid growth over 2–4 weeks, a central keratin plug and spontaneous resolution over 2–12 months, leaving a depressed scar (Fig. 21.10).

Classically, KA is seen in light-skinned individuals on hair-bearing, sun-exposed skin (or UV light exposure, e.g. from sunbeds), especially on the face, neck, and hands. It is slightly more common in males and its incidence increase with age. Peak incidence is between 50–70 years, rare before 20 years.

Usually solitary. Rarely, giant or multiple forms of KA are seen.

Aetiology remains unknown. Sunlight and chemical carcinogens have been implicated in its pathogenesis. Clinically, KA is commonly classified as benign or low-grade malignant tumours. Clinically and histologically, KA is difficult to differentiate from SCC. In view of this, despite its good prognosis, many pathologists report it as a variant of a well-differentiated SCC.

Usual presentation

- Initially begins as a smooth, dome-shaped papule that rapidly expands over a few weeks into a 2-cm skin-coloured or slightly erythematous lesion often with a central brown or black keratin-filled crater ('horn')
- If patients present later in the development, they may report that lesion is not growing or starting to resolve

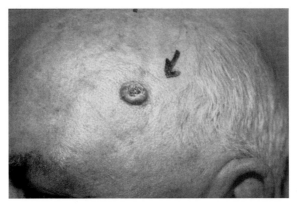

Figure 21.10 Keratoacanthoma.

- Non-tender, firm lesion with a hard central core
- Lies within skin, mobile over deeper structures
- Regional lymph nodes are not involved

Treatment

- Although these lesions have a natural history of spontaneous resolution, treatment, usually with complete excision, is recommended as there are no reliable criteria to confidently differentiate KA from SCC. Other forms of treatment include cryotherapy, curettage and cautery, radiotherapy, laser therapy, and Moh's micrographic surgery. (Shave or punch biopsy are insufficient to accurately differentiate KA from SCC.)
- Lesions are also commonly on exposed areas and patients may favour excision for cosmetic reasons. The scar that develops as a result of treatment usually has a better appearance than when KA regresses spontaneously
- Complete removal of the lesion is required to avoid recurrence post-treatment

Actinic/solar keratosis

Develop due to exposure to ultraviolet radiation and is usually found on skin commonly exposed to the sun—dorsum of hand, face. They are more common with age and usually affect fair-skinned individuals who are exposed to UV radiation repeatedly.

If untreated—may regress, persist or in up to 10% progress into SCC.

Usual presentation

- Flat or thickened, yellow/brown, rough , scaly
- Often multiple
- May develop into a cutaneous horn—catch on clothes

Treatment

- Prophylaxis—avoid sun exposure, use protective sunscreen and clothing
- Surgical—cryotherapy, curettage, shave excision, conventional excision
- Topical—useful for large areas, 5-fluorouracil, imiquimod, or photosensitizing agents
- Regular review to assess change

Intraepidermal carcinoma (Bowen's disease) (see Fig. 21.11)

This is a squamous carcinoma in situ (has not breached the basement membrane) which develops due to long-term sun or UV light exposure. In 5% , it may progress to invasive SCC.

Most commonly seen on sun-exposed areas or areas exposed to UV light on the fair-skinned. Its incidence increases with age.

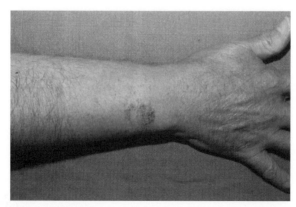

Figure 21.11 Bowen's disease. Also see Colour Plate 19.

It is more commonly seen in women, especially on the lower legs. In men, it is more often found on the head and neck.

Presentation

- Small red scaly plaques up to a few centimetres
- Slowly growing
- A fifth of patients have >1 lesion
- Change in appearance—bleeds, ulcerates, enlarges—may signal progression to SCC

Bowen's disease of the glans penis is called erythroplasia of Queyrat.

Bowen's disease is usually diagnosed with a biopsy as it may be difficult to differentiate clinically from some skin conditions (discoid eczema, psoriasis).

Treatment

Recommended as there is a small risk of progression to invasive SCC

- Prophylaxis—avoid sun exposure, use protective clothing and sunscreen
- Surgical—cryotherapy, curettage, excision
- Topical—5-fluoruracil, imiquimod, photodynamic therapy

Malignant skin lesions

Skin cancers are broadly divided into melanocytic cancers—malignant melanoma (4%), and non-melanocytic cancers—basal cell carcinomas (BCCs, 76%) and squamous cell carcinomas (SCCs, 20%)

Basal cell carcinoma/rodent ulcer (see Fig. 21.12)

BCCs are the commonest type of skin cancer and its incidence is continuing to increase. The estimated lifetime risk of BCCs in white populations is between 25–33%.

BCCs are epithelial tumours which arise from the basal layer and can invade dermis. They are typically slow-growing tumours which rarely metastasize but are locally invasive and can cause significant destruction to surrounding tissue if allowed to develop.

These tumours commonly occur on sun-exposed skin, especially on the head and neck. Cumulative sun exposure is a risk factor in the development of BCCs. They are usually seen in fair-skinned individuals and are more common in males and with increasing age. Immunosuppression, predisposing conditions (e.g. xeroderma pigmentosa) and exposure to UV rays (e.g. from sunbeds) or arsenic are also recognized risk factors.

Development of one BCC puts the patient at increased risk of developing subsequent BCCs at other sites. The presence of multiple BCCs is a feature of Gorlin's/basal cell naevus syndrome.

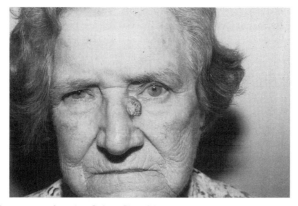

Figure 21.12 Basal cell carcinoma. See also Colour Plate 20.

BCCs are twice as common in males as compared to females and its incidence increases with age. They can occur on any part of skin but has a proclivity for certain sites:

- Majority (>70%) occur on the head and neck—especially on the face above a line drawn from the angle of the mouth to the external auditory meatus. Common sites include the peri-orbital region, around the naso-labial fold and on the forehead
- On the trunk (25%)— incidence of truncal BCCs are increasing
- In the perianal region or around the penis/vulva (5%)

Presentation

- Slowly-growing, non-healing lesion on sun-exposed skin
- Non-tender lesion usually small (but can grow into large lesions if not treated)
- Confined to skin—mobile over deeper structures

Subtypes

- **Nodular**—commonest variety:
  - ◆ Raised, rolled, pearly edge with fine telangiectasia
  - ◆ Centrally depressed ulcer with adherent crust
- **Cystic**—become tense and translucent and demonstrate cystic spaces histologically
- **Multicentric**—superficial, often multiple, plaque-like lesions often seen on the trunk.
- **Morphoeic**—Sclerosing (scarring) variant with a white-yellow morphoea-like plaque and central depression

Diagnosis

- Usually clinical (especially for the nodular subtype)
- To confirm diagnosis or if diagnosis unclear—lesion should be biopsied
- Shave biopsies are adequate for diagnosis and will also provide information about subtype
- Skin biopsy may be curative if lesion completely excised

High-risk features

Management options are determined by risk of tumour recurrence. The following factors increase the risk of BCC recurrence:

- Incomplete excision
- Increasing size
- Poorly defined margins
- Site—on the T-zone of the face or around the ears
- Aggression—perineural or perivascular involvement
- Recurrent tumours are at higher risk of recurrence
- Immunosuppression

Patients with lesions suspicious of BCC, particularly if there are high-risk features, should be referred to a rapid access skin cancer clinic.

Management

Treatment can be divided into surgical or medical. Surgical management is further divided into destructive methods (unable to confirm histological clearance) or excision of lesion

- **Excision:**
  - ◆ For 95% clearance, aim for:
    - At least a 5mm macroscopic peripheral clearance for small lesions <2cm
    - 5–10 mm clearance for small recurrent lesions <2cm
    - For larger lesions >2cm aim for 15mm clearance
  - ◆ Ideally extend excision into subcutaneous fat
  - ◆ Low recurrence rate if lesion completely excised with deep and peripheral microscopic clearance

- **Moh's micrographic excisional surgery:**
  - ◆ Used for high-risk, primary, and recurrent lesions—especially for facial lesions
  - ◆ Involves serial excision of tumour which is examined microscopically to confirm clearance before closure
- **Destructive techniques**—should only be used for primary low-risk lesions as there will be no histological evidence of clearance:
  - ◆ Curretage and cautery
  - ◆ Cryosurgery
  - ◆ CO_2 laser surgery—uncommon
- **Non-surgical techniques:**
  - ◆ Imiquimod—useful for primary superficial lesions, may have a role to play in the treatment of primary nodular lesions
  - ◆ Photodynamic therapy—useful for primary superficial lesions, may have a role in the treatment of primary nodular lesions
  - ◆ Radiotherapy—useful treatment for primary BCCs and has a role to play in the treatment of recurrent (but not radiorecurrent) lesions

Prognosis

5-year survival is 100%.

Prophylaxis

Avoid sun exposure, use protective sunscreen and clothing.

Squamous cell carcinoma (SCC) (see Fig. 21.13)

SCCs are the second commonest skin malignancy (after BCC) and its incidence is continuing to increase. It arises from keratinizing cells of the epidermis or its appendages. SCCs are capable of locally infiltrative growth, spread to regional lymph nodes (<6%), and also have a low but significant potential for distant metastases.

Its incidence increases with increasing age and it is more common in males and fair-skinned individuals. Although uncommon in dark-skinned individuals it is the commonest form of skin malignancy in this group.

Aetiology

- Typically occurs on sun- or UV-irradiation damaged skin. People with fair skin or those with predisposing conditions (e.g. albinism, xeroderma pigmentosa) are particularly prone to SCCs. Cumulative sun exposure is an important risk factor for the development of SCCs

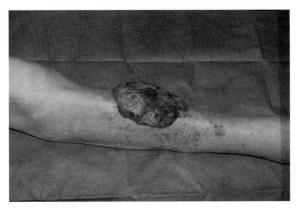

Figure 21.13 Large squamous cell carcinoma in a patient with surrounding Bowen's disease. See also Colour Plate 21.

- Immunocompromised patients
- Exposure to carcinogens—ionizing radiation, arsenic, human papillomavirus (HPV), tar
- Marjolin's ulcer—ulcerating SCC in a chronic wound or scar—e.g. long-standing venous ulcers, poorly-healed burn wounds, sinuses from chronic osteomyelitis, post-radiotherapy scars. The latency period is usually 25–30 years. A high index of suspicion is needed and any change in chronic wounds or scars should be biopsied early—usually a wedge biopsy of the margin. These SCCs tend to be slower growing, painless with later lymphatic spread (due to destruction of local lymphatics) than classical SCCs. Other features may also be masked by the pre-existing wound. These SCCs should be treated vigorously as they can sometimes be aggressive and may have a poor prognosis
- Pre-malignant conditions—Bowen's disease, solar keratosis

Clinical features

Most SCCs are found on sun-exposed sites—face, lips, ears, pre-auricular region, forehead, scalp (70% occur on the head and neck) dorsum of hands, forearms, or lower legs.

They vary in size from a few millimetres to several centimetres in diameter. They usually grow slowly in size over months to years.

Presentation

- Slowly progressive, non-healing ulcerative lesion on sun-exposed skin
- Usually small (but can grow into large lesions if not treated)
- Confined to skin—mobile over deeper structures
- Usual presentation—hyperkeratotic, crusty shallow ulcerated lesion with raised, everted edges and central keratotic plaque
- May also present as plaque-like or exophytic lesions (especially with peri-oral or anogenital SCCs)
- May be preceded by the development of actinic keratosis or develop in a pre-existing scar or ulcer
- Examine regional lymph nodes for lymphadenopathy (most commonly affected are the parotid and cervical nodes)

Assessment and diagnosis

- Usually clinical (especially for nodular subtype)
- To confirm diagnosis or if the diagnosis is unclear—a full-thickness biopsy should be performed at the periphery of the lesion with some normal skin for comparison. Ideally, biopsies should be performed parallel to Langer's lines
- Small lesions in non-critical areas may be amenable to excisional biopsy (diagnostic and curative). Otherwise, an incisional or punch biopsy may be more suitable
- Biopsy report should also provide information about subtype, degree of differentiation, tumour depth, level of dermal invasion, evidence of perineural/vascular/lymphatic invasion
- Assessment of cranial nerves (CN)—most frequently involved CN are CN V and CN VII
- Enlarged nodes—further evaluated with FNA or nodal biopsy
- Imaging (CT or MRI) to evaluate extent of disease

High-risk features

High-risk lesions have a poorer outcome in terms of recurrence and cervical metastases. Features of high-risk lesions include:

- Size– the most important determinant of outcome:
  - Width >2cm
  - Depth >4mm
- Location:
  - Ear or preauricular region—may invade the parotid gland
  - Lip—nodal involvement, may warrant prophylactic neck dissection in some cases

- ◆ Non sun-exposed sites
- ◆ Marjolin's ulcers
- Histological features:
  - ◆ Perineural invasion
  - ◆ Lymphovascular invasion
  - ◆ Poorly differentiated grade
- Recurrent lesions—higher risk of recurrence or more aggressive lesion
- Immunosuppression

The extent of nodal disease (especially if not palpable) in patients with high-risk SCC can be evaluated with any of the following methods: PET scan, US-guided FNA or sentinel lymph node biopsy.

Patients with lesions suspicious of SCC, particularly if there are high-risk features, should be referred to a rapid access skin cancer clinic.

Management

The goal of treatment is complete removal or destruction of the SCC and any spread, preferably with histological confirmation. The choice of treatment will be determined by the site and size of the tumour. Surgical excision or Moh's micrographic surgery are the ideal methods of choice. In addition, SCCs may give rise to 'local' metastases. These in-transit lesions are discontinuous with the primary tumour and will also need to be excised or destroyed as incomplete treatment will lead to early recurrence. Tumour positive nodes should also be managed contemporaneously, usually by regional node dissection.

- **Surgical excision**—treatment of choice for majority of SCCs
  - ◆ Allows histological examination of tumour and evaluation of adequacy of treatment
  - ◆ For well-defined, low-risk tumours <2cm in size—aim for a minimum 4mm peripheral clearance; for high-risk tumours or tumours >2cm in size—aim for a minimum 6mm peripheral clearance (for complete excision in >95% of cases)
  - ◆ Large, aggressive lesions often have extension beyond the macroscopic superficial boundaries and wider surgical excision may be warranted
  - ◆ If in-transit lesions are present—wider surgical excision is necessary
- **Moh's micrographic surgery:**
  - ◆ Used for high-risk, primary, and recurrent lesions—especially for difficult sites
  - ◆ Involves serial excision of tumour which is examined microscopically to confirm clearance before closure
  - ◆ Allows precise definition of clearance and hence has a low risk of recurrent disease
  - ◆ Not appropriate for large or aggressive lesions—surgical excision is the ideal in these cases
- **Destructive techniques**—should only be used for small (<1cm) biopsy-confirmed primary low-risk lesions. No histological evidence for adequacy of treatment is possible with these techniques. Not appropriate for recurrent or high-risk lesions:
  - ◆ Curretage and cautery
  - ◆ Cryosurgery
- **Radiotherapy:**
  - ◆ As a primary form of treatment for patients who are unable to undergo surgical excision
  - ◆ Curative in >90% of cases
  - ◆ Avoid at some sites—dorsum of hand, abdominal wall, lower limb or if bone or cartilage involved
  - ◆ May also be used as an adjuvant to surgery for high-risk tumours
- **Lymph node dissection:**
  - ◆ In patients with nodal involvement—excision of primary lesion and lymph node dissection (periauricular area, frontotemporal scalp and mid face drain via parotid nodes—hence the parotid is the most frequently involved site for extra-lesional spread)
  - ◆ Elective lymph node dissection has been proposed for SCC >8mm (>6mm if on the lip) but the evidence for this is weak

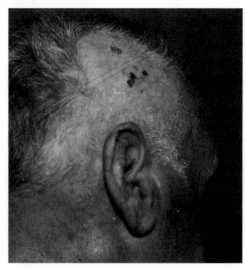

Figure 21.14 Malignant melanoma. See also Colour Plate 22.

Prognosis

Overall, 5-year survival of adequately treated SCCs is 85% (low-risk lesions close to 100%, high-risk lesions 73%).

Prophylaxis

Avoid unprotected sun exposure, use protective sunscreen and clothing.

Malignant melanoma (MM) (see Fig. 21.14)

*MM is an important skin malignancy (significant associated with mortality, morbidity, and public health issues) and hence is discussed in some detail below.

Introduction

 MMs is an invasive malignant epidermal tumour with a significant metastatic potential. It arises from melanocytes located predominantly in skin (95%) but also found in the GI tract and anogenital, oral, nasal, and ocular membranes. MMs may progress radially (within the epidermis) or vertically (dermal extension). Vertical phase MMs tend to progress rapidly and is more commonly associated with metastasis. Satellite lesions may occur in more aggressive MMs. MMs may cease to grow or regress naturally.

 MMs are the least common skin cancers although the incidence is increasing faster than any other cancer. It currently accounts for up to 4% of all skin cancers, but are the major cause of skin cancer mortality, accounting for >75% of skin cancer deaths. In the UK, the incidence is currently 3500/year with a mortality rate of 800 deaths/year. Lifestyle changes, particularly increasing recreational sun exposure (e.g. sunbeds, holidays in the sun), have been speculated to play a major role in the rising incidence of MMs.

 Unlike most solid tumours, MMs are notorious for affecting young and middle-aged individuals. Its incidence increases in a liner fashion from 15–50 years with approximately half the incidence of MMs in individuals aged 35–65 years. The age-standardized incidence of MMs is slightly higher in women than men (1.3:1). The most common areas for developing MMs are on the back in men and the limbs in women. MMs are 10 times more often seen in fair-skinned individuals than darker-skinned individuals, presumably related to the higher sensitivity of fair skin to sun exposure. Plantar MMs have a similar incidence in both white and non-white populations, while non-cutaneous MMs are more commonly seen in dark-skinned populations.

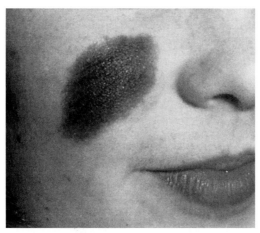

Figure 21.15 Congenital naevus. From *Training in Surgery*, Gardiner and Borley (2009), with permission from Oxford University Press.

Risk factors

Exposure to UV radiation

Unprotected intense exposure to UV radiation is an important risk factor for developing MMs especially in individuals with fair skin, skin that tans poorly, light-coloured hair and light-coloured eyes, or those with predisposing conditions (e.g. xeroderma pigmentosa, albinism). The risk is further exacerbated in at-risk populations living in lower latitudes with increased sun exposure as well as in regular sunbed users. In contrast to non-melanotic skin cancers, the development of MM is related to intermittent intense sun exposure (marked by the number of sunburnt episodes) rather than regular exposure. Childhood exposure also increases the risk of developing MMs later in life.

*The general population should be educated on the risk factors of MMs and on primary prevention, especially sun-protective measures (sunscreen, protective clothing).

Benign and congenital naevus (see Fig. 21.15)

Twenty-five per cent of MMs develop in conjunction with pre-existing benign naevus. Markers of increased risk of MMs in individuals with benign naevus include the presence of multiple benign naevus (risk raised if >10 naevi), large naevi (risk raised if >5mm), dysplastic naevi, and personal or familial history of MMs. The presence of 1–4 atypical naevi (irregular colour and border, erythema, accentuated skin markings) or change in size of a naevus also raises the risk of developing MMs.

Patients with a giant congenital naevi (>20cm maximum diameter at term) have an increased of malignant change and MMs in these individuals tend to develop earlier than *de novo* MMs.

Personal and familial history

Ten per cent of patients with MMs have a positive family history of MMs. Patients with a first-degree relative with MM is at a two times increased risk of developing MM than the general population. A personal history of MMs also increases the risk of developing further MMs.

Immunosuppression

The risk of MMs is raised in immunosuppressed individuals such as patients with AIDS, haematological malignancies, or patients on immunosuppressants post-organ transplantation.

Classification

There are four common clinicopathological subtypes of MMs and the types and their characteristics are shown in Table 21.1.

Table 21.1 Types and characteristics of malignant melanoma

Feature	Superficial spreading melanoma	Nodular melanoma	Lentigo maligna melanoma (LMM)	Acral lentiginous melanoma
Frequency	70%	10–15%	5–10%—incidence is increasing	2–8% (30–70% of MMs in dark-skinned populations)
Clinical features	Flat or slightly elevated (thin), irregular border, variegated colour	Thick, darkly pigmented nodule. May ulcerate or bleed. 5% of lesions are amelanotic[1]	Arises from lentigo maligna[2]—progression to LMM (dermal invasion) is characterized by the development of raised nodules	New pigmented lesion on non-hair-bearing surfaces. Often has a delayed diagnosis and consequently a worse prognosis
Median age (yrs)	30–50	40–60	50–60	60–70
Location	Any site—proclivity for the trunk in males, legs in females	Any site—legs and trunk	Head, neck and arms	Palmo-plantar, subungual[3], mucous membranes
Typical size (cm)	2.5	1–2	3–6	3
Precursor naevus	Common (20–30%)	Less common (8%)	Uncommon (3%)—usually a large, long-standing lesion	Uncommon
Duration of radial growth phase (years)	1–7	Months–2 years, progresses rapidly to vertical growth phase (high-risk lesion)	5–15, slow growth	1–3
Regression	Common	Uncommon	Common	Common
Actinic damage	Slight	Slight	Marked	None—not related to sun damage

[1] *Amelanotic melanomas* account for <5% of MMs and present as a non-pigmented pink or flesh coloured lesion. These lesions are most commonly nodular MMs or melanoma skin metastasis, with poorly differentiated cells unable to synthesize melanin. Not uncommonly amelanotic MMs may be misdiagnosed as a BCC or SCC.
[2] Lentigo maligna/Hutchinson's lentigo are large (usually >3cm), brown to black pigmented macules. Hypopigmented areas are also common. This lesion is confined to the epidermis and is a precursor to LMM.
[3] Pigment spread to the proximal or lateral nail folds is termed Hutchinson sign, which is a hallmark of acral lentiginous melanoma.

Diagnosis

A new or changing pigmented lesion is the most common warning sign for MMs. Well-established and easy to use guides for clinical assessment of pigmented lesions are the ABCDE mnemonic (Box 21.1) and the Glasgow 7-point checklist (Table 21.2).

The **'ugly duckling sign'**—lesions which deviate from the common characteristics of a person's other skin lesions. The ugly duckling sign is a useful guide to aid self-diagnosis and community assessment of suspicious lesions. Dermatoscopy improves diagnostic accuracy in the hands of trained users.

If a suspicious lesion is identified:

- Examine the rest of the patient's skin for other lesions
- Examine draining lymph nodes
- Referral for specialist opinion
- Biopsy of lesion for histopathological excision –ideally an **excision** biopsy with a 2-mm circumferential margin. This will allow assessment of the entire lesion and direct wound closure without compromising subsequent wider surgery. For large lesions (e.g. lentigo maligna

---

Box 21.1 ABCDE mnemonic

- A—**A**symmetry
- B—irregular **B**order
- C—**C**olour variegation (especially if >3 colours)
- D—**D**iameter >6mm
- E—**E**volving (any change in colour, size, shape, surface or symptoms)

Table 21.2 Glasgow 7-point checklist—if >3 points, high risk of MM and warrants specialists assessment

Major features (2 points each)	Minor features (1 point each)
Change in:	Inflammation
• Size	Crusting or bleeding *(late sign)*
• Shape	Sensory change—itch, altered sensation *(late sign)*
• Colour	Diameter >7mm (beware lesions with vertical growth)

melanoma) or lesions in surgically difficult areas (e.g. eyelids, toes), an *incisional* full-thickness biopsy of the most abnormal area may be undertaken, preferably by a specialist. Shave biopsies should never be used to biopsy suspicious pigmented lesions

Extent of tumour and staging

Extent of tumour

Besides confirming the presence of melanoma and determining subtype where possible, the biopsy result will also provide the following information

- Maximum tumour thickness (Breslow's thickness)
- Level of invasion (Clark's levels)
- Presence of ulceration
- Circumferential margins—microscopic clearance
- Lymphovascular invasion
- Growth phase—radial vs. vertical
- Microscopic satellite lesions

Breslow's thickness– has been validated as one of the three most important prognostic histological factors in MMs (the others being *T stage* and the presence of *ulceration*). It is also a useful means of predicting lymph node disease.

Clark's levels—describes the anatomical level of MMs invasion. It should be used in conjunction with Breslow's thickness. It has a lower predictive value and is currently mainly used in *thin MMs* (Breslow thickness <1mm).

- Level I: confined to epidermis/above basement membrane (melanoma in situ)
- Level II: invasion into papillary dermis
- Level III: invasion to the junction of the papillary and reticular dermis
- Level IV: invasion into reticular dermis
- Level V: invasion into subcutaneous fat

Nodal and metastatic disease

All patients with confirmed melanoma should have a clinical examination of lymph nodes. Patients with palpable lymph nodes either at first presentation or subsequent visits should have histological evaluation of their lymph nodes either with FNAC or nodal biopsy.

Elective lymph node dissection is no longer advocated in the management of patients with MMs. However, current American Joint Committee on Cancer (AJCC) guidelines recommend sentinel lymph node biopsy (SLNB) for staging MMs >1mm thickness or thin MMs <1mm with high-risk features (Clark level 4, lymphovascular invasion, high mitotic rate). Sentinel node status is the most important prognostic factor for recurrence and is the most powerful predictor of survival in melanoma patients.

Imaging studies (CT, USS, or PET scan) are not routinely indicated in the initial assessment of primary melanoma unless the patient has a high-risk lesion or signs and symptoms suspicious of metastases. Patients with recurrent disease should routinely be imaged to assess for metastases.

Staging

The most widely used staging system for melanoma is the AJCC TNM staging (*5-year survival with treatment):

- Stage 0: melanoma in situ (Clark level 1)—almost 100% 5-year survival*
- Stage I: invasive melanoma—85–99% 5-year survival*
  - Non-ulcerated or ulcerated melanoma <1mm thickness ($T_{1a/b}$) OR non-ulcerated melanoma <2mm thickness (T_{2a})
  - No evidence of nodal or distant spread
- Stage II: high-risk melanoma—40–85% 5-year survival*
  - Ulcerated lesion <2mm thickness (T_{2b}) OR non-ulcerated or ulcerated melanoma <4mm thickness ($T_{3a/b}$) OR non-ulcerated or ulcerated melanoma >4mm thickness ($T_{4a/b}$)
  - No evidence of nodal or distant spread
- Stage III: regional metastasis—25–60% 5-year survival*
  - Any tumour thickness with or without ulceration (typically thick MM)
  - Positive regional lymph nodes AND/OR regional skin/in-transit metastases
- Stage IV: distant metastasis—9–15% 5-year survival*
  - Any tumour thickness and nodal status
  - Distant metastasis—lung, liver, brain, or distant skin metastasis

Management

Ideally, patients with Stage IIB or more advanced MMs should be managed in a specialist melanoma centre by a MDT. The team should include a dermatologist, surgeon, oncologist, pathologist, radiologist, specialist nurse, and palliative care nurse.

Excision of lesion

Surgical excision is the principal mode of treatment for cutaneous melanoma. Even if the lesion has been completely removed at biopsy, further wide local excision is required to reduce the risk of recurrence. Thicker tumours are associated with a worse prognosis and hence wider excision margins are recommended. However, the most efficacious margins have yet to be determined. Current recommendations are as listed in Table 21.3.

Excision margins wider than 2cm does not confer any added advantage in terms of recurrence, relapse, or survival. It is recommended that the depth of excision should extend up to, but not include, the deep fascia.

Most wounds are amenable to direct wound closure. For larger lesions, however (e.g. lentigo maligna melanoma), a referral to specialist centres for wide local excision and reconstructive procedures such as

Table 21.3 Recommended excision margins

Breslow thickness	5-year survival	Recommended surgical margins of excision
Melanoma in situ	95–100%	5mm
<1mm (pT$_1$)	95–100%	1cm
1–2mm (pT$_2$)	80–95%	1–2cm
2–4mm (pT$_3$)	60–75%	2cm
>4mm (pT$_4$)	50%	2cm

skin graft may be necessary. Moh's micrographic margin-controlled surgery is a useful technique for excision of thin MMs in areas where tissue-sparing is necessary (e.g. around the eye, on the face). This is usually carried out in specialist centres.

Management of regional lymph nodes

Regional lymph node metastases are associated with poor prognosis, with a 5-year survival of between 25–60%. The risk of developing nodal metastases increases with the thickness of the primary lesion. Nodal metastases is rare in lesions <1mm thick but affects 25% of patients with lesions between 1.5–4mm and >60% of patients with lesions >4mm thick.

The presence of positive lymph node/s (either from FNAC, nodal biopsy or SLNB) implies advanced stage disease and is an indicator for radical dissection of that lymph node basin. Therapeutic lymph node dissection of all draining nodes is required to control locoregional disease and for full pathological examination. The number of involved nodes is of prognostic significance.

Adjuvant treatment

At present, there are no routinely used adjuvant treatments for patients with high-risk or recurrent disease in the UK, other than in a trial setting. Clinical trials involving chemotherapy, radiotherapy and immunotherapy have so far not produced results to support routine clinical practice. The most promising results so far stem from large randomized controlled trials of adjuvant interferon-α (IFN-α) which have demonstrated longer disease-free interval after surgery but no significant overall survival benefit. However, concerns about toxicity of high doses of IFN-α have prompted several trials to test lower doses. However, this has been found to be less efficacious at delaying progression. Other potential agents include melanoma vaccine and monoclonal antibody, bevacizumab.

Advanced (Stage IV) disease

Prognosis for patients with distant metastases is poor and survival time is usually between 6–9 months. Management options for patients with advanced disease are largely palliative and include metastectomy (if appropriate), single-agent chemotherapy with dacarbazine or temozolamide, and radiotherapy for bone or brain metastases. None have been found to prolong survival significantly. Poorer survival is observed in patients with initial metastases to liver, bone, or brain, involvement of more than two primary site, visceral metastases, and poor performance status. All patients with advanced melanoma require a multidisciplinary management with input from a specialist palliative care team for symptom control and support.

Locoregional recurrence

Locoregional recurrence is defined as recurrent melanoma in the anatomical region of the primary site to the regional lymph nodes, after apparent complete excision. Surgery, where possible, is the treatment of choice for recurrent lesions or the involved nodal basin. Postoperative adjuvant radiotherapy may be considered if there are adverse features, although the value of this remains contentious. Patients with multiple local metastases in a limb should be managed in a specialist centre by a MDT where isolated limb perfusion with melphalan, CO_2 laser ablation, and/or the local use of other chemotherapeutic agents may be considered.

Prognosis

Prognosis of MMs is multifactorial and is primarily dependent on:

- Breslow thickness (see Table 21.3)
- Presence of ulceration—adverse factor
- Stage of disease—as detailed above
- Regional lymph nodal involvement (Stage III)—most important determinant of survival
- Prognosis is worse if:
  - ◆ Higher number of nodes involved
  - ◆ Macroscopic nodal involvement
- Distant metastases—<20% 5-year survival

Other factors which determine prognosis include Clark's level, type of melanoma, location of lesion, and presence of recurrence.

Surveillance

All patients with invasive melanoma should be followed-up to allow detection of recurrences and second primaries. Patients should also be educated on sun-protective measures (sunscreen, protective clothing) and self-examination techniques to prevent recurrence, or failing that, minimize the consequences by early detection.

Scenario

Scenario 1

Examination of a skin or subcutaneous lump

This is Mrs Jones. Please examine this lesion on her left arm. You may explain to me your steps and describe your findings as you go along. Please do not take a history but you may ask the patient a few pertinent questions. You have 5 minutes.

Answer

Scenario 1

- Wash your hands
- Introduce yourself. Ask permission to examine patient
- Expose adequately
- 'Can you point to the lump that you are concerned about?' 'Does it hurt?'
- If you are allowed to ask questions:
  - 'How long has it been there?'
  - 'Has it changed since you first noticed it?'
  - 'Do you have any other similar lesions?'
  - 'Are you otherwise well?'
- Inspect:
  - Size—define it in at least two dimensions (length × breadth) in units, preferably centimetres. If the lesion is raised, define its height from skin surface
  - Shape, symmetry, border—well defined/poorly defined
  - Site—use a fixed landmark, bony prominence
  - Skin changes—red, warm, indurated, discoloured, ulcerated, excoriated, pus, pointing, punctum
  - Scar
- Palpate:
  - Tender:
    - ALWAYS ASK PATIENT ABOUT PAIN BEFORE YOU EXAMINE!
    - Ensure that you WATCH THE PATIENT'S FACE (not your hands) as you examine the lump so you can instantly see if you are causing the patient any discomfort
  - Temperature—with dorsum of hand
  - Surface—smooth, lobulated, bosselated, rough
  - Edge/margin—well-defined, diffuse
  - Consistency—soft, rubbery, firm, spongy, stony-hard
  - Surrounding area—oedema, ischaemia, venous changes, inflammation, induration
- 'Press':
  - Pulsatility—expansile—arterial malformation or aneurysms, transmitted (i.e. adjacent to an artery)
  - Compressibility—disappears on pressure and reappears on release—fluid-filled
  - Reducibility/cough impulse—disappears on pressure, reappears on increasing compartmental pressure (coughing/ gravity)—hernia

- ◆ Fluctuation—fluid or low density tissue, i.e. fat (fluid thrill)
- Layer of origin:
  - ◆ Mobility in two planes—horizontally and vertically
  - ◆ Fixation to skin—intradermal, moves with skin (e.g. sebaceous cyst). If deep to skin—skin moves over lump
  - ◆ Fixation to muscles—test by checking mobility before and after contracting the muscle beneath, lump becomes less prominent or mobile when muscle contracted.
  - ◆ Fixation to surrounding structures—i.e. move the nearby structures—sticking out your tongue to assess connection with thyroid, neurofibromas are more mobile across the line of the nerve that along it
  - ◆ Fixation to bone—bony-hard consistency and does not move independently to the underlying bone
- Special tests (if indicated by signs elicited earlier in examination):
  - ◆ Transilluminate—e.g. hydrocoele
  - ◆ Palpate for thrills– if pulsatile (AV fistula)
  - ◆ Auscultate for bowel sounds (hernia) or for bruits (AV fistulas/aneurysms)
  - ◆ Neurovascular
- Regional lymph nodes
- Thank the patient, cover them (especially if you have had to expose them for the examination), check they are comfortable

Inspect

- Size
- Shape
- Site
- Overlying skin changes
- Scar

Palpate

- Check for tenderness
- Temperature
- Surface
- Margins
- Consistency
- Surrounding area

Finishing touches

- Assess mobility/layer of origin
- Special test if indicated
- Palpate regional lymph nodes

'Press'

- Pulsatility
- Compressibility
- Reducibility
- Fluctuation

*Note: many examiners prefer that you explain your steps and findings as you go along. I would encourage you to get into the habit of doing that as it gives the examiner and opportunity to give you marks as you go along. This way even if you don't get to the end of the examination or haven't formulated a differential yet, you would have still gained marks for your technique and your findings. In addition, you may also find that it helps you to focus your thought and actions during the examination.

*Note: do not repeat your steps again and again just because you are unsure what your findings are—it is unlikely that you are going to glean any further information from that part of the examination and you risk hurting the patient, irritating the examiner, and running out of time for the rest of the examination. It is better to continue with the examination, collate your findings and perhaps repeat the step at the end if absolutely vital.

PART 3
APPLIED SURGICAL SCIENCES AND CRITICAL CARE

Section 2 **Applied surgical physiology and critical care**

Introduction

This section, by far the largest, deals with every aspect of physiology, pathology, and surgical sciences as applied to the patient. Examples of scenarios are given based on the subject that is dealt with. The answers appear at the end of the scenarios. The reader is encouraged to work out the answer and write it down within 9 minutes—the duration at each station; once that is done, the reader should then look at the answer. This would turn out to be an excellent form of self-assessment.

Chapter 22 **Basic cellular physiology**

This chapter helps you to understand the concept of 'the cell' and its function. The part on ECF is very important from the examination point of view and may be asked in the station on 'Applied surgical science'. The scenarios are typically encountered in your practice as surgical trainee and therefore can easily crop up in any of the stations in the examination.

Introduction

The aim of this chapter is to explain how cells function as microscopic, independent, but cooperative entities to produce vital body functions such as thinking, circulating the blood, and producing musculo-skeletal movements. The first part concerns general functions which are common to most body cells. The rest of the chapter describes how groups of cells with the same basic properties can be highly specialized in order to carry out the function of their organ. The aim is to emphasize simple but crucial aspects of cellular physiology which experience shows that candidates need, but often fail to understand thoroughly.

Varieties of cells

The general concepts are the basis for understanding the specialized functions in different tissues. This variety is remarkable, from sophisticated cerebral neurons with negligible ability to store energy sources, to multicellular skeletal muscle fibres with major stores of both carbohydrate (glycogen) and fat. Dimensions also vary hugely. The main cell bodies of larger cerebral neurons are about 15 times the diameter of red blood cells and are just big enough to be visible to the naked eye (several times smaller than the full stops in this book). Although skeletal muscle cells have a tiny diameter, they can have lengths measured in tens of centimetres. The axons of neurons can measure up to a metre in length.

The concept of the cell

One possible diagram of the human cell would consist of many small circles within a rectangle (see Fig. 22.1). The interior of the circles could have one colour—say black—and the rest of the area within the rectangle could have a different colour—say grey. Black would represent intracellular fluid and grey extracellular fluid (ECF). Cells contain a variety of subcellular organelles surrounded by intracellular fluid of a fairly uniform composition. Intracellular fluid is an aqueous solution rich in potassium cations and relatively poor in sodium cations. The anions consist mainly of quite large phosphate and protein

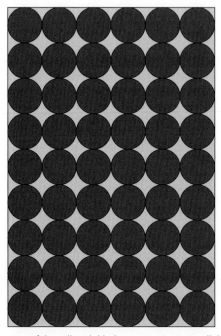

Figure 22.1 A diagram of the concept of the cell, with black representing intracellular fluid and grey ECF.

molecules, with a relatively low level of chloride ions. The extracellular fluid surrounding the cells (their internal environment within the human body) is an aqueous solution with the high levels of sodium and chloride ions and the relatively low level of potassium ions familiar to you from routine reports of plasma analysis.

The extracellular fluid

ECF can be subdivided into plasma (intravascular) and the rest of the ECF (extravascular, interstitial fluid). These two components of ECF are separated by the capillary wall which is freely permeable to electrolyte ions and many other small uncharged particles, such as glucose and urea. They therefore have the same composition with respect to these vital contents, the plasma proteins being an exception—they are largely retained in the circulation due to their large molecular size. Thus plasma levels give a vital window into the composition of the ECF which is the immediate environment in which body cells function. Since water also passes the capillary membrane freely, the two sides must be in osmotic equilibrium and so plasma osmolality equals interstitial fluid osmolality. In fact, because the cell membrane also is freely permeable to water (but not to ions and many other small particles), plasma osmolality also equals intracellular osmolality. Both intracellular fluid and ECF have an osmolality just under 300 milliosmoles per litre and this is also the normal osmolality of plasma.

You will recognize that this is also similar to the osmolality of normal saline—check an infusion bag if you haven't recently done so. The common IV fluids, normal (0.9%) saline and 5% dextrose are both isotonic with the body fluids. This means that these infused fluids do not disturb body cells, including the blood cells and endothelial lining they come into immediate contact with. Much more concentrated fluids (such as 20% dextrose for nutrition) tend to draw fluid out of cells causing serious local irritation at the point of infusion, which is the reason why these concentrated fluids are given by central line. Note that the number of dissolved particles determines osmolality. Since glucose has a molecular weight of 180, and the average ionic weight of sodium and chloride is around 30, the mass of glucose in an isotonic solution is approximately six times that of sodium chloride in an isotonic solution.

One of the main aspects of body cells to be considered shortly is how they maintain the dramatic difference in ionic levels on each side of their outer cell membranes, and how this difference is essential for function.

General properties of body cells

Let's now consider functions which are common to most body cells. This involves functions of the nucleus, the cell membrane, and the intervening cytoplasm, which in many cells is substantial and contains various subcellular organelles. Since cells are controlled by the nucleus, it is reasonable to start here.

The nucleus of body (somatic) cells contains the 46 chromosomes (44XX for female, 44XY for male). These giant molecules with their constituent genes contain an awesome amount of stored information, approached for compactness only in recent years by miniature computer storage systems. The chromosome molecules provide templates for synthesis of enzymes which control cell and organ function in response to external signals. These signals are received by specific receptors on molecular structures floating in the lipid cell membrane. The link with the interior of the cell usually involves a series of chemical events (second messenger systems).

Thus hormones acting on gut cells stimulate the cells to produce digestive secretions at appropriate times. A hormone such as gastrin can stimulate (via a detailed pathway not considered here) the nuclei of parietal cells in the stomach to produce enzymes which favour the generation of hydrogen ions within the parietal cells and the secretion of hydrogen and chloride ions into the gastric lumen. Again the hormone aldosterone can stimulate the nuclei of renal tubular cells to produce chemicals which lead to increased absorption of sodium and chloride ions from the renal tubule lumen, and increased secretion of hydrogen and potassium ions into it. Another very different function of these renal tubule cell nuclei is to produce enzymes for the synthesis of erythropoietin when the ambient oxygen concentration falls below a critical level.

The parietal cells in the first example are being influenced by events within the gut. The renal cells in the second example are influenced by changes in the circulation and its electrolyte content. In the final example it seems that cellular hypoxia directly influences the nucleus in its control of erythropoietin formation and secretion. In all cases control is by a series of events which fit response to body requirements. Thus the cell nucleus controls critical cell activities via internal chemical changes which ultimately affect body function such as digestion and maintenance of an appropriate level of circulating haemoglobin.

In general cells have a limited range of major activities. Parietal cells specialize in secreting hydrochloric acid, with a hydrogen ion concentration around a million times that in the body fluids (pH in the cell vicinity around 1). Renal tubular cells can generate a urinary hydrogen ion concentration around a hundred to a thousand times that in the general tissues (minimum urinary pH around 4–5). Secretory cells in particular often have a series of chemical synthetic reactions taking place in a part of the cell known as the endoplasmic reticulum. This is a cell organelle with an ability to hold synthetic enzymes for the efficient production and initial storage of the secretion.

Remarkably, all body cells have the same chromosomes containing the same genes. This may seem to be contradicted by the fact that the genes concerned with formation of hydrochloric acid are highly active in parietal cells in the stomach, but not in brain cells. Similarly genes concerned with mechanisms to absorb nutrients are highly active in jejunal mucosal cells, but are dormant in many cells elsewhere in the body.

However, inactive genes have not disappeared, but remain dormant and may be activated in certain circumstances. One situation is when cells undergo cancerous change. Some lung cancer cells, for example, secrete hormones such as antidiuretic hormone/vasopressin. This may lead to an inappropriately high level of the hormone, which causes renal collecting ducts to reabsorb excess water back into the circulation, so that the body is swamped with water, and cells swell. This is particularly dangerous in the brain since it raises intracranial pressure, depressing neuronal function and leading to impaired consciousness and risk of death.

Another outcome of the full preservation of chromosomes and their genes in somatic cells is the potential for cloning an individual from non-germ cells.

In order to provide the necessary energy for their varied activities, cells have other specialized structures known as **mitochondria**, which have a highly developed compact double membrane structure to hold the many enzymes concerned with progressive and efficient generation of energy from the oxidation of substrates, particularly glucose and fat. These chemical reactions been intensively studied, producing the complex diagrams of the Krebs cycle, not considered in detail here. The membrane structure of organelles such as mitochondria is similar but not identical to outer cell membrane.

The energy thus derived is used to build up chemicals, such as adenosine triphosphate (ATP), with its high-energy phosphate bonds. Such chemicals then circulate in the cell to areas demanding utilization of energy for chemical synthesis and particularly for energy-consuming ionic pumps such as those in most outer cell membranes. These pumps are rich in the enzyme ATPase. They move huge amounts of sodium, potassium, and other ions across the cell membrane. Throughout the body they account for something like half of the resting energy use and hence oxygen consumption of the resting individual. One of their major roles is to maintain the high internal potassium and low sodium ionic levels needed for essential cellular electrical activity. Another role is the secretion of hydrogen ions against huge concentration gradients in stomach and kidney, and also the secretion of bicarbonate ions in the exocrine pancreas and in the duodenum.

Some aspects of the **outer cell membrane** will now be considered in more detail. We start with an explanation of how the membrane is essential for the electrical activity of cells. Such electrical activity is essential for neurological, skeletal muscle, and cardiac function, together with many other bodily functions, such as glandular secretions and smooth muscle activity.

The nature of the cell membrane is critical for two reasons. Firstly it functions for most of the time as an effective electrical insulator. Secondly, it can intermittently, under strictly controlled circumstances, release a sudden pulse of electricity. We shall now consider how these functions are achieved.

The insulating properties of the cell membrane rely on its basic structure which is a thin layer of lipid, relatively impervious to most molecules, and particularly to charged particles such as sodium ions. This allows the sodium pumps to keep the intracellular sodium ion concentration much lower than the extracellular concentration. The ability of the extremely thin membrane to retain cellular contents is related to the tiny scale of cell size, minimizing the effect of gravity. Even so, cells require appropriate supporting tissue; for example the brain would collapse to its destruction from the effect of gravity were it not floating in cerebrospinal fluid in a rigid container.

Vital floating structures which span the full width of the membrane are the **ionic channels**. These channels are complicated proteins which in the 'open' state allow specific ions to 'flow' along their concentration gradients. Another type of channel in the renal collecting ducts allows water molecules to flow along an osmotic gradient from the lumen of the nephron to the hypertonic interstitium of the kidney. This hypertonicity is generated by membrane pumps in the ascending limbs of the loops of Henle and the channels are opened by the presence of antidiuretic hormone (vasopressin).

Let's return to the **sodium channels** which have both dramatic and widespread effects. They are responsible for the rapid upsweep of depolarization in the action potentials without which cerebral, peripheral neuronal, skeletal and cardiac muscular activity would be impossible. The channels are called **fast sodium** channels because of the rapidity of the entry into the cell of sodium ions through them, compared for example with 'slow' calcium channels. These fast sodium channels are opened when the transmembrane potential is reduced (depolarized) from an initial value of around −70mV to −90mV to a threshold value of around −55 mV. This initial relatively gradual depolarization may be produced by a spreading electrical current from a nearby action potential, or by a chemical transmitter, or 'ligand'. Channels which are opened by a change in potential (voltage) are referred to as voltage gated channels. Those opened by a chemical ligand are referred to as ligand gated channels.

The rapid depolarization upsweep carries transmembrane potential from the negative threshold value to a positive value (reversed polarity) of around +30mV. The fact that the upsweep continues while polarity is reversed shows the crucial role of the sodium ion concentration gradient in generating this rapid upsweep (or depolarization). The rate of change of voltage is impressive—around 100mV (one tenth of a volt) in less than a millisecond. The upsweep ends abruptly because the channels are programmed to close in less than a millisecond, before the potential reaches the equilibrium value for sodium ions of about +60mV, when entry of sodium would cease. The brief but powerful inward surge of sodium ions has already achieved its purpose, which depends on the cell type. In a myelinated neuronal axon this is to propagate the nerve impulse to the next segment. In cardiac muscle it initiates myocardial contraction. At the neuromuscular junction of skeletal muscle, it triggers release of packets of acetylcholine to promote a spreading muscle action potential to activate contraction of the muscle. This action of acetylcholine in opening sodium channels in the postsynaptic muscle membrane is an example of ligand gating.

The brief, programmed, opening of the sodium channels leading to rapid depolarization is an interesting example of the body's economical and efficient functioning. A depolarization of about 100mV is clearly effective in producing the required 'switch on' effect. If the gate remained open for, say, twice as long, sodium ions would continue to pour in until slowed by the equilibrium potential of sodium. If twice as many sodium ions entered, then twice as many sodium ions would have to be pumped out, requiring twice the energy expenditure on what is already one of the major energy requirements of the cell.

Very different subcellular organelles are **lysosomes**. These are vesicles bound by intracellular membrane and containing enzymes (lysozymes) which can dissolve and destroy living tissue. This is how phagocytic white cells destroy invading organisms they have engulfed. Such enzymes are present in most cells where they may play a role in the destruction and disposal of cells when they are surplus to requirements. The process is called **apoptosis**, derived from a Greek word meaning plants shedding their petals or leaves. Apoptosis is important during fetal development by causing cell destruction which helps to sculpt the developing tissues. Thus, development of digits in the spade-like fetal hand is achieved by apoptosis (self-destruction) of linear columns of cells so that clefts are formed to reveal the developing digits.

Cellular self-destruction mechanisms may also have a part in the suppression of cancerous cells. Apoptosis involves the programmed synthesis of a variety of destructive enzymes within the cell. It has been called 'cell suicide' and a major stimulus for it to occur seems to be withdrawal of the normal stimuli from outside the cell which stimulate the cell's normal function. It seems to be an ultimate example of **disuse atrophy**, whereby cells whose activity is severely reduced lose their ability to function at a high level. Two very different examples of disuse atrophy are the loss of skeletal muscle bulk with bed rest, and adrenal cortical atrophy during steroid therapy. The cellular basis in each case is the loss of bulk of critical chemicals, such as the contractile proteins, or the enzymes which synthesize cortisol. There seems be an intriguing parallel between cellular apoptosis and human society, where withdrawal of 'encouragement' and loss of worth of the self, such as with unemployment, or severe social disapproval can increase the risk of the individual's suicide. But back to the cell!

Cells have the ability to expel a small amount of their cytoplasm, or to take into their cytoplasm some external material. Expelling a small amount of cell content is called **exocytosis** (externalization). The reverse is called **endocytosis** (internalization), when a 'bite' of material is taken into the cell, initially forming a membrane-lined vesicle. An example of endocytosis is when an invading organism or other foreign material is phagocytosed by a neutrophil or macrophage. An example of exocytosis is when the action potential arriving at the neuromuscular junction of skeletal muscle leads to fusion of acetylcholine vesicle membrane with the external cell membrane, forming an opening through which the acetylcholine molecules diffuse towards their receptors at the motor end plate. Blockade of this activation at the motor end plate is the mechanism of muscle relaxation during surgery.

Adaptation of cellular physiology to specific functions

We now look at some cell properties which are highly developed in certain cells. Consideration of such cellular functions is important in the understanding of the organs involved. Many of the drugs used in the treatment of organ disorders act at a cellular level, often either by blocking or stimulating cell receptors. Consideration of these special cellular functions also highlights what occurs in a more limited way in other cells.

The **brain** is the dominant organ of the body in a number of ways. It ultimately controls the major body systems. With serious loss of brain function, not only is the personality lost, but other body systems collapse. Logically, the brain is the most pampered organ in the body and all physiological compensations are directed towards its continued function, regardless of temporary loss of function in other systems. Thus with severe loss of blood, the circulation to skin, muscles, kidneys, and gut is seriously and deliberately impaired (largely by sympathetic vasoconstrictor effects) while circulation to the brain is maintained at a relatively normal level.

This special treatment of the brain is related to the special needs of the brain cells as well as their role in central body control. Brain cells, with relatively minor fluctuations, are active, day and night, throughout life. Automatic functions such as breathing must be maintained and during sleep higher centres are involved in complicated activity which comes to light in dreams recalled on wakening. The brain cells (probably more in number per person than the total world population of over seven billion—around 10^{10}) are connected to one another in complex networks. Each cell is connected to many other cells, perhaps something like everyone in the world being in phone contact with up to 100 other people.

An insight into the activity of the brain during sleep is given by the **electroencephalogram** (EEG). The EEG is recorded from the body surface (scalp), as with the surface electrocardiogram but the net electrical activity is much smaller than that recorded from the heart, being measured in microvolts rather than millivolts. Logically one might expect all the electrical potentials produced in the brain to cancel out, but this is not so, with recognizable waves during wakefulness (alpha and beta waves) and much bigger slower waves (delta waves) during sleep. Thus the electrical activity is in some way synchronized to produce waves which are larger during deep sleep, but revert to smaller waves during the rapid eye movement (REM) phases particularly associated with dreaming. Clearly in sleep the need for action by the ionic pumps is maintained, and hence oxidation of substrate and production of energy must continue more or less unchanged.

All this cerebral activity depends on two major outputs of brain cells –chemical and electrical. The chemical activity consists of small packets of transmitters, such as catecholamines, acetylcholine, serotonin, and endorphins, released at the ends of axons closely applied to other neurons. These transmitters traverse a small gap (synaptic cleft) to cause ligand gated ion channels to open and produce changes of a few millivolts in the post synaptic membrane around the synapse. A transmitter which opens sodium channels leads to a brief local inrush of sodium ions which causes a local temporary depolarization, or decrease in the negative potential. This moves the local potential towards the threshold voltage for opening the voltage gated channels. This small voltage change is called an **excitatory post-synaptic potential**. In contrast, a transmitter which opens either potassium or chloride ion channels produces the opposite effect—either potassium ions leave the cell, removing positive charges and increasing the negative potential, or chloride ions enter the cell (again due to their concentration gradient from outside to inside the cell) and again increasing the internal negative potential. This effect is an **inhibitory post-synaptic potential**.

At any time a given neuron is bombarded by many such potentials. If the excitatory potentials win, the firing threshold is reached at a crucial region of the neuron around the base of its major efferent axon. Once the firing threshold is reached, a massive sodium inrush occurs and generates a full action potential (around 100mV) which carries a signal from that particular neuron to other neurons in its network. Thus each neuron acts as an integrator of various inputs. As long as the overall effect is below threshold the neuron is quiescent. When the threshold is exceeded an action potential is transmitted and releases transmitters to the neurons in its network.

As mentioned earlier, all this activity depends on chemical and electrical events. The chemical transmitters must be synthesized in the neuron and transported to the synaptic endings where they are stored in vesicles ready for release. In addition, membrane ionic channels must be maintained, and above all the sodium/potassium gradients across the cell membrane must be preserved by membrane pumps so that channel opening can produce the precise electrical events required. As mentioned earlier, these pumps contain an ATPase which liberates the energy required for ionic movement against a concentration gradient.

Neurons consume large amounts of oxygen to generate the necessary ATP and this is reflected in their high content of mitochondria. Despite weighing only about 2% of total body weight, the brain receives about 15% of the resting cardiac output. Brain cells extract much more of the available oxygen, around two-thirds, than most other body cells at rest (cerebral venous blood has a dark bluish hue). So the brain consumes about 100ml of oxygen per minute, or about 40% of the total resting oxygen consumption of 250ml/min. Most of this is used to oxidize substrates to provide the energy required by the ionic pumps.

All this energy production requires a large and steady provision of substrate. What substrates are used, and are there significant intracellular stores? The answers are that *usually* the brain relies almost entirely on glucose as a substrate, and there are no significant intracellular substrate stores. The evidence for reliance on glucose is that if an individual is given a dose of insulin which lowers the circulating blood glucose level to around a quarter of normal (severe hypoglycaemia), brain cell function is rapidly depressed so that unconsciousness of the individual results, and a further drop in blood glucose can result in death.

This is a major hazard for people taking insulin for their diabetes mellitus. Their lives depend on recognition (by friends and relatives in some cases) of the early signs of hypoglycaemia which include inappropriate behaviour due to impaired brain function, plus signs of reflex sympathetic activity to combat the hypoglycaemia by mobilizing liver glycogen. These signs include tremor, sweating, and tachycardia. The sufferer from hypoglycaemia must be given promptly either something orally such as a sugar lump, or, if unconscious, IV glucose to supply the necessary substrate for the starved brain cells.

Since cerebral neurons cannot store substrates, it is not surprising that their membranes are not influenced by the substrate-storing hormone insulin. The role of insulin is to promote intracellular uptake of glucose and other small nutrient molecules into storage sites, particularly in skeletal muscle and fat cells.

Although the brain *usually* relies totally on glucose as a substrate, there is a situation as far as substrate is concerned when the brain can obtain significant energy from oxidation of the ketone metabolites of fat. This can occur during prolonged fasting, when body carbohydrate stores are depleted and fat is being used at the main substrate throughout the body. A variant of this situation has been seen in very active people carrying out strenuous exertion with limited availability of food. Men crossing Antarctica towing their own food supplies had a daily metabolic rate *several times* the sedentary rate and this outstripped their copious intake of fat rich food. At the end of their trip, not only had they exhausted normal body energy stores, but they had metabolized much of their previously excellent skeletal muscle bulk.

Their blood glucose levels were found at this stage to be inadequate to support consciousness in normal people, but they remained conscious. It seems their brains were relying heavily on ketone substrates.

Neurons in the rest of the nervous system function in similar ways but with less complicated networks and lower energy requirements. An interesting way in which energy requirements are reduced in peripheral nerves is the conduction of impulses along large myelinated axons. The electrically insulating Schwann cells, which surround these axons, allow action potentials to occur only at infrequent, short, non-insulated segments (nodes). The action potential at one node induces adequate depolarization at the next node to trigger a further action potential. So, fewer sodium ions cross the axonal membrane to enter the interior of the axon, and less energy is needed to pump them out again. This mode of conduction is referred to as **saltatory** (leaping) conduction, since the impulse leaps from node to node. With large axons it is also a faster method of conduction than the alternative steady progression of the action potential along an unmyelinated axon.

The next cell specialization to be considered is that of **skeletal muscle**. Skeletal muscle has to fulfil a demanding specification—it must be powerful enough to move the human body, it must produce extremely rapid contractions (the time window for movements to maintain balance during running and dodging is a tiny fraction of a second), and the whole muscle must contract almost synchronously even though its length is measured in tens of centimetres, thousands of times the length of most cells. The answer is to have a multicellular syncytium formed by thousands of cellular units fused together, to make use of linear molecules which can almost instantly ratchet over each other to produce macro shortening of the multicellular fibre, and to have a system of membranes which can conduct action potentials to all parts of the muscle within a fraction of a second. Much of this is achieved by adaptation of cellular mechanisms already discussed.

Muscle fibres consist of a multinucleated strip of vast numbers of segments end to end. Each segment contains parallel molecules of the linear proteins actin and myosin and each segment shortens when activated. As muscles grow in length, they acquire more and more segments. The multiple nuclei control the maintenance of the actin and myosin from their location just under the cell membrane which surrounds the actin and myosin and also the many mitochondria required.

A major role of the nuclear chromosomes and their component genes is to synthesis enzymes to repair the protein of the actin and myosin molecules which are constantly shedding amino acids. It's not surprising that actin and myosin suffer constant wear and tear in view of their vigorous activities. In fact, after a bout of strenuous exercise, such as running the marathon, muscle contents, including enzymes, rise considerably in the circulation, to a level which does indeed suggest muscle damage, fortunately repairable. This vigorous activity of the cells requires very strong protective muscle fascia and tendons, in which extracellular collagen is vital.

Speed and synchrony of contraction are achieved through skeletal muscle's own internal nervous system. The outer membranes of the muscle fibres are able to conduct muscle action potentials at the necessary velocity to produce virtually synchronous contraction of all the fibres of the muscle. There are also branch invaginations of membrane which distribute the stimulus into the central parts of the fibre. The muscle action potentials then release calcium ions from intracellular membrane-bound stores to raise the cytoplasmic ionic calcium environment of the contractile proteins, actin and myosin, far above its very low resting value. This triggers the sliding of the sliding filaments like interdigitating fingers moving together so that the whole muscle shortens powerfully. This whole system is elaborately controlled by central nervous system reflexes for skilled rapid tasks. For this to be effective, skeletal muscle must have a swift switch off at cellular level as well as a rapid switch on.

The switch off is achieved in a series of events of remarkable brevity. As soon as the brain switches off activity in a particular motor neuron, there is no further stimulus for the release of acetylcholine at the motor end-plate. Because the already released acetylcholine must pass through a network rich in acetylcholinesterae, the remaining acetylcholine is almost instantly destroyed, and electrical activity in the muscle ends. The calcium is rapidly taken up into its stores, and the muscle proteins slide back into their relaxed state, reversing the muscle shortening.

The demands of the muscle mitochondria for oxygen to provide energy for muscle contraction dominate the entire circulation during maximal exercise, when the oxygen consumption increases tenfold in a fairly average young person, or as much as 15–20-fold in exceptionally fit individuals such as national and international level sports people. This is achieved at circulatory level by a 3–4-fold increase in cardiac output and at muscle cellular level by a huge increase in the rate of oxygen extraction from the capillary circulation rushing though the muscles. The secret again is concentration gradient. The mitochondria are so active that their oxygen pressure falls to almost zero so that about 80% of the oxygen reaching the muscle is extracted from the blood perfusing it. The oxygen carrying pigment myoglobin also plays a part in providing an intracellular pool of oxygen. It has a high affinity for oxygen and helps in the extraction of oxygen from the circulating haemoglobin. With the extremely low mitochondrial oxygen pressure, the oxygen can easily pass to the sites of oxidation during activity.

In order to achieve this huge flow to muscle, the circulation to other tissues actually falls (rather as it does as a consequence of haemorrhage). The losers are the viscera—kidneys, gut, and liver. In contrast, the heart receives increased cellular oxygen for its increased activity. As the brain is at its maximal level of activity in coordinating maximal exercise, it requires a modest increase in oxygen and hence blood flow.

Energy production in skeletal muscle fibres differs dramatically from that in cerebral neurons in some fundamental ways. Firstly, skeletal muscles have large stores of intracellular carbohydrate in the form of glycogen granules. Secondly, they also have substantial intracellular lipid stores. Thirdly, they are highly sensitive to insulin, which favours intracellular uptake of glucose and lipids, which in turn favours deposition in stores. Fourthly, their energy requirements are normally met by metabolism of a blend of carbohydrate and fat in approximately equal proportions. These differences are appropriate for tissues which are highly intermittent in their cellular activity, in contrast to brain cells which show only small variations in activity by day and night.

Muscle intracellular energy stores undergo a cyclic variation. During digestion of a meal, the insulin level is high, and glucose and other substrates consequently pour across the cell membrane to be stored in the muscle cells. During exercise the glycogen and fat stores provide substrates for a considerable amount of activity, particularly bursts at maximal levels. These stores increase with time during the increased muscle fitness produced by training, and contribute to supremacy in prolonged endurance activity such as running the marathon. At these times muscle cells have the adequate glucose metabolism to maintain the Krebs cycle efficiently and also use significant amounts of energy-rich lipid substrate. Oxidation of lipid releases about twice the amount of energy as oxidation of the same mass of carbohydrate.

Lactate formation builds up as a normal individual increases the rate of exertion towards the maximal possible. In fact, one of the signs that an athlete has reached maximal exertion (during measurement of **maximal oxygen consumption** which is the gold standard of physical fitness) is that the blood lactate level has risen to 5–10 times the resting level. Such a rise occurs as the individual reaches peak exertion during a test involving progressively increasing exertion. The reason for the lactate formation is that the person has reached maximal oxygen consumption involving aerobic metabolism (oxidation) of glucose. A little more effort can still be wrung from the near-exhausted muscles by **anaerobic metabolism** of glucose. This involves breakdown of glucose not involving oxidation but leading to lactate as an end product. The use of glucose in this way is very inefficient as the amount of high energy phosphate produced is only about 5% of that produced by aerobic metabolism. However in life-threatening situations (or during sporting activities!) the extra spurt of running speed could have a highly desirable effect.

It is interesting to compare the lactic acidosis of athletes with that of desperately ill people fighting for life. In the former the acidosis indicates the extra supreme effort which may mean an Olympic gold medal. In the latter, **lactic accumulation** indicates that the patient has reached the limits of survival where the cells in **hypoxic tissues** are just able to maintain function and hence life. This final common pathway of tissue hypoxia occurs with severe anaemia (anaemic hypoxia), inadequate saturation of haemoglobin (hypoxic hypoxia), or local or general circulatory failure (stagnant hypoxia).

The effects of tissue hypoxia are relevant in two other settings. The first such setting is **sudden occlusion of the circulation (ischaemia)** due to vascular thrombosis or embolism. This may occur in the myocardium, a limb, usually the leg, and in the gut. Pain develops rapidly in the heart, where myocardial cells must continue to function and lactic acidosis develops rapidly. In the conscious patient, ischaemia in a limb causes no symptoms initially, but then gradually increasing pain develops due to an increasing level of lactic acid and other metabolites.

The second such setting is when a **limb tourniquet** is applied, for example, to obtain a bloodless field during knee replacement surgery. The tissues, particularly skeletal muscle, rendered ischaemic, gradually develop hypoxia and subsequently gradual damage. The damage must be balanced against the requirements of surgery, but the duration of ischaemia is of critical importance. Up to an hour or so the effects are mild, but after that they steadily increase. As time goes by, potassium leaks out of the muscle as its membrane pumps become ineffective. In addition the intracellular myoglobin begins also to leak out. With release of a tourniquet after prolonged ischaemia, the sudden surge into the circulation of potassium and lactic acid in particular may cause serious malfunction in cells in the rest of the body, and the circulating myoglobin tends to accumulate in renal tubules producing serious damage.

Such effects occur on a much more severe scale when a victim is trapped under rubble with significant amounts of tissue (often in the legs) rendered ischaemic for many hours. The effects of suddenly restoring the circulation to such tissue may be fatal for the above reasons, and amputation of the part may be necessary to save life.

The **heart** provides further variations of cellular activity, with some similarities to skeletal muscle cells and also (in the conducting Purkinje tissue) some similarities to nerve cells. Cells in the heart must provide the following functions: firstly, produce a clear regular electrical signal to initiate the heart beat; secondly, provide for central (brain) modification of this heart rate; thirdly, cause the ventricles to contract from apex to base for efficient ejection of blood; and fourthly, allow the ventricles to contract much more rapidly and forcefully as heart rate increases. All these functions are served by various modifications of cardiac muscle cells, together with the sympathetic and parasympathetic nerves which supply the heart.

Initiation of the heart beat is provided by the sinoatrial node cells in the right atrium. These modified cardiac cells have their outer membranes relatively permeable to several ions, so that sodium, potassium, and calcium ions leak across the membrane through channels which remain open permanently. Since the movement of sodium ions dominates, this results in gradual depolarization, with movement of the internal potential towards the threshold potential for full opening of sodium channels. With full opening of these channels, the rapid upstroke of an action potential occurs, and this impulse is transmitted throughout the atrial muscle and, via the atria-ventricular node and the conducting Purkinje tissue, to the ventricular muscle. As the sodium channels close, the potential falls below the threshold voltage and the procedure is repeated.

In the absence of a nervous input, impulses are generated around 100 times per second. Activity in the right vagus, parasympathetic, nerve releases acetylcholine, which decreases the rate of ionic passage through the channels. The overall effect is to reduce the rate of automatic depolarization and hence the rate of spontaneous action potentials and hence the heart rate. Vagal slowing reduces the resting heart rate to around 60–70 beats per minute in most people. The slowing can be much more marked in the resting athlete's heart. In certain circumstances vagal slowing can be very potent. It is one component of vaso-vagal syncope in which people may faint with certain disturbing experiences, such as viewing surgery for the first time! During certain surgical manipulations, there may even be the risk of cardiac arrest. In the opposite direction, circulating catecholamines and noradrenaline from sympathetic nerves can speed up ionic movement, increase the spontaneous depolarization slope of the pacemaker cells and increase the heart rate up to a maximum of around 200 per minute in normal young adults.

Effective ventricular contraction requires a wave of contraction to start at the apical region, followed by a wringing kind of peristaltic activity expelling blood rapidly from the ventricles. This is achieved by conduction through modified cardiac myocytes which have more of the properties of nerves than contractile tissue. This Purkinje conducting tissue picks up the impulse from the atria at the atrioventricular node and conducts it faster than autonomic nerves to the apex of the heart, whence the impulse spreads back towards the base.

In both atria and ventricles the myocardium has a resting membrane potential that is stable over time (like muscles and nerves) and which is activated to produce a sudden upsweep with the opening of sodium channels. Again, with both atrial and ventricular myocytes, the action potential peaks rapidly and begins to decline as the sodium channels revert to their closed state. However, particularly in the ventricles, calcium channels are opened by the sudden change in local potential. These are called *slow calcium channels* and allow calcium ions to enter relatively slowly but for a prolonged period. Their entry prolongs the ventricular action potential hugely beyond the duration of somatic nerve action potentials (about one millisecond) to around 300 milliseconds, after which, aided by opening potassium channels, the potential rapidly declines, then gradually stabilizing around the resting membrane potential. This potential, at around −80 mV, is quite similar to that of nerves. The duration of the cardiac action potential determines the duration of systole, since the onset of the action potential triggers systole and the rapid decline triggers diastole.

Cardiac cells have regular bundles of actin and myosin much like those in skeletal muscle which allow for prompt forceful contraction. However their structure differs in that there are more definite divisions into individual segments/cells each with a central nucleus. This difference makes them resemble in some ways visceral smooth muscle cells (e.g. intestinal) which also have individual nuclei and function by transmitting a similar but much slower wave of contraction (peristalsis) for bulk movement of contents. The various muscle types have been tabulated below with the speed of contraction decreasing from left to right: Note that cardiac muscle at a high heart rate, say 180 beats per minute (as seen around maximal sympathetic drive during maximal physical exertion) behaves very differently from the resting heart— the entire cardiac cycle must be completed three times per second! In the diagram below, reading from left to right, decreasing speed of contraction is accompanied by decreasing energy cost.

Fast skeletal muscle	Endurance skeletal muscle	Cardiac muscle high rate	Cardiac muscle low rate	Visceral muscle

Fast skeletal muscle fibres are used for brief explosive activity, as in weight lifting and the hundred metres dash. Slower fibres are used for sustained activity, such as longer distance cycling or running, including the marathon.

Visceral muscle is not only the slowest muscle in the above scheme (its contractions last for seconds or minutes rather than fractions of a second) but is the only type of muscle in the table which does not have regular bundles of actin and myosin. Hence it is referred to as smooth rather than striated muscle. However it does contain less highly organized actin and myosin. Smooth muscle cells tend to have less explosive electrical activity and depend on slower calcium ionic movements than the rush of sodium ions through their fast channels.

The next type of specialized cell to be considered is the **nutrient absorbing cell**. This type of cell is found in the jejunum, where most nutrients are absorbed from the gut and where it is called the **enterocyte**. Very similar cells are found in the **proximal convoluted tubule** of the nephron, where they have a rather parallel function to the enterocytes. Both cells avidly absorb glucose. Both also absorb a high proportion of the water and electrolytes presented to them. In view of these similar functions, it is not surprising that their structures and cellular function are remarkably similar. Both have an increased surface area to speed absorption. This is provided by microvilli on the luminal cell surface. Both have clefts in the opposite surface to facilitate the pumping of ions towards nearby capillaries.

In fact, in both cells the active absorption of salt is linked with and facilitates the absorption of glucose. This is the cellular basis of **oral rehydration therapy**, in which roughly equimolecular quantities of common salt and glucose are given by mouth and rapidly absorbed in the jejunum.

Both the enterocytes and the proximal convoluted tubule cells are more or less columnar, abundant in cytoplasm, and with much endoplasmic reticulum for enzyme synthesis and many mitochondria for production of energy. Both have prominent central nuclei for control of these activities. They also appear to be biochemically similar with their glucose absorption blocked by the same chemical.

Activity in the nutrient absorbing cells in the gut occurs episodically with the pattern of meals to be absorbed. In contrast renal tubular cells are very active day and night, as they must absorb most of the filtered water and electrolytes and all the glucose in the glomerular filtrate. This may be one reason why these cells are also the source of **erythropoietin**, the hormone which stimulates increased activity in the blood-forming red bone marrow. Since their activity requires a constant rich supply of oxygen they are in a position to recognize a consistent fall in oxygen supply due to either anaemia or a central cyanotic condition. In both these situations, erythropoietin formation is stimulated, so that either anaemia is corrected or secondary polycythaemia (increased haematocrit secondary to impaired saturation with oxygen of arterial blood) is produced in chronic cyanotic lung disease or at high altitudes. Another variation on this theme is that some renal tumours secrete inappropriately large amounts of erythropoietin, again leading to polycythaemia.

A further group of specialized cell consists of the various cells concerned with **bones**. These include **osteocytes**, which maintain bone structure, **osteoblasts**, which lay down new bone, and **osteoclasts**, which reabsorb bone. Among them, these cells control the extracellular bone matrix, with its blend of complex calcium phosphate molecules for strength in compression, and tough collagen fibres for tensile strength. Osteoclasts have an unusual role in that they are particularly stimulated by parathyroid hormone when the circulating calcium level falls. This stimulus activates release of enzymes which dissolve the calcium phosphate matrix, thereby promptly raising the calcium level towards normal. In the longer term, deposition of matrix is stimulated by weight bearing exercise such as walking and stair climbing, which can be particularly helpful in resisting osteoporosis in older people.

Weakening of the collagen matrix is an adverse effect of therapy with glucocorticoid steroids as these hormones and synthetic analogues favour conversion of amino acids into glucose. Thus the repair of bone collagen fibres, like the repair of skeletal muscle, is hindered, leading to weakening of both. Strictly speaking, loss of the calcium matrix is described as osteomalacia (malacia implies softening), and loss of collagen is described as osteoporosis (brittle porous bone), but all forms of bone weakening, including that associated with ageing, tend to be described loosely as osteoporosis.

Another variant of cells working in conjunction with a non-cellular matrix is found in the **thyroid** gland. The endocrine cells which produce thyroxine and triiodothyronine are grouped around the outside of little spheres (follicles) with the centre occupied by a protein matrix, thyroglobulin. This matrix, synthesized by enzymes from the surrounding cells, is used as a scaffolding upon which molecules of tyrosine are joined into pairs and then have iodine atoms added (three for triiodothyronine, T_3, four for thyroxine, T_4). In order to provide the iodine, thyroid cells have the ability to pump iodine into the follicle (iodine trap). This can be taken advantage of using radioactive iodine to visualize the thyroid for diagnostic purposes and has also been used in higher doses for destructive purposes in the treatment of overactive or cancerous thyroid glands.

Thyroid follicular cells have all their activities (iodine pumping, hormone synthesis, and hormone release into the circulation) increased through cell receptors sensitive to **thyroid stimulating hormone** (thyrotropin, or TSH) released from the anterior pituitary. The pituitary cells themselves decrease their activity in response to negative feedback from circulating thyroid hormones and increase activity through an over-riding action of **thyrotropin releasing hormone** (TRH) passing from the hypothalamus via the hypothalamic-pituitary portal system. This activity illustrates an endocrine ability of neurons. Hypothalamic neurons release TRH as a local hormone passing to the anterior pituitary via a limited portal circulation. Other hypothalamic neurons have axons which terminate in the posterior pituitary and there release vasopressin and oxytocin, hormones which circulate in the general systemic circulation. These activities can be regarded as extensions of the usual neuronal action of releasing a chemical transmitter to act very locally at receptors on innervated organs. In the case of sympathetic neurons, noradrenaline can overflow into the general circulation to become a hormone acting on distant organs, including the heart.

Fat tissue, consisting of **adipocytes,** constitutes a hugely variable mass of stored energy and also a rapidly increasing source of technical problems with anaesthesia and surgery. Each cell has a large mass of membrane-bound fat, dwarfing the peripheral nucleus and other organelles. When dietary energy intake exceeds energy expenditure the action of insulin leads to deposition of the surplus substrate by increasing the large intracellular fat deposits in the adipocytes. These huge deposits of fat contrast with the relatively minute deposits of fat which are part of the normal energy stores in striated muscle.

In circumstances of episodic energy availability fat stores would tend to increase in times of plenty, to be used in times of relative famine, even though excessive reliance on lipid for cellular energy production leads to impaired function due to a degree of ketoacidosis. However, now that most major nations have surplus available food, excessive fat deposits constitute not only a mechanical but a metabolic problem and a major health risk. Surgery is sometimes called on to reduce food intake, for example by reducing stomach size by stapling, or to reduce stored fat by removing subcutaneous deposits, particularly in the anterior abdominal wall.

Brown adipose tissue is a variant of the adipocyte and is found in babies. It is very different from the adult adipose tissue in that the cells are adapted to rapid utilization of the fat to generate heat at a stage in life when heat loss is a major problem, and heat production by shivering is not yet possible due to undeveloped cerebral control of skeletal muscle. The brown adipocytes have the appearance of active cells, with small dispersed fat globules, many mitochondria, and a rich sympathetic nerve supply. Their fat globules are more like those in skeletal muscle, used to maintain a high rate of metabolism for a moderate period.

Scenarios

Scenario 1

A patient with lung cancer and metastases has developed hot flushes and bouts of malignant and uncontrollable high blood pressure. Please explain to this actor (who is playing a medical student) why this has happened.

Scenario2

You have been summoned to the Coroner's Court to give evidence on the death of a patient who has come through the Emergency department. He was brought in by the police after a fight when he suffered a head injury. He was still violent in the Emergency Department where he was sedated. He slipped into coma and died shortly afterwards, before you actually had a chance to see him. In retrospect it was discovered that he was an insulin dependant diabetic. The post-mortem showed no obvious cause for the sudden death. The actor here is the Coroner. Please explain to him what you think may have happened.

Scenario 3

The actor in this scenario is acting a top-level athlete who wants to ask you some questions about training. He specifically wants to try to understand aerobic and anaerobic respiration.

Candidate: 'I am Dr. Smith and I have come to try to answer your question about training.'
Actor: 'Doctor I am a long-distance runner. Can you explain to me what limits the speed at which I can run?'

Scenario 4

The actor is an elderly lady who has slipped and suffered a fractured neck of femur. She has been told that she has osteoporosis and wants to ask you what this is, how do the doctors know that she has this diagnosis and what she can do about it.

Answers

Scenario 1

Candidate: 'As you know all cells have a nucleus which contains a complete set of genes. Most of these are switched off leaving only those functioning which control the cell's correct specialist function. So the cells making up this patient's tumour were originally lung cells and were differentiated to do this job. Most of the genes in a lung cell like any other differentiated cell are turned down or switched off completely, so that it can focus on its function as a lung cell. When a cell becomes malignant many of the controls on the genes are lost. The cells of the cancer start dividing more rapidly than they should. At the same time the cells de-differentiate, losing their special structure and function as the controls on the genes are lost. In some cases, genes become active which previously had been suppressed and cells start producing substances in an uncontrolled way, which they should not be producing at all. If these agents are biologically active (like adrenaline, or vasopressin) the patient will have far too much of these hormones in the blood stream and their homeostatic mechanisms will be thrown into disarray. The patient will experience symptoms relating to excess production of these hormones. These are the symptoms which this patient is showing. This is going to make their preparation for surgery difficult because the hormones produced by the tumour cells will throw out of balance the normal homeostatic mechanisms which the body uses to return to optimal physiological condition. Only when the tumour has been removed will their physiology have a chance to return to normal. This is going to make the job of the anaesthetist very difficult.'
Actor (student): 'What happens once the tumour is removed? Does the patient return to normal?'

Candidate: 'In some cases this may indeed happen, but two problems can arise. The first is that the glands which normally produce that hormone may have been switched off by the high level of hormone being produced by the tumour. Over a period of time this will lead to atrophy of the gland, so that it is no longer capable of producing enough hormone when it is again required to do so. It may therefore be necessary to tide the patient over this critical period with supplements of the hormone. This is especially the case with steroids produced by the adrenal cortex. If patients have been on high doses medicinally and these are suddenly stopped when they are nil-by-mouth during surgery, then an Addisonian crisis will result if supplements are not given to tide them over the stress of the surgery.'

Scenario 2

Candidate: 'Hello, I am Dr Anwar and I believe that you have asked me to come to the court to answer some questions about the death of a patient in our Emergency Department.'

Actor: 'Doctor. I believe that you were on duty on the night that this patient died but did not have a chance to see or treat him before he suffered a cardiac arrest and died. Could you tell us what you think is the likely explanation of his death?'

Candidate: 'This patient was brought to hospital following a head injury. He was violent. It is not clear whether the violence was the cause of the head injury or whether the head injury itself has caused him to become violent. The differential diagnosis of a patient who is violent is a broad one. The patient may have had a legitimate grievance which we do not know about. He may also have a personality disorder or indeed have a full-blown psychiatric disorder which made him behave inappropriately. He may also have been under the influence of alcohol or drugs. The head injury itself may have caused him to have become confused and because he was not understanding properly what was going on around him, he became violent. However, the diagnosis which may fit in this case relates to his diabetes. We now know that he was an insulin-dependant diabetic. This means that his body was no longer producing any or adequate amounts of insulin to enable him to manage the sugar levels in his blood and the amount of sugar taken in to act as food for his body's cells.'

Actor: 'So why should this make him violent or indeed cause him to die?'

Candidate: 'Brain cells are especially reliant on a constant supply of glucose for them to maintain their high metabolic rate. If a patient who is on insulin does not receive enough insulin, then their blood sugar rises. In normal healthy people the amount of insulin released by the pancreatic gland fluctuates throughout the day. After a meal a large amount of insulin is released to hold the blood sugar levels from rising. At night and between meals the insulin level falls to allow the blood glucose level to stay up at its correct level.'

Candidate: 'If you have insulin-dependant diabetes you have to be careful with your diet and inject yourself with the correct amount of insulin at the right times of day so that your blood sugar neither goes too high nor falls too low. Blood sugar levels in a diabetic patient can fall if they take too much insulin, or if they miss a meal. Ingestion of alcohol especially on an empty stomach or a bacterial infection can also disturb the balance between plasma sugar and insulin needed to keep a patient conscious and healthy. Because brain cells are so reliant on a high and constant supply of glucose, they are the first to suffer if the blood glucose level falls. The patient is likely to become confused and classically may become quite violent in their twilight conscious state.'

Actor: 'So why do you think this patient died?'

Candidate: 'It is very difficult to assess or treat a violent patient and the temptation is to sedate them to prevent them and the staff looking after them from getting hurt. In this case sedation is the worst thing that you can do, as you further reduce the function of the brain cells without addressing the underlying cause. If it had been recognized that the violent behaviour might be the result of hypoglycaemia, then a sugar solution given to the patient to drink or intravenously (if they will not/cannot drink) would have brought about an instant and dramatic improvement in conscious state and behaviour. Sedation, however important for the safety of the patient and staff, will have had exactly the opposite effect and in this case may have hastened his death.'

Actor: 'So was the sedation an overdose?'

Candidate: 'Not necessarily. The dose given might have been quite appropriate for a patient with a normal blood sugar but in this case would simply have pushed the patient into an even deeper coma.'

Scenario 3

Candidate: 'I am Dr. Smith and I have come to try to answer your question about training'

Actor: 'Doctor I am a long distance runner. Can you explain to me what limits the speed at which I can run?'

Candidate: 'When you are running, the muscles (of your legs mainly) are doing a lot of work. In order to do this they need oxygen to be carried to them. They use this to burn the carbohydrate and lipid stores which they have in the muscles to create adenosine triphosphate (ATP) which they use to contract the muscles. They also need the breakdown products of that work to be carried away again. Finally you need a good volume of muscle tissue to be able to drive your legs quickly. The system needed to support the muscles is complex. First of all your lungs need to be expanding well and to have a good circulation so that oxygen can diffuse into the blood stream. The blood needs to have good quantities of haemoglobin in it to carry the oxygen away from the lungs and to the muscles. Then the heart needs to be pumping that blood as fast as possible. In the muscles, the arterioles need to be fully dilated to accept the maximum amount of blood into the muscle tissue that is possible. In the other direction carbon dioxide and waste products of metabolism need to be removed from the muscles and carried away to the lungs and liver as quickly as possible. Each person grows up physiologically slightly different, and it is likely that the maximum speed of distance running will be held-down by whatever is the rate-limiting step in this complex process.'

Actor: 'So what happens in training?'

Candidate: 'In training the body responds to hard exercise by improving the performance of each part of the energy transfer process. Muscles may get larger and the blood supply may improve also. The body's tolerance to the pain caused by the build of waste products in the muscle seems to modify with training too.'

Actor: 'So what about anaerobic respiration? Why don't I use that when running?'

Candidate: 'Anaerobic respiration occurs when tissues need more oxygen than is being made available for them. They can then by pass the Krebs cycle and so do not need to use oxygen. Instead of creating ATP by burning glucose to carbon dioxide and water they metabolize it to lactate. The problem with anaerobic respiration is that for each molecule of glucose burnt only 5% of the amount of energy is produced so it uses up the body's stores of energy very quickly indeed. It also produces large quantities of lactate which then have to be eliminated from the muscles. The build up of lactate actually causes pain and so can only be used for short periods. It is of little use to you as a long-distance runner.'

Scenario 4

Candidate: 'Hello, I am Dr Jones. I believe that you have some questions for me about how you broke your hip?'

Actor: 'Yes. I want to know why my hip broke, when it was only a minor fall. In fact I think the hip may have broken before I fell. The fracture of the hip caused the fall, and was not a result of it.'

Candidate: 'I understand that you have been told that you have osteoporosis?'

Actor: 'Yes that is right. I had a bone scan.'

Candidate: 'Bone is a material made of a mixture of materials. Calcium phosphate salts make up most of the mineral structure while there is also a mesh of collagen fibres which give the structure flexibility. There are cells inside the bone some of which are eating bone away and others laying down new bone to replace the bone which has been removed. This means that bone is continually being refreshed. However, as we get older the cells eating bone away appear to get ahead of those laying bone down, so that our bones get thinner and thinner. In women this change is especially noticeable especially after the menopause. Testosterone and oestrogen stimulate new bone formation and the reduction in oestrogen levels with age in females can lead to serious osteoporosis or thinning of the bone. Because the bone is turning over more slowly the crystals making up the structure of the bone become more brittle and subject to fatigue. So for many reasons your bones are less able to support your body or to resist a fall.'

Actor: 'So what can I do about it? Should I change my diet?'

Candidate: 'Unless your diet is very poor it is likely that you are eating more than enough calcium to look after your bones, and that the vitamins you eat (especially vitamin D) are also adequate. Hormone replacement therapy should prevent the further thinning of your bones but will not stimulate the laying down of new bone. There are some drugs which can stimulate your body to lay down more bone, and it may be that it would help if you were treated with some such as bisphosphonates. You would need to discuss this with your GP.'

Chapter 23 **Managing the critically ill surgical patient**

Introduction

As a surgical trainee you will certainly be involved in the management of critically ill surgical patients. These patients will largely fall into three groups:

- Acutely unwell patients presenting to A&E
- Inpatients who suffer acute deterioration
- Patients recognized as being unwell who require re-evaluation

With the Working Time Directive and current shift work pattern, you may be asked to review unwell surgical patients with whom you are unfamiliar. It is vital that you develop a systematic logical approach when managing these patients. Using a system that you are familiar and comfortable with will ensure that important steps do not get missed out both in your day-to-day practice and the MRCS OSCE exam.

Under normal circumstances, patient assessment involves taking a systematic history, a full examination, arranging appropriate investigations, formulating a differential diagnosis, and initiating management. However, this is not practical and may be unsafe when assessing the deteriorating or critically ill patient. Assessment and management in this situation must be carried out simultaneously, often before a diagnosis is reached as these patients may be in extremis or at risk of deteriorating very quickly. Initiating definitive management early can prevent deterioration and save lives.

In the examination

In the exam, you may be given a scenario of an unwell patient and asked to:

- Assess/manage the patient
- Make a telephone call to your consultant asking for advice on the management of an unwell patient
- Document your entry into the notes/write a referral letter after assessing an unwell surgical patient
- Speak to relatives

The last three scenarios will be discussed briefly here and explored further in the communication section.

> It is worth bearing in mind that, in practice and in the exam, surgical patients do not suffer exclusively from surgical problems and may be unwell from medical problems as well. These may be either from pre-existing comorbidities, due to their medication or a 'new' medical problem. Hence, it is important to consider these in your differential diagnosis and management plan.

In this OSCE station you will likely be given a scenario of an unwell patient. This may be supplemented with:

- Clinical charts which may include:
  - ◆ Observation chart
  - ◆ Fluid balance chart
  - ◆ Blood sugar chart
- Investigation results which may include:
  - ◆ Haematology or biochemistry results
  - ◆ Radiology results
  - ◆ Microbiology results

The skills assessed here are largely twofold

1 Ability to recognize the unwell or potentially unwell patient
2 Ability to prioritize and initiate your immediate management

In practice, both these skills will be in use simultaneously but here we will discuss them separately.

> **Box 23.1 Surgical patients at risk of physiological deterioration**
>
> - Emergency admissions (e.g. pancreatitis, GI haemorrhage)
> - Patients at extremes of age (children, elderly)
> - Patients with comorbid disease or on specific medication
> - Patients undergoing complex surgery
> - Patients in the immediate post-operative period (general anaesthesia)
> - Patients who are failing to progress despite treatment
> - Patients who have developed complications
> - Patients returning from critical care wards

Recognizing the critically ill patient

Recognizing the critically ill patient early and instituting preventive intervention early is more effective than trying to salvage at a later stage. Waiting till these patients are on ICU/HDU is often too late. Most critically ill patients demonstrate signs and symptoms of decompensation (tachypnoea, tachycardia, hypotension, decreased consciousness, oliguria, pyrexia) which should alert you to their deterioration long before they need higher dependency care. Worsening respiratory, cardiovascular, and neurological systems are good indicators of impending critical events and simple, logical steps such as regular vital sign measurement and chart review is fundamental to the early detection and management of an acute illness.

Within the surgical cohort, some patients are more at risk of deterioration (Box 23.1) and it is important to recognize these patients early so appropriate measures can be put in place to prevent any possible complications.

Assessing and managing the critically ill surgical patient

If, in the examination, you are asked to assess or manage an unwell surgical patient, ensure that you employ a systematic logical approach to your assessment. We suggest one such framework here as a guide.

You will most likely be given specific information about the 'patient' in the exam, which will lead on to the specific area being examined (see clinical examples). Each case will have a different focus and as a result you will have to modify your system slightly. However, the main focus of this station, and indeed the exam, is to ensure that you are able to maintain patient safety.

Step 1: preparing for the station

You may be given a few minutes to read the scenario at the start of the station. Ensure that you read the scenario carefully and use the information given to start to focus your thoughts. Ask yourself the following questions:

- How old is the patient?
- When was the patient admitted? What was the diagnosis?
- Have they had an operation? If so, what and when?
- What is the current problem?
- How quickly have they deteriorated?
- What are their vital signs?

The answers to these questions will help you to start to formulate a differential diagnosis as well as to mentally 'triage' the patient.

On a minor note, if you are provided the patient's name in the scenario, try to remember the patient's name and use it during the station. This is not essential but just makes you look slick and prevents repetition and time-wasting during the station.

Step 2: initial management

The priority here is to make the patient safe and initiate clinical improvement rather than making a diagnosis. Most patients start to improve with prompt recognition and correction of common problems (hypoxia, dehydration) with simple logical steps (oxygen, IV fluids, analgesia).

Deal with the patient in this station the same as you deal with ill patients on the job.
Initial resuscitation should consist of

- ABCDE—simultaneous assessment and management. Always correct life-threatening or serious problems at each stage before moving on to the next stage
  - If the patient is in respiratory/cardiac arrest, follow the resuscitation guidelines
- Bedside monitoring—oxygen saturations, respiratory rate, heart rate, blood pressure, temperature, urine output, fluid balance and blood glucose
  - Set parameters which are 'acceptable', beyond which further resuscitative measures will need to be taken
- Start simple resuscitation early—oxygen, IV fluids, analgesia
- 'Do I need help?'—call for help early. Even if you are confident in your assessment and management of the patient, consider calling for help at early as two pairs of hands (and two heads) are always better than one
- Re-assess—have the measures you put in place made any difference? Is the patient improving? If not, start your assessment again

> In practice and in the exam, ensure your safety, safety of other members of the team and that of the patient. You should wear personal protective clothing (aprons, gloves) to reduce contamination from secretions and blood, dispose of needles and other sharps safely, take note of environmental hazards—fluid spillages etc.—practice aseptic techniques for invasive procedures, and ensure you practice good hand hygiene.

Step 3: definitive management

The steps above will usually result in some clinical improvement and act as a holding measure to allow you to gather more information about the patient and work out a definitive diagnosis and management plan:

- Take a history from the patient (if able) or from staff/relatives
- Remember to ask about comorbid conditions and drug history as these can have a significant impact on a patient's response to critical illness and must not be overlooked.
- Full physical examination
- Review notes, charts, and investigations
  - Clinical notes available
  - Drug chart—look at current medication (prescribed and check if administered), remember also to look for drugs that have been omitted, look at the PRN sheet—has the patient been requesting analgesia more frequently recently?
  - Observation chart—look at absolute values and trends. Trends are often more useful in these situations as they reflect temporal progress/deterioration
  - Fluid balance chart—make sure you look at all input (oral, enteral, IV) and output (urine output, diarrhoea, stoma, vomiting, pyrexia, drains, etc.) charts. When reviewing output, it is also useful to review the nature (colour, consistency) of the output, if, available.
  - Review available haematological, biochemical, microbiological, and radiological investigations

Using all available information, formulate a diagnosis or differential diagnosis and institute investigations and definitive management, which may include urgent surgery, as required.

Step 4: summing up

Re-assess the patient. If the patient is failing to progress or deteriorating, start your assessment again and get help quickly. You may have missed something or the patient may have developed a complication.
  Once the patient starts responding appropriately to your management and is stable:

- Document your entry into the patient's notes detailing the:
  - Patient's condition when you arrived
  - Patient's response to treatment

- ◆ Current plan
- ◆ Clinical parameters to aim for, and
- ◆ Plan in case of deterioration
- Ensure your documentation is legible, timed, dated, and signed with your contact details
- Communicate events, diagnosis and plan to patient and/or relatives
- Consider if the patient needs a higher level of care or advice from your consultant /other specialities. The key here is good, effective communication
- When making the call, ensure that you have all the information you need. Get the message across in the first 20 seconds:

Hello, this is Ms Smith, the on-call surgical registrar. I apologize for disturbing but Mr. Brown has deteriorated and I think he needs an operation/HDU care/I would value your advice. I would like you to come and see him

- We suggest using the RSVP format:
  - ◆ R: reason for calling
  - ◆ S: story
  - ◆ V: vital signs (initially and after treatment)
  - ◆ P: make a plan together of the next steps

Summary

In the exam, if you have a station on the assessment or management of a critically ill surgical patient, you will most likely be given a scenario and either be asked to discuss your management plan with the examiner or perform your clinical assessment on a simulated patient or manikin.

- It will likely be focused on specific parts of the assessment/management (you won't have enough time to carry out a full assessment and management in 9 minutes). Listen to the instructions carefully and only do as asked.

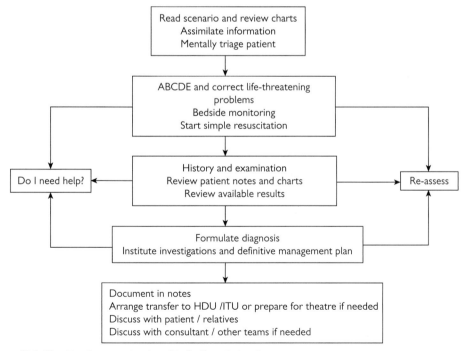

Figure 23.1 Algorithm for managing the critically ill surgical patient.

- Don't rush or try to get through the whole framework. Be systematic and methodical. It is essential that you are able to perform a rapid assessment of the patient and concurrently administer potentially life-saving treatment. Sort out each 'problem' before moving on to the next system
- Use all the information provided on the scenario and charts that you have in front of you
- Remember, the most important message here is to keep the patient safe

With a few exceptions, most acute illnesses develop in a timely, predictable, and reproducible manner. Here we provide you with a simple, systematic framework which will allow you to manage any scenario competently even under stressful circumstances—see also Fig. 23.1.

Chapter 24 **Shock and haemorrhage**

Blood

Functions, components, and properties

The functions of blood are to:

- Transport dissolved water-soluble nutrients and metabolites or chemically-bound molecules, e.g. O_2 and CO_2
- Transport hormones to their target sites
- Transport of heat for heating or cooling the body
- Transport of water-insoluble substances
- Buffer body fluids
- Effect an immune defence
- Provide the plasma oncotic pressure

In adults, blood constitutes about 6–8% of the body weight (4.2–5.6L). It is composed of two major components: plasma, which is an aqueous solution of proteins, mineral salts, and other small organic molecules, and a cellular component, the red blood corpuscles (or erythrocytes), the white blood cells (or leucocytes), and platelets (see Table 24.1). These two components can be clearly identified if blood is either centrifuged or allowed to sediment. The percentage fraction containing the red blood cells is called the haematocrit. This is usually around 45%, the white blood cells and platelets comprise some 0.5–1.0% with the supernatant plasma the remainder. One litre of plasma will contain around 70g of plasma proteins and 9g of electrolytes, mainly sodium, chloride and bicarbonate. There will also be a few grams of small organic molecules such as glucose ($\approx$1g), nitrogenous waste products, mainly as urea (250mg), and a few grams of lipids in the form of triglycerides, phospholipids, and cholesterol.

Red blood corpuscles

These cells are anuclear, bi-concave discs 2μm thick with a diameter of approximately 8μm. They are extremely deformable with a large surface to volume ratio. Their ability to deform means that they can pass through blood vessels with a smaller diameter than their own. The high fluidity of their contents and

Table 24.1 Blood constituents

		Function
Haematocrit (%)	46 (male) 41 (female)	
RBC (N°/μl)	5.4×10^6 (male) 4.8×10^6 (female)	Oxygen carriage
WBC total (N°/μl)	$7–7.5 \times 10^3$	Defence
Granulocytes (N°/μl)	4.5×10^3	Phagocytic
Monocytes	300	Phagocytic
Eosinophils	150	Bactericidal
Basophils	40	Histamine releasing
Lymphocytes	2.5×10^3	Immune response
Platelets (N°/μl)	$1.5–3 \times 10^6$	Clotting
Plasma protein g/L	65–74	
Plasma proteins g/L	Albumin 46–48	Oncotic pressure and binding
	α_1-globulin 2–4	Transport of lipids and hormones
	α_2-globulin 4–7	Transport of lipids and hormones
	β-globulin 6–11	Transport of lipids and hormones
	γ-globulin 6–12	Immunoglobulins
	Fibrinogen $\approx$2.9	Clotting

cell membrane means that when blood is fast flowing it behaves more like an emulsion than a cell suspension and the viscosity of blood will not be much greater than that of plasma alone. Their production is mainly controlled by the hormone erythropoietin and they have a life span of around 120 days and some 3×10^9 cells are produced per day for each kg of body weight. Aged red blood corpuscles are removed, degraded, and approximately 30% of the iron from the haemoglobin is recycled (see Chapter 30).

The total body content of iron (in the ferrous state) is some 3.4g in males and 3.5g in females. Of this 60–70% is bound in haemoglobin, 10–12% is found in myoglobin and iron-containing enzymes, and the remainder 16–29% is bound intracellularly to ferritin. The daily intake of iron is around 11–18mg (a little higher post-menstruation), most (80%) passes straight through the intestine and is voided in the faeces, and the remainder is absorbed in the duodenum. This absorbed iron takes two routes:

- It binds to mucosal transferrin and is transferred to ferritin in the mucosal cells where it is stored until it is used or lost when the mucosal cells slough off, or
- It diffuses into the plasma and binds to the iron-transporting protein apotransferrin to give transferrin which is transported in the plasma to cells in the spleen, liver, bone marrow, heart, and muscle to be stored with the intracellular ferritin. This keeps the iron as a soluble non-toxic store which can be released in a controlled fashion when needed

The daily requirement for iron is around 1mg and the daily excretion of iron, excluding that which is not absorbed, is around 1mg. Iron requirement can vary markedly, especially in pregnancy, following childbirth (blood losses), and with the menstrual cycle (11–29mg). A deficiency of iron can lead to anaemia or can occur with vitamin B_{12} or folic acid deficiencies. These vitamin deficiency anaemias are characterized by enlarged red blood cells, and that the decrease in cell number is greater than the decrease in haemoglobin concentration. One common cause of this latter type of anaemia is an insufficient production of intrinsic factor from the parietal cells in the fundus and body of the stomach necessary for absorption of vitamin B_{12}. Another is malabsorption of folic acid. Because of the large store of vitamin B_{12} in the liver, some 7–8mg compared to the daily requirement of 1mcg, anaemia generated by this deficiency will take a long time to appear. For folic acid the timescale is much faster, the daily intake is some 50mcg compared to tissue stores of around 5–10mg.

This shows that for a life expectancy of 120 days then to be in 'blood-balance' the body has to replace approximately 35ml of blood per day. Thus any loss of blood greater than this can be expected to cause problems. If, however, a person donates some 500ml of blood then very little physiological effect is seen. The 'medication' for such a procedure usually consists of a small glass of fruit juice or a cup of tea so that, in the short term, the body has enough reserves of iron and blood cells to sustain a small amount of blood loss.

White blood cells (leucocytes)

These cells can be divided into two groups on their staining properties with haematoxylin and eosin and also on the structure of their nuclei as:

- Multilobed nuclear cells (polymorphonuclear leucocytes) with obvious cytoplasmic granules (granulocytes) the neutrophils, basophils, and eosinophils, and
- Those with simple nuclei (mononuclear leucocytes) with no apparent cytoplasmic granules (agranulocytes), the lymphocytes, monocytes, and macrophages

Neutrophils account for 58% of the population of white blood cells. Their major function is to phagocytose (eat) bacteria and infectious fungi. They invade infected tissue, 'gorge' themselves, die, and form pus.

Basophils release histamine as part of the inflammatory response (<1% of leucocytes).

Eosinophils (3.5%) attack larger parasites and play a role in allergic inflammatory responses.

Lymphocytes, some 28% of the population, release antibodies and aid activation of T cells:

- *T helper cells* are involved in the activation and regulation of T + B cells
- *Cytotoxic T cells* attach to virus infected and tumour cells

Table 24.2 Circulatory vessels

	Aorta	Arteries	Arterioles	Capillaries	Venules	Venous branches	Large veins	Venae cavae
Number	1		0.16×10^9	5×10^9	0.5×10^9			2
Diam (cm)	2.6	0.8-0.06	0.002	0.0009	0.0025	0.15-0.7	1.6	3.2
Area (cm²)	5.3	20	500	3500	2700	100	30	18
Vol (cm³)	180	250	125	300	550	1550	900	250
Pressure mm Hg	100		30		15			4

- *Suppressor T cells* restore the function of the immune system after an infection and prevent autoimmunity

Monocytes comprise some 6% of the population. These cells migrate into tissues and form tissue resident macrophages, e.g. Kupffer cells in the liver.

Macrophages phagocytose cellular debris and pathogens and also activate immune cells that respond to pathogens. They have a similar role as neurophils but have a longer lifespan and present fragments of pathogens to T cells so that the pathogens can be subsequently recognized and destroyed.

Dendritic cells are antigen presenting cells which activate T cells

Blood flow and its distribution

On the systemic (left) side of the circulation, blood flows from arteries to arterioles to capillaries to venules and then to veins. It is a high-pressure system with a systolic pressure of some 120mmHg and a diastolic pressure of 80mmHg giving a mean pressure of around 100mmHg (= diastolic + one-third of the systolic/diastolic difference). If we look at the structure of this multibranching tubular system then some interesting facts arise (see Table 24.2).

The pressure in the aorta and major arteries is pulsatile but the elasticity of the arterial walls will smooth this out and at the arterioles the pressure will be steady. The pressure difference across the different compartments will determine the overall flow according to a simple flow equation:

$$\Delta P = CO \times TPR$$

where ΔP = pressure difference, CO = cardiac output, TPR = total peripheral resistance.

The flow will be the same entering and leaving each circulatory compartment. This means that the cardiac output will be equal to the venous return. The velocity of flow, however, will be different in each of the compartments because it is proportional to the total cross-sectional area of the blood vessels. From Table 24.2 it is clear that the velocity of flow is lowest in the capillary beds. This increases the dwell time of blood in the capillaries to enhance exchange of substances between blood and interstitial fluid. Just imagine the flow of water out of a reservoir; in the outflow pipes the flow is dramatic whereas nothing much seems to be happening in the reservoir. The pressure drop across the arteries and arterioles accounts for about 50% of the TPR. Therefore, in the arteries the pressure is dependent upon the cardiac output and TPR, in the veins the pressure is mainly determined by blood volume and capacitance.

The capillary bed, with an enormous number of tubes in parallel will only account for some 25% of the TPR. This is aided by the fact that the viscosity of blood changes depending upon the radius of the tube. Blood has an anomalous viscosity in that its 'apparent' viscosity decreases as the size of the tubes decrease.

Overall the relatively low velocity of flow, together with their structure (thin and permeable walls allowing water and small dissolved molecules to freely cross through the gaps between the endothelial cells) plus their huge surface area (some 300m²) allows the capillary beds to behave as very efficient exchange surfaces. Any concentration difference between the blood and interstitial fluid will allow

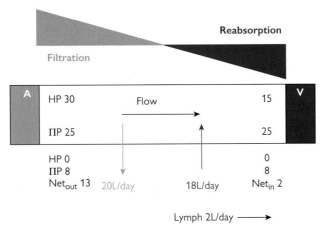

Figure 24.1 The forces in the capillary bed driving the exchange of water from the intravascular compartment to the intercellular compartment. A, arteriolar end of the capillary; V, venular end; HP, hydrostatic pressure; πP, oncotic pressure in mmHg. Tissue hydrostatic pressure is usually at or near zero and the non-protein osmotic pressure is identical in the capillaries and the interstitial space. All pressures are given in mmHg.

diffusional exchange to occur so that nutrients and O_2 can be delivered to the tissues and the products of metabolism and CO_2 will be taken up by the blood. Dissolved particles will be pulled along by the movement of water (solvent drag) but the over-riding exchange is diffusional (see Fig. 24.1).

This figure is for a hypothetical capillary bed. In life the capillary beds can be shut down, when required, by pre-capillary sphincters or bypassed by arteriovenous shunts. It is important to see how this exchange can be upset to produce tissue oedema:

- In theory an increase in arteriolar pressure will drive more water out, however patients with essential hypertension, mean blood pressures of 150mmHg or greater do not tend to be overly oedematous. The arterial/arteriolar vessels have a high resistance and the pressure drop across them will not alter the entry capillary pressure very much. Changes can occur, however, in severe hypotension
- If the oncotic pressure decreases, as in malnutrition or liver disease, then oedema will result
- Any factors which influence the venous pressure will give rise to oedema. Because the resistance of the venous side of the circulation is very low any rise in venous pressure will be translated as a large rise in capillary pressure at its venular end. These include an increase in venous pressure due to heart failure, to blockage of the venous drainage as occurs in DVT, inactivity (failure of the muscle pump to empty the veins adequately or even sitting cross-legged compressing the veins in the upper leg against the bottom leg)
- Any factors which decrease the lymph outflow such as inactivity or blockage of lymph nodes due to infection or tumour
- Any factors which influence capillary permeability. Trauma, e.g. bumps, lead to lumps especially in young children. Histamine release near a capillary bed also gives rise to swelling. Infection can lead to dramatic increases in capillary permeability. Burns (chemical, electrical, and thermal) can destroy them to produce a massive loss of plasma, just think of the blisters superficial burns can produce and the massive fluid loss in partial thickness burns. Full thickness burns 'cook' everything (proteins taken above 40°C will coagulate) so the total destruction of all tissues means that no blood will flow into the wound, hence no exudates except at the edges of the burnt area

Normally any excess fluid produced by capillary exchange will be returned to the circulation via the thoracic duct. Human thoracic duct lymph contains a fairly large amount of protein which leaks out across the capillary wall amounting to approximately 32g/L. This is composed mainly of albumin 20g/L and globulin 12g/L plus all of the clotting factors.

One dangerous condition can arise if the oedema is confined within a fascial compartment which can lead to compartment syndrome. Because the connective tissue defining the compartment will not stretch, an initial oedema caused by increased capillary permeability as a result of trauma of inflammation can lead to a cycle of events that leads to a pressure increase sufficient to compromise venous and lymphatic outflow causing a vicious cycle of more capillary fluid loss giving a steadily increasing pressure rise which will eventually collapse the arterioles and produce tissue ischaemia. If the pressure rises to a level such that diastolic pressure exceeds compartment pressure by less than 30mmHg it is considered a medical emergency.

The pressure at the venous end of the circulation serves as the primary force to deliver blood back to the left ventricle which has an initial filling pressure of around 0. The blood is aided by gravity to drain blood from all structures above the level of the heart. Blood returning to the heart from below this level is aided by muscular activity and the negative pressure in the thorax during inspiration. Taking the figures for volumes of the various blood vessel compartments it can be seen that around 79% of the blood is contained within the venous vasculature which leads to them being termed capacitance vessels. This store of blood can be immediately mobilized when required, e.g. in exercise.

Control of the circulation

The circulation is regulated to provide adequate tissue oxygenation over a wide range of normal demands from rest to heavy exercise. This entails:

- Maintaining an appropriate blood flow to all organs
- Regulating blood pressure and maintaining an appropriate peripheral resistance, and
- Regulating cardiac output

Regulation of blood flow

The state of contraction of the smooth muscle in the vascular wall is the principal way by which blood supply to organs can be effectively controlled. This is achieved in three ways; by local effects, neural activity, and hormonal activity.

Local effects

- **Myogenic** Flow is controlled in some organs by a direct contraction of the arteriolar smooth muscle to stretch, e.g. in the kidneys
- **O_2 deficiency** An oxygen deficiency usually causes vasodilatation except in the lungs where local oxygen lack causes local vasoconstriction to shunt blood to other parts of the lung where conditions for oxygen uptake are more favourable
- **Metabolites** Local high concentrations of CO_2, H^+, K^+, ADP, and AMP can cause a local vasodilatation which serves to wash them from the tissue. Cerebral and coronary blood flow is mainly controlled by O_2 deficiency and local metabolites
- **Vasoactive substances** Local release of 'tissue hormones' such as bradykinin and histamine (vasodilators) or angiotensin II (vasoconstrictor) are sometimes released to local stimuli

The reactive hyperaemia seen after, for example, removing a tourniquet is as a result of these mechanisms.

Regulation of blood pressure

Neural control

Figure 24.2 shows a number of potential circulatory regulation paths:

Temperature—information from the thermoreceptors in the skin is conveyed to the cerebral cortex and the hypothalamus via the spinothalamic tracts. This information can be used to entrain complex behavioural and autonomic changes. The cerebral cortex controls and integrates all motor behaviour and the hypothalamus performs the same function for the autonomic system. For example, if you feel cold you shiver, adopt all the necessary tactics to avoid heat loss such as putting on more clothing or finding a heat source and the blood vessels to the skin vasoconstrict. The reverse is seen if you feel hot—less

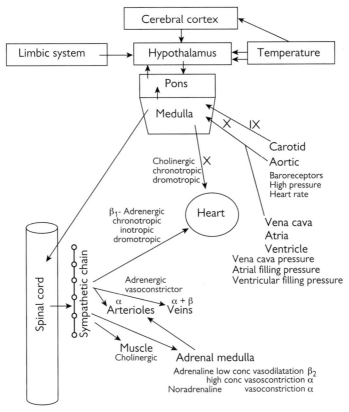

Figure 24.2 Schematic diagram of the neural control of the circulatory system. Arrows show flow of information, for further details see text.

clothing, finding a cool place, cutaneous vasodilatation, plus sweating. The hypothalamus acts as a thermostat to keep core temperature around 37°C. In fever, circulating pyrogens can reset this to a higher level. This central higher 'set point' then conflicts with the thermoreceptor input and starts activity to increase the temperature so you feel chilled and shiver. As the fever subsides the set point returns to normal but as the body is too warm the conflict results in vasodilatation and sweating.

High pressure receptors are located in the aortic arch and carotid sinus. Sensory input is conveyed to the medulla and pons via the vagus (aortic) and glossopharyngeal (carotid sinus) nerves. There is an area which is concerned with blood pressure and heart rate regulation stretching from the middle of the pons to the obex. One area of this, in the lateral reticular formation in the rostral medulla, when activated increases blood pressure and heart rate, and a more central and caudal area has the reverse effect. These areas show some overlap. The sensory information signals both diastolic and systolic pressures from which the central nervous system can gain additional information such as the rate of change of pressure and heart rate. The outflow from these areas have both a direct path to the heart, the vagus via the nodose ganglion, and an indirect path via the spinal cord, sympathetic chain and sympathetic ganglia to the heart and blood vessels. The vagus modifies the action of the heart by altering the rate of change of the pre-potential in cells of the sinoatrial node altering the heart rate (chronotropic effect) and by altering the speed at which impulses are generated by cells in the atrioventricular node (dromotropic effect). These are mediated by the parasympathetic (cholinergic) part of the autonomic nervous system. Sympathetic (adrenergic) activity acts in an identical, but opposite, way and in addition, can alter the contractility of the cardiac muscle (inotropic effect). Thus increased vagal activity will decrease heart rate and vice versa. Increased sympathetic activity will have the reverse effect. Since the pathway from the pressure controlling centres is fairly direct via the vagus and less so from the sympathetic system the initial changes in the reflex controlling deviations of blood pressure from its set point (120/80mmHg) will occur via the parasympathetic route, the multineuronal route taken by the sympathetic system will occur later and last longer (the half-life of adrenaline is greater than the half-life of acetylcholine). The viability of the baroreceptor 'reflex' can easily be checked in patients by asking them to stand up from the sitting or lying positions. There will be an immediate decrease in venous return, due to gravitational pooling of venous blood in the legs, which if not rapidly corrected will result in syncope (fainting). Therefore if a patient can stand and remain vertical the reflex is working. This is usually an extraordinarily fast response with an initial reduction in vagal discharge giving an increased heart rate and by a sympathetic resetting of the entire vascular system to compensate for the postural change. It is not quite so simple as this because the nervous system predicts the standing and will, to a certain extent, prepare for the change in activity. The speed of action of both of these pathways can easily be checked by measuring heart rate and blood pressure after a subject sits down heart rate rapidly (≈30 seconds) decreases but blood pressure from a longer lasting arteriolar vasoconstriction takes some 3–5 minutes to be reset to an appropriate value for sitting (see Fig 24.3).

The major action of the sympathetic control is not just to keep blood pressure at the correct level but to redistribute blood according to need. Regional blood flow varies over an enormous range. Table 24.3 shows approximate blood flow at rest and during maximal activities as well as the blood flow related to organ weight. From these values it is obvious that blood flow to some organs will have to be decreased or increased according to activity and this appears to be a prime function of the hypothalamus. Blood

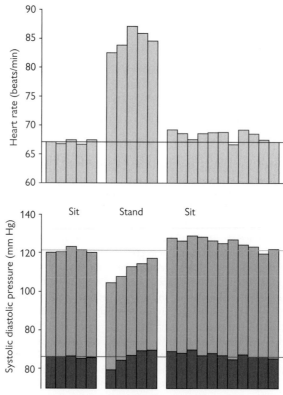

Figure 24.3 This shows the averaged values of blood pressure and heart rate in a 72-year-old man (10 trials) on medication for essential hypertension (nifedipine 10mg, two times daily and ramipril 2.5mg daily) to show the efficacy of cardiac control exerted on blood pressure when changing from a sitting to standing (keeping still) back to a sitting position. Each block shows the averaged values in a 30-second time period. NB In this case the normal sympathetic vasoconstrictor regulation will be both truncated and sluggish.

Table 24.3 Regional blood flow values

Organ	Resting flow mL/min	Maximum flow L/min	Resting mL/min/g
Brain	750	2.0	60
Heart	200	1.2	800
Kidneys	1200	1.5	4000
GI Tract	750	5.5	500
Liver	500	3.0	40
Muscle	750	15.0–25.0	5
Skin	200	3.5	15

flow patterns will be different in the awake or asleep states, when sitting, standing or running and flow to the GI tract will increase when digesting a meal. The blood flow to certain organs is autoregulated, in the brain and heart mainly by local metabolic activity and in the kidney to sympathetic (pre-glomerular) and myogenic (post-glomerular) mechanisms. Nervous control of the other organs is regulated by their sympathetic innervation via α1 receptors (vasoconstriction) or β2 receptors (vasodilatation). The proportion of these two receptors varies in different organs α receptors predominate in kidney and skin, stomach and intestine have about equal numbers of each and in skeletal muscle there are more β than α receptors. Muscle also possibly has a cholinergic innervation of the arteriovenous anastomoses which may act to cause an increase in blood flow in preparation for exercise. Skeletal muscle, however, is controlled more by circulating adrenaline than nervous activity. In essential hypertension the excess pressure is not signalled as such. The pressure slowly increases over a long period and the baroreceptors appear to change their mechanical linkage to the arterial walls and become less sensitive so that the central nervous system gets a false reading of the correct pressure. In the veins the α and β adrenergic receptors control their diameter but here the major effect is to change their volume (capacity) and blood can be 'mobilized' or 'stored' according to demand. The adrenal medulla releases a mixture of adrenaline (80%) and noradrenaline (20%) when pressures fall to a low level or when the body is stressed, physically or psychically. The circulating catecholamines mimic the activity of the nervous system but give a more pronounced and longer-lasting effect. In stress conditions these catecholamines mobilize stored energy supplies, glycogen via glycogenolysis produces glucose and fat via lipolysis produces fatty acids. They also promote the cellular uptake of glucose.

Low pressure receptors are located in the vena cava, atria, and ventricles; these are activated mainly by the filling activity of the heart. Their action in direct nervous control of the circulation is poorly understood. In experimental conditions a sudden increase in venous return, such as occurs with a rapid IV infusion, gives a rise in heart rate via decreased vagal activity which is called the Bainbridge reflex.

Hormonal effects (see Fig. 24.4) respond to a decrease in blood volume by conserving salt and water, acting on the kidney either directly or indirectly. The fluid exchange across capillary beds will, with a decreased blood pressure, automatically lose much less water—as much as 1L of water can be retained in the vascular volume per hour. The haemodilution that this gives lowers blood viscosity, haematocrit, and plasma oncotic pressure aiding blood flow and allowing less water to be lost from the plasma. The effects of the various hormones released are dealt with in Chapter 28. They exert their effects over a slow timescale; days rather than minutes or hours. Figure 24.4 is shown for completeness. There is one extra feature and that is the influence, by barely understood mechanisms, of angiotensin II to produce a sensation of thirst and hence a drive to increase water intake.

Control of cardiac output

There are two ways that cardiac output can be altered—altering heart rate and/or stroke volume. The heart muscle gets its blood supply during diastole. On increasing heart rate the diastolic duration decreases and thus there is an upper rate at which the heart can beat before running into oxygen supply problems. Apart from the effects, on contractility of the cardiac muscle, of the sympathetic activity,

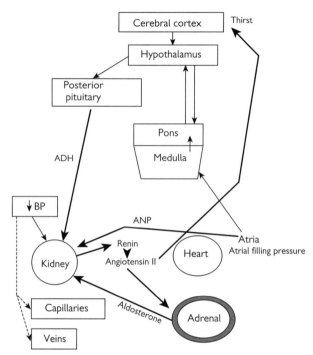

Figure 24.4 This shows the actions of various hormones released when blood pressure falls to restore blood volume.

directly or via secretion from the adrenal medulla, there is a mechanism which produces a force proportional to the length of the cardiac muscle fibres, which can be translated, for a spherical shaped object, as its volume. Figure 24.5 shows the relationship between end diastolic volume and stroke volume. This is shown as a single curve but it has to be remembered that the real relationship is a series of curves depending upon sympathetic activity. Usually there is some basal activity which can be either increased or decreased, thus the relationship can shift up or down. As in all muscle fibres if the stretch is too much then the active tension generated will fall and in this case give heart failure.

Shock

This condition can be defined as an inability to provide oxygen and nutrients to tissues. Initially the anoxia will cause a failure of cells to produce ATP so all cellular pumping mechanisms will be compromised and cellular function will be perturbed due to inappropriate movement of electrolytes and water. They will also start to derive energy by anaerobic cellular respiration. This will produce lactic and pyruvic acids which will lead to systemic metabolic acidosis. This will lead to hyperventilation to restore blood pH (see Chapter 26) and the body will entrain all its nervous and humoral mechanisms to restore blood pressure (see above). (*The renin–angiotensin mechanism will also be activated but this will take some time to become effective and does not play a major role in the initial compensatory mechanisms.*) If the cause of the shock is not treated then the compensatory mechanisms start to fail. Increasing acidosis will cause smooth muscle to relax and pre-capillary arterioles will lose their resistance, causing pooling of blood in the capillaries and increased capillary hydrostatic pressure. This will favour capillary filtration and large amounts of fluid will be moved into the interstitium, and the blood will have an increased viscosity impeding flow. Vital organs will start to fail, further worsening the shock. Thereafter there will be complete failure of the vital organs and death will ensue rapidly.

Attempting to classify the various types of shock is difficult and Table 24.4 attempts to do this in two ways, firstly by trying to broadly categorize them into types (left hand column) and secondly by varieties

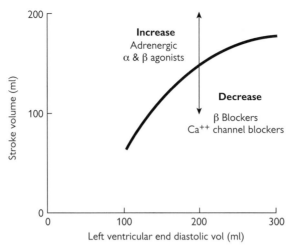

Figure 24.5 Shows the relationship between left ventricular filling and stroke volume.

(in bold) as shown in Table 24.4. For example, distributive shock could be considered as a form of 'effective' hypovolaemia because it presents as a form of inadequate circulatory volume. Distributive shock usually leads to true hypovolaemia because of decreased arteriolar tone and increased capillary permeability. The type of shock causing decreased venous return or cardiac output could be considered as cardiogenic. It is convenient to present their signs and symptoms in tabular form (Table 24.5).

Management of shock

Shock is a condition that requires immediate treatment. First you have to stabilize the patient: ensure an adequate airway, give oxygen to restore oxygen delivery to the tissues, insert two wide-bore needles intravenously and give saline (approximately 1L over a 10-minute period). This is a very efficient way of increasing the cardiac output (by increasing pre-load, see Fig. 24.4). This will always give a breathing space for properly addressing the problem. Enough of 1L of saline will remain in the intravascular compartment for approximately 30 minutes. The cause of the shock then has to be determined and its cause identified, if a patient is bleeding then the bleeding must be stopped. If the patient is in cardiac failure you address this problem first, etc. The next stage is to restore the patient back to 'normal'. Subsequent management depends upon the type of shock.

One part of the treatment for any type of shock is to restore circulatory performance with an appropriate fluid. Three types of solution can be used, crystalloid, colloid, or oxygen-carrying blood substitutes, to either restore intravascular volume, to increase cardiac performance, or to suspend packed red blood cells for transfusion:

- **Crystalloids** In general, large volumes of crystalloid (0.9% saline or Ringer's lactate) should be avoided since they are not retained for very long in the intravascular compartment, colloid osmotic pressure is reduced so fluid is lost to the interstitial space, and their overuse could cause pulmonary oedema
- **Colloids** Colloid solutions last longer in the intravascular compartment with a consequent prolonged effect on cardiovascular function and they maintain oncotic pressure. However, in shock with an increased capillary permeability they can leak out into the interstitium and enhance oedema formation and, in addition, they can inhibit saline diuresis allowing build up of unwanted waste products and restrict the kidneys ability to address the problem of metabolic acidosis by secreting H^+. Colloid solutions used are fresh frozen plasma which is pooled from multiple donors and therefore represents a real risk of containing sources of infection, particularly hepatitis. Plasma protein fraction can be used instead but is very expensive. Dextrans, polymolecular polysaccharides in either 5% dextrose or saline can be used. They have a powerful osmotic effect

Table 24.4 Categories and types of shock

Type	System upset			Main causes
Hypovolaemic	Decreased circulating volume	Loss of blood	Externally	Trauma
			Internally	Haemothorax Ruptured aneurism Intestinal ulceration
		Fluid loss	Externally	Vomiting Diarrhoea Excessive sweating Burns
			Internally	Leaky capillaries Intestinal obstruction
Cardiogenic	Pump failure			Myocardial infarction Arrhythmias Cardiomyopathy Congestive heart failure Air embolism
Obstructive	Impeded flow	Decreased venous return		Cardiac tamponade Tension pneumothorax Pulmonary embolism
		Impeded ventricular outflow		Aortic stenosis
Distributive	**Septic**	Sepsis		Gram −ve endotoxins Gram +ve endotoxins
	Anaphylactic	Reaction to incompatible molecules		Drugs Dyes Foodstuffs Foreign proteins
	Toxic	Sepsis		Non-sterile tampons
	Neurogenic	Decreased sympathetic control		Central nervous system and spinal cord damage or transection
Endocrine		Hormonal imbalance		Hypothyroidism Thyrotoxicosis Acute adrenal insufficiency

Table 24.5 Signs associated with different types of shock. The table entries in **bold** are an attempt to differentiate the types. Further information is given in the text

Shock	CNS	BP	HR	PP	CR	Skin	RR	T	JVP	Ha	UO
Hypovolaemia	↓	↓	↑	↓	↓	**CC**	↑	↓	↓	–	↓
Cardiogenic	↓	↓	↑	↓	↓	**CC**	↑	↓	↑	**Y**	↓
Obstructive	↓	↓	↑	↓	↓	**CC**	↑	↓	↑	–	↓
Septic	↓	↓	↑	↓	↑	**WS**	↑	↓	↓	–	
Neurogenic	↓	↓	↓	↓	↑	**WD**	V	↓	↓	–	–
Anaphylactic	–	↓	↓	↓	–	**Rash**	**Noisy**	–	–	–	–

CNS, central nervous system; BP, blood pressure; HR, heart rate; PP, pulse pressure; CR, capillary refill; RR, respiratory rate; T, temperature; JVP, jugular venous pressure; Ha, heart arrhythmias; UO, urine output. ↓, decreased; ↑, increased; CC cold and clammy; WS, warm and sweaty; WD warm and dry; V, varies, Y, yes and -, not seen or not a real sign.

and cause fluid resorption from the interstitial space expanding the intravascular volume by approximately twice the volume infused, decreasing the viscosity of the intravascular fluid but also decreasing the elasticity of the red blood cell membranes making them less flexible and restricting their ability to flow through small capillaries. They also cause renal damage if used in doses >1.5g/kg body weight. Gelatin readily cross the glomerular membrane so that its half-life is only some 2–3 hours and it can cause a diuresis, not what you want when trying to expand intravascular volume. Hydroxyethyl starches are also used. These are fairly expensive and give a volume expansion more or less equal to the volume infused. If all this is confusing then listen to what your consultant suggests, this will be a choice of experience—better than any textbook!

- **Oxygen-carrying blood substitutes** Recently some oxygen-carrying blood substitutes have been introduced to clinical practice, mainly fluorocarbon emulsions using a detergent as the emulsion stabilizer which can cause problems, added to which their affinity for oxygen is high and they do not last long in the intravascular compartment

Hypovolaemia due to fluid loss

Vomiting

The stomach can contain around 1L of fluid after a meal which can be spectacularly evacuated! The real danger of vomit is if it is aspirated which can lead to respiratory complications and, if not noticed, death. Usually those patients prone to vomiting (those on chemotherapy and radiotherapy) are given anti-emetic drugs and clear information on how to manage themselves. If it is excessive, patients present with hypovolaemia coupled with a metabolic alkalosis (see Chapter 28).

Diarrhoea

The intestinal tract can produce up to 6L of secretion per day and loss of this fluid plus its electrolytes (Na^+, 45–85mmol/L; K^+, 1–11mmol/L; Cl^-, 64–110mmol/L; and HCO_3^-, 8–41mmol/L) can produce, if not treated (bacterial or amoebic) with an appropriate antibiotic (ciprofloxacin, metronidazole) a life-threatening condition. Outbreaks of *Escherichia coli* infection although rare in the UK usually lead to some deaths. In developing countries it is a major cause of death (1.5 million under the age of 5 annually according to UNICEF) it can also seriously threaten the life of children anywhere. Children can lose around 10–14% of their body water very quickly. The underlying dehydration can be effectively reversed by the use of rehydration solution given orally. This contains glucose 75mmol/L, sodium chloride 36mmol/L, tri-sodium citrate 16.2mmol/L plus potassium chloride 27.6mmol/L and is a cunning example of the use of information obtained from physiological research since all the ingredients play a role in its action.

- Na^+ provides the energy for the carrier mediated glucose transport which will transfer glucose plus a large quantity of water into the bloodstream as well as a source of sodium chloride to replace losses
- Citrate will provide ATP via the Krebs cycle to pump Na^+ out of the cell so that NaCl will be transported with water into the bloodstream
- K^+ will allow the transfer of KCl into the bloodstream to replace its loss

Sweating

In combination with respiratory water loss this can become problematic in long-distance runners and exacerbated by the increased lactic acid production can lead to problems. Usually this is easily remedied by a little oxygen and a bottle of proprietary sports drink—an expensive version of rehydration fluid.

Burns

After making sure that respiration is adequate you have to make an informed opinion of the likelihood of development of upper airway (singeing of nasal hairs, presence of soot, etc.) or lung damage (nature of the fire situation whether there would have been a possibility of inhaling industrial chemicals such as ammonia, sulphur dioxide, or chlorine). Careful monitoring will be required. Burns victims will also require adequate analgesia. Initial fluid replacement follows a strict guideline related to percentage of surface area burnt and body weight. Erythematous changes without blistering will require no intervention they usually resolve themselves. Apart from the initial fluid loss in blisters or overt leaking of fluid from the burnt surface there will probably be a large loss of plasma. The Mount Vernon formula estimates the amount of plasma required:

$$\text{Volume of plasma to be infused} = [\% \text{ burnt area}] \times [\text{weight in kg}/2]$$

The calculated volume of fluid to be given (per period) is infused in successive periods of 4, 4, 4, 6, 6, and 12 hours. For a patient with 30% burns weighing 70kg this amounts to a volume of about 1L with a total volume of 5L.

Or the Parkland formula for those who initially resuscitate with crystalloid:

$$\text{Volume of fluid to be infused} = 4\text{mL Ringer lactate} \times \% \text{ burnt area} \times \text{weight in kg}$$

The total volume, for the same patient will amount to 8.4L. Half in the first 8 hours, the remainder in the next 16 hours. Surface area is computed using the 'rule of nine', see Table 24.6. Fluid resuscitation is titrated with patient urine output which has to be >0.6mL/kg/h.

Hypovolaemia will be compounded by tissue oedema. Initially because capillary beds under and around the burnt area will become leaky due to thermal injury and the subsequent release of vasoactive substances. Later oedema will be caused, in all tissues, because of the hypoproteinaemia. However, by this time the patient will have been moved to a burns unit.

Hypovolaemia due to blood loss

This is categorized by cold, clammy, possibly cyanosed skin with increased capillary refill time, oliguria or possibly anuria, tachycardia, and, in severe cases, confusion and restlessness. The large increase in sympathetic activity produces generalized vasoconstriction to maintain blood pressure with decreased tissue perfusion. The degree of shock can possibly be roughly estimated because the skin changes occur more proximally the greater it is. Hypotension may not be present because pressure can be maintained even with blood loss as great as 25%. The goal is to give appropriate fluid resuscitation until tachycardia, urine output, and capillary filling are restored toward normal levels and sweating stops. Patients are often tachypnoeic which must be carefully monitored because if it persists it can be an indication that the patient is developing something nasty, e.g. ARDS.

Blood transfusion

The choice of fluid for resuscitation you would think would be blood as soon as it becomes available. However, blood transfusion has some problems. Rarely, inappropriate blood group can be given, see Table 24.7. Other dangers may be due to pyrogens or transmissible infections.

Other potential dangers are:

- **Hypothermia** Blood is stored at 4°C, with massive transfusions this could drop core temperature. Cold fluid will cause venoconstriction slowing transfusion rate and can cause dysrhythmias. The solution is to warm the blood before use
- **Microemboli** Stored blood can contain microaggregates of dead platelets and white cells. The majority of these will not be removed by the filters in normal blood giving sets (pore size 120μm).

Table 24.6 Percentage area of body regions

Region	Adult (%)	Child (%)
Head	9	14
Chest + abdomen	18	18
Back	18	18
Arm	9	9
Leg	18	16
Genitals	1	

Table 24.7 Shows the various simple blood groups and their distribution. Rh +ve blood transfused into Rh −ve recipients makes the latter produce anti-Rh +ve antibody. Rh −ve mothers with a Rh+ve baby will develop anti Rh +ve antibody on their first pregnancy which will put babies of subsequent pregnancies at risk. *You have to excuse the somewhat politically incorrect mention of the distribution of blood groups, it is included because a common question is about their distribution. The answer to this question should commence with where in practice it is—an appropriate answer from this table!*

Group	Antigen cell	Antibody plasma	Distribution (%) White English	Chinese	Hindu
A	A	Anti-B	42	25	19
B	B	Anti-A	9	35	41
AB	A+B	—	3	10	9
O	—	Anti −A +B	47	30	31
Rh +ve	Rh +ve	—	88	98	81
Rh −ve	—	—	17	2	9

These are considered, by some authorities, to be a potential contributory factor in the development of ARDS in patients receiving massive blood transfusions and they suggest filters with a pore size of 40μm be used, others maintain that ARDS develops because the hypoxaemia in trauma victims is proportional to its nature and extent

- **Coagulopathy** Stored blood has no platelets and is deficient in clotting factors. This can be remedied by giving fresh frozen plasma. If there is an identified lack of Factor VIII cryoprecipitate can be given. There is an added complication in the modern world because elderly trauma victims can be on all sorts of medication. If they are hypertensive they will be on medication, usually calcium channel blockers, ACE inhibitors plus low dose aspirin, these must be taken into account in their management. In addition some patients may be on warfarin (vitamin K reversible over 1–2 days) or heparin (protamine sulphate reversible over 1–4 hours) to counter ongoing coagulopathy or cardiac problems

- **Metabolic alkalosis** Patients receiving massive transfusions often develop a metabolic alkalosis after 1–2 days. This is possibly due to metabolism of the citrate used to prevent the stored blood coagulating and will be exacerbated if any preceding acidosis has been corrected with IV bicarbonate

- **Hypocalcaemia** The citrate in stored blood is used to bind calcium to prevent clotting. Transfused citrate will probably lower the ionized calcium in the recipient. If necessary, but not routinely, this can be remedied by giving 10ml of 10% calcium chloride IV

- **Oxygen affinity** The amount of 2,3-DPG in stored blood is reduced, the oxygen dissociation curve is shifted to the left, and the ability of haemoglobin to release oxygen is reduced. Warming the blood is usually sufficient to increase the metabolism of the red blood cells and restore the correct level of the 2,3-DPG

- **Hyperkalaemia** Na^+ is usually removed from red blood cells in exchange for K^+ by an active ATPase pump which requires oxygen and glucose. This reaction will slow down and stop for three reasons. First the oxygen and glucose will be rapidly used up by the red blood cells and secondly the blood is stored at 4°C. Chemical reactions have a Q10 of approximately 2, that is a 10°C fall in temperature will halve the reaction rate so that close to a 40°C drop in temperature will mean that the reaction rate automatically falls to 1/16th of its normal rate so the membrane ion exchange pumps will effectively stop. Red blood cell membranes will then behave passively and normal diffusional exchange of Na^+ and K^+ will take place with Na^+ moving into the cell down its concentration gradient and K^+ moving in the opposite direction—see Table 24.8. There will undoubtedly be some lysis of the red cells when suspended in saline/colloid for transfusion but the majority of the K^+ will come from cellular loss in storage. Storage at a cool temperature will

Table 24.8 Changes in red blood cell electrolyte concentrations as (mmol/L) in stored blood

Day	0	10	20	30	40
K$^+$	90	75	68	60	53
Na$^+$	18	25	30	37	42

have one beneficial effect—the life cycle of the cells will be prolonged. Warming the blood and infusing it into an environment with more oxygen will restart the membrane pumps and the cells will quickly achieve the normal Na$^+$/K$^+$ distribution

Large transfusions will undoubtedly be accompanied by plasma or plasma substitute to maintain an adequate volume. However, there may be a benefit to limited haemodilution in that a decrease in haematocrit to 25–30% helps because the decreased oxygen delivery can be offset by an increased cardiac output and better flow rates of less viscous blood.

To assess whether massive/large transfusions underfill or overfill the patient then central venous pressure measurements can be used. The absolute measure is not very helpful but the trend in pressure seen after a 250-ml bolus of saline is very helpful. In the underfilled patient the pressure will show a transient increase which will return to normal in a few minutes, overfilled patients will show a maintained increase in pressure; those correctly filled will show an initial rise which slowly returns to normal over several minutes as the venous capacity adapts to a small but acceptable volume increase.

Cardiogenic shock

This type of shock shows the same signs as hypovolaemic shock with an added component of raised jugular venous pressure (JVP). The initial management is to increase cardiac output by increasing venous return. Thereafter the cardiac defect must be addressed. Cardiac effects are not only confined to those patients with an overt cardiac problem but can also occur as a consequence of severe hypovolaemic or septic shock. Severe metabolic acidosis may impair cardiac contractility and if blood Ph is <7.2 then 10-ml doses of sodium bicarbonate in small aliquots (50ml 8.4%) can be administered with careful monitoring of the pH. If preload adjustment and blood pH adjustment do not produce an adequate response then myocardial stimulants may be employed.

Inotropic drugs

- **Adrenaline's** effect is dose dependent. With low doses its β-receptor effects predominate, giving chronotropic and dromotropic actions with a decrease in peripheral resistance. At higher doses its α-receptor effects dominate and it also acts as a +ve inotrope and causes an increase in peripheral resistance. As the dose increases its vasoconstrictive actions can cause problems. Reduction in renal flow causes oliguria and can precipitate renal failure, and its chronotropic action can cause large increases in heart rate, therefore the dose has to be carefully titrated for best effect
- **Isoprenaline** stimulates β-receptors and shows both chronotropic, dromotropic, and inotropic effects. It also reduces peripheral resistance by dilating skin and muscle vessels. However, its cardiac effect is mostly chronotropic which limits its use
- **Dopamine** in low doses acts mainly as a +ve inotrope and decreases peripheral resistance by dilating renal and splanchnic vessels thereby improving renal and hepatic function. However, as the dose is increased it releases noradrenaline which increases peripheral resistance and thus afterload
- **Dobutamine** acts in a similar way to dopamine as a +ve inotrope and decreases peripheral resistance

Overall dobutamine is the drug of choice for cardiogenic shock and cardiac failure whereas dopamine is the drug of choice for other types of shock because of its renal and hepatic action. However, all these agents if used in patients with additional respiratory failure increase venous admixture either by opening pulmonary vessels or by reversing the hypoxic vasoconstrictor effect.

In some cases it may be necessary to decrease the after load in order to achieve an increase in stroke volume. Reference to Fig. 24.4 shows that, for those patients with impending cardiac failure, the flat part of the curve, cannot increase their stroke volume with an increased venous return. Such an approach is potentially dangerous and has to be carefully monitored. Sodium nitroprusside dilates arterioles, venous capacitance vessels, and the pulmonary vasculature and as a consequence will decrease pre-load and after-load in both ventricles which can improve cardiac output and decrease the myocardial demand for oxygen. Gross over-dosage with this drug will lead to cyanide poisoning so care has to employed, if it is administered, with continuous careful monitoring of the patient's haemodynamic status.

For obstructive shock the treatments for tension pneumothorax and PE have been dealt with in Chapter 26. In the case of cardiac tamponade the signs are a raised JVP, hypotension and muffled heart sounds. The immediate treatment is to remove the fluid in the pericardial cavity. Thereafter the patient will be transferred to a specialist unit.

Septic shock

Initial resuscitation is the same as for hypovolaemic shock. Then the source of infection has to be found and dealt with. There may be an accumulation of pus somewhere, e.g. an intra-abdominal abscess. Blood samples will need to be sent off for culture to determine appropriate antibiotic therapy; in the interim broad-spectrum antibiotics can be used. The early signs are peripheral vasodilatation due to opening of arteriovenous shunts, peripheral resistance is low, and both cardiac output and capillary flow will be high. Circulating endotoxins will depress cellular oxygenation. Later accumulation of metabolites and release of vasoactive substances (see Fig. 24.6) relax capillary arterioles leaving capillary venules constricted. Blood will accumulate in capillaries favouring fluid filtration leading to oedema, haemoconcentration, and increased blood viscosity and hypotension. Pulmonary hypertension may be seen (see Fig. 24.5). There may also be the start of reversible aggregation of red blood cells and platelets. This further reduces blood flow and increases viscosity. The release of ADP from platelets augments platelet aggregation. Cell damage, caused by endotoxins and a decrease in PGI2 production (inhibits platelet aggregation normally, see Fig. 24.5) enables even greater aggregation of platelets. Factor XII may also be activated by endotoxins. Therefore, there is a high risk of disseminated intravascular coagulation (DIC)

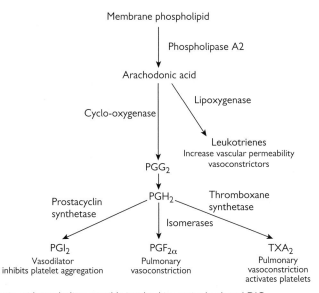

Figure 24.6 Arachidonic acid metabolites possibly involved in septic shock and DIC.

occurring. Capillaries blocked by clots, and the tissues they supply, will start to die further enhancing oedema.

Disseminated intravascular coagulation

DIC, also known as consumptive coagulopathy, leads to the formation of blood clots. These clots will use all the available coagulation factors and platelets leading to abnormal bleeding. The dying cells will release tissue factor (TF), a transmembrane glycoprotein present on the surface of endothelial cells. TF is also released from cells exposed to endotoxin. When TF binds with coagulation factors, intrinsic and extrinsic coagulation pathways will be activated. This leads to excess amounts of circulating thrombin and it acts to converts fibrinogen to fibrin, forming clots. This excess thrombin also converts plasminogen to plasmin resulting in fibrinolysis the breakdown products of fibrin have powerful anticoagulant properties. The clots can block micro- and macrovessels leading to a potential for gangrene, especially in the extremities. DIC is not confined to patients with sepsis; any form of shock can produce it but its occurrence in sepsis is more common.

Septic shock will therefore show three stages an early stage when the patient feels warm and is normotensive, followed by a stage where they are warm and hypotensive and then cold (excess sweating) and hypotensive. Septic patients are also subject to nausea and vomiting.

Anaphylactic shock

Severe anaphylaxis is usually triggered by exposure to injected proteins (insect bites), ingestion of foodstuffs (peanuts), drugs (penicillin), dyes (fluorescein), and occasionally pollens. After an initial exposure to these allergens, the immune system develops a sensitivity to them and subsequent exposure causes an 'allergic' reaction which is sudden, severe, and involves all body systems. The allergic reaction is generated by immunoglobulin E-induced release of histamine and other substances from mast cells. The effects of histamine are to cause bronchospasm, arteriolar dilation, and increased capillary permeability. Thus patients presenting with an anaphylactic reaction have difficulty breathing (wheezing), hypotension, hypovolaemia, and possibly pulmonary oedema. They can also display rashes, flushing, and swelling of the lips. The allergic reaction can occur with extreme speed and is a life-threatening scenario because of the rapid constriction of the airways. The primary treatment is the immediate administration of adrenaline which has a very powerful action on β2-adrenergic receptors in the lung causing bronchodilation. Its β1-adrenergic action on the heart has both a chronotropic and inotropic action improving cardiac output. People with established allergies usually carry a 'pen' containing adrenaline which can be used for the immediate effects allowing time to get to a hospital if their 'attack' is really serious. When they arrive antihistamines are administered (diphenhydramine, chlorphenamine) to counter the effect of circulating histamine but are usually not sufficient so are accompanied with high doses of IV corticosteroids (dexamethasone or hydrocortisone). The hypotension is treated with IV fluids. To continue medication for the bronchospasm salbutamol is used. Because of the possibility of a rebound reaction patients are carefully observed for 4 hours and if they have recovered can be allowed home.

Neurogenic shock

Here I am making the assumption that the initial resuscitation, attention to respiration, and appropriate immobilization has occurred at the site where the injury occurred and that after appropriate initial hospital resuscitation they will be transferred speedily to a specialist neurological injury unit.

Severe damage to the brain or spinal cord will result in 'spinal shock' which will shut down much of its function with a timescale dependent upon the degree of injury. Sympathetic outflow will cease and there will be a sudden decrease in peripheral vascular resistance. Patients will present with bradycardia, hypotension, warm dry extremities due to peripheral vasodilatation with no sweat gland activation, venous pooling, and will be unable to maintain their core temperature (they will become poikilothermic). Large volumes of fluid may be needed to maintain their circulation with the addition of inotropes and vasopressors. If possible, dependent upon their injury, elevating their legs above their heads can aid venous return.

Scenarios

Scenario 1

A 40-year-old man has been brought in to A&E following a RTA in which he sustained a blunt injury to the chest. He was the driver and was not wearing his seat belt. He is gasping for breath, his systolic blood pressure is 80mmHg and there is air entry into both lungs. What would you suspect and how would you manage his condition?

It's obviously not a tension pneumothorax so you would suspect a cardiac tamponade.

Signs (Beck's triad):

- Raised jugular venous pressure (JVP)
- Low systolic blood pressure
- Muffled heart sounds

Take care though:

- Raised JVP may not be present because of his hypovolaemia
- Muffled heart sounds are sometimes hard to hear in a busy A&E department
- Hypotension is most often caused by hypovolaemia

Scenario 2

A young lady has been admitted after a RTA, obviously in shock but with no sign of external bleeding. The car she was driving had skidded on an icy road and collided with a tree. She was wearing her seat belt and the car's air bags had deployed.

Signs and symptoms:

- Tachypnoea
- Dyspnoea
- Decreased breath sounds on the right side
- Tracheal deviation to the left
- Dull resonance on percussion
- Unequal chest rise
- Tachycardia
- Hypotension
- Narrowing pulse pressure
- Pale, cool, and clammy skin
- Prolonged capillary refill

Answers

Scenario 1

Management

Investigation required is an echocardiogram as quickly as possible.

Do not delay treatment if the patient is unstable and not responding to resuscitation. This case warrants an active intervention—in this case pericardiocentesis.

Pericardiocentesis

Under local anaesthesia a wide-bore needle is inserted to the left of the xiphisternum between the xiphisternum and the ribcage. The needle is advanced towards the tip of the scapula into the pericardial space. An ECG electrode attached to the needle will indicate when the heart is touched by an increased T-wave and needle induced dysrhythmias.

Withdrawal of 15–20ml of blood may result in an immediate improvement. An experienced cardiac surgeon whom you called when starting the pericardiocentesis should have arrived and will consider the advisability of an open pericardiotomy.

Scenario 2

The signs for this patient all indicate blood loss into the pleural cavity, i.e. a haemothorax. Remember that each side of the thorax can hold up to 30–40% of a person's blood volume.

Treatment and management

Fluid resuscitation plus high-flow oxygen. The blood must be drained from the thoracic cavity by inserting a chest drain on the patient's right-hand side. Usually the bleeding will stop after a drain is inserted and the lung re-expands. The drain has to be carefully managed because the blood in the pleural space is liable to clot and clog the drain. The patient has to be carefully monitored to check that the bleeding has stopped.

Chapter 25 Sepsis and multiorgan failure

Introduction

Sepsis and its management is a vital aspect of a surgeon's professional life. A surgical trainee will be called upon to manage patients with sepsis mostly in an emergency. In some situations one may be aware that sepsis is the primary reason for presentation whilst in others, sepsis has occurred as an unexpected complication.

As a surgical trainee, the ability to manage sepsis is paramount. Otherwise a preventable cause of death might be missed. It is essential to be able to diagnose the presence of sepsis, ascertain the source of sepsis, and finally treat the condition with, if necessary, senior help. The management may turn out to be a multidisciplinary team effort with the involvement of the microbiologist, radiologist, and intensive care specialist.

> The examination candidate may come across the topics of sepsis, multiorgan dysfunction syndrome (MODS), and multiple-organ failure (MOF) in 'Applied surgical science and critical care' stations, both generic and specialty context; also in certain communication stations such scenarios may be present, e.g. phoning the consultant about a post-operative problem or a diagnostic conundrum, management in post-operative pyrexia.

> After a brief discussion of sepsis in general, several scenarios will be given. The reader is expected to make the diagnosis, think about the investigations, and then formulate a management. To make this chapter an interesting challenge, at the end of all the scenarios, a list of the diagnoses is given in the form of an extended matching questions (EMQ) exercise. The answers to each of the scenarios are given at the end of the chapter.

> The examiner is looking to see if the candidate is on the correct diagnostic pathway, if a systematic assessment is carried out, if the candidate seeks help in case of doubt as in the telephone conversation station, and if the candidate has a fair idea about the overall management of the problem

Clinical situations

In surgical practice, sepsis may be encountered when a patient on the ward, usually post-operative, fails to progress. On the other hand, a septic patient may be seen, for the first time, as an emergency. In both situations the cause is to be determined by investigations followed by the appropriate treatment. One must be aware that on occasions there may be a patient whose sepsis is the result of a hospital acquired infection (nosocomial infection).

Clinical features

There should always be a high index of suspicion, for this diagnosis, particularly in the post-operative patient who has had an operation for abdominal sepsis such as acute perforated appendicitis, perforated diverticulitis, and emergency bowel resection. Patients with a CVP line, an indwelling urinary catheter, and those with pre-operative comorbid respiratory diseases are particularly vulnerable to infection. The common clinical pointers are:

- Fever, rarely hypothermia
- Tachycardia
- Tachypnoea and hypoxia
- Altered mental state
- Oliguria
- Obvious suspected source: a post-operative patient

A full clinical examination is carried out. When a patient is admitted with clinical features of sepsis without any obvious cause, pathology should be sought in the GU, GI, and biliary tracts. Renal cell carcinoma and urothelial cancer may sometimes present with 'pyrexia of unknown origin'.

Investigations

Laboratory

- Blood cultures; these may be sterile as the symptoms may be due to mediators and not from the presence of bacteria themselves
- Full blood count: PMN leucocytosis (rarely leucopenia)
- Specimen of urine (midstream or from catheter)
- Sputum

Imaging

- CXR
- USS
- CT scan
- MRI

The imaging technique used will depend upon the clinical suspicion. Resuscitation should not be delayed by the need for investigations. The two should run in parallel.

General measures

Once sepsis is suspected and the appropriate investigations are set in motion, immediate resuscitation is started in the form of IV fluids, oxygen, and 'best guess' antibiotics. The latter is changed according to the blood cultures (which if possible, should be taken before antibiotics are started). Once the source of infection has been found, specific measures such as surgery or interventional radiology need to be considered.

Terminology

If clinical sepsis is accompanied by any two or more of the following, then **SIRS** (systemic inflammatory response syndrome) is diagnosed: pyrexia of <36°C or >38°C, tachycardia of >90/min, tachypnoea of >20/min, WBC count >12,000/mm³ or > 10% of immature neutrophils. SIRS is caused by any condition giving rise to prolonged or inadequately treated infection, trauma, burns, and severe acute pancreatitis.

Sepsis syndrome is a diagnosis made when SIRS is accompanied by a confirmed infectious process and where there are signs of at least one organ dysfunction. Examples are: CNS (confusion), respiratory system (pneumonia/ARDS), cardiovascular system (arrhythmia/hypotension), the liver (jaundice), the kidneys (oliguria), haematological system (coagulopathy) or severe metabolic acidosis. In cases with sepsis syndrome, **septic shock** is diagnosed when hypotension is not responsive to intensive care therapy with inotropes. This is only one step away from **MODS** a precursor of Multiorgan failure (**MOF**) which leads to death.

Multiple organ dysfunction syndrome (MODS)

MODS can be defined as a syndrome characterized by failure of two or more organ systems. This occurs following severe shock where there is hypoperfusion. The sequence of events may be as follows: functioning organ → insult → organ dysfunction → organ failure. Thus MODS can lead to MOF, the ultimate outcome in untreated or uncontrolled infection (Fig. 25.1).

The organ systems that might fail are: cardiovascular, respiratory, renal, haematological, GI, and neurological. These organs are interdependent and the result is progressive physiological failure due to hypoxia and hypotension.

In cardiovascular failure the patient may have hypotension requiring inotropes; respiratory failure may need ventilation; renal failure may require dialysis, haematological failure causing disseminated intravascular coagulation (DIC) needing platelet infusions; GI failure causing ileus and stress ulcerations may need parenteral nutrition and H₂ receptor antagonists; finally neurological failure is diagnosed where the GCS score is <15 (in the absence of head injury) requiring overall supportive therapy.

The summary of management of MODS is: control the cause, prevent tissue hypoxia, institute correct metabolic support, prevent nosocomial infections, and modify and control the acute inflammatory response. The prognosis worsens when more organs are involved and longer the condition lasts.

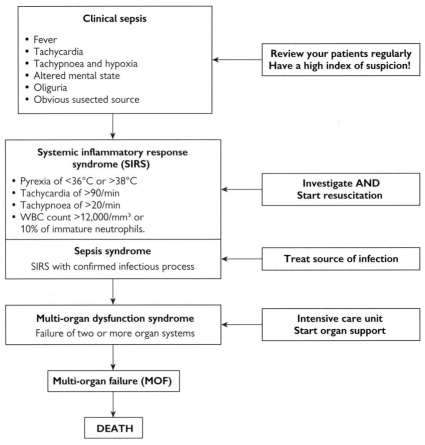

Figure 25.1 Progression of untreated/uncontrolled infection.

(Acknowledgement: Smith SM and Bihari DJ (1997) Multiple-organ failure, in Goldhill D and Withington S (eds.) *Textbook of Intensive Care*. London: Chapman & Hall.)

Scenarios

The remainder of the chapter is devoted to clinical scenarios. In the examination stations these would be shown to the candidate. The candidate should read the scenario and talk it through in his/her mind about the cause of sepsis, investigations, and overall management.

The scenarios will be given first with all the answers at the end of the chapter. In order to give the reader a good academic exercise in self-assessment, the answers will not be in order but 'jumbled' to make it an exercise in EMQs.

Scenario 1

A 60-year-old woman has been admitted as an emergency with a 4-day history of severe right upper quadrant pain, vomiting, jaundice, and intense pruritis. She is very toxic—high temperature with rigors and hyperdynamic circulation. What is your diagnosis? Outline the management plan.

Scenario 2

A 70-year-old man has been admitted as an emergency with severe right loin pain, dull in nature, without any radiation. It has been present for 8 hours. He applied a hot water bottle to the area, took several strong analgesics, and when the pain became unbearable he consulted his GP who sent him in after injecting him with morphine. The GP has made a diagnosis of 'renal colic' as the patient had dysuria and frequency.

On examination he has tachycardia of 90/min, tachypnoeic, pyrexia of 40°C, fullness in the right loin with overlying oedema and redness from the hot water bottle and extremely tender.

Scenario 3

A 65-year-old lady has been admitted with dull aching pain in her left iliac fossa coming in spasms. In between the spasms she is left with discomfort which at times is 'agony'. She normally suffers from constipation, having a bowel action every 2 or 3 days. She is apyrexial with some tenderness in the left iliac fossa.

She has been treated as constipation from 'diverticulitis' with analgesia. After 2 days her pain is much worse. She has pyrexia of 39°C, and is extremely tender. You can feel a boggy mass and some local distension. She does not like to move because of the pain.

Scenario 4

A 50-year-old patient underwent an emergency cholecystectomy for a gangrenous, perforated gall bladder 5 days ago. The operation was commenced laparoscopically but was converted to an open procedure as the dissection was difficult. The procedure was completed through a midline incision and a drain was left in Morrison's pouch. Post-operatively there was hardly any drainage and the drain removed after 3 days.

From the 5th day onwards he became very toxic, with a temperature of 40°C. He became very tender in the right upper quadrant at the site of the drain and complained of pain in his right shoulder tip. He has signs of fluid in the right lung base and is quite dyspnoeic.

Scenario 5

A 70-year-old man underwent an anterior resection for rectal cancer 6 days ago. He progressed uneventfully for about 5 days. Thereafter his abdomen started to get distended, he became oliguric, tachypnoeic, and tachycardic; his blood pressure was 90/60mmHg. He was apyrexial. The abdomen was tender all over with rebound and rigidity.

Scenario 6

Following an abdomino-perineal resection (A-P resection), a 66-year-old patient started getting rigors after 48 hours. At the height of his rigors his temperature was 39°C. His chest is clear and he has no untoward abdominal signs. His abdominal and perineal wounds are fine.

Scenario 7

A 45-year-old man was admitted with gradual onset of severe abdominal pain radiating to the back. It had been present for 4 hours. The pain spread all over the abdomen and was associated with severe vomiting of clear fluid. On examination he had tachycardia, tachypnoea, dehydration, and a blood pressure of 100/60mmHg. Abdominal examination showed generalized tenderness, rigidity, signs of peritonism, and bluish discoloration around the umbilicus.

He was resuscitated with full supportive measures and his serum amylase came back as 3000IU. He was treated as acute pancreatitis. After further investigations he was transferred to the HDU. Four days after his admission he developed a temperature ranging from 38–40°C and slight jaundice. His abdomen continued to be distended but was not as tender as before, probably because of his good pain control.

Scenario 8

A 25-year-old lady was admitted with typical features of acute appendicitis, her symptoms lasting for well over 24 hours before operation. A perforated gangrenous appendix was removed. She was discharged home 5 days later.

She returned after 3 days with fever and rigors, generally feeling unwell. On examination she looked toxic with lower abdominal tenderness. Her incision site was fine. She was very uncomfortable on vaginal and rectal examination.

Scenario 9

A 55-year-old lady who is known to suffer from large bowel Crohn's disease was admitted with a foul smelling vaginal discharge for 3–4 weeks' duration. She has been developing temperature on and off during this period. In general she has been feeling very unwell. On examination she looks ill with obvious signs of weight loss, pyrexia of 39°C and generalized abdominal tenderness. There is a midline scar of a previous hysterectomy.

Scenario 10

A 72-year-old man, a chronic smoker, underwent a left hemicolectomy for colon cancer 4 days ago. He now feels increasingly breathless, looks cyanosed and his pulse oximeter shows an oxygen saturation of 92%. The air entry into both lung bases is poor. He is on nasal oxygen. There are no untoward signs in his abdomen.

The diagnoses in the 10 scenarios above are given below in a jumbled order for you, as the reader, to match them as an exercise in 'Extended Matching Questions'. The answers for each scenario are given in the way you should answer them.

Choose your answers from the following diagnoses

A	Urinary infection
B	Chest infection
C	Leaking large bowel anastomosis
D	Subphrenic abscess
E	Colovaginal fistula
F	Pelvic abscess
G	Diverticular abscess
H	Acute pyonephrosis
I	Acute cholecystitis and cholangitis
J	Acute pancreatic necrosis

In the oral examination remember to answer in 'first person singular' For example: 'I would make a diagnosis of…. my investigations would be… I would treat the patient with…'.

Answers

Scenario 1

I Acute cholecystitis and cholangitis

- With these clinical features, my diagnosis in this 60-year-old lady would be acute cholecystitis with acute cholangitis because she has high temperature with rigors and obstructive jaundice causing pruritis. The hyperdynamic circulation—bounding pulse, large pulse pressure—means that she is in the early stages of septic shock. I would also like to exclude co-incidental acute pancreatitis
- I would now investigate her, confirm my diagnosis, and then institute my definitive treatment
- I would send blood cultures and start the patient on IV fluids and 'best guess' antibiotics. FBC may show PMN leucocytosis; LFTs would show deranged liver function with raised alkaline phosphatase, prolongation of prothrombin time, and there may be an increase in serum amylase
- I would do an urgent USS of the liver and biliary tract to look for gall stones particularly in the CBD. If the CBD is dilated and no stones can be seen because of overlying bowel gas, then I would get a magnetic resonance cholangiopancreatography done
- Once stones are confirmed in the CBD, I would get an endoscopic retrograde cholangiopancreatography and endoscopic papillotomy done. This would be followed by laparoscopic cholecystectomy at the same admission
- While all this is going on, I would give the patient 5% dextrose, the appropriate antibiotics according to the blood cultures and vitamin K. I may consider giving the patient mannitol to prevent hepatorenal syndrome causing renal failure
- Should the patient have acute pancreatitis, then I would concentrate on that first by stratifying the severity and go on from there

Scenario 2

H Acute pyonephrosis

- This patient has acute pain in his right renal region with toxic features. The fullness in the loin and extreme tenderness with overlying oedema points to a diagnosis of acute pyonephrosis
- I would give him morphine as an analgesia and start IV fluids. Having sent bloods for culture, FBC, and U&Es, I would also start him on broad-spectrum antibiotics
- I would ask for an urgent USS of his kidneys. This would show the right renal pelvis to be a bag of pus (pyonephrosis). The interventional radiologist would at the same time do a percutaneous nephrostomy and drain

the pus. The catheter would be left in place in the renal pelvis until the patient recovers from this acute phase which may take up to a week
- An antegrade pyelogram is then done to see the site and cause of the ureteric obstruction. I would ask for an isotope renogram to see the exact amount of function in that kidney, at the same time making sure that the other kidney is functioning normally
- If the kidney function is >20% then the kidney is salvaged by removing the cause which may be a stone or congenital hydronephrosis (to be treated by pyeloplasty—Anderson–Hynes or endopyelotomy)
- If kidney function is <20% then the patient should undergo a subcapsular nephrectomy

Scenario 3

G *Diverticular abscess*
- The history of this 65-year-old lady is typical of acute diverticulitis to start with. While in hospital she deteriorated and developed a full-blown pericolic abscess
- I would resuscitate this patient with IV fluids and analgesia. Having sent all the bloods for FBC, U&Es, and blood culture, I would start the patient on broad-spectrum antibiotics
- I would have the patient imaged by USS or CT scan, the latter being much more accurate although it has the drawback of radiation. This would confirm an abscess
- An abscess would be drained by US or CT guidance. The patient's condition would improve greatly although she has a high chance of developing a faecal fistula. This should be treated conservatively
- After 4–6 weeks the patient should be thoroughly imaged: a flexible sigmoidoscopy or colonoscopy should be performed to exclude an unsuspected carcinoma within the diverticular segment. This may not be successful because of the diverticular stricture. A CECT scan of the left colon should also be performed with a fistulogram and barium enema if necessary
- I would expect the faecal fistula to have dried up after a couple of months or so. After all the investigations are at hand, the patient should have a sigmoid colectomy

Scenario 4

D *Subphrenic abscess*
- As the patient had a difficult emergency cholecystectomy as evidenced by the conversion, I would suspect a fluid collection in Morrison's pouch. He has all the classical features of the saying 'Pus somewhere, pus nowhere, pus under the diaphragm'
- I would resuscitate the patient by full supportive therapy—IV fluids, analgesia, and broad-spectrum antibiotics. All routine blood tests need to be done including blood cultures
- I would get an USS and/or CT done. This should be accompanied by drainage under US or CT guidance
- As a subphrenic abscess can be multilocular, the procedure may have to be repeated. In rare instances because of the thick nature of the pus and multiple loculi, an open drainage by the extraperitoneal route may be necessary

Scenario 5

C *Leaking large bowel anastomosis*
- As this patient had an anterior resection, I would have the diagnosis of anastomotic leak very high in my index of suspicion. My patient is very ill with respiratory, renal, and cardiovascular problems. Therefore something very serious has happened, such as breakdown in the anastomosis
- After doing all the routine blood tests, I would have a contrast CT done which would confirm if a leak has occurred. If the complication is confirmed, the patient needs thorough optimization for theatre
- I would ask the anaesthetist's help in resuscitating him, reserving a bed in the ICU and arranging theatre
- At operation I would expect my consultant to dismantle the anastomosis, bring out a terminal left iliac end colostomy, close off the rectum as a Hartmann's procedure, and finish the operation by thorough pelvic lavage with several litres of warm normal saline
- I would expect this patient to have a very stormy post-operative period

Scenario 6

A *Urinary infection*
- As every patient undergoing an A-P resection has an indwelling catheter for a few days post-operatively, I would suspect urinary tract infection (UTI) as the first cause of pyrexia in the absence of chest and wound infection. The 2nd day post-operatively is really too early for a wound infection to be the cause of his problems

- I would send off a catheter specimen of urine (CSU) for culture and blood cultures. I would replace the catheter and wash out the bladder with warm normal saline. The patient is put on the appropriate antibiotic. Bladder washouts may be done twice daily for 3–4 days

Scenario 7

J Acute pancreatic necrosis (Fig. 25.2)

- This patient has acute pancreatitis. The fact that as a patient with acute pancreatitis he has been transferred to the HDU after more investigations means that he is suffering from severe acute pancreatitis. The subsequent investigations were done to determine the grade of severity of the disease
- I would now wish to find out the cause of his pyrexia. In this situation the patient needs an urgent CECT to look for pancreatic necrosis. If the presence of pancreatic necrosis is confirmed, the radiologist would then perform a CT-guided FNAC to see if the necrotic tissue is infected
- If infected necrosis is confirmed, the patient should be started on broad-spectrum antibiotics. I would subject the patient to a laparotomy with a view to pancreatic necrosectomy
- This is carried out with a roof-top (bilateral Kocher's) incision. The lesser sac is entered, all the debris is removed, thorough washout of the area performed, and two wide-bore drains are left in place. Any biliary pathology is dealt with at the same time followed by a feeding jejunostomy. The wound may be closed as a laparostomy as such a patient may require further explorations for more necrosectomy.
- The patient is transferred to the ICU. The patient should have further CECT carried out at intervals. The drains may be used to do further washouts in the ICU

Scenario 8

F Pelvic abscess

- This patient, who has had an appendicectomy for acute perforated appendicitis, has developed post-operative pyrexia. In such a patient, I would always bear in mind the possibility of an intra-abdominal abscess. As she is toxic with discomfort on internal examination, she is most likely to have a pelvic abscess
- I would give her a broad-spectrum antibiotic, IV fluids, and full supportive therapy to prevent her from going into septic shock
- I would have her urgently imaged by pelvic, transvaginal, and/or transrectal US to confirm the abscess. Ideally, this should be done under an anaesthetic when also EUA (examination under anaesthesia) is carried out. At the same time the abscess is drained transvaginally. If the abscess is large with several loculi, this would require a formal laparotomy

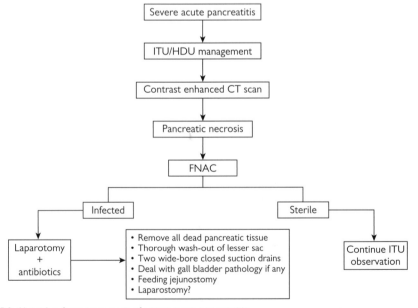

Figure 25.2 Algorithm for management of severe acute pancreatitis.

Scenario 9

E Colovaginal fistula

- This 55-year-old lady is a known patient of large bowel Crohn's disease. This condition is notorious for forming fistulae. It is apparent that she has a foul smelling vaginal discharge. I would strongly suspect that she has developed a colovaginal fistula, particularly in view of the fact that she had a hysterectomy in the past
- I would involve the gastroenterologist and the gynaecologist at an early stage as management of this patient requires a team approach
- I would do all the blood tests—blood culture, FBC, U&Es, LFTs, C-reactive protein (CRP). I would send a vaginal swab for culture and sensitivity (C&S). She needs imaging and an EUA along with a gynaecologist. This patient is ideally managed along with a gynaecologist
- Colonoscopy and biopsy of the area of Crohn's is done as malignant transformation in colonic Crohn's can occur. CECT of the pelvis is done to view the fistulous tract
- I would also consult the gastroenterologist with regard to the best drug treatment; whether an immunosuppressive should be used. The patient should be optimized prior to consideration for surgery where the affected segment of bowel will have to be removed and the vaginal fistula closed

Scenario 10

B Chest infection

- This patient who has had a major bowel resection for cancer is hypoxic and liable to develop post-operative chest infection in view of his smoking habit. His clinical features and the low oxygen saturation show that his respiratory function is compromised
- I would send sputum for C&S, do ABGs, and ask for a CXR. The patient would have respiratory acidosis. The CXR may show diffuse changes, bilateral basal bronchopneumonia, and pleural effusion; empyema, lung abscess or acute respiratory distress syndrome (ARDS) may supervene later. I would transfer the patient to the HDU
- I would start the patient on humidified oxygen, physiotherapy, and antibiotics on empirical grounds. I would involve the anaesthetist at an early stage just in case the patient should deteriorate rapidly and may require ventilation
- If there is evidence of atelectasis, vigorous physiotherapy should be instituted. If this is unsuccessful, bedside flexible bronchoscopy by the anaesthetist is carried out. As a last resort the patient may require bedside mini-tracheostomy by the Seldinger technique

Chapter 26 **Respiratory system in critical care**

Introduction

The principal task of the lungs is respiration, which means, for the purposes of this chapter, the exchange of oxygen (O_2) from the inhaled air into the bloodstream and of carbon dioxide (CO_2) from the blood to exhaled air. To achieve this, the respiratory system needs:

- An airway to conduct atmospheric air into the alveoli and alveolar air out of the lungs
- A mechanism to produce the forces required to move gases into and out of the lungs
- An exchange surface to allow the O_2 into the bloodstream and CO_2 out
- A system to transfer inhaled O_2 to the tissues and the CO_2 from tissue metabolism to the alveoli to be exhaled
- A control system to adjust respiratory effort to changing demands
- Apart from these functions the lungs play a 'metabolic' role
- A vital role in acid–base regulation (see Chapter 28)

Airway

Structures involved

Air is conducted to the lungs via the nasal and oral cavities to the pharynx and into the trachea. The trachea branches into two bronchi, one supplying each lung. These then divide repeatedly, some 16 times, giving rise to the terminal bronchioles. Those with a few alveoli in their walls, the respiratory bronchioles, lead to the alveolar ducts and have at their ends the alveolar sacs (approximately 3,000,000 in total). Gas exchange is limited to the alveolar portion of the system which has an approximate surface area of $100m^2$ and a total volume of some 3.0L. The exchange, alveolar, surfaces of the lungs are in close apposition with the capillaries from the pulmonary circulation. These alveolar capillaries form an interconnecting network giving an almost continuous sheet of vessels on the alveolar walls. The non-exchange surface of the lung, the bronchial tree, is supplied with blood from the bronchiole arteries arising from the aorta with a flow of some 50ml per minute.

Function of the airway

In its passage to the alveoli the inhaled air is heated to 37°C, saturated with water vapour, and cleansed. Large particles of dirt (>20μm) are filtered by the nasal hairs—useful for recognizing potential inhalational damage in burns victims; moderate to small sized particles (>10μm) collide with the walls of the bronchi (particles tend to travel in a straight line and in a multibranched system will hit the walls) and are trapped in a layer of mucus. These trapped particles are either phagocytosed by macrophages or are propelled in the mucus secretion towards the glottis by the ciliated epithelial cells lining the bronchial tree at a rate of around 1cm/min. About 10–100ml of mucus is produced per day, depending upon a variety of factors such as local irritants e.g. cigarette smoke and parasympathetic (vagal) activity. This mucus film is usually swallowed when it reaches the glottis. In diseased states there is an excessive production of mucus which needs to be removed by coughing. Particles (0.1–10μm) deposited on the alveolar wall are taken up by macrophages which either migrate towards the bronchial tree or enter the lymphatic drainage of the lung.

Control of the airway

Because the bronchioles are firmly anchored in the surrounding lung tissue their diameter increases as the lung inflates. Patients with diseased airways and an increased airway resistance, e.g. bronchial asthmatics, often breathe with an increased lung volume at rest which reduces the airway resistance. Another important control is the overall tone of the bronchial musculature which is controlled by the autonomic nervous system. Sympathetic activity causes bronchodilatation whereas parasympathetic activity causes bronchoconstriction. Sympathetic activity is effected by an action on β receptors. β2 agonists such as salbutamol, which has a prolonged action, are used to control the bronchoconstriction seen in asthmatic patients, usually by means of an inhaler. The nebulizers used to deliver a drug in this manner need to be carefully designed to give droplets of the correct size so that they can reach the smaller bronchioles before settling on their walls. Other factors which lead to bronchoconstriction are a fall in pCO_2 due to hyperventilation or a local reduction in pulmonary blood flow, possibly via a direct action on the bronchial smooth muscle. Bronchoconstriction can also be caused reflexly by stimulation of receptors in the trachea and large bronchi by irritants such as cigarette smoke, inhaled dust, cold air, or by noxious gases.

Obstruction of the upper airway by foreign bodies, trauma, burns, tumours, haematomas (particularly after thyroid surgery), laryngeal oedema, stenosis after endotracheal intubation, or tracheostomy can lead to dyspnoea (respiratory distress) with inspiratory stridor and wheezing. This sound is caused by an increased turbulence in the air-flow. Patients compensate, initially, with increased inspiratory effort. However, if it persists the patients become exhausted and deteriorate rapidly and need to have an assisted airway—intubation or tracheostomy. Both these procedures will result in a dramatic decrease in the humidification and warming of the inhaled air which means that the air they breathe must be artificially warmed and humidified. In addition the normal means of removing the mucus flow from the bronchial tree will not exist and their mucus will need to be removed by suction.

Mechanics of respiration

Basic physiology

The structure of the lung parenchyma which contains both collagen and elastic fibres plus the surface tension of the thin layer of fluid covering the external surface of the alveoli will act together to give a force which will make the lungs tend to collapse. The pleural cavities (one for each lung), consist of the layer lining the chest wall (parietal pleura) and that applied to the lungs (pulmonary or visceral pleura) and the gap between them is filled with a small amount of fluid. At a fixed temperature fluids will not expand and the action of the elastic forces acting on the pleural cavity results in a negative pressure of around $-3cmH_2O$ preventing the lungs from totally collapsing. On inspiration the diaphragm contracts and moves downwards by some 7cm. This action increases the negative pressure in the pleural cavity to around $-6cmH_2O$. The decreased pleural pressure will generate a small negative pressure in the thoracic cavity which will drag air into and inflate the lungs (see Fig. 26.1).

Diaphragmatic contraction alone is responsible for around 75% of the inspiratory volume increase. The rest of the volume expansion is accomplished by contraction of the external intercostal muscles.

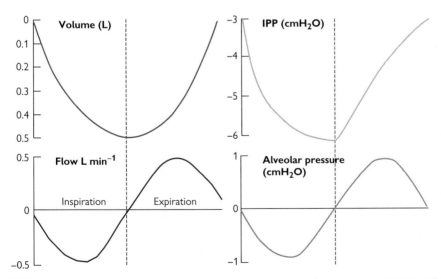

Figure 26.1 This shows the change in lung volume (Volume), the change in intrapleural pressure (IPP), the difference in lung pressure generated by the IPP (Alveolar pressure), and air flow (Flow) during a single respiratory cycle in the resting subject.

These are mechanically linked with the ribs to move the rib cage upwards. This action pushes the sternum upwards and outwards and increases the anterior–posterior diameter of the rib cage. Movements generated by either the diaphragm or the rib cage can sustain adequate respiration at rest. If the movement of the diaphragm is impeded, as in late pregnancy, ventilation on exercise will not be adequate. This is obvious when a heavily pregnant woman is carrying heavy shopping or walking upstairs. For resting respiration, expiration is a passive process governed by the elastic recoil of the lungs, the return of the rib cage to its starting position as the intercostal muscles relax and the return of the diaphragm to its original position. During exercise or forced inspiration the accessory muscles come into play. The scalene muscles elevate the first two ribs and the sternocleidomastoids move the sternum outwards. A very strong inspiratory effort can reduce the pleural pressure as low as $-40\text{cmH}_2\text{O}$. During exercise, expiration is aided by contraction of the internal intercostal muscles whose insertion acts on the rib joints to pull the rib cage down and decrease the chest wall expansion.

The presence of a negative pleural pressure poses potential dangers. If, for whatever reason, air or blood enters the pleural cavity the pressure will immediately decline towards zero and the lung will collapse.

Types of pneumothorax.

A primary spontaneous pneumothorax **can** develop, for no apparent reason, in young adults (<40 years of age) developing usually via a tear in the apex of the lung, releasing alveolar air into the pleural cavity. This condition has symptoms of sudden pain on the affected side, which becomes more severe on inspiration, and is accompanied by breathlessness. Secondary spontaneous pneumothorax can develop in patients with existing lung disease, e.g. emphysema, when the lung can rupture into the pleural cavity. Treatment depends upon the severity of the pneumothorax. Conservative management consists of careful patient monitoring and allowing the air to be absorbed into the bloodstream. Alternatively a needle can be inserted into the pleural cavity and via a suitably valved syringe the air can be sucked out. For a severe pneumothorax a chest drain needs to be inserted. Other causes of air leaking from the lungs into the pleural cavity are barotrauma either as a result of an explosion or positive pressure artificial ventilation or as a consequence of inserting a central venous line.

An open pneumothorax occurs when there is a penetrating injury to the chest wall. In this case the pleural cavity pressure will immediately become zero (that of the atmosphere) and the lung will totally collapse due to the parenchymal elastic fibres and the surface tension of the fluid lining the alveolar wall. Gas exchange of the lung on the unaffected side will be compromised because:

- Air will be exchanged, in part, with the collapsed lung on breathing out
- The weight of the collapsed lung will impede full inflation of the remaining lung, and
- The abnormal pressure in the pleural cavity presses the mediastinum onto the healthy side

This condition is treated by repairing the wound to stop any haemorrhage, repairing the hole in the chest wall, and inserting a chest drain. The same change in intrapleural pressure will occur if there is haemorrhaging into the pleural cavity. The differential diagnosis between a pneumothorax and a haemothorax is relatively simple and can be explained by the difference in sound you hear when striking a tin can full of fluid, a dull resonance compared to an empty one, a hyper-resonance.

Some penetrating injuries can result in a wound with a tissue flap which allows air into the pleural cavity on inspiration but does not allow its outflow on expiration. In this case the pressure in the pleural cavity will become increasingly positive. There will be a distinct mediastinal shift to the opposite side usually big enough to push the trachea towards the unaffected side. As the pressure increases the resultant hypoxia causes vigorous ventilation and the intra-pleural pressure can rapidly rise to 2.7–4.0kPa (20–30mmHg). The pressure in the inferior vena cava is around $5\text{cmH}_2\text{O}$ (3.8mmHg) so that small rises in pressure can collapse this vessel resulting in a considerable decrease in venous return. The life-threatening nature of this condition is readily apparent when you take into account that the pulmonary circulation has a systolic pressure of 25mmHg. Thus speedy treatment, by inserting a wide-bore needle into the second intercostal space is vital. Once in place there will be an audible hiss as the compressed air is released. The wound needs to be sealed and a chest drain inserted and the patient carefully monitored.

There is one more condition which can have a major effect on lung ventilation: this occurs when a rib or ribs each suffer multiple fractures. This condition is described as flail chest and is easily recognized because the affected part of the rib cage will move inwards on inspiration. Therefore, the lung under this part of the chest will deflate upon inspiration and upon expiration the neighbouring parts of the lung will inflate the affected part of the lung. A volume of gas will be shunted back and forth between adjacent parts of the lung(s) and play no part in respiratory exchange with atmospheric air. Treatment is to put a large sticking plaster over the affected area to anchor normal and abnormal chest wall together to restore the appropriate movement and hence appropriate respiration.

Respiratory parameters

At rest the respiratory rate is between 12 to 16 breaths/min. (*Most 'normal' data has been obtained from American medical student laboratory classes and pertains to fit, healthy people, around 20 years of age with a mean weight of 70kg.*) Obviously parameters change with age; new born babies have a respiratory rate of 44 breaths/min which declines steadily to adult rates. The volume of air inspired is around 500ml (tidal volume) which gives a total rate of change of some 6–8L/min (respiratory minute volume). Not all of this gas is involved in alveolar gas exchange a certain amount of inspired air will remain in the air passages, around 150ml (anatomical dead space) which amounts to approximately 2.2ml/kg body weight. On exercise the total ventilation can go as high as 160L/min. If a young fit adult is asked to breathe in as deeply as possible after a normal expiration, a single inspiration can move 3.5L into the lungs. Thus an extra 3L of air (3.5–0.5L tidal volume) can be drawn into the lungs and constitutes the inspiratory reserve volume. If asked to make a forced expiration a volume of 1.5L can be breathed out (expiratory reserve volume). Thus a total volume of 4.5L can be exchanged in vigorous breathing (vital capacity). Even after a forced expiration some air still remains in the lungs and this amounts to some 1.5L (residual volume see Fig. 26.2).

A much easier determination of respiratory capability is to measure the volume of air that can be forcibly exhaled in 1 second—the FEV_1. If this is expressed as a percentage of the volume of air that can be expelled as hard and as far as possible after a full inspiration the forced vital capacity (FVC) (usually to determine the vital capacity the subject has to strain hard to achieve the maximum volume possible and thus most patients will not give, or be able to give their all in this manoeuvre) then this value can be used as a diagnostic tool. Normally the relative FEV_1 (FEV1/FVC) is >80% at 20 years, >75% at 40 years,

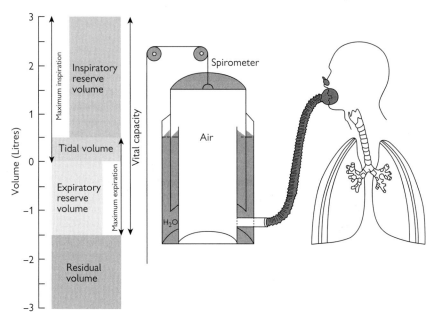

Figure 26.2 Measurement of lung volumes with a spirometer.

Table **26.1** Proportion of gases in room air, the alveoli, and expired air. All values expressed as kPa (mm Hg)

Gas	Room air	Alveolar air, kPa (mmHg)	Expired air
O_2	21.17 (158.8)	13.33 (100.0)	15.33 (115.0)
CO_2	0.03 (0.23)	5.20 (39.0)	4.40 (33.0)
H_2O	–	6.27 (47.0)	6.27 (47.0)
N_2	80.1 (601.0)	76.50 (574.0)	75.33 (565.0)

and >70% at 60 years. In restrictive pulmonary disease, e.g. pulmonary oedema, both FEV_1 and FVC are reduced and the ratio tends to give normal values. The ratio is reduced in obstructive pulmonary disease, e.g. asthma and emphysema. Needless to say a single measure of respiratory capability is not of much use. It is more enlightening to take serial measures when the disease process can be examined to detect changes.

The respiratory exchange surface

Gaseous exchange

First we have to look at Dalton's law: *in a mixture of gases the partial pressure of each gas is equal to the total gas pressure times the fractional concentration of the gas. At sea level air has a mean barometric pressure of 101.3kPa (760mmHg).* Using this relationship the proportion of gases in room air, the alveoli, and expired air are shown in Table 26.1.

Gas exchange only occurs in the alveolated portion of the lung which comprises a volume of roughly 3L. The walls of the alveoli form a barrier between the capillaries comprised of: a) an alveolar epithelial cell covered by a thin layer of fluid containing pulmonary surfactant, b) an interstitial layer, and c) a capillary endothelial cell . This barrier is <0.5μm thick in places. The combination of a large surface area and small thickness are ideal characteristics for diffusional exchange across the alveolar walls.

Blood is delivered to the alveolar capillaries which form a dense network and give an almost continuous sheet on the internal alveolar wall. In maximal respiratory effort some 80% of the total alveolar wall area is made available for gaseous exchange. Air is delivered to the alveoli by flow through the bronchioles but the exchange of gases in the blind alveoli into and out of the blood takes place by diffusion alone. Gases will diffuse across the barrier (i.e. liquid/alveolar cell/interstitial fluid/capillary epithelial cell) from regions of high to low partial pressure. Diffusion through a barrier will depend upon many factors, the principle ones of which are its area and thickness, the molecular weight of the diffusing molecule, and the solubility of the gas. In this case diffusion is proportional to the solubility of the gas in saline divided by the square root of the gas molecular weight. Comparing the quotients of the molecular weights of CO_2 (MW 44) and O_2 (MW 32) means that CO_2 diffuses 20% slower than O_2 because of its molecular weight. However, CO_2 is approximately 24 times more soluble than O_2 so that its diffusion rate is overall 20 times that of O_2.

The exchange is, however, a bit more complicated than these figures would suggest. Gases have to exchange between the alveoli and the bloodstream so that the diffusional path will be considerably longer than the 0.5μm liquid/cellular structural barrier. The gases will have to diffuse through the plasma and across the cell walls of the red blood corpuscles. The O_2 will have to react with the haemoglobin which takes a finite time, approximately 200msec and a similar limit will occur with CO_2 removal because the reactions are equally complex. These include the exchange of chloride and bicarbonate ions across the red cell membrane, the conversion of bicarbonate to CO_2 and H_2O in the red blood cells catalysed by carbonic anhydrase, the decoupling of carbamino compounds and the diffusion of the CO_2 produced out of the red blood cells. All of these reactions occur with approximately the same speed with which O_2 reacts with haemoglobin. Under normal conditions there will be a considerable safety margin for these reactions since the pulmonary venous blood is in contact with the alveoli for around 750msec. The quantities of gas/liquid interplay are shown in Fig. 26.3.

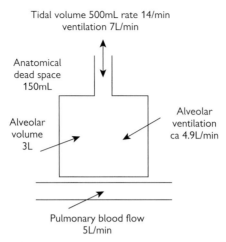

Tidal volume 500mL rate 14/min
ventilation 7L/min

Anatomical
dead space
150mL

Alveolar
volume
3L

Alveolar
ventilation
ca 4.9L/min

Pulmonary blood flow
5L/min

Figure 26.3 Quantities of gas and fluid involved in respiratory exchange at rest. Comparison of the vital capacity (ca. 4.5L) and tidal volume indicates that only some 9% of the lung is used at rest.

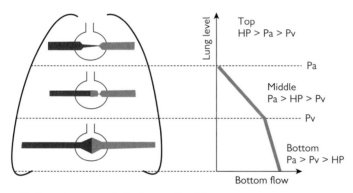

Top
HP > Pa > Pv

Pa

Middle
Pa > HP > Pv

Pv

Bottom
Pa > Pv > HP

Bottom flow

Figure 26.4 Effect of hydrostatic pressure in the lung on blood flow.

Pulmonary circulation

The lung receives the entire cardiac output from the right ventricle. With a pulmonary systolic arterial pressure of 3.33kPa (25mmHg) and a diastolic pressure of 1.07kPa (8mmHg) this gives a mean pulmonary arterial pressure of around 2kPa (mean pressure = DIASTOLIC +1/3[SYSTOLIC − DIASTOLIC]). The capillary pressures will be somewhat less around 1.6kPa (12mmHg) at the arteriolar end and 1.07kPa (8mmHg) at the venular end (all pressures measured at the level of the pulmonary valve). However, in an upright lung there will be a difference in hydrostatic pressure between top and bottom. For a lung 30cm in length, top to bottom, this will give a column of fluid of 30cmH₂O (23mmHg). Thus to push the blood to the top of the lung the pulmonary pressure would have to be at least 23mmHg. Clearly from the above figures blood flow through the upper third of the lung will be negligible, that in the lower third will be continuous and aided by the hydrostatic pressure and that in the middle third will be somewhere in between (see Fig. 26.4). This will give rise to a gradient of perfusion and a difference in the ability of the lung to undertake gaseous exchange. This gradient of usability of the lung is described as the physiological dead space. Effectively the top part of the lung will be ventilated but underperfused or not perfused at all, in the middle the flow will be governed by how much the capillary arteriolar pressure exceeds the hydrostatic pressure and in the lower third flow will be normal and proportional to the arteriolar/venular difference.

It is not known, with any certainty, how much filtration occurs across the walls of the capillary bed. Normally this is governed by the arteriolar pressure (12mmHg) and the colloid osmotic pressure

(28mmHg) so that theoretically the capillaries should suck water out of the interstitial space. However, the normal filtration parameters will be perturbed by the hydrostatic pressure difference in the lung and the effect of a negative intrathoracic pressure. It is probable that net outward filtration (pulmonary lymph) occurs at a rate of approximately 20ml/hour which is around 10% of that seen on the higher pressure systemic side of the circulation.

For average values of alveolar ventilation 4.9L/min and a blood flow of 5L/min the ventilation perfusion ratio will be around 1. If ventilation ceases totally the ratio will be 0 and if perfusion ceases the ratio approaches infinity. In the upright resting lung this ratio varies between 3.3 at the apices and 0.63 at the bases. During physical exertion these differences become less marked. The lung does, however, possess a mechanism to prevent marked changes in the ratio. Hypoxia leads to constriction of the afferent alveolar blood vessels (hypoxic vasoconstriction) causing a decreased blood flow. As a consequence alveoli receiving little oxygen are bypassed whereas the better functioning alveoli will be relatively hyperperfused.

Physical properties of alveoli

The lung is essentially a system of millions of interconnecting bubbles. This means that the normal physics of bubbles has to be manipulated. The pressure inside a bubble is proportional to the surface tension of the bubble divided by its radius. Thus small bubbles will have a higher internal pressure than bigger bubbles. The outcome of this is that smaller bubbles will collapse and inflate even further the bigger bubbles. The lungs deal with his by using a chemical which reduces the surface tension in a bubble as it gets smaller—the pulmonary surfactant. Its composition is not known with certainty but it is a phospholipid with as its major constituent dipalmitoyl phosphatidylcholine mixed with a small amount of protein produced by the type 2 alveolar cells. The effect on the surface tension of the alveoli is inversely proportional to its concentration. With a fixed amount per alveolus its concentration in the surface fluid layer will become higher the smaller the radius. The surfactant has two effects:

1 It will allow the alveoli to inflate more easily than if they were just bathed in a thin layer of saline, and
2 It will stabilize alveolar size

Surfactant is produced in the later stages of fetal development. In premature infants its lack causes respiratory distress because of the inability of the baby to inflate its lungs. Even a full-term newborn has a problem taking its first breath—intrapleural pressures as low as -100cmH$_2$O can be generated in their first breath.

Respiratory distress

Taking all these factors together it is apparent that respiration can be impaired via a variety of causes:

- A reduction in blood flow
- A reduction in ventilatory capability
- An increase in the diffusional path for gases

These can occur individually but, most often, in a variety of combinations. For example, in the early stages of hypovolaemic shock pulmonary blood flow can be markedly reduced, ventilation can be severely impaired by obstruction of the airway, and lung oedema will give a large decrease in gaseous diffusion.

One particularly dangerous condition is lung sepsis which can lead to acute respiratory distress syndrome (ARDS). This is identified as a sudden onset of respiratory distress (dyspnoea, commonly called breathlessness or shortness of breath by patients) with increased respiratory rate (tachypnoea) and cyanosis and is refractory to increased O$_2$ supply, i.e. little or no improvement of blood O$_2$ saturation level is seen with high flow O$_2$. A CXR will show pulmonary oedema which will not be cardiogenic in origin and diffuse bilateral infiltrates.

As with most diseases ARDS is a multifactorial disruption:

- Sepsis will give a raised body temperature increasing both the demand for O$_2$ and the production of CO$_2$ resulting in an extra respiratory demand

- The resultant release of all sorts of inflammatory agents will make capillaries more leaky leading to fluid extravasation, impaired fluid drainage from the lungs, and impaired perfusion
- As the disease progresses cells and inflammatory exudate will enter the alveoli giving rise to an increase in the diffusional path for gaseous exchange and leading to a further increase in respiratory demand
- Oedema leading to dilution of pulmonary surfactant will cause many alveoli to collapse or flood. This reduction in fully functional alveoli can cause a large intrapulmonary blood shunt. The effects on pulmonary surfactant will cause a major decrease in the ease with which the lungs can be inflated (compliance)

Management is: a) to treat the cause of the sepsis and b) increase the FiO_2, since P_aO_2 values of 60mmHg are commonly seen. To maintain acceptable gas exchange patients need to be mechanically ventilated with oxygen given with some form of pressure ventilation. This latter measure is needed to both increase alveolar O_2 pressures and to force open as many alveoli as possible.

Respiratory failure

Broadly speaking this condition exists when a patient cannot maintain levels of blood oxygen and blood carbon dioxide at their normal levels, i.e. P_aO_2 >8kPa (60mmHg) and P_aCO_2 <6.7kPa (45mmHg). Two types of respiratory failure can be recognized.

Type I respiratory failure is caused by factors which results in a ventilation perfusion mismatch, e.g. parenchymal disease, vasculature upsets resulting in a right–left shunt such as pulmonary embolism and interstitial lung disease such as ARDS and pneumonia. The patients become hypoxic P_aO_2 <60mmHg whilst P_aCO_2 remains normal or becomes slightly hypocapnic ≤ 45mmHg. The hypocapnia results from the patients becoming tachypnoeic (increased respiratory rate) with a small tidal volume, i.e. they hyperventilate.

Type II respiratory failure is seen whenever alveolar ventilation is impaired, e.g. depressed respiratory effort seen after anaesthesia and with opiate administration, disease giving an increased airway resistance such as asthma, and diseases giving a decrease in the amount of lung tissue available for gaseous exchange as is seen in emphysema. These patients show hypoxia P_aO_2 <8kPa (60mmHg), hypercapnia P_aCO_2 >6.7kPa (45mmHg), and show a decreased pH (<7.38).

No matter what the cause of respiratory insufficiency, oxygen will have to be administered to restore P_aO_2 to normal levels or a blood saturation >84% (with a normal haematocrit). In the majority of cases all that is required will be supplemental oxygen given either by a simple face mask or nasal prongs. The inspired oxygen concentration (FiO_2) will depend upon many factors such as the rate of oxygen flow, how well the mask fits, and the patient's respiratory volume. It is estimated that with an oxygen flow rate of 6L/min the FiO_2 varies between 35–55%. If a more accurate FiO_2 is required then tight-fitting face masks or venturi masks can be used. Patients on mechanical ventilation will normally have their oxygen delivery carefully monitored and maintained at an appropriate level.

Gas transfer

Oxygen

Oxygen can be carried in the blood in simple solution in extra- and intracellular water. Normally this represents a small fraction (1/70th or approximately 3mL/L) of the total of oxygen carried in the blood (210mL/L). The reaction between oxygen and haemoglobin is an oxygenation, the iron in the haem moiety of the molecule exists in the ferrous state. If the iron becomes oxidized (ferrous → ferric) then the haemoglobin is transformed into methaemoglobin which has no oxygen carrying capability. Haemoglobin is a globular (roughly spherical) protein with four haem units attached and has a molecular weight of around 64,800 Daltons. Each of the haem moieties can react with one molecule of oxygen. The oxygenation reaction is not straightforward. The first oxygen molecule attaches with difficulty, once attached this enhances the affinity of the second haem moiety for oxygen, etc. Once the fourth oxygen molecule is attached the haemoglobin can accept no more. The haemoglobin cannot be fully saturated at normal O_2 concentrations: full saturation occurs if the O_2 concentration in the alveoli reaches 20kPa. This chain of

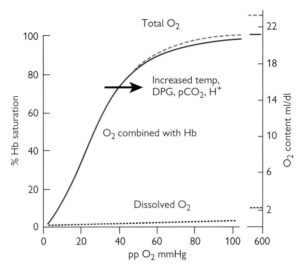

Figure 26.5 Oxygen–haemoglobin dissociation curve

events gives the oxygen/haemoglobin saturation curve its distinct sigmoid shape. It has to be remembered that in life this saturation curve cannot be represented by a single line. The reaction can be shifted to the right or the left by varying conditions seen in blood giving a real saturation curve that departs from the classic textbook figure. The affinity of haemoglobin for oxygen can be increased, (shifted to the left) by a decrease in blood CO_2, temperature or 2,3-diphophoglycerate (2,3-DPG) or by an increase in pH and the affinity decreased (shifted to the right) by the reverse changes of these factors. Thus the affinity of haemoglobin for oxygen is potentiated in the lungs ($<P_aCO_2$, $>$pH) giving an increase in oxygen uptake and diminished in tissues ($>P_aCO_2$, $<$pH) allowing more oxygen to be released (see Fig. 26.5). The effect of pH on haemoglobin is the Bohr effect.

One gram of haemoglobin can carry approximately 1.38mL O_2, with an average normal concentration of 150g/L of haemoglobin 1L of blood can carry some 210mL of O_2 and hence a normal cardiac output can supply slightly more than 1L of oxygen per minute to the body tissues. Myoglobin has a much greater affinity for O_2 than haemoglobin and will start to release its bound oxygen at P_aO_2 levels <40mmHg. The affinity of haemoglobin for carbon monoxide is much greater than that for oxygen and at partial pressures of around 1kPa can totally displace all the oxygen loosely bound to it. This can pose a threat to life for people rescued from burning buildings.

Carbon dioxide

The end products of aerobic metabolism are principally CO_2 and H_2O. The CO_2 diffuses out of the cells into the plasma and then into the red blood cells forming carbonic acid where approximately 80% is rapidly converted to HCO_3, an action which is sped up by the presence of carbonic anhydrase in the blood corpuscles:

$$H_2O + CO_2 \leftrightarrow H_2CO_3 \leftrightarrow H^+ + HCO_3^-$$

The hydrogen ion is mainly buffered by the haemoglobin in the red blood cells whereas the bicarbonate ions diffuse out of the cells into the plasma down its concentration gradient. To maintain the electroneutrality of the red blood cells an equivalent amount of chloride ion passes into the cells. The relatively small amount of hydrogen ions which diffuse out of the red cell reduces the pH of the blood from 7.4 to 7.36. (pH is a logarithmic scale so a change of 0.04 of a pH unit represents a rise in hydrogen ion concentration of some 10%). The buffering capacity of the haemoglobin within the red cells is augmented at the tissue level because deoxygenated haemoglobin is a much better buffer than the oxygenated variety. This buffering action of the haemoglobin plays a helpful role because it will drive the reaction of CO_2 and H_2O to the right allowing more HCO_3^- to be formed. In addition some of the CO_2 entering the

Table 26.2 Distribution of CO_2 in blood (ml/L)

	Solution	HCO3⁻	Carbamino
Arterial plasma:	16.6	312.8	2.4
Red blood cells	11.9	154.1	26.1
Blood	28.5	466.9	28.5
Venous plasma:	19	338.9	2.4
Red blood cells	14.2	170.6	33.2
Blood	33.2	509.5	35.6
AV difference	4.7	42.6	7.1

red cells will form carbamino compounds with the protein moiety of haemoglobin and some of the CO_2 in the plasma will form carbamino compounds with the plasma proteins. To form these compounds the amino groups of the protein react with CO_2.

$$Pr\text{-}NH_2 + CO_2 \leftrightarrow Pr\text{-}NHCOO^- + H^+$$

Table 26.2 shows the distribution of CO_2 in blood as ml/L., assuming a haemotocrit of 45% and that 1mmol of CO_2 occupies 23.7ml at 37°C.

From this it can be seen that of the percentage of exhaled CO_2 9% is carried in solution, 78% as bicarbonate, and 12% as carbamino compounds (roughly 80% in association with haemoglobin). With a cardiac output of 5L/min a normal person, at rest, will exchange approximately 0.27L of CO_2/min from venous blood to alveolar air.

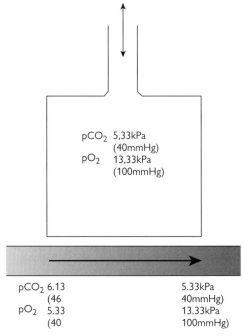

pCO₂ 5,33kPa
      (40mmHg)
pO₂   13,33kPa
      (100mmHg)

pCO₂ 6.13   5.33kPa
     (46   40mmHg)
pO₂ 5.33   13.33kPa
     (40   100mmHg)

Figure 26.6 Gaseous exchange in the lungs for a normal subject at rest.

The changes in gas concentrations in alveolar air and the pulmonary circulation are shown in Fig. 26.6.

At rest the rate of O_2 utilization is approximately 0.3L/min and CO_2 production 0.27L/min. Oxygen utilization ranges from 1.0L/min in moderate, to 1.5L/min in mild, and to 2L/min in severe exercise.

Types of hypoxia

Gaseous exchange in the body tissues are under the same constraints as is the exchange in the lung. Arterial blood supplies the tissue with O_2 and the CO_2 produced by tissue metabolism is removed in the venous blood. A lack of oxygen supply to tissues is sometimes called anoxia, this literally means no oxygen at all, the correct term is hypoxia which means less oxygen. Four types of tissue hypoxia can be recognized clinically.

Hypoxic hypoxia

This is the condition when there is an inadequate O_2 supply to the lungs and hence a reduced amount of oxygen in arterial blood. Causes are:

- Low atmospheric pressure—high altitudes
- Hypoventilation—respiratory depression as in paralysis of respiratory muscles, a depressed respiratory drive, airway obstruction, or a collapsed lung (atelectasis)
- Alveolar to capillary diffusion block—pulmonary oedema or pneumonia
- Ventilation/perfusion imbalance—emphysema

Anaemic hypoxia

This is caused by any process which lowers the oxygen carrying capacity of the blood. Causes are:

- From blood loss, decreased red blood cell count (decreased production or increased destruction)
- Reduced haemoglobin concentration—iron deficiency leading to hypochromic anaemia
- Abnormal haemoglobin—sickle cell anaemia
- Altered haemoglobin oxygen affinity—carbon monoxide poisoning, methaemoglobinaemia

Ischaemic or stagnant hypoxia

This is seen during shock, heart failure, or intravascular obstruction. The local pO_2 falls to low levels and tissues will respire anaerobically until the circulation is restored.

Histotoxic hypoxia

Seen when tissues cannot use O_2 for oxidative processes, e.g. cyanide poisoning.

The effects of hypoxia depend upon its severity. For example, in cardiac arrest unconsciousness can occur within 15 seconds, irreversible cell damage in 2–3 minutes, and cell death in 4–5 minutes. Lesser degrees of hypoxia are signalled by alteration in respiratory frequency, confusion, and disorientation.

Control of respiration

Respiration can be controlled by a wide variety of stimuli both external and internal. Basic respiratory pattern is controlled by what are termed the respiratory centres in the pons and medulla. However, the term centre is somewhat misleading, plotting the locations of the various centres, e.g. respiratory and cardiac, and the location of the ascending and descending reticular activating system, shows that there is a wide degree of overlap. It is better to refer to them as the respiratory controllers as part of an integrated system to exert an integrated control of and interplay between all of these functional controllers. In that way it makes sense of the changes in all systems (respiratory, cardiac, motor, and vegetative) that occur prior to, during, and after changes that demand an integrated and to some extent a predictive control, e.g. changes of posture, moving, sleeping, and waking. For example, when you get out of bed after waking up your body is prepared for the change in posture before you stand up.

There are six aggregations of neurons in the pons and medulla (three on each side; see Fig. 26.7A) which show activity related primarily to the respiratory cycle.

1 The dorsal respiratory groups (DRG) located in the ventrolateral portion of nucleus tractus solitarius which sends efferent axons to a ventral group of cells (see below) and downwards to the phrenic and thoracic motoneurons. The cells in this group are mainly active during inspiration and, from their behaviour appear to control the timing and force of inspiration

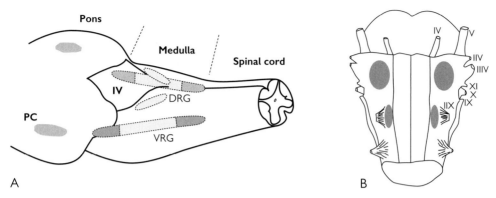

Figure 26.7 A) A diagrammatic representation of the groups of cells in the pons and medulla controlling respiration. DRG, dorsal respiratory group: IV, fourth ventricle; PC, pneumotaxic group; VRG, ventral respiratory group. B) A diagrammatic representation of the locations of the central chemosensory cells on the ventral surface of the medulla.

2 The ventral respiratory group (VRG) located in the nucleus retroambigualis, nucleus ambiguus, nucleus para-ambiguus, and the pre-Boltzinger complex. Cells in these locations show activity in both inspiration and expiration. Their efferent axons project to the thoracic motoneurons. Their activity indicates that they control the force of both inspiration and expiration. Expiratory muscular activation becomes necessary when respiratory minute volume exceeds 40L/min

3 There is another group of cells located in the dorsolateral part of the pons termed the pneumotaxic group mainly in the nucleus parabrachialis. Cells located here are active in either inspiration, expiration, or throughout the respiratory cycle. Their action seems to be to inhibit inspiration by their action on cells in the DRG and VRG and are involved in the fine tuning of inspiration

Cells in the DRG and VRG receive an input from the pulmonary stretch receptors via their nerve fibres which travel to the medulla in the vagus. These receptors signal the degree and rate of lung inflation and their input is used to aid the switching off of inspiration. In vagatomized animals respiration becomes slower with an increase in tidal volume.

Respiratory demand to artificially controlled chemical stimuli shows that:

• The effect of oxygen lack is very small until the P_aO_2 falls to <50mmHg after which there is dramatic rise in respiratory minute volume of some 18L/min
• There is a linear increase in respiratory minute volume from 5 to 80L/min as P_aCO_2 increases from 40 to 70mmHg
• The effect of changing pH is not very marked until the pH falls to around 7.1 after which the respiratory minute volume increases to 30L/min

Comparing these different artificially manipulated effects show that they are additive since their total is the same (80+30+18 = 128) as that seen in exercise giving comparable changes in arterial CO_2, O_2 and pH levels, see Fig. 26.8.

The increased respiratory drive to increasing levels of CO_2 is produced by the increase in activity of groups of cells located on the ventral surface of the medulla (see Fig. 26.7). These cells do not detect CO_2 levels per se but respond to pH changes in the cerebrospinal fluid (CSF). Hydrogen ions do not cross the blood–brain barrier but CO_2 does. Once in the CSF CO_2 reacts with water to produce H^+ and HCO_3^- ions. Since CSF has very little buffering capacity, compared to blood, larger pH changes will occur which serve to stimulate these cells which, in turn, influence the activity of the cells in the respiratory controller groups giving the required changes in frequency and depth of respiratory activity.

The effect of O_2 lack is sensed by the activity of peripheral receptors located in the carotid and aortic bodies. Sensory fibres from the carotid bodies are carried in the carotid sinus nerves which join the

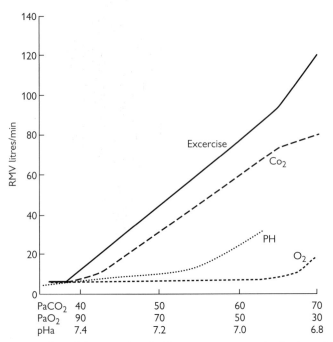

Figure 26.8 This shows the effect of altering and artificially maintaining various levels of arterial pH, O_2, and CO_2. Responses are compared with the maximal ventilation the subject can attain by transient voluntary effort. The subject showed normal compensatory adjustments so that the responses to O_2 and pH were obtained as P_aCo_2 was falling. (Redrawn from Patton HD, et al. (eds) (1989). *Textbook of Physiology*, 21st Edition. Philadelphia, PA: Saunders.)

glossopharyngeal nerve (cranial nerve IX) and those from the aortic bodies are carried in the vagus (cranial nerve X). These signals are thus lead directly into the medulla and pons to influence the respiratory controller cells. The carotid bodies have a blood flow which is extremely high (2100mL/100g/min, in the cat) which is about 40 times that supplied to the brain. They also have a very high O_2 consumption, around 9ml O_2/100g/min, and so any decrease in P_aO_2 will have a marked effect on their behaviour. Studies on the differential effects of increasing P_aCO_2, decreasing P_aO_2 and decreasing pH on the activity of the sensory fibres from these structures show that all three stimuli activate the sensory cells but that they show a rapid rise in activity at levels of P_aO_2 which stimulate respiratory drive.

In patients with chronic CO_2 retention the medullary cells become less sensitive to CO_2 levels so that P_aO_2 becomes the principle drive for their respiration. If such patients are placed upon high flow O_2 their respiratory drive will become diminished or abolished. This results in apnoea, coma or death. The resulting rise in P_aCO_2 means that CO_2 levels in the brain could rise high enough for it to act as an anaesthetic. Such patients, therefore, should only be given enriched air (*ca.* 28%) to breathe and be carefully monitored.

That hypoxia stimulates respiratory drive via the peripheral chemoreceptors is shown by the fact that if their influence is removed hypoxia depresses respiration. Prolonged hypoxia, however, can cause mild cerebral acidosis which can stimulate respiration. Although the effect of transient hypoxia, under laboratory conditions, is quite modest, people ascending to high altitudes show a large and persistent increase in ventilation even at modest altitudes. A possible reason for this is that initial hyperventilation to a reduced P_aO_2 will reduce P_aCO_2 and CSF will become alkalotic. This removes a CO_2 drive so people will not hyperventilate as much as they should. However, after a day or so CSF pH will be reduced by outward movement of HCO_3^-; 2–3 days after this blood pH will return to normal levels because of renal secretion of HCO_3^-. Thus the true sensitivity of the peripheral chemoreceptors may be masked.

The effects of increasing hydrogen ion concentration in blood also has to be signalled to the central nervous system by the peripheral chemoreceptors since H^+ cannot cross the blood–brain barrier.

Other factors influencing respiration are:

- Cutaneous cold receptors—people tend to gasp if they are drenched with cold water and hold their breath if their face is immersed in cold water
- If core temperature rises it will lead to an increased metabolism with ensuing changes in O_2 demand and CO_2 production
- Activities such as coughing, hiccoughs, yawning, swallowing, and sighing all affect respiration. Sighing may play a role in redistributing pulmonary surfactant
- Joint receptors in the limbs can stimulate respiration. Passive movement of a joint gives an increase in respiratory minute volume
- Hormones—particularly those which have an effect on metabolism
- Drugs such as opiates and general anaesthetics
- Changes occur on going to sleep and waking up
- Marked changes occur when speaking and particularly when singing or playing a wind instrument. Here the problem is less of getting air into and out of the lungs but keeping a constant flow of air whilst the chest volume is changing. To acquire any of these skills takes a lot of training to precisely control the diaphragm and develop and control the intercostal musculature
- Breathing is under voluntary control. You can, if you wish, hold your breath. Incidentally if you wish to see the powerful drive CO_2 exerts stand in front of a mirror, hold your breath, and see whether you can hold it long enough to become cyanotic

Metabolic function of the lung

In addition to their function in gas exchange the lungs also have some important metabolic functions.

- Angiotensin I is converted to angiotensin II by the angiotensin converting enzyme (ACE) produced by the vascular endothelial cells. Angiotensin II has a much more powerful vasoconstrictor action than its precursor and also releases aldosterone from the adrenal cortex
- The lungs deactivate some vasoactive substances. The potent vasodilator bradykinin is deactivated by ACE. The products of arachidonic acid metabolism derived from membrane phospholipids such as prostaglandins E_2 and $F_{2\alpha}$ and leukotrienes are removed. Other products such as leukotrienes (LTB_4, LTC_4 and LTD_4) are implicated in the brochoconstriction seen in asthma
- Pulmonary surfactant is produced by type II pneumocytes
- Lung tissue is continuously being broken down and resynthesized

Clinical scenarios

There are, of course, many reasons why patients have a challenged respiration, they have either:

- Had a lengthy operation and are liable to post-operative complications
- Have had chest trauma
- Suffer from sudden respiratory distress

General principles

The basic task is to restore respiration to normal, deciding from the signs and symptoms what is causing the problem, to manage the patient, in the short term to keep them alive and then having thoroughly investigated to remove/treat the cause. Thereafter they have to be managed back to health.

A common complication of surgery is post-operative hypoxia from a variety of causes. Surgical patients most at risk of post-operative hypoxia are: smokers, those with chronic pulmonary disease, the elderly, the obese, those who have received pre-operative opiates and sedatives, those who have undergone abdominal emergency surgery, and those who have had orthopaedic surgery.

The dangers of post-operative hypoxia include: obtunded pain sensation, post-operative confusion, tachycardia, myocardial ischaemia, hyperpnoea, respiratory muscle inadequacy (from morphine, anaesthetics, painful wound), renal failure, reduced immunoprotection, reduced platelet function, coagulation problems, and impaired wound healing.

Table 26.3 Common causes of respiratory compromise

Sudden respiratory distress	Post-operative complications	Thoracic trauma (those marked * for a complete picture)
Spontaneous pneumothorax	Absorption atelectasis	Chest wall:
Disturbances of bronchial tree:	Acute atelectasis	Flail chest
Bronchial blockage:	Adult respiratory distress syndrome	Sternal injury
Aspiration	Barotrauma	Shoulder girdle injury
Food	Iatrogenic simple pneumothorax	Pleuro-pulmonary:
Near drowning	Inability to ventilate properly	Haemothorax
Bronchospasm:	Immobility	Lung contusion
Asthma	Consequences of massive blood transfusion	Lung laceration
β-blockers		Blast injury
Insect bites/stings	Pulmonary embolus	Burns victims:
Post exercise	Pulmonary oedema	Hot air
Underlying disease:	Pulmonary thromboembolus	Toxic fumes
Chronic obstructive disease	Sepsis	Carbon monoxide
Chronic atelectasis		*Mediastinal injury:
Emphysema		*Cardiac tamponade
Infection		*Cardiac contusion/rupture
Pulmonary embolus		*Great vessel injuries:
Acute pancreatitis		*Aortic rupture
Carbon monoxide inhalation		*Arch vessel injuries
Complications after childbirth		*Venous injuries
Hysterical hyperventilation		Tracheo-bronchial injury
Inhalation of toxic vapours or gases		Oesophageal injury
		Ruptured diaphragm
		Stab injuries
		Gunshot injuries

In all cases an arterial oxygen tension (P_aO_2) of >8kPa must be attempted.

Common causes of respiratory compromise can be listed (somewhat artificially) as shown in Table 26.3.

Scenarios

Scenario 1

A 60-year-old man has had a right hemicolectomy. On the 1st postoperative day he has developed a temperature of 39°C, is very short of breath, and looks slightly cyanosed; his oxygen saturation is 92%. What will you suspect and how will you manage the condition?

The clinical signs are:

- Tachypnoea
- Pyrexia
- Productive cough
- Cyanosis
- Dullness on percussion

Scenario 2

A 65-year-old lady had a hip replacement 10 days ago. She is ready to be discharged. She went to the toilet just prior to leaving the ward for home. She collapsed in the toilet. What is your diagnosis and management?

Clinical signs are:

- Dyspnoea—low blood oxygen saturation
- Tachypnoea
- Tachycardia—hypotension
- Chest pain on inspiration
- Small haemoptysis
- Calf tenderness and swelling

Scenario 3

A fit young man was thrown off his motorbike and brought into A&E with severe shortness of breath; his airway is fine but he is gasping for breath and becoming progressively more 'air-hungry'. The pulse oximeter shows an O_2 saturation of 90%. What would you suspect and how will you manage the problem?

Clinical signs are:

- Chest pain
- Air hunger
- Respiratory distress
- Tachycardia
- Hypotension
- Tracheal deviation
- Unilateral absence of breath sounds
- Neck vein engorgement
- Hyper-resonant chest on percussion
- Cyanosis—late sign

Answers

Scenario 1

These signs suggest that he is suffering from pulmonary collapse which is commonly referred to as atelectasis. Any blockage of air transport to the alveoli will result in the air being absorbed but as it is not being replaced the alveoli will collapse and/or become filled with fluid. (This collapse will be faster if the alveoli are filled with O_2—enriched air, O_2 is absorbed faster than N_2.)

Management

The pyrexia should be treated with an antibiotic, e.g. amoxicillin. Infection with consolidation supervenes with the organisms being *Haemophilus influenza, streptococcus pneumoniae, coliform, MRSA*, and *Pseudomonas*

- Oxygen therapy should be administered with an inspired concentration of 30–40% with humidification to help make the secretions more fluid
- Vigorous physiotherapy should be given with or without doxapram. Because of the reduced ventilation of the lung bases it will result in accumulation of bronchial secretions
- There could be basal, segmental, lobar, or complete lung collapse. The degree of hypoxia depends upon the extent of collapse
- Urgent fibreoptic bronchoscopy. He might have 'swallowed' something which is blocking a bronchus or there may be a compression of a bronchus
- Minitracheostomy may be necessary to get an adequate amount of oxygen into his bloodstream

Continue with antibiotics, physiotherapy, and monitor blood gases aim for oxygen tension to be no less than 10kPa also continually monitor blood saturation with pulse oximetry.

Scenario 2

Her clinical signs are all suggestive of a pulmonary embolus (PE) possibly due to embolization of fat (orthopaedic surgery) although the timescale and the presence of calf tenderness and swelling points to a more probable cause, that the embolus is a result of a thrombus (blood clot) from the deep veins in the legs, i.e. venous thromboembolism. This is a severe case indicated by the sudden collapse.

Management

Management in general is to:

• Resuscitate
• Investigate
• Treat

Management, however, will depend upon whether the patient is stable or unstable.

The stable patient

• An ECG
• CXR
• Blood gases
• VQ scan
• Duplex Doppler US of leg veins
• Pulmonary angiogram
• Contrast venography and plethysmography

The unstable patient

• Echocardiogram will show right heart function impairment. An indication that the pulmonary artery is severely obstructed
• CT pulmonary angiogram with radiocontrast will show filling defects of the pulmonary arteries. An ordinary CXR will not be normal but will not show the presence of a PE

Treatment depends upon the severity; in this case severe:

• Anticoagulation therapy (heparin for a quick effect, warfarin for a prolonged effect)
• An emergency embolectomy may be required in this case a certainty
• Inferior vena cava filters can be implanted if anticoagulation therapy is not effective and/or to prevent new emboli entering the pulmonary circulation after a post-pulmonary embolectomy
• Thrombolysis—in a haemodynamically unstable patient with refractory shock, a thrombolytic can be administered either intravenously or by pulse spray directly into the embolus if embolectomy is contraindicated

Scenario 3

This is in all probability a tension pneumothorax.

Management is to immediately decrease the tension in his thorax by inserting a wide-bore needle in the 2nd intercostal space in the midline position on the affected side. The needle will be in the correct position when you hear a distinct hiss as the air under pressure is released. The needle should be left in position, possibly with a valve, until you have located and repaired the sucking wound site.

Chapter 27 **Cardiovascular system in critical care**

Introduction—critical challenges to the cardiovascular system

In a surgical crisis requiring critical care, the circulation is a major focus at the initial assessment and throughout management. In such a critically ill patient the cardiovascular system is responding to a variety of challenges. These can include circulatory failure of central origin (direct traumatic damage to the heart), and circulatory failure of peripheral origin (various forms of shock, including haemorrhage and burns). There is often also a demand for increased oxygen delivery and hence increased cardiac output to support the body's response to injuries in other organs. There may also be regional problems due to impairment of the local circulation. The outcome is determined by the severity of the challenge and the ability of the patient's cardiovascular system to respond to the challenge indicated in the following equation:

Severity of cardiovascular challenge versus **cardiovascular response**

If, in an often complex situation with multiple critical injuries, the left side of the above equation dominates, then death is due at least in part to failure of the cardiovascular response. The aim of management is to support the response so that it is adequate to meet the challenge.

The cardiovascular response involves autonomic sensory nerves, control centres in the brain, autonomic motor nerves and circulating hormones, and the heart and blood vessels themselves. Appropriate management requires a thorough understanding of the mechanisms involved, thus working with the body's physiology to secure a favourable outcome. Maintenance of appropriate body fluids, especially in the circulation, is essential, and the presence of drugs and toxins must also be taken into account.

Previous cardiovascular fitness

The outcome of a specified challenge (e.g. 40% full thickness burns of the skin) is clearly related to the patient's previous fitness, age being a major marker for this. The age-related loss of ability to respond to such challenges involves all body systems, but loss of cardiovascular fitness is a major component. It is helpful to consider in detail how cardiovascular fitness can be assessed, not because the results of such assessments are likely to be available for the patient admitted to critical care, but because such studies give essential insight into how the cardiovascular system works. The quantitative information they give, and consideration of the mechanisms involved are the foundation of appropriate management. They are particularly relevant to understanding and using quantitative information on the cardiovascular system during critical care monitoring.

Measurement of physical fitness

The gold standard test of physical fitness is measurement of the **maximal oxygen consumption** which the individual can achieve. In this test, the person often runs or walks on a treadmill while oxygen consumption and cardiovascular parameters are closely monitored. In practice the speed of the treadmill, and in some cases its slope, are increased steadily so that exercise reaches a maximum in around 10–15 minutes. The time is kept reasonably short to avoid fatigue preventing maximal activity being reached.

How is it known when maximum activity has been reached? As well as aiming for the point at which the person genuinely cannot further increase the level of exercise, a useful quantitative test is measurement of the lactic acid (lactate) level in a small earlobe sample. At maximal exertion, the recruitment of anaerobic glycolysis for energy results in a lactate level some five to ten times the resting level. It is a curious coincidence that this corresponds to the lactate level found in the severely hypoxic patient fighting for life in intensive care. Again, the patient's life-supporting energy requirements can only be met by anaerobic glycolysis.

Relationship between maximal oxygen consumption and the heart

Why should measurement of maximal oxygen consumption throw light on the cardiovascular system? It does so because oxygen consumption depends on oxygen delivery and oxygen delivery depends crucially on cardiac output. In health, cardiac output can be increased at least severalfold during exercise, whereas the other components of oxygen delivery cannot vary appreciably, provided they are initially normal. Consider the formula below for calculating the amount of oxygen delivered to the entire body by the circulation each minute (ignoring the normally very small amount of dissolved oxygen):

Oxygen delivery = [cardiac output] × [oxygen content/L of arterial blood]

The oxygen content of blood is determined by its haemoglobin content and by the degree of saturation. For a healthy individual the haemoglobin content is around 150g/L, and this haemoglobin is virtually fully saturated in arterial blood. Since each gram of haemoglobin can hold about 1.33ml of oxygen, a litre of arterial blood normally carries about 200ml of oxygen. Thus the only change that can increase oxygen delivery is an increase in cardiac output. A high maximal oxygen consumption indicates, as well as a high level of general physical fitness, an effective cardiovascular system, and particularly a heart that can pump a large amount of blood per minute.

Comparison of different levels of cardiac fitness

Moving to maximal cardiac output as an indicator of cardiovascular fitness, some typical values to be expected in healthy people are given in Table 27.1 for various levels of fitness. Values are shown for people aged 20–25 years with similar body masses, so they have similar resting oxygen requirements and hence similar resting cardiac outputs. Heart rate (HR), stroke volume (SV), and cardiac output (CO) are shown. SV is expressed as ml, and CO as litres/minute.

Some typical values for **heart failure** are given for comparison at the bottom of the table. Notice that they represent a level of cardiac output below the normal range, particularly during exercise, which becomes more and more limited as heart failure progresses.

Notice the results for very high fitness. It is largely the ability to reach such a high cardiac output that determines the ability to become an Olympic champion in many areas.

Two features of the results show a progressive change from low to very high fitness states. The resting heart rate slows and the maximal cardiac output rises. The resting stroke volumes also rise progressively with increasing fitness. In all cases, stroke volume increases moderately from rest to exercise. The heart rate at maximal exercise, however, is the same for all the individuals. Maximal heart rate is determined by the ability of the cardiac tissues to perform at very high speeds and this is a function of age, such that in general:

Maximal heart rate = 220 − age in years

What is the basis for these patterns, and what light do they throw on cardiac function? The constancy of the heart rate at maximal exercise is a robust finding for people of a given age. The effect is similar in males and females. Thus at age 20, the maximum rate to be expected is a remarkable 200 beats per minute. Such a rate is commonly found briefly during sporting activities requiring sudden bursts of speed and it is also another indication in the measurement of maximal oxygen consumption that the person

Table 27.1 Components of cardiac output (CO, litres/minute) at various levels of fitness. Typical heart rate per minute (HR) and stroke volume in ml (SV) are given; CO is the product of HR and SV

	Rest			Maximal exercise		
Fitness level	HR	SV	CO	HR	SV	CO
Low	80	60	4.8	200	75	15
Moderate	70	70	4.9	200	90	18
High	55	90	4.95	200	120	24
Very high	40	125	5.0	200	150	30
Heart failure	80	45	3.6	90	50	4.5

has indeed reached maximal effort. Naturally people vary, but at age 20 the usual maximum would be around 180–210 beats per minute.

The decline with age is not surprising when we consider the amazing phenomenon of all the events of the cardiac cycle being completed in 0.3 seconds (300 milliseconds). Body tissues become stiffer with age—the effects on skin and joints are examples of this. The biochemical efficiency of cardiac muscle also declines with age, as with other tissues. Thus in the average 80-year-old person, the maximal heart rate would be 140. The values in the above table would correspond to people aged about 20.

Next let's turn to the values for stroke volume. In Table 27.1 we see that this increases at rest with the level of fitness. In other words, the fitter the person, the more blood the heart pumps with each beat. In simple terms, very fit people have larger than usual hearts for general body size. This explains why their hearts don't need to beat so frequently at rest to maintain the necessary output per minute.

Ejection fraction during exercise

A second feature of the stroke volume patterns is that the volume increases moderately from rest to maximal exercise. At rest the normal heart expels around 60–65% of the end diastolic volume during systole. This value is called the **ejection fraction** and is a useful measurement in heart failure, since it falls steadily with progression of the failure as considered below. During exercise the heart contracts more forcefully. The end diastolic volume does not usually increase, but more of it is expelled so that the ejection fraction increases to around 75%.

Because the stroke volume increases only modestly with exercise (by about a quarter to a third) it follows that the main component increasing cardiac output is the heart rate. This is where the very fit person scores, as the resting heart rate is so slow. The two extreme examples in the above table have the same exercising heart rate, but because the resting heart rate varies twofold, the least fit person increases heart rate by a factor of 2¼ and the most fit by 4½. This explains most of the difference in cardiac output and hence oxygen delivery and oxygen consumption.

Neural control mechanisms of the cardiovascular system

Now let's look at the mechanisms which move normal hearts from the resting state to that of maximal effort. The changes are controlled by the brain so that cardiac output is closely matched to the needs for oxygen delivery to the muscles. Muscle receptors ('metaboreceptors', i.e. receptors for metabolism) detect the metabolic state and provide fine tuning to provide for the metabolic requirements of the highly active muscles.

The brain component controlling the circulation during exercise can be described loosely as the **exercise centre**. This concept refers, however, not to a precise location in the brain, but to a network which links the commands issued by the motor cortex to appropriate commands to the cardiovascular system, particularly the heart. Thus cardiac output is closely related to the severity of the exercise taking place at a particular time. The need for precise matching of exercise level and cardiac output is seen by considering the effects of inadequate or excessive cardiac output in relation to the level of exercise, and is an application of the basic relationship:

Arterial blood pressure = [cardiac output] × [total peripheral resistance]

Total peripheral resistance falls inevitably and dramatically under the control of peripheral metabolic changes produced in exercising muscles. Therefore if cardiac output is inadequate at this point, arterial blood pressure will fall, brain perfusion will fail, and the individual will faint. Although this can occur, it is extremely rare in healthy people. In the opposite direction, if cardiac output is excessive, arterial blood pressure will rise to levels risking vascular damage and haemorrhage.

The anatomical basis for this cerebral control of the circulation is the autonomic nervous system, particularly the sympathetic subdivision.

This can be explored by comparing the situation in the resting person with the heart beating about once a second, with the situation in maximal exercise in a 20-year-old, with the heart beating 200 times per minute. The changes in the heart's activity at maximal exercise depend on two fundamental changes—a change in the rate of impulse formation in the sinoatrial node, and a change in the speed and force of cardiac muscle contraction.

The **sinoatrial node** is a collection of cells in the right atrium, and is the pacemaker of the heart. It regularly generates impulses even if its vagal and sympathetic innervations are severed, as in the transplanted heart. The impulses are generated by ionic movements through a mixture of sodium, calcium, and potassium channels, in which the sodium channels are particularly important so that there is a constant tendency for the membrane potential to become less negative, reach the threshold firing voltage, and trigger, at regular intervals, an action potential. Vagal fibres to the node release acetylcholine which tends to suppress all this activity, so that the rate at which the impulses (action potentials) are formed falls. Sympathetic fibres release noradrenaline, with the opposite effect. Circulating catecholamines, adrenaline, and noradrenaline, augment the sympathetic effect.

Without nerves, the denervated node sends out impulses at the intrinsic heart rate of around 100–120 beats per minute. Thus it is clear that the resting heart rate can only occur due to steady vagal activity and this steady (tonic) activity is referred to as the resting vagal tone. A cholinergic blocker such as atropine can remove this effect. A beta 2 adrenoceptor blocker will remove sympathetic effects, but these are usually small at rest. As expected, removal of autonomic inputs to the heart leads to a rate at the intrinsic level. It is also clear that a heart rate of around 200 beats per minute can only occur in the presence of a very high level of sympathetic activity.

The brain links the skeletal muscle activity, which it originates, with the autonomic activity, which it also controls, so that at rest there is dominant strong vagal activity and at maximal exercise there is dominant strong sympathetic activity. During moderate exercise, with an intermediate heart rate, little neural activity is required.

There is a further refinement to the control of the heart rate. The impulse to the ventricles must pass through the **atrioventricular node** in the fibrous junction of atria and ventricles. This node receives parallel autonomic nervous input to the sinoatrial node. With dominant vagal activity, the atria contract at a relatively slow rate, say 60 per minute. With parallel vagal activity to the atrioventricular node, the impulse is *slowed* as it passes through the node, allowing appropriate time for final filling of the ventricles by the contracting atria. Thus *at rest* there is economy of effort with the cardiac cycle occurring in relatively slow motion, adequate for the circulatory needs at rest, and with minimal cardiac energy requirements.

During maximal cardiac effort, everything is speeded up (three- to fourfold in young adults) by the withdrawal of vagal tone and the imposition of maximal sympathetic tone. The effects can be subdivided into two main components—*chronotropic* (increasing the heart rate) and *inotropic* (increasing the force of cardiac muscle contraction).

As discussed earlier, the **chronotropic** effect is achieved by withdrawal of vagal tone, and by the steady increase in sympathetic tone. Drugs which block cholinergic effects tend to lead to a higher resting heart rate. Drugs which block beta adrenergic effects tend to slow the heart rate, and particularly prevent it reaching its usual maximum.

Inotropic effects are also achieved by sympathetic beta effects. These effects are produced by the combination of release of noradrenaline by sympathetic nerves in close contact with cardiac muscle fibres and also arrival at these fibres of circulating noradrenaline and adrenaline. These are released from the adrenal medulla, which has been likened to a sympathetic nervous system where glandular cells have replaced the post-ganglionic sympathetic fibres. Much circulating noradrenaline is also derived from released but not fully taken up noradrenaline from sympathetic postganglionic endings throughout the body. In all cases these catecholamines (adrenaline and noradrenaline) act through beta 1 receptors in cardiac muscle. Drugs which stimulate beta 1 receptors tend to increase the heart rate. Drugs which block beta 1 receptors, and general beta blockers tend to prevent the heart rate reaching its potential maximum. This can be helpful if high heart rates are a problem, for example by increasing cardiac oxygen requirements in disease states where coronary artery disease limits oxygen delivery. Such drugs can be unhelpful if they slow the normal heart and limit the person's ability to exercise normally.

Frank/Starling effects

Frank and Starling both discovered and described these effects, though Starling often gets the sole credit. Essentially, it was shown that the force of cardiac contraction is related to cardiac fibre length at the time contraction begins. The cardiac fibre length is in turn related to the content of the cardiac chamber at the time of contraction. This critical content is the end diastolic volume. The relationship has been studied particularly for the left ventricle, the ultimate expeller of blood into the circulation. So if in a particular left ventricle the end diastolic volume is 130ml, then the fibres are more stretched and the force of contraction is greater than with an end diastolic volume of 120ml. This relationship is altered by beta 1 stimulation, as considered later.

Cardiac muscle is not unique in such effects. They are found also in skeletal muscle. Here also the force of the muscle action increases as the initial fibre length increases. In both cardiac and skeletal muscle this can be explained by the sliding filament mode of contraction they both rely on. When the muscle fibres are near minimal length, the amount of overlap between the orderly arrangement of actin and myosin is high, with little scope for development of movement and strength. As the fibres are stretched, the overlap decreases, and more power can be developed. In theory with marked stretch the overlap can become too small to allow development of as much power, and decline in the force of contraction could occur. With skeletal muscle this commonly occurs. However with cardiac muscle, the heart in normal circumstances is not capable of sufficient distension to reach this point, thus preventing a potentially disastrous decline in stroke volume.

The Frank/Starling relationship at rest in shown (Fig. 27.1). Various units can be used in the vertical axis, including stroke volume, but the most fundamental term is cardiac work, which depends not only on stroke volume, but also on the speed with which stroke volume is expelled and on the resistance to expulsion of the stroke volume into the aorta. This resistance is itself related to arterial blood pressure and distensibility of the aortic wall, which is relatively elastic in young people, and more rigid in older people.

On this curve, the point X represents the amount of work done by the normal resting left ventricle, with the normal amount of ventricular filling and hence fibre length. Points A and B are theoretical, as the normal ventricle is not subject to such gross underfilling or overfilling.

In normal life, small beat-to-beat variations in filling can be compensated by this mechanism. Slightly increased filling and hence distension would slightly increase stroke volume, bringing filling back to normal. The reverse would happen with slightly decreased filling.

What happens to the relationship in strenuous exercise? At first sight it might seem that mechanisms for an increased ventricular end diastolic volume would increase cardiac muscle stretch and hence stroke volume. However, increased ventricular filling would tend to delay the onset of systole and slow the heart rate so that little if anything would be gained in terms of cardiac output. What is required is a more powerful and more rapid ventricular contraction which would, firstly, maintain stroke volume in the lesser time available for the cardiac cycle at a higher heart rate, and, secondly, would increase stroke

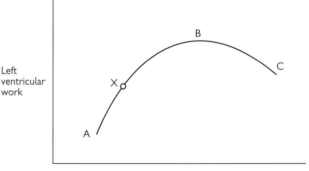

Figure 27.1 Frank/Starling relationship at rest.

volume by an increase in *ejection fraction*. In practice this is what happens and this is precisely what the beta 1 effects of the sympathetic nervous system produce. Cardiac muscle *changes its behaviour*, so that contraction occurs much more powerfully and rapidly. The sliding filaments of actin and myosin oscillate back and forth up to and beyond three times a second and the product of a modestly increased stroke volume and a markedly increased heart rate give a cardiac output to meet the demands of the exercising muscles.

The greatly altered cardiac function in strenuous exercise is due to a dramatic change in the Frank/Starling relationship as shown in Fig. 27.2.

In strenuous exercise, intense sympathetic activity has changed the whole curve, from AXBC to AEXD, the second **EX** denoting the new position of the ventricle on the new Frank/Starling curve. Notice that the curve has moved dramatically upwards and to the left (Fig. 27.2). The new **EX** is high above and slightly to the left of the old X, indicating hugely increased ventricular work at a slightly lesser degree of stretch. The heart is keeping ahead of the now torrential venous return by contracting at a slightly smaller end diastolic volume than before.

In the situation of vigorous exercise, the work of the heart is considerably assisted by at least two extra physiological pumps in series with the heart. The first is the **muscle pump**. Exercising limb muscle compresses, during dynamic activity at least (running, rowing, swimming), the deep limb veins. Valves prevent serious retrograde flow, so the blood is propelled towards the heart with each 'beat' of the, usually, rhythmically exercising limb muscle.

The second ancillary pump is the **respiratory pump**. The respiratory muscles, unlike the cardiac muscles, increase both their rate of contraction per minute and the volume shifted per breath. Tidal volume can increase from about half a litre to four or five litres. Respiratory rate can increase to about one per second. These huge flows are driven by huge changes in thoracic and abdominal pressures. During inspiration, blood is sucked into the heart through the inferior vena cava by the strongly negative intrathoracic pressure and transmitted through to the ventricles for expulsion through the aorta.

How do these mechanisms translate through to the cardiovascular system in critical care? In critical care the individual is quiescent, so the **muscle pump** is not working. The effect of the **respiratory pump** is relatively small, but helpful. If its action is nullified by positive pressure artificial ventilation, venous return is reduced and stroke volume and hence cardiac output tend to fall. In many critical care situations,

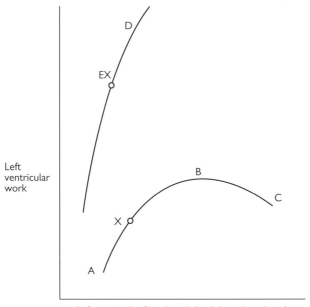

Figure 27.2 Frank/Starling relationship at rest and during strenuous exercise.

the circulating blood volume is reduced, so, again, cardiac filling is reduced and stroke volume falls. This situation is considered in detail in the chapter on haemorrhage (Chapter 24). Peripheral vasoconstriction and redistribution of blood are of great importance. The role of the heart is to help maintain cardiac output as near normal as possible by increasing heart rate and stroke volume. This is achieved by removal of vagal tone and by moderate sympathetic activity so that heart rate is increased. The second component of cardiac output, stroke volume, is raised from a depressed value towards an adequate value to keep cardiac output, still below normal, but high enough to maintain brain and other vital functions.

In this situation, the heart is driven, not by the 'exercise centre' linked to conscious muscular activity, but by autonomic reflexes at brain stem level. These are in turn regulated particularly by arterial baroreceptor activity in the carotid sinus and aortic arch to maintain arterial blood pressure at or approaching normal levels. In this situation, different from the exercising state, venous return tends to be low, and the high rates of 180–200 often seen in healthy young adults, are not appropriate. The tachycardia is often around the intrinsic heart rate, at which the increased cardiac work and hence increased oxygen requirements are much more modest, in keeping with the severely limited capacity to provide oxygen.

Circulatory failure

At this point it may be helpful to consider circulatory failure in relation to the Frank/Starling curves above. Circulatory failure can be central or peripheral in origin. Central circulatory failure implies defective cardiac function, e.g. congestive cardiac failure due to valvular disease or to myocardial damage from coronary artery narrowing and infarction. In peripheral circulatory failure the problem is usually a reduction in circulating blood volume as in shock due to haemorrhage. In septic shock the problem is inappropriate vasodilation, but again the problem is peripheral, with a disproportion between circulating blood volume and vascular capacity.

The Frank/Starling relationship is shown for the two kinds of failure (Fig. 27.3).

In **peripheral circulatory failure** the heart is not directly affected, so its Frank/Starling curve remains AXB. However, because of the impaired venous return produced by an inadequate circulating blood volume, cardiac filling is reduced and the heart functions at the lower point X_{pf}, still on the normal curve. Note that both point X_{pf} and X_{cf} indicate impaired cardiac work (with reduced stroke volume). However for the peripheral failure, cardiac size is reduced, whereas with central failure cardiac size is increased.

In **central circulatory failure** the heart is less efficient than normal, so the curve is moved downwards and to the right, from AXB to A X_{cf} B$_{cf}$. For any degree of stretch, the fibres perform less work. The movement is the opposite to that seen with sympathetic stimulation in exercise. Thus the basic heart activity moves from X to X_{cf}. Note the typical effect of heart failure—the heart is dilated, but stroke volume is impaired. As heart failure gets worse, the curve moves further down and the point X_{cf} moves down and to the right as indicated by the point X_{scf} for severe cardiac failure.

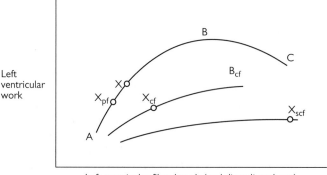

Figure 27.3 Frank/Starling relationship in circulatory failure. cf, central failure: pf, peripheral failure: scf, severe central failure.

Filling pressure of the heart

The heart can only pump out the blood it receives back from the body in the venous return. At rest the venous return is such that the heart is appropriately filled for systole once per second. With strenuous exercise, the blood is pouring back to the right atrium at several times the resting rate. If the heart continued pumping as at rest, a huge backlog would develop in the systemic veins between heartbeats and at the same time pressure in the aorta would slump shortly after each ejection of blood from the left ventricle. The heart's action is coordinated in exercise so that the very rapid pumping keeps the blood flowing round the system.

With central circulatory failure the heart falls behind in this task and the output is reduced. Consequently the pressure in the great veins does indeed rise, giving the congestive aspect of congestive heart failure. In contrast, with peripheral circulatory failure the impaired circulatory volume leads to impaired venous return, the heart is not adequately filled and, as a consequence, stroke volume and cardiac output fall.

Measurement of central venous pressure

CVP can be assessed clinically (more accurately for a raised pressure than a reduced pressure) but knowing the precise value is important for assessment and management in critical care. As there are no valves between the right atrium and the great central veins in the thorax, they form a common chamber for cardiac filling, and pressure measured in the superior vena cava, for example, indicates CVP, which is the filling pressure of the heart. A cannula placed in the superior vena cava can be connected to a pressure manometer to indicate the CVP. This is often expressed in the height of the column of fluid above heart level, for example 5cm of fluid. Since the pressure is measured within the thorax, it naturally shows respiratory fluctuations, falling during inspiration and rising during expiration. The presence of these fluctuations confirms that the cannula tip is indeed in the thorax and also that the cannula is not blocked.

For diagnosis, a raised central pressure is a strong indicator of the presence of central circulatory failure, and a reduced pressure suggests peripheral failure. During management a central pressure rising above normal is a serious warning that the heart is failing (perhaps because of pre-existing disease) to cope with the circulatory volume, and further fluid infusion could precipitate severe cardiac failure. Conversely, a falling central pressure in the presence of signs of poor cardiac output in an otherwise healthy heart suggests that the infusion rate should be increased promptly.

This can be explored further using a **fluid challenge** of infusion of a bolus of IV fluid to assess the circulatory state. If the fluid challenge leads to signs of improved cardiac output with prompt return of the raised filling pressure (due to the bolus infusion) towards normal, it is likely that increase of the rate of infusion is required. If, on the other hand, the filling pressure remains elevated, then it is likely that the heart would not cope with a significantly raised circulatory volume, and the rate of infusion should be reduced.

Ejection fraction in heart failure

Measurement of the ventricular ejection fraction is a helpful quantitative measure of the severity of heart failure:

$$\text{Ejection fraction} = \text{stroke volume/end diastolic volume}$$

As heart failure progresses, the features of low output (pale, cold, perhaps bluish peripheries) and congestion (raised venous pressure, hepatomegaly, and cardiomegaly) both develop. Both features tend to reduce the ejection fraction—stroke volume falls while end diastolic volume increases. Ejection fraction can be **measured** by transoesophageal echocardiography (TOE), using ultrasound. The cross-sectional area of the left ventricle can be measured at end diastole and end systole and the chamber volume computed. In a heart with end diastolic volume 100ml and end systolic volume 40ml, the stroke volume is 60ml. Ejection fraction is 60/100, 60% or 0.6. A value below 50% warns of a significant degree of failure, around 30% indicates severe failure, and in terminal heart failure the value can fall as low as 10%.

How does the ratio fall as low as 10%? The answer is that it is due mainly to a dramatic rise in the end diastolic volume. Stroke volume cannot fall markedly, since a value much below normal would not maintain life. Typically a ratio of 10% would be derived from a fraction of 50/500 with maintenance of a just viable stroke volume and gross distension of a feeble heart whose Frank/Starling curve is indicated in Fig. 27.3.

If this pathetic curve is contrasted with the near vertical line for the highly athletic heart in strenuous exercise, it is not surprising that the patient with heart failure may not survive even mild trauma or other circulatory challenge, whereas the young fit heart may come through severe procedures without apparent difficulty.

Measurement of the ejection fraction is thus a useful quantitative measure of the cardiac state. A reduced value suggests increased operative risk, with the risk increasing severely at low levels. The decision to proceed with anaesthesia and surgery is based on a balance between the perceived risk and the value (perhaps life saving) to be gained from potentially dangerous procedures.

Measurement of cardiac output

Consideration of this physiological measurement serves two purposes. It is a key cardiovascular functional measurement in critical care, and the various methods give useful insight into cardiological function.

Oxygen Fick method for cardiac output

The method described by Adolph Fick remains the gold standard for measurement of cardiac output. It is derived from the self-evident principle that if an organ takes up from or adds a substance to the circulation, then the amount taken up (or added) must equal flow through the organ multiplied by the arteriovenous **concentration** difference for the organ. Fick applied the principle to estimating cardiac output by measuring the blood flow per minute through the pulmonary capillaries. This value is closely similar to the cardiac output into the systemic circulation by the left ventricle. The indicator substance used was oxygen. Applying the Fick principle to flow through the lungs:

Oxygen uptake = [flow] × [arteriovenous concentration difference].

From the equation and related assumptions, we can say:

$$\text{Cardiac output} = \frac{[\text{oxygen uptake}]}{\text{arteriovenous oxygen concentration difference}}$$

Mixed venous blood must be sampled from the pulmonary artery, because only there are the different streams coming into the right atrium (from superior and inferior venae cavae and coronary sinus) properly mixed.

We can insert values into the equation by assuming a resting oxygen consumption (and hence uptake) of around 200ml/min for an adult female and 250ml/min for a male. Blood oxygen **concentration** is expressed in ml oxygen per unit volume of blood (partial pressure units are not appropriate). If we assume both male and female have an arterial oxygen concentration of 200ml/L, and a mixed venous concentration of 150ml/L (25% oxygen extraction by circulation), then for both the arteriovenous oxygen difference is 50ml/L. Work out cardiac output from the above formula. You should find, for the female, cardiac output = 200ml/min divided by 50ml/L = 4L/min. For the male, the result = 5L/min. The reason for the low overall resting oxygen extraction at rest is that much of the resting circulation passes through regions such as kidneys and skin where hardly any oxygen is extracted, so venous blood is bright red.

For someone exercising strenuously (stair climbing 5–10 floors at a good rate), oxygen uptake can be eight times the above resting rate, i.e. 2000ml/min. Arterial oxygen concentration remains at 200ml/L, but the **mixed venous concentration** falls to around 75ml/L. This is because most of the venous return now comes from exercising leg muscles which extract most of the oxygen flowing through them. Thus the arteriovenous oxygen content difference is 125ml/L and cardiac output = 2000ml/min divided by 125 ml/L= 16L per minute. In this example, the increased oxygen uptake depends on the following changes from the resting state: Firstly, oxygen delivery to the systemic circulation is approximately trebled because cardiac output has trebled (mainly due to increased heart rate). Secondly oxygen extraction has increased from 25% to 62.5%.

Other methods for measuring cardiac output

Although the oxygen Fick method is very reliable, it is highly invasive and quite complicated. Other methods can be useful when serial measurements are used to indicate trends. They are technically simpler and less invasive, particularly when they make use of equipment already in position to treat or monitor seriously ill patients. The **carbon dioxide Fick method** can be used when a patient is being ventilated and expired carbon dioxide values monitored. This method substitutes carbon dioxide for oxygen in the equation given previously. It can be applied in someone who is being ventilated and monitored for carbon dioxide levels. The required values for carbon dioxide can be calculated from the routine measurements, with the addition of a short period of rebreathing to estimate alveolar carbon dioxide content and hence mixed venous concentration of carbon dioxide.

The **indicator dilution method** relies on adding an indicator bolus to the blood and monitoring indicator concentration as it passes a downstream sampling point. This gives a curve of rising concentration followed by a fall. The indicator dilution gives the volume of blood passing the observation point over a certain time and hence the flow rate per minute. The **thermal dilution** method can be used in patients who have a cannula in the pulmonary artery. An injection of cold saline is given proximally in the pulmonary artery and blood temperature is measuring distally.

Ultrasound (US) can be used in a variety of ways. As for measuring flow in any blood vessel, a probe can be directed to one of the great vessels carrying the cardiac output (pulmonary artery or proximal aorta). Scanning gives the vessel diameter. Use of the Doppler principle (change in frequency of US waves reflected from approaching red blood cells) gives blood flow velocity. Combining the results gives blood flow volume per minute.

Another use of US scan is to visualize a cross section of a ventricle before and at the end of systole. Calculation can estimate ventricular volume at these times, and hence stroke volume. Multiplying by heart rate gives the cardiac output.

The transoesophageal approach brings the probe very close to the heart. **TOE** is being used increasingly for preoperative screening and perioperative monitoring in critical situations.

Cardiac cycles

The cardiac cycle relates various synchronous measurements which illustrate interrelated events in the heart. It is often depicted in the normal resting state, but this is rather like studying a high performance engine at low speeds. Two cardiac cycles, at rest and during maximal exercise, are shown (Fig. 27.4) for a fit young adult, corresponding to the person of greatest fitness in Table 27.1. The selected measurements illustrate the dramatic changes seen in maximal exercise in fit individuals.

Notice firstly the changes in the **electrocardiogram** which is a surface record of the electrical activity initiating cardiac contraction. At rest the briefer atrial systole (corresponding to the PR interval) is followed by the longer ventricular systole (RT) and then there is a pause (isoelectric line) indicating common diastole before the next atrial systole. With maximal exercise, the situation is very different. At over 200 beats per minute, there is less than one third of a second (around 300 milliseconds) for the entire cardiac cycle, so the duration of events reduces severely. With the P wave following immediately after the T wave there is no appreciable period of general diastole, but rather atrial and ventricular systole alternate fierce powerful brief ejections of slightly more than the resting stroke volumes.

This leads to corresponding rapid fluctuations in **ventricular volume**, so that almost immediately the volume reaches its minimum, it begins to climb steeply to the next peak. Ventricular and arterial pressures show similar rapid fluctuations. Notice in particular the timing of the arterial pressure rise, so that just as arterial pressure reaches a pressure around the resting diastolic value, it soars up to a value which would indicate serious hypertension were it to occur at rest.

Such extreme activity of the heart at 200 beats per minute has been discussed to indicate the capability of the very fit heart, but even in health maximal activity cannot be maintained for long. The critical care scene generally requires more moderate but sustained activity and compensatory tachycardia is usually intermediate between the two extremes shown in Fig. 27.4, e.g. 120–150 beats per minute. Interestingly this more moderate activity requires relatively little nervous activity to the cardiac autonomic nerves, with the vagal tone switched off and sympathetic tone at a modest level.

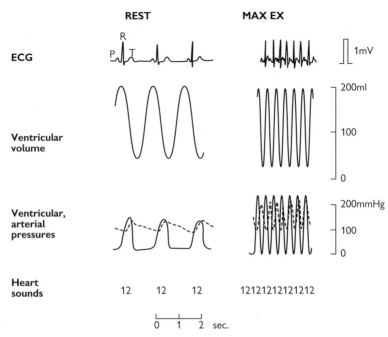

Figure 27.4 Cardiac cycles in an extremely fit young adult.

Problems of ischaemia

We now turn to the peripheral circulation to consider the problems of regional ischaemia.

The effects of ischaemia are related to a lack of oxygen and substrates arriving in the region involved, and to an excess of carbon dioxide, lactic acid and other metabolites and chemicals which accumulate. These changes are detected by local sensory nerves, particularly pain endings, and can lead to **severe pain**, as in myocardial infarction due to coronary occlusion, or in a limb, commonly the leg, with local arterial occlusion due to thrombosis or embolus. As the oxygen level falls, and toxins accumulate, **failure of function** in the region develops, for example muscular paralysis.

Another feature of loss of local blood flow in a limb, whether due to vascular occlusion or to a severe fall in arterial blood flow due to reflex vasoconstriction of the arteriolar resistance vessels, is unusual **coldness** to the touch. Normally the skin, particularly in the hands and feet, acts like a domestic heating radiator, releasing heat when flow through it is increased. In the peripheries of the body, local metabolism is normally too low to generate appreciable heat; so the reason they are usually above ambient temperature is that they receive considerable flow of blood from the core of the body, where the temperature is around 37°C.

Regional blood flow must equal perfusion pressure divided by regional vascular resistance. Perfusion pressure equals arterial inflow pressure minus venous outflow pressure. Alternatively, if pressure in the region exceeds venous outflow pressure, perfusion pressure is arterial pressure minus regional pressure. Examples are the reduction of perfusion pressure when intracranial pressure rises, and reduction of perfusion pressure in the left ventricle in systole due to myocardial contraction around the regional blood vessels. Again, when a weight-lifter holds aloft a heavy weight, the contracting muscles supporting the weight develop a very high internal pressure. During this **static work**, the cardiovascular system generates very high mean arterial pressures (BP around 250/150mmHg) to maintain flow. The stress on the heart and on the muscles and other supporting tissues is enormous.

In situations where an organ, such as a muscle, is in a **restricted compartment** the entry of blood through a patent circulation is restricted by the pressure in the compartment, and ischaemia develops (**compartment syndrome**). This is an analogous situation to the above examples, with developing pain, paralysis and cold indicating the need for urgent surgical relief of the increased compartment pressure.

Venous occlusion, for example due to DVT, also impairs the circulation by reducing the perfusion pressure. The local discomfort and swelling (often in the calf) are related in this case to leakage from capillaries which now have increased intraluminal pressure transmitted back from the obstructed veins. This situation is, of course, particularly serious because of the risk of clot breaking off, returning to the heart, and causing obstruction in the central circulation by lodging in the larger pulmonary arteries (pulmonary embolism).

Pulmonary embolism impairs filling of the left side of the heart, leading to an impaired cardiac output. At the same time, the pulmonary artery obstruction places strain on the right ventricle, which may lead to its failure. When the entire pulmonary artery is obstructed, there is total failure of the central circulation and cardiac arrest.

Scenarios

Scenario 1

A patient underwent a total gastrectomy for curative resection for carcinoma. In the HDU 12 hours after the operation his systolic is 90mmHg, tachycardia of 120/min and no urinary output over the preceding 3 hours. As the duty ST1, you have been called to see this patient at 2am. What is your management?

Scenario 2

A 73-year-old patient who is an ASA 3 category risk underwent an emergency closure of a perforated duodenal ulcer. On the first postoperative day his systolic is 80mmHg, tachycardia of 110/min and is tachypnoeic. What is your management—assessment, investigations, and diagnosis?

Answers

Scenario 1

I would strongly suspect **post-operative hypotension due to slipped left gastric artery ligature**. This patient needs to have blood cross-matched and arrangements for theatre made forthwith. I would inform my consultant and the anaesthetist on call. The patient would undergo a laparotomy at once for re-ligature of the left gastric artery at its source from the coeliac axis.

Scenario 2

This patient was ASA category 3 meaning that he had comorbid disease. Closure of a perforated duodenal ulcer will not have any chance of post-operative bleeding. Therefore his hypotension must be from a **myocardial infarction.**

The management would be as follows:

- Patient already has a drip
- ECG—ST elevation in precordial leads
  - Development of new Q waves—wide and/or deep
  - T-wave inversion
- Pulse oximeter
- Blood for:
  - CK-MB (creatine kinase, membrane bound)
  - ALT (alanine aminotransferase)
  - AST (aspartate aminotransferase)
  - LDH (lactic dehydrogenase)
  - Troponin T assay

Transfer to CCU. At this stage I would expect the patient to be under the care of the cardiologist.

CCU management:

- CVP
- Consider PAFC

- O$_2$ therapy
- Aspirin
- Nitrates, ACE inhibitors and opiates
- IV beta blockers
- Consider reperfusion strategy

Chapter 28 **Renal system in critical care**

Introduction

The principal functions of the kidney are to maintain the volume of body water and the osmotic pressure of the various body water compartments, excrete the end products of nitrogen metabolism, hormone production, and to fine-tune body pH and the level of various electrolytes such as potassium.

Volume and osmotic regulation

Body compartments

There is a daily mandatory requirement for water to maintain an exact balance between the amount of water lost and the amount gained. Failure to get the balance exact means that people would become dehydrated or overhydrated which are both life-threatening states. The daily requirement for a normal 70-kg person with a core temperature of 37°C, in an ambient temperature of 20°C and in salt (NaCl) balance is 2.5L. Of this, 1.5L is taken in as water, 1.2L is taken in with food, and 0.3L is gained from the oxidative metabolism of the food constituents such as carbohydrates and fats. The daily loss of water is 1.4L as urine, 0.1L is lost in faeces, and 1L as insensible losses of which roughly 0.5L is lost in respiration and 0.5L as sweat. Every household in the world has a pot of salt in the kitchen, for cooking purposes, and dining tables will have a salt cellar. The daily requirement for salt is around 6g (≈260mEq sodium) but intake is usually between 8–15g depending upon diet. The majority of this salt is deliberately added to the food we cook or, on demand, sprinkled on the food we eat. A similar quantity of potassium is gained automatically from the food we eat. Water intake is normally controlled by 'thirst' under the control of the osmoreceptors located in the hypothalamus.

Some 60% of body weight (42L) is composed of water. This is distributed in the intracellular compartment (25L), and in the three extracellular compartments: the interstitial fluid bathing the tissue cells (13L), the plasma (3L), and in the transcellular compartments, e.g. respiratory and intestinal tracts (1L). These water compartments have different compositions when they are analysed, shown in Table 28.1

Looking at this table it can be seen that the body has to maintain its hydration at a correct level to prevent shifts of water between compartments allowing water to be lost if the body is overhydrated or retained if the body is dehydrated. It also has to maintain the ionic concentrations at the correct levels by losing excess or trying to retain an ion if there is a deficit. For example, supposing that you were unable to regulate your sodium chloride concentration then ingesting your daily salt 'allowance' of 6g would mean you would have to retain 666.7ml of water to keep the salt concentration in plasma isotonic

Table 28.1 Concentration differences in the three major fluid compartments. Concentrations expressed as mmoles/kg water. Osmolarity expressed as mOsmoles/kg water

	Plasma mmol/L	Interstitial mmol/L	Intracellular mmol/L
Na^+	150	144	10
K^+	5	5	160
Mg^{2+}	2	2	28
Ca^{2+}	3	3	
Cl^-	110	114	3
HCO_3^-	27	28	10
Protein	17	4	65
Phosphate^{2-}	2	2	100
Sulphate^{2-}	1	1	20
Organic acids	4	4	
Osmolarity	285	285	285
pH	7.4	7.4	7.1–7.2

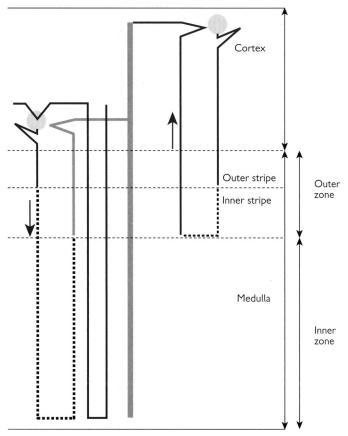

Figure 28.1 Showing a highly schematic diagram of the cortical (right) and juxtamedullary (left) nephrons. The labels 'Outer stripe' and 'Inner stripe' refer to the divisions of the outer zone of the renal medulla. Thin dark blue lines: proximal convoluted tubule and thick descending limb; dotted line: the thin parts of the loop of Henle; thin light blue lines the thick ascending limb and distal convoluted tubule; thick light blue line the collecting tubule. The black lines indicate the extent of the post-glomerular capillary bed. In the medullary part the capillaries form the vasa recta. The arrows indicate the flow of tubular fluid.

(normal saline is a 0.9% solution of salt in water). Examining the packaging of ready meals in my local supermarket shows that each meal contains 40–80% of the daily recommended salt allowance which can lead to real problems in maintaining a correct intake.

Functional kidney unit—the nephron

The functional unit of the kidney is the nephron (Fig. 28.1) of which there are some 2.4 million in the, normally, two kidneys. The kidneys can be divided macroscopically into two major zones; an outer cortex and an inner medulla. This latter can be further divided histologically into two: an inner zone and an outer zone. The nephron is composed of several histologically different parts. Essentially the nephron is a bent tubular structure with a bulbous Bowman's capsule surrounding a capillary tuft—the glomerulus. Following the capsule the tube is coiled up—the proximal convoluted tubule after which the tube dips down into the medulla and then ascends upwards to the cortex—the loop of Henle, it then has another coil—the distal convoluted tubule and finally joins with a collecting duct.

- **Capsule and glomerulus** The capillary bed surrounded by, and in close association with, the wall of the capsule forms a narrow barrier between the blood plasma and the fluid in the tubule. The capillary endothelial cells have gaps of 50–100nm between them and are separated from the cells lining the capsule, the **podocytes,** by a basement membrane. The podocytes have closely interdigitating appendages, the pedicels, with slit-like spaces between them covered by a membrane with pores of 5nm in diameter. This structure serves to filter the plasma allowing all the components in the blood, except blood cells and large molecules with a molecular radius of ≥4.4nm and a molecular weight of some 80,000. There is another constraint for large molecules, e.g. plasma proteins and that is they have a charge. For example, plasma albumin has a molecular radius of 3.5nm but is negatively charged so normally, only some 0.3% will be filtered. Overall the function of this filtration system is to produce an ultrafiltrate of blood. Filtration is aided by the fact that the capillary bed is fed from an afferent arteriole and drained by an efferent arteriole, with a smaller diameter, giving a higher hydrostatic capillary pressure that that seen in the capillary beds in the rest of the systemic circulation

- **Proximal convoluted tubule** Near the nephron the next part of the tube takes a somewhat convoluted path—hence its name. The cuboidal cells have a brush border on the surface bathed in filtrate and an elaborately folded basal and lateral membrane in contact with capillary endothelial cells. The cells in this part of the tubule contain numerous mitochondria. Their structure and contents would suggest that they have a high metabolic activity and this, together with the extensive surface areas on both luminal and basolateral parts, suggests that they have a resorptive and/or secretory function

- **Loop of Henle** The extent of the loop which dips down towards the renal papillae distinguishes the nephrons into two types. Those with a long loop reaching downwards as far as the renal papillae are situated near the corticomedullary boundary—the juxtamedullary nephrons, and comprise about 20% of the total population. The remainder have a shorter loop which only extends through the outer medullary zone. A further structural distinction can be made. Juxtamedullary nephrons have a thick-walled initial descending portion followed by a thin-walled descending portion then thin and thick ascending portions. The loops of the cortical nephrons have a thick wall on the descending loop followed by thin- then thick- walled ascending portions

  (Wherever in the body you get two closely apposed tubes with fluid flowing in opposite directions you get the potential for a counter current exchange. For example, arteries and veins transfer heat between them such that the blood flowing back in the veins from a cold extremity, e.g. fingers, is warmed before it gets back to the heart. Think of the extreme case when a penguin is sitting on ice at −30°C in a howling blizzard!)

- **Distal convoluted tubule** When the ascending limbs of the loops of Henle arrive back in the renal cortex they form another convoluted tube near their parent capsule. The tubule wall in this part of the nephron, where they are in contact with their parent glomerulus, contain special cells—the macula densa. After this part of the nephron several of the tubules will connect with a collecting duct which conveys any fluid contents to the renal papillae and pelvis to be passed down the ureter into the bladder

- **Capillary system** The efferent arterioles from the glomeruli give rise to a capillary system which is closely apposed to the proximal and distal convoluted tubules which are located near their parent capsule and follow the path of the tubules in the loops of Henle (the vasa recta). When they reach back into the cortical region they form venules and then connect into the venous drainage of the kidney

Renal blood supply

The kidneys receive blood directly from the descending aorta via two short renal arteries. These branch to form the arcuate arteries coursing through the boundary between the cortex and medulla. The inter-lobular arteries, which supply the cortex are branches of the arcuates. Total blood flow is around 20% of the cardiac output ≈1.2L/min. Renal plasma flow is unequal in the various layers of the kidneys: 500ml/min in the cortex, 120ml/min in the outer medulla, and 20ml/min in the inner medulla. The kidney blood flow shows autoregulation; changing the mean pressure over a range from 11–27kPa (80–200mmHg) shows almost no change in flow or the glomerular filtration rate. This autoregulation occurs in dener-vated kidneys and is probably a function of changes in afferent and efferent arteriolar resistance. Renal O_2 consumption is around 18ml/min. The O_2 consumption of the cortical layer is some 20 times higher than that in the inner medulla.

Filtering capacity

This is measured as the volume of plasma that can be filtered per minute termed the glomerular filtration rate (GFR). To determine this you need to use a substance that is:

- Not metabolized by the kidney
- Not secreted by the kidney
- Not reabsorbed from the filtrate, and
- Does not affect the function of the kidney

One suitable substance is the polyfructose inulin which can be infused to give a fixed concentration in the plasma. If the concentration of the marker is measured in the urine and the flow of urine is measured then the GFR is determined by:

$$GFR = \frac{\text{concentration in urine} \times \text{urine flow as ml/min}}{\text{concentration in plasma}}$$

Supposing that the plasma concentration of a substance is 2mg/ml, and its urine concentration is 240mg/ml and urine flow is 1ml/min then the quantity excreted must have been contained in 120ml of plasma. Therefore GFR = 120ml/min which is, purely by coincidence, the normal average value. This gives a daily filtration volume of 172.8L. This means that, theoretically, all the extracellular fluid can be filtered 10 times per day. With an average urine output of 1ml/kg/h (the standard value) then urine output per day is around 1.7L which is approximately 1% of the filtrate. In practice the creatinine clearance is used clinically to estimate the GFR since it is produced by the metabolism of creatinine phosphate, in a normally nourished person its production is fairly constant (about 2g/day) and its plasma concentration is fairly stable. There is a slight drawback—creatinine is actively secreted into the urine in the terminal parts of the proximal convoluted tubule but at a much slower rate than its filtration. Estimates of GFR with this 'natural' marker are approximately 10% too high. There is also a website that lets GPs roughly estimate the GFR from plasma creatinine concentration alone. The results obtained in this way for GFR can only be used as suggestive of a kidney problem not definitive.

If the plasma marker is both filtered and secreted and neither metabolized nor reabsorbed then its filtration volume can be used to determine the volume of plasma flowing through the kidney and knowing the haematocrit, the renal blood flow.

Functions of the different parts of the nephron

Glomerulus and capsule

As mentioned above, the structure of the interface between the glomerular capillaries and the capsule wall has an extensive surface area, a short path for solvent and solute transit from tubule to capillary, and a barrier with small holes would suggest a simple filtration system. The pressures inside the capillary bed (see Table 28.2) are such that 120ml of isotonic fluid filtrate are produced per minute.

The pressure in the Bowman's capsule is generated by the large volume inflow into a small tube and is necessary to drive the fluid through the tubular system. Note that in this capillary bed with arterioles at both ends there is a net hydrostatic pressure pushing fluid out and an insufficient, opposing, oncotic (colloid osmotic) pressure to suck it back in. It must also be pointed out that if the relative diameters of the afferent and efferent arterioles change then the hydrostatic pressures in the capillary will alter

Table 28.2 Pressures in the glomerular capillary bed (mmHg). The hydrostatic pressures have been estimated by extrapolation of data from animals. Net = (Hydrostatic – Oncotic) – 20

	Start	End	Ave	Capsule
Hydrostatic	61	59	60	20
Oncotic	25	37	31	0
Net	16	2	9	

considerably, a mechanism probably used to keep the filtration pressure normal if blood pressure changes. A rise in blood pressure will make the afferent arterioles constrict thus reducing capillary pressure and decreasing the rate of filtration. A fall in blood pressure is probably sensed by the cells in the macula densa which somehow constricts the efferent arterioles and the resultant decrease in blood outflow from the glomerulus will maintain capillary pressure which will, in turn, maintain the rate of filtration. No urine will be produced if the mean systemic blood pressure falls below 60mmHg. The filtering capacity of the kidneys will also be dependent on the total filtration surface area (number of active nephrons) and also the number and size of the endothelial fenestra. Both of these factors can be changed by disease.

Proximal convoluted tubule

The fluid passing to this part of the nephron is an ultrafiltrate of blood which contains all of the free ions and small molecules present in the plasma and with which it is almost isotonic. These constituents of the tubular fluid have to be removed and returned to the plasma. Approximately two-thirds of the sodium is absorbed in the proximal tubule—75% as sodium chloride and 25% as sodium bicarbonate. There are a variety of mechanisms that can achieve this including active transport, carrier mediated transport, solvent drag (the ability of water to drag solutes with it), and passive diffusion.

If we first consider the reabsorption of sodium. This is the most important active process throughout the entire nephron and accounts for the major part of the oxygen consumption in the kidney. Because of the large concentration gradient from extracellular to intracellular for Na^+ and the large transmembrane potential difference (-60 to -80mV) sodium ions will tend to diffuse into the tubule cells. Once inside they will be removed by the Na^+/K^+ ATPase exchange pumps located on the basolateral membrane of the tubular cells (Fig. 28.2).

In the first part of the tubule some sodium movement is coupled to carrier mediated transport systems for glucose and amino acids. All of the filtered glucose and most of the L-amino acids will be removed from the filtrate in the proximal convoluted tubule with Cl^- and water following the Na^+ via the leaky 'tight' junctions between the tubular cells. Ions and molecules will have a water shell so that some transfer of water will automatically occur. The leaky tubular epithelium means that it is extremely permeable to water, its hydraulic conductivity is higher than found in any other leaky epithelium and the resorption of solute will cause a very small decrease in the osmolality of the tubular fluid, a very small change in osmolality 5–20mOsmol/kg H_2O will be sufficient to achieve the water transfer seen. (*Pure water has a concentration of 55.6 M, 18g in 1L, adding solute to water decreases the water concentration so that the concentration gradient for water increases as a solution becomes more dilute.*) Because the reabsorption of glucose and amino acids is limited by the number of carrier molecules available it means that there is a limit to the amount that can be removed from the tubular fluid. This is referred to as the Tm or transport maximum. Normally blood glucose concentration is between 3.6–5.8mmol/L (mean 5.0mmol/L) the maximal concentration that can be completely cleared from the filtrate is around 10mmol/L. Blood glucose concentration can vary markedly throughout the day e.g. in a fasting state (low), post meal (high) or post 'snack' (high to very high), during exercise (high), or post stress (high to very high). Glucose will not normally appear in the urine but does so under two conditions; first if plasma glucose concentrations reach abnormally high levels, e.g. in diabetes mellitus, and secondly if there if there is a defect in the

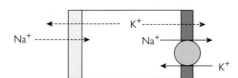

Figure 28.2 Shows the basic ionic exchange across all cells in the body. Na^+ diffuses into the cell down its chemical and electrical gradient, in this case from the luminal side and is pumped out by the Na^+/K^+ ATPase exchange pump on the basolateral surface (3Na^+ out for 2K^+ in). By swapping the egress of Na^+ with the ingress of K^+ there will be a saving of 2/3rds of the energy needed to transfer these ions against their electrical gradients. This gives a net transfer of Na^+ into the blood and the K^+ can move out either into the lumen or into the blood depending upon prevailing chemical gradients or the charge in the luminal fluid. *In this and subsequent figures the luminal surface is on the left; passive solute flow is shown as dashed lines and active movement is shown as solid lines.*

glucose carrier, e.g. in renal glucosuria a rare hereditary disorder. Almost all of the plasma L-amino acids are reabsorbed, only some 0.5–2.0% of the total filtered load appears in the urine (see Fig 28.3).

Some of the passive ingress of Na^+ results in an exchange for intracellular H^+, derived from carbonic acid or intracellular metabolism. H^+ secretion into the tubular lumen takes place via the Na^+/H^+ antiport or countertransport system. If the H^+ is derived from the conversion of intracellular CO_2 then the bicarbonate ion formed will exit across the basolateral membrane of the cell via a carrier mediated process in which the exit of three HCO_3^- ions is coupled with the exit of one Na^+. The other Na^+ will be actively pumped out of the cell. In the lumen the H^+ will react with HCO_3^- forming CO_2 which will diffuse in to the cell to form HCO_3^-. The net result will be to transfer $NaHCO_3$ from the tubular lumen into the peritubular space and then into the peritubular capillaries. The tubular cells contain relatively large amounts of carbonic anhydrase (see Fig. 28.4).

As a result of the transfer of HCO_3^- from the lumen its concentration falls from 25mEq/L to 3.8mEq/L and the luminal concentration of Cl^- increases from 105mEq/L to 126mEq/L. This will provide a sufficient drive for diffusional absorption of sodium chloride. This passive process also drives the reabsorption of KCl and some 60% of the filtered K^+ load is removed from the filtrate and its concentration in the filtrate reaches almost the same as its concentration in the plasma. Urea is also passively transferred from the filtrate. At the start of the tubule its concentration is some 4mmol/L and at the end it is about 6mmol/L meaning that slightly less than 50% is reabsorbed. Both phosphate and sulphate are reabsorbed in the proximal tubule. Phosphate transfer is under the control of parathyroid hormone and so the amount excreted or absorbed shows considerable variation. Sulphate has a maximal rate of re-absorption and renal excretion is the main regulator of its plasma concentration. Albumin appears in the filtrate at around 1% of its concentration in plasma, 30mg/dl. If all this albumin were to be excreted in the urine the albumin loss per day would amount to some 54g/day (300mg/L × 180L/day). This does not occur because the kidney reabsorbs most of it via a Tm limited process, for this molecule by pinocytosis, normally the loss is only some 150mg/day. If the plasma albumin concentration goes above 60–70g/L the rate of albumin excretion increases markedly. Oligopeptides in the filtrate, e.g. molecules such as the hormones insulin, glucagon, calcitonin, ADH, and angiotensin, are removed by peptidases located on the brush border of the tubule cells. The resultant amino acids are transported into the cell and thence to the blood stream. Renal metabolism of filtered hormones is a primary route for their normal turnover.

A large number of organic acids and bases, including potentially harmful substances, are rapidly removed from the blood by active secretion into the proximal tubule. Many drugs are removed from the

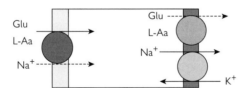

Figure 28.3 The active reabsorption of glucose and L-amino acids is as a result of coupling inward Na^+ diffusion with a specific carrier molecule for the glucose or the individual L-amino acid. The potential energy for the entry of Na^+ is maintained by the ATPase exchange pump and the basolateral membrane has a facilitated diffusion mechanism to allow the organic molecules to pass into the blood.

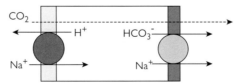

Figure 28.4 This illustrates the mechanism of HCO_3^- reabsorption in the proximal convoluted tubule. Active H^+ secretion is coupled to Na^+ entry by an exchange diffusion mechanism. The extruded H^+ reacts with luminal HCO_3^- to produce CO_2. The HCO_3^- disappearing from the lumen is accompanied by an equal amount of HCO_3^- leaving the cell across the basolateral membrane.

circulation in this manner sometimes aiding their action, e.g. the most widely used diuretics can reach clinically desirable concentrations in the tubular fluid, without needing potentially harmful plasma concentrations, to exert their effects. Conversely, some drugs, e.g penicillin-like antibiotics, are rapidly cleared from the blood stream.

There are two ways in which the absorption in the proximal convoluted tubule can be manipulated for clinical benefit. A carbonic anhydrase inhibitor such as acetazolamide will disrupt the transfer of sodium bicarbonate and its accompanying water and give a diuresis but the effect is relatively small and such inhibitors will have the side effect of metabolic acidosis. A better way to produce a diuresis is to use a molecule which is freely filtered but poorly reabsorbed such as mannitol. The majority of the filtered load ($\approx$95%) is maintained within the tubular system and both Na^+ and water re-absorption will be decreased giving a large diuretic effect. Na^+ transfer will be decreased because of the dilution with the water retained in the tubule and hence a significant amount of back diffusion, from plasma to luminal fluid, will occur.

Limb of Henle

Overall the ability of the kidney to produce concentrated or dilute urine is very simple to understand. There is a very large difference in osmolality from the start of the limb of Henle from 280–1200mOsmol/kg H_2O at the tip of the long loops. Turning on the water permeability of the collecting duct cells allows water to be 'sucked' out of the fluid exiting the nephron giving a concentrated urine and turning it off allows the fluid to exit as hypotonic urine. This is dependent upon several differential properties of the ascending and descending limbs and their anatomical arrangement:

- The flow of fluid is in opposite directions
- The limbs are in close apposition
- The thick part of the ascending limb actively pumps NaCl and KCl out of the fluid
- The descending limb is highly permeable to water but not solute, and
- The ascending limb is permeable to solute but not water

Thus for short-limbed loops, those descending to the outer zone/inner zone boundary of the medulla, fluid entering the thick part of the limb will become dilute due to the transfer of K^+, Na^+, and $2Cl^-$ via a special carrier molecule. The Na^+ is then pumped out of the cell by the Na^+/K^+ ATPase exchange pump with the Cl^- following passively. The K^+ diffuses back into the luminal fluid. This produces a hypotonic intra-tubular fluid and a hypertonic extracellular fluid. This draws water from the descending limb and the concentration of the fluid increases to $\approx$600mOsmol/kg. As the fluid flows back up solute, is actively removed. Therefore we have the basis for a counter-current multiplier. In the nephrons with long loops the established concentration gradient will be maintained and amplified because of the leak of water from the descending limb and in the ascending part will become less concentrated because of the outflow of solute (see Fig. 28.5).

An additional component for helping to produce and maintain this enormous concentration is the role played by urea. In protein-deficient conditions which leads to a decrease in urea production the osmolality gradient is decreased. The concentration of urea entering the thick ascending limb is around 20mM. This remains unchanged as the fluid flows through the distal convoluted tubule and connecting tubule

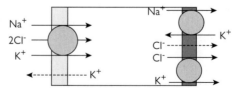

Figure 28.5 Illustrates the active reabsorption of NaCl. The movement of Na^+, $2Cl^-$, K^+ ions is via a co-transport molecule on the luminal surface. The Na^+ is extruded across the basolateral membrane by the ATPase exchange pump. Cl^- leaves passively via Cl^- channels and by co-transport with K^+. The K^+ can also re-enter the luminal fluid using normal K^+ channels.

into the collecting duct. All of these regions have a low urea permeability. In the presence of ADH water is removed and the urea concentration increases to around 100mM. The collecting duct becomes permeable to urea in the inner part of the medulla. This causes an increase in the NaCl concentration in the water permeable thin descending limb and in the ascending limb this NaCl leaks out passively thus replacing the active transport of NaCl in the thick ascending limb to maintain a horizontal osmotic gradient. The whole process is 'kick-started' by the active extrusion of NaCl from the thick ascending limb and then amplified and maintained by differences in osmolality in the interstitium aided by the differential water/solute permeabilities of the ascending and descending limbs plus the continual flow of liquid. The loop diuretic furosemide acts by stopping the active extrusion of NaCl causing the entire medullary osmotic gradient to vanish within minutes.

The final part of the maintenance of the osmotic gradient is that played by the capillaries. These also have descending and ascending parts closely apposed and help to maintain the gradient by allowing passive diffusion of water and solute as they pass through the medulla. The additional osmotic effect of the plasma proteins in the ascending capillaries helps to stabilize the gradient by returning the net efflux of water and giving a further saving of water.

Distal convoluted tubule, connecting tubule, and collecting duct

These three components of the nephron complete the conversion of the tubular fluid into urine. This includes reabsorption of virtually all of the Na^+, K^+, 60% of the urea, and up to 15% of the remaining filtered water. The composition of the fluid reaching the distal convoluted tubule will, of course, be dependent on the lengths of the loops of Henle in the individual nephrons.

Na^+ will be taken from the filtrate in the distal convoluted tubule and the connecting tubule by a carrier mediated process transporting Na^+ and Cl^- together. The Na^+ is then removed by the Na^+/K^+ ATPase pump Cl^- following passively. This Na^+/Cl^- co-tranporter carrier can be blocked by the thiazide class of diuretics. Because of their low permeability to water the filtrate osmolality and electrolyte concentration will both be lowered. The low urea permeability means that its concentration will remain unaltered. Na^+ enters the cells of the collecting tubule down its electrochemical concentration gradient and is then pumped out followed by a passive flux of Cl^-. This exchange is dependent upon aldosterone levels. The water permeability of the collecting duct cells is regulated by antidiuretic hormone (ADH) as is urea permeability in the later parts of the ducts. With a maximal secretion of ADH the permeability to water is very high so water leaves the ducts via the osmotic gradient of the medulla to give a minimal excretion of water (water excretion can rise as high as 7–10% of the glomerular filtrate in the absence of ADH). ADH secretion is controlled by the osmoreceptors located in the supra-optic and paraventricular nuclei of the hypothalamus. These receptors respond to a change in osmolality as low as ≈3mosm/kg H_2O. The cells in these nuclei synthesize ADH which is then transported down their axons to the posterior pituitary and released by action potentials. The action potentials in this region are long lasting ≈10msec to give an adequate release of the hormone. ADH gains access to the systemic circulation because the blood brain barrier for vessels leaving the posterior pituitary is 'leaky'.

Hormonal control of kidney function

There are four other hormone systems which act upon the kidney; aldosterone, atrial natriuretic hormone, parathyroid hormone, and calcitonin.

Aldosterone increases the ability of the kidney to retain sodium by increasing the luminal permeability of apical cells in the distal convoluted and collecting tubules to both K^+ and Na^+ and activates the basolateral Na^+/K^+ ATPase pump thus transferring Na^+ (and Cl^-) into the capillaries and the increased intracellular K^+ concentration to the urine. It may also act on the central nervous system to increase ADH secretion and thereby to conserve water as well as Na^+. The amount of aldosterone release appears to be directly related to plasma K^+ concentration, increased angiotensin and ACTH levels, and decreased atrial natriuretic hormone levels.

Atrial natriuretic hormone is released by myocytes in the right atrium possibly in response to stretch caused by an increase in blood volume. It acts to dilate the afferent arterioles to the glomerulus which will give an increase in GFR. Blood flow through the vasa recta will also be increased so that the amount of electrolytes washed out of the medullary interstitium will be increased. It also decreases sodium

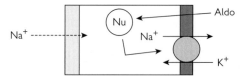

Figure 28.6 The action of aldosterone (Aldo) is to act on the cell nucleus (Nu) to increase the expression of ATPase exchange carriers. The increase in carrier numbers will augment the extrusion of Na^+ and ingress of K^+.

Table 28.3 Approximate daily amounts reaching the capsule (Caps), the descending limb (DL), the distal convoluted tubule (DCT) the collecting duct (CD) and exiting from the papilla (Pap) and the % amount excreted (% Load). The calculations were made assuming that 1M NaCl contains 23g of sodium, 1M KCl contains 39.1g of potassium, 1M of urea contains 60.1g, and that 50% of the plasma calcium is bound and that its plasma concentration is around 50mg/L. The data assumes the hypothetical person is in salt, water, and potassium balance and has the correct daily protein intake. All figures are approximate and serve to illustrate the parts of the nephron in which major changes occur

Subs	Caps	DL	DCT	CD	Pap	% Load	Units
Water	173.0	52.0	20.7	12.1	1.4	0.8	L/day
Urea	52	26		52	20.8	40.0	g/day
Na^+	575	207	46	41.4	4.6	0.8	mEq/day
K^+	28.2	11.4	2.4	3.1	3.9	14.0	mEq/day
Ca^{2+}	9	3.6	0.9	0.9	0.2	2.0	g/day

reabsorption in the distal convoluted and collecting tubules and inhibits both rennin and aldosterone secretion.

Parathyroid hormone stimulates the active reabsorption of Ca^{++} from the filtrate as it passes through the thick ascending limb and the distal convoluted tubule. It also reduces the excretion of phosphate. Thus its effect is twofold retaining body calcium directly and indirectly changing the calcium:phosphate ratio to give a greater proportion of free ionized Ca^{++} in the plasma. **Calcitonin** has the reverse action.

The overall function of the kidney for the major body ions, urea, and water is shown in Table 28.3. These values can be compared with the overall behaviour of the ion and water exchanges in the nephron (Fig. 28.7).

Finally, the urine is passed via the ureters to the bladder. The composition of the urine is not altered at all by these structures. The cellular lining of the bladder is impermeable to water and urea.

Clinical conditions affecting urine output

Urine output can be altered in three major ways due to pre-renal factors, renal factors, and post-renal factors. Generally renal function is considered abnormal if the rate of urine production falls below 0.5ml/kg/h.

Pre-renal causes—this is seen in any clinical condition which influences blood pressure and renal perfusion. These include a direct decrease in renal perfusion as for example in renal arterial stenosis. Decreased blood pressure can be as a direct influence of alteration of sympathetic activity, e.g. in spinal shock or epidural anaesthesia or to conditions which influence blood volume, e.g. loss of blood—haemorrhage, loss of plasma—burns, loss of fluid—diarrhoea or vomiting, loss of water—sweating as a result of fever or a hot environment, hyperventilation, and diabetes mellitus or insipidus. An increase in body water, hypervolaemia, is another condition which is clinically dangerous. This can occur due to excessive fast water intake, excessive ADH secretion, and water translocation in surgical procedures. For example, transurethral resection of the prostate can lead to TURPs syndrome. To keep the operating field clear

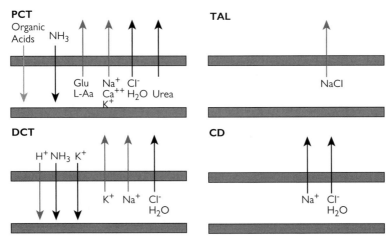

Figure 28.7 Diagram showing the movement of ions and water in the different parts of the nephron. Black arrows indicate passive diffusion, blue arrows active and carrier mediated transports. CD, collecting duct; DCT, distal convoluted tubule; PCT, proximal; TAL, thick ascending limb.

and to allow the diathermy current to take the correct path the bladder is flushed continually with an isotonic solution of an organic solute, e.g. glycine or sorbitol. This solute, together with water, gets absorbed down a very large concentration gradient, and can give a dangerous dilution of the plasma, extracellular, and intracellular fluids. The danger mainly lies in the time lag between ingestion, maximum ADH plasma concentration, and maximal effect on the kidney. The maximal effect on the kidney, i.e. the time required to completely remove a modest load of 1.4L consumed over a 30-minute period takes 3.5 hours. During this time there can be considerable shifts of fluid from the extracellular to the intracellular compartments leading to major changes in cellular function. TURPs is further exacerbated in that the large quantities of glycine can, albeit rarely, produce a large increase in plasma ammonia leading to cerebral oedema. The consequences of drinking large volumes of water over a short time scale can be coma, convulsions, and death.

Any large increase in venous pressure e.g. congestive heart failure can affect the filtration process in the kidney:

- **Renal causes** include any circumstance that allows delivery of toxic substances to the kidney either from endogenous sources, e.g. haemoglobin from lysis of red blood cells after a large transfusion, myoglobin from muscles after a crush injury, or exogenous chemicals given as drugs, e.g. non-steroidal anti-inflammatory drugs (aspirin, ibuprofen, and diclofenac) can disrupt the function of the distal convoluted tubule, aminoglycoside antibiotics (gentamicin) can affect the function of the proximal convoluted tubule, and β-lactam antibiotics (vancomycin) can lead to the development of acute tubular nephritis. Any infection of, or disease of, the kidney can lead to changes in urine output
- **Post-renal causes** include any conditions which block the entry of urine to the ureters—urinary calices, the transfer of urine down the ureter—kidney stones or compressing tumours and any condition which impedes outflow of urine from the bladder such as an enlarged prostate or quite commonly a blocked urinary catheter

Hormones produced by the kidney

Renin

This hormone is secreted from specialized cells in the juxtaglomerular nephrons, the juxtaglomerular apparatus. This is comprised of the macula densa cells of the distal convoluted tubule and the granular cells located in the afferent arteriolar wall of the tubule's parent glomerulus. The stimulus for this secretion is:

- A decrease in arterial blood pressure caused by hypovolaemia and/or hypotension (possibly detected by the granular cells)
- A decrease in NaCl levels in the filtrate reaching the distal convoluted tubule which is possibly detected by the macula densa cells, or
- By sympathetic nervous system activity (renal nerves) mediated by β_1 receptors

The released renin hydrolyses angiotensinogen in the plasma to produce the vasoconstrictive deca-peptide angiotensin I, this is then converted by the endothelial cells in the lung to the much more potent octapeptide angiotensin II. Angiotensin II can give a large rise in systemic peripheral resistance and a consequent rise in systemic blood pressure. The vasoconstrictive action on the afferent arteriole will reduce renal blood flow and glomerular filtration leading to salt and water retention. On a longer tim-escale angiotensin stimulates thirst and salt appetite, leading to increased salt and water uptake and stimulates release of aldosterone which also acts to increase salt and water retention.

Erythropoetin

Ninety per cent of erythropoietin is produced in the kidney glomeruli (the remainder in the liver) in response to chronic cellular oxygen deficiency. This hormone controls the production of red blood cor-puscles. The production of the hormone ceases when the mass of red blood cells is capable of reducing the oxygen deficiency.

1,25-dihydroxycholecalciferol

Vitamin D is hydroxylated in the liver to produce 25-hydroxycholecalciferol. In the kidney it is fur-ther hydroxylated, under the control of parathyroid hormone, to produce the more active agent 1,25-dihydroxycholecalciferol. This acts to increase the absorption of Ca^{2+} from the intestine.

Acid–base balance

The body produces approximately 15–20L of normal acid from the production of carbon dioxide and 190mM of acid from protein metabolism: hydrochloric acid from arginine, lysine, and histidine, sulphuric acid from methionine and cysteine, and phosphoric acid from nucleotides.

Of this some 130mM are used up in the metabolism of amino acids, e.g. glutamate and aspartate and some in the metabolism of other dietary organic anions, e.g. lactate. This leaves some 60mM of non-vola-tile acid which is removed by the kidney. The large amount of acid produced as carbon dioxide will be lost from the body in respiration. The reaction between CO_2 and H_2O is reversible and the production and loss of acid (H^+) will depend upon the concentration of CO_2 in the aqueous phase of the plasma.

$$CO_2 + H_2O \leftrightarrow H_2CO_3 \leftrightarrow H^+ + HCO_3^-$$

The reaction between carbon dioxide and water is catalysed by the enzyme carbonic anhydrase. Enzymes only increase the rate of a chemical reaction—they do not affect its equilibrium point. However, it is readily apparent that if the concentration of CO_2 increases it will drive the reaction to the right and if it decreases it will drive the reaction to the left.

In spite of the need to transport a large quantity of acid the pH of the plasma stays reasonably constant at 7.4 ± 0.15. A pH of 7.4 represents a H^+ concentration of some 40nM/L (4×10^{-8}M/L). Remember that pH is a logarithmic scale so that a change in pH of 0.15 units represents a 40% change in H^+ concentration (the antilog of 0.15 = 1.41253). Normally the H^+ concentration, and hence pH are kept fairly constant by the buffer pair CO_2 and HCO_3^-. The activity of this buffer pair can be described by the Henderson–Hasselbach equation.

$$pH = pk + \log_{10} \frac{[HCO_3^-]}{[CO_2]}$$

The the pk is a constant pH at which the reaction of the buffer pair is 50% complete and for this buf-fer pair has a value of 6.1.

The concentration of CO_2 is the actual concentration times its solubility coefficient.

(*In any titration of buffer acid versus buffer base the curve of change in pH is sigmoid which means that the rate of change of pH is bell-shaped with the pH at the top of the bell equal to the pk. Because the rate of change is lowest at the 50% titration point it means that there is a zone in the reaction at which pH will not change by very much and H^+ concentration will be fairly stable.*)

The HCO_3^-, CO_2 buffer pair is not a very good buffer; for the body it would be desirable to have a buffer pair with a pk of 7.4. However, the concentrations of the reactants is fairly large and their quantity in the body is sufficient for them to be used as the main buffering system in the plasma plus the $[CO_2]$ can be manipulated by the respiratory system.

The importance of the Henderson–Hasselbach equation is that it is the ratio of the concentrations of CO_2 and HCO_3^- ($[CO_2]$ and $[HCO_3^-]$) which determines the pH. Normally the $[HCO_3^-]$ is 24mmol/L and that for $[CO_2]$ is 1.2mmol/L giving a ratio of 20 the log10 of which is 1.3 and thus the pH will be 7.4. If this buffer were in a closed system ($[CO_2]$ fixed) an addition of 2mM H^+ would result in a change in $[HCO_3^-]$ from 24 to 22mmol/L and a change in $[CO_2]$ from 1.2 to 3.2mmol/L changing the ratio and pH to 6.93. However, the body is an open system and the $[CO_2]$ is continuously regulated by respiration and if $[CO_2]$ rises the excess is removed in the lungs. Thus for the above example the $[HCO_3^-]$ would still fall to 22mmol/L but the $[CO_2]$ remains the same at 1.2mmol/L and the pH would only change to 7.36. If H^+ from a source other than carbonic acid were to be added to the plasma, e.g. from the production of non-volatile acids from metabolism ≈60mM/day, this would require the removal of an equivalent amount of HCO3- from the plasma, equal to approximately 17% of the HCO_3^- contained in the extracellular fluid. To achieve the efficient removal of this non-volatile acid the kidney is used. In the kidney for each hydrogen ion that is removed one bicarbonate ion is generated. The HCO_3^-/CO_2 buffer accounts for approximately 67% of the buffering capacity of the blood. The remaining third is accounted for by the non-bicarbonate buffers. It should be noted that when excess HCO_3^- is formed by buffering alkali then the kidney can increase its rate of HCO_3^- secretion.

Normally the total buffering capacity is 75mmol/L/ΔpH and the total buffering base concentration is around 48mEq/L. This latter is the sum of all the buffering forms that can accept H^+, e.g. the bicarbonate buffer HCO_3^- and the non-bicarbonate buffers Hb, HbO_2, diphosphoglycerate, plasma proteinate, HPO_4^{2-}, etc. The phosphate buffer with a pk of 7.1 is the most important tissue intracellular buffer because its buffering capacity is not CO_2 dependent and its pk is close to ideal.

Role of the kidney in acid–base balance

Hydrogen ion secretion takes place in the proximal convoluted tubule via a H^+/Na^+ common carrier on the luminal surface of the tubule cells (one H^+ out for one Na^+ in) the Na^+ is then extruded across the basolateral surface by the Na^+/K^+ ATPase exchange pump. Normally most of the 60mM excess acid is excreted. The pH value of urine can drop as low as 4.0, i.e. an acid concentration of 0.1mmol/L which means that only 2.5% of the acid load can be excreted as acid per se. A much larger quantity is excreted as 'titratable acid' 80% as phosphate, 20% mainly as uric and citric acids. Phosphate is mainly in blood as HPO_4^{2-} and in the urine as $H_2PO_4^-$ this will automatically take H^+ out of the filtrate. Some 170mM of phosphate is filtered per day 80–95% of this is reabsorbed giving a net loss of 9–30mM/day. 80% is excreted as $H_2PO_4^-$ giving an excretion of 8.5–27mM of H^+ per day. There is an added benefit because most of the phosphate in plasma is in the form of Na_2HPO_4 and in urine as NaH_2PO_4 it means that for each H^+ excreted in this way one Na^+ is transferred back into the plasma. Additionally the kidney can excrete NH_4^+ derived, possibly, from glutamine deamidation in the tubule cells. This reaction requires H^+ and is an indirect way of secreting this ion. NH_4^+ and HCO_3^- are metabolized in the liver to form urea which is another indirect way to remove the non-volatile acid load. The remainder of the non-volatile H^+ excess (8.5–34mM/day) is removed as other titratable acids.

Disturbances in acid–base balance

When plasma pH falls below 7.35 a state of **acidosis** is said to occur and if it rises above 7.45 **alkalosis** is seen. Changes primarily in $[CO_2]$ can be regarded as a **respiratory** cause and changes in $[HCO_3^-]$ can be regarded as a **metabolic** cause. These disturbances can either be **compensated** or **uncompensated**.

Another measure which is useful to distinguish whether an acid/base imbalance is caused by a respiratory, metabolic or mixed respiratory/metabolic cause is the base excess. This refers to the amount of acid–base equivalents which are required to return the pH of blood to a value of 7.4. Normally the range is between −5 and +3, with +ve values indicative of alkalosis and −ve values acidosis. Clinically the value can be determined by the empirical formula:

$$\text{Base excess} = 0.93([HCO_3^-] - 24.4 + 14.8(pH - 7.4))$$

assuming a Hb value of 150g/L.

Metabolic acidosis

This condition is categorized by a low pH and a low $[HCO_3^-]$. Common causes include:

- Failure of the kidney to excrete the normal acid load
- Ingestion of acid, e.g. citrus fruit juices
- Excess production of acid can occur in diabetes mellitus or starvation. The ketoacids produced are from incomplete metabolism of fats
- Anaerobic metabolism producing lactic acid from incomplete metabolism of carbohydrate
- A high protein diet can lead to production of hydrochloric and sulphuric acids
- Loss of HCO_3^- as in diarrhoea

Central chemoreceptors will cause hyperventilation to remove excess CO_2 (respiratory compensation) and the kidney will excrete more H^+, forms more HCO_3^-, and excretes more NH_4^+. When acidosis develops less HCO_3^- is available for urea formation in the liver (needs NH_4^+). The secretion of H^+ via NH_4^+ can account for an extra secretion of H^+ of up to 300mM per day.

Metabolic alkalosis

This condition is accompanied by both a high pH and a high $[HCO_3^-]$. Common causes include:

- Ingestion of HCO_3^-
- Metabolism of lactate and citrate to produce H_2O and CO_2 which produces H^+ and HCO_3^-
- Loss of H^+ from vomiting
- Loss of H^+ from an increased renal secretion of H^+ as a consequence of hypokalaemia

Hypoventilation may occur to try to compensate for this condition but the ensuing hypoxia limits this mode of compensation. Renal excretion of HCO_3^- rises and that of H^+ decreases. Metabolic acidosis reduces the amount of free Ca^+ in the plasma which can lead to tetany. Indeed a common test to see if a patient is becoming hypocalcaemic is to ask them to hyperventilate and see if they develop tetany (carpal spasm = Trousseau sign). There is also a danger of central nervous irritability which may produce convulsions.

Respiratory acidosis

A condition in which there is a low pH and a high pCO_2. This occurs whenever respiratory effort to remove CO_2 is impaired:

- Chronic obstructive airways disease with impaired sensitivity to CO_2
- Reduction of functional pulmonary tissue as in tuberculosis and pneumonia
- Reduced ventilation as occurs with post-operative pain, morphine administration, or fractured ribs
- Abnormalities of the rib cage, e.g. scoliosis

In this state the restricted respiration gives an elevated pCO_2 and lowers the pH. The H^+ excess is buffered by the non-bicarbonate buffers as a result of which a small amount of HCO_3^- will be formed but is not sufficient to alter the ratio of $[HCO_3^-]$ to $[CO_2]$ which remains below normal leading to the low pH. Renal excretion of H^+ will therefore become important to compensate for the acidosis. In the process of H^+ secretion the kidney will generate HCO_3^-; this coupled with the excretion of H^+ as NH_4^+ and as $H_2PO_4^-$ returns the pH to near normal levels. However, this change in renal activity takes 1–2 days to develop fully so that an acute respiratory acidosis is poorly tolerated compared to that seen in a chronic respiratory acidosis.

Respiratory alkalosis

Categorized by a high pH and a low pCO_2 develops whenever there is excessive ventilation. This excessive ventilation can be voluntary, due to a stressful situation, or when there is an oxygen deficiency such as at high altitudes. This causes a shift in the non-bicarbonate buffers equilibrium condition which releases H^+ which react with HCO_3^- to slightly lower the concentration of this latter ion. The kidney decreases its secretion of H^+ and increases HCO_3^- secretion. This gives a sufficient reduction in plasma $[HCO_3^-]$ to return the ratio of $[HCO_3^-]$ to $[CO_2]$ to a normal value and hence returns the pH towards normal.

Scenarios

Scenario 1

A 40-year-old man has been brought in from a building site after a wall collapsed trapping him by the legs. He was trapped for 90 minutes before members of the fire service managed to extricate him. He has no broken bones but two very badly bruised, grazed, and swollen legs. What are your initial concerns and how would you manage this patient?

Scenario 2

A 79-year-old man had undergone a transurethral prostatectomy with a spinal anaesthetic. The operation was complex and took 100 minutes to complete. Three hours after returning to the ward the nurses said that he was confused, tachycardic (HR 92 beats per minute) and hypotensive (90/55). A blood sample was taken which showed a plasma Na^+ concentration of 117mmol/L. How do you treat this patient?

Answers

Scenario 1

Crush injuries can lead to:

- Metabolic acidosis
- Hyperkalaemia
- Initially hypocalcaemia followed by hypercalcaemia
- Rhabdomyolysis

There will be a large fluid shift from the intravascular compartment into the interstitial and intracellular compartments (damaged muscle will swell). The initial management will be fluid resuscitation, 6–12L of saline in the first 24 hours. The muscles in the leg will have been anoxic so will release lactic acid, potassium, and myoglobin into the bloodstream, when circulation is restored, resulting in metabolic acidosis, hyperkalaemia, and the potential to produce tubular necrosis from deposition of myoglobin and possibly uric acid in the nephron. Hence there is a need to carefully monitor cardiac function (ECG) and to check plasma K^+ concentration. There is a need to monitor the degree of rhabdomyolysis by measuring blood kinase levels, values above five times the normal upper limit are an indication, levels up to 100,000 times are sometime seen. If hyperkalaemia becomes a problem then an insulin/dextrose solution may be employed to increase cellular uptake of potassium. An adequate urine flow is mandatory and can be achieved by administering a loop diuretic to try to 'flush' away myoglobin and uric acid. The iron from the haem moiety of the myoglobin can produce free oxygen radicals, which are highly cytotoxic, and can lead to acute renal failure 1–2 days after the initial muscle damage. There is also the possibility of compartment syndrome so it would also be advisable to measure interstitial pressure, values of 30–50mmHg (4–6.5kPa) would indicate a need for fasciotomy

Scenario 2

The irrigation fluid used for the operation was an isotonic solution of sorbitol to allow a focused cauterization. This will lead to an absorption of the solute and accompanying water, in this case giving a fluid overload resulting in encephalopathy, and an increase in circulating blood volume which can push the patient's 'Starling curve' into a potential heart failure scenario (see Chapter 24, Fig. 24.5; remember that muscle when overstretched beyond its optimal length will contract less). Treatment will consist of IV fluid such as Hartmann's plus a diuretic, either furosemide or amiloride. The resultant diuresis can lead to hypokalaemia hence the need to deliver both Na^+ and K^+ in the IV fluid. Use of amiloride gives a lesser loss of K^+ compared to furosemide. The patient will need careful monitoring (ECG and blood pressure and mental state) and serial blood samples taken until plasma Na^+ and K^+ concentrations are returned to normal (Na^+ 150mmol/L, K^+ 5mmol/L).

Chapter 29 **Gastrointestinal system in critical care**

Introduction

The aim in this chapter is not to discuss the many acute surgical problems which arise from disease or injury of the gut, but to consider how the gut is affected by critical situations in general, and how disturbance of its function affects recovery.

An immediate sacrifice

When someone is suffering from life-threatening critical problems, normal activity in the gut is suppressed. Appetite is lost, replaced by nausea and a tendency to vomit. Blood flow to the gut falls to a level insufficient to maintain normal function in the cells lining the lumen. These events are produced by brain stem control mechanisms induced by the stress of the critical incident, such as severe burns or injury. The mechanisms are immediate neural reflexes and more sustained hormonal surges.

A major reflex in this situation is the **baroreceptor reflex** which detects falling arterial pressure, particularly with loss of blood. The sense organs are stretch receptors in the internal carotid arteries (carotid sinuses) and aorta. They send **afferent** impulses to the brainstem centre, so with lower blood pressure and a weaker pulse, fewer action potentials pass along the afferent nerves to the reflex centre in the brainstem In response, this centre alters its output along **efferent** autonomic nerves to effectors which determine arterial blood pressure—the heart, which produces the cardiac output, and peripheral resistance vessels (arterioles), which together make up the peripheral vascular resistance:

$$\text{Arterial blood pressure} = [\text{cardiac output}] \times [\text{total peripheral resistance}]$$

Stimulation of the heart tends to raise cardiac output, including restoring a failing output level. The sympathetic output to peripheral resistance vessels is selective—arterioles in the brain and heart are not caused to constrict, but rather, arterioles in non-vital regions do so. The non-vital regions include particularly the skin and the gut.

The vital cerebral and cardiac blood flows can thus be relatively well maintained by a relatively adequate arterial blood pressure and by local vasodilation (autoregulation, or local 'self-regulation' in contrast to regulation by nerves controlled by the reflex centres). For example, if carbon dioxide accumulates in the brain due to inadequate flow, this leads locally to arteriolar dilation which favours restoration of a more normal level of flow.

Thus blood flow to the **splanchnic** (visceral) region in the abdomen, involving the gut and accessory organs such as liver and pancreas is sacrificed to maintain flow to the vital regions. Intense **vasoconstriction** in the presence of normal or moderately reduced arterial pressure leads to severe reduction in blood flow in this region, particularly in the gut. A severe reduction in flow which impairs function and threatens local tissue survival is referred to as **ischaemia**.

Gut function is also limited by reflex nausea and vomiting produced by the critical conditions of the patient. Reflex vomiting is part of the response to severe stimulation of pain endings. The afferent part of the reflex thus consists of the pain pathway in the spinothalamic tracts which pass to the thalamus and stimulate the nearby vomiting centre. At this stage, the vomiting reflex will be considered in some detail.

The vomiting reflex

Vomiting is controlled from the medulla oblongata and is a coordinated activity in response to a variety of stimuli. Vomiting is a dramatic means of ejecting the gastric contents from the body. It is achieved by relaxing smooth muscle tone in the upper gut, particularly the lower oesophageal sphincter, so that the normal barrier to gastric reflux is removed. Gastric contents are then actively expelled by the **Valsalva manoeuvre**. This is a widely used physiological action which greatly raises pressure in the abdomen and chest. Not only does this expel gastric contents when the upper exit is open, but it is also involved in childbirth when the way out of the uterus is fully dilated, and it aids expulsion of urine and of faeces, again when the relevant sphincters are relaxed. It can be carried out voluntarily.

The **Valsalva manoeuvre** starts with a deep inspiration. The glottis is then closed, retaining the air in the lungs. A powerful forced expiratory movement is then carried out by the powerful anterior abdominal muscles. With expiration prevented, this greatly raises pressure in both abdomen and thorax, thus expelling gastric or other contents as explained above.

The high abdominal and thoracic pressures prevent normal venous return so that the face becomes flushed and the neck veins are distended, particularly if the manoeuvre is carried out voluntarily for more than a few seconds. The manoeuvre is also involved when weight-lifters hold weights above the head, as it gives a firm muscular base for supporting the weight.

The most obvious and appropriate trigger for the vomiting reflex is when **ingestion of irritating material** has occurred. Food poisoning is also associated with infective and toxic irritation of the gut. In these cases expulsion of the offending material is therapeutic.

Another logical stimulus is the presence of **acidosis** as in diabetic ketoacidosis or severe renal failure. Here the loss of the powerful gastric acid at least reduces the body's acid load, though more specific measures are needed to cure the underlying condition.

A variety of chemicals can initiate vomiting; these include drugs such as morphine and a variety of poisons. These agents act in the vicinity of the vomiting centre in the medulla at a site known as the **chemoreceptor trigger zone.**

Severe pain as considered earlier is one of a number of **highly disturbing states** which are conveyed to the individual by various receptors, including visual scenes of horror. Severe disturbance of the organs of balance has given us the origin of the word 'nausea'. It has the same origin as 'nautical'—travel in ships has for millennia been recognized as a cause of nausea and vomiting.

The effects of **vomiting in the unconscious person** can be life threatening, because cerebral suppression prevents the part of the vomiting reflex which protects the respiratory tract. Normally the larynx is elevated during vomiting—just as it can be seen to be elevated during swallowing. Elevation of the larynx presses its obliquely forward-facing entry against the back of the tongue, which acts as a safety barrier. When this fails, corrosive gastric acid with a pH around 2 can enter and seriously damage the respiratory tract. The damage is augmented by pepsin and by pathogenic organisms from recently taken food. The gastric acidity is normally a powerful defence mechanism against pathogens ingested with food. When gastric reflux in the unconscious is seen as a serious hazard, the gastric acid secretions can be reduced by H_2 **receptor blockers** to block hormonal and nervous stimulation of the acid-producing **parietal cells** of the stomach. Secretion of acid can be blocked directly by **proton pump inhibitors**, so named from the fact that proton is an alternative term for a hydrogen ion. The proton pump inhibitors block the pump which pumps the hydrogen ions from the cell to the gastric lumen (against a pH gradient of approximately 6, which corresponds to a millionfold hydrogen ion concentration!).

Returning to general impairment of gut function it can be noted that the splanchnic region also experiences suppression of blood flow and function during strenuous exercise, such as running a marathon. Even with this much lesser interference with blood flow, there can be nausea and diarrhoea in some people. With major threat to life, in the critical situation the suppression of gut circulation and function is more severe and continues much longer. It can eventually lead to serious and potentially fatal problems. The situation of suspending normal gut function, or 'gut sacrifice' can help to save life by preserving vital cerebral and cardiac function, but in the long term it can itself be fatal.

The mechanisms of this impaired gut function are outlined in Fig. 29.1.

Problems with gut sacrifice

When blood flow to the gut is greatly reduced, the cells in the gut, particularly metabolically active mucosal cells, experience a serious deficiency of oxygen and energy substrates, particularly glucose and fatty acids. It can be shown that blood flow is inadequate to maintain normal resting function. This can be monitored by probes in the gut which show developing cellular acidosis. This acidosis is partially respiratory in type (caused by carbon dioxide accumulation) and partly metabolic acidosis due to lactic acid produced by anaerobic metabolism. Such studies demonstrate not only gut dysfunction but can also be used as a monitor, indicating how severely circulation to the gut is threatened. The greater the threat to the circulation, the greater will be the compensatory vasoconstriction in the gut and the greater the cellular acidosis.

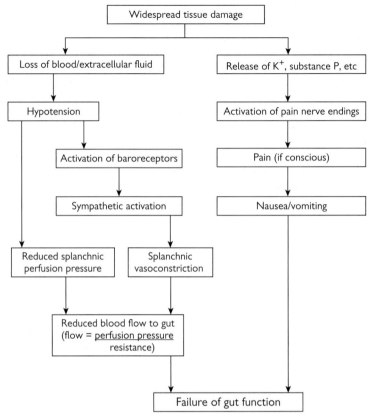

Figure 29.1 Some factors leading to impaired gut function in the critical care situation.

Progressive loss of gut integrity

When ischaemia is present for hours and days there is significant deterioration of cells and function in the gut. This effect is augmented in the long term by disuse atrophy of the mucosal cells, following the basic physiological principle that 'if you don't use it you lose it' (whether applied to skeletal muscle, the heart, or endocrine glands). This is one of the disadvantages of prolonged IV nutrition, where the digesting and absorbing functions of the gut may be bypassed for days or weeks.

Effects of loss of gut integrity

Firstly, **loss of normal nutrition** has an obvious but very important effect. Only regular normal ingestion, digestion, and absorption of a normal balanced diet can maintain normal nutrition. Life can be maintained with only water by mouth for some weeks, due to normal extensive stores of fat. However, the person's state soon becomes suboptimal, with serious lack of mental and physical capacity, due particularly to absence of a regular glucose source (hepatic and muscle glycogen stores are largely depleted after a day or two), and, more gradually, due to lack of adequate protein, vitamins and trace elements.

Artificial IV (**parenteral**) **nutrition** can be a very helpful but inferior source of nutrition. Firstly, there are the demanding problems of preparing the appropriate mix of an elemental diet. This requires a large amount of glucose, plus fat and a spread of amino acids, mainly the 'essential' ones, together with a potentially huge number of trace elements and vitamins. Secondly, the solvent water must be limited to prevent overload of the circulation. Thirdly, the high concentration of glucose must be administered to a large central vein to avoid rapid termination of the infusion by hyperosmolar irritation of peripheral veins. Fourthly, great care must be taken to avoid infection of the catheter—the gut's defences (acid, antibodies, digestive enzymes) have been bypassed. In addition, delivery into a central vein avoids the normal regulation of insulin secretion by gut hormones, and the passage of nutrients through the liver.

A further distinct problem is erosion of the mucosal barrier to absorption of pathogenic organisms and their toxins from the gut lumen to the circulation. This **loss of mucosal integrity** relates to progressive physical damage to the mucosal cells and loss of immunological defences. The problem applies particularly to lower parts of the gut where bacterial numbers are largest.

Entry of pathological organisms and toxins to the circulation and body generally produces widespread damage (multiple organ damage and failure) with accompanying hypotension, known as the **toxic shock syndrome**, where hypotension is caused mainly by relatively low peripheral resistance rather than reduction in blood volume. This condition leads to widespread breakdown of normal body function and, not surprisingly, it carries a high mortality.

Nutritional requirements in critical care

One of the problems with the above suppression of gut function is that the need for nutrition is increased at a time when gut activity is suppressed as part of the battle to remain alive.

Hormonal surges

A marked and prolonged surge in efferent sympathetic nervous activity has been discussed above. The sympathetic system itself includes an endocrine component—the adrenal medulla—from which there is a surge in the hormonal catecholamines adrenaline and noradrenaline. These raise the metabolic rate and need for nutrition.

Of the various other hormonal surges which also occur, a surge of cortisol (from the adrenal cortex) is particularly prominent and, indeed, essential for survival in severe physical stress. As with the surge of adrenaline, the cortisol surge is controlled from the brain. The **hypothalamus** has a central role in nutrition and metabolism. The appetite and satiety centres are found here and are regulated by afferent inputs from the gut (an empty stomach favours hunger, a full stomach favours satiety) and also by less understood inputs indicating the state of energy stores. It is thus appropriate that the hypothalamus has a major input to the pituitary which controls various endocrine glands and functions related in various complicated ways to body metabolism and hence nutritional requirements. Such functions include basal metabolic rate (thyroid controlled) and reproductive activity which in the female is related to the level of body energy reserves.

Also included is control of the adrenal cortical hormone **cortisol** which has profound and essential effects in critical life-threatening situations. A surge of cortisol is essential during major stress, including major surgery, to maintain adequate arterial blood pressure. It also has profound metabolic effects which are essential for survival. Prominent here is cortisol's stimulation of **gluconeogenesis**. This term implies diversion of other nutrients, particularly amino acids, to the formation of glucose.

As mentioned earlier, tissues require glucose along with the more abundantly available fat in order to carry out their functions. In critical situations there is need for an **increased metabolic rate** above the normal resting value to provide for life-saving activity which uses energy in the various responses needed for survival. In the healthy person resting in bed, energy is required to maintain breathing and cardiac activity, together with chemical synthesis to maintain cellular function and integrity. Also, about half the resting metabolic rate is used in maintaining ionic gradients. These gradients across the cell membrane are essential for activation of most cells, particularly nerve and muscle cells. Maintenance of the gradients requires use of energy by the relevant ionic pumps. In the critically ill person lying in bed, much activity occurs over and above the basic normal level.

Synthesis of clotting factors must be maintained in face of their use at sites of injury and bleeding. Repair of vital tissues must occur. The presence of infection may require increased antibody synthesis.

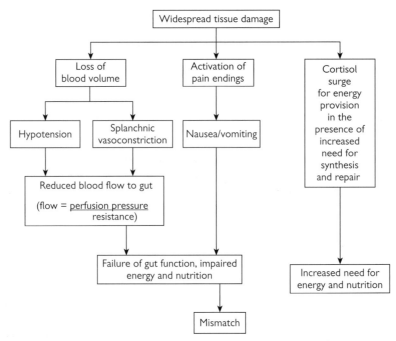

Figure 29.2 Factors leading to mismatch of nutritional needs and provision in the critical situation.

Cardiac work is likely to be increased and there is increased activity in the nervous system involving the reflexes already discussed. Measurements have shown that the metabolic rate in the critical situation is well above the normal resting value, widespread severe burns being a notable example.

Without appropriate intervention, there is a serious **mismatch** between **nutritional needs and nutritional provision** in someone fighting to survive critical stress such as multiple trauma. This is summarized in Fig 29.2.

A major task of management in this situation is therefore to provide the increased nutrition needed during the critical period. This is difficult with the body's (necessary) responses opposing such provision. In severe cases where life cannot be maintained in the face of overwhelming challenge, failure to reverse the mismatch between energy and nutritional requirements and their provision may be one of the factors leading to death.

Depending on the patient's state, in cases of lesser severity, nutrition can be provided where possible by the normal **oral** route, palatability of the food offered being of prime importance. This is the optimal solution to the problem. In some cases where the oral route is impossible, including with the unconscious patient, **parenteral nutrition** by tube into the stomach or duodenum is the next best option, as the fluid nutrient can be digested by the gut, whose integrity is thereby supported. The **enteral nutrition** option, as discussed above, is a difficult and less satisfactory option, but is the only one when gut failure is complete.

Nutrition and energy balance

The opportunity is taken at this stage to review this topic in general and then apply the principles to the critical care situation. We start by examining the normal physiological events associated with a meal and the subsequent metabolism over some hours. We then apply these principles to four quite different individuals who face severe injuries requiring critical care. First considered is a fairly sedentary individual, followed by a very fit active individual, followed by an elderly frail person; finally people with serious anorexia are considered.

Basic physiological principles

Food intake by healthy people is determined by at least four physiological influences and one environmental factor:

1 Appetite centres in the hypothalamus
2 Satiety centres in the hypothalamus
3 Physical activity
4 Cerebral cortical activity which favours variety of diet
5 Available food supplies

At a time when world population is at a record level, food supplies have also reached record abundance in the more developed parts of the world, while other parts suffer severe limitation and episodic famine. When food is abundant, people give considerable thought (cerebral cortical activity) in planning their menu and thus obtain a varied diet, likely to contain necessary vitamins and trace elements.

Sedentary individual

A sedentary individual with abundant available food is unlikely to experience the level of hunger which causes marked activation of the hunger centre. Eating is likely to be initiated mainly by habits related to the time of day and terminated by the satiety centres. The level at which these satiety centres become active is highly significant in determining the presence or absence of progressive obesity. Strong satiety centre activity (as in anorexia nervosa) leads to nausea and an inability to eat more. If substantially more is eaten despite the opposition of the satiety centre, vomiting is likely. Failure of the physiological controls, often supported by considerable cortical effort is indicated by the large number of people who cannot overcome obesity and increasing numbers who combat severe obesity with the help of surgery.

In the early stages after starting a meal, nervous and hormonal influences cause a surge of insulin which coincides with the surge into the circulation of absorbed nutrients. Release of insulin is induced partly by vagal activity to the endocrine pancreas, partly by the rising levels of glucose and other absorbed basic nutrients required for anabolism—amino acids, fatty acids, and potassium ions. Also insulin release is induced partly by the same gut hormones which stimulate digestive secretions and gut movements.

Insulin acts as an **anabolic** hormone by favouring the entry of nutrients into **skeletal muscle** in particular. Here glucose builds up energy stores in the form of glycogen in muscle glycogen granules; fat is also stored in muscle fat droplets. Amino acids help to maintain muscle protein depleted by wear and tear and potassium ions contribute to the intracellular fluid contents. Energy stores are gradually used up, after absorption ceases, by the limited amount of exercise taken by the sedentary person. A combination of glucose and fat is oxidized in the biochemical production line (Krebs cycle) of the mitochondria to generate high energy phosphate bonds in adenosine triphosphate (ATP). ATP then circulates within the cell to provide energy for muscle movement and for membrane ionic pumps. At the same time, ATPase enzymes break down ATP to adenosine diphosphate (ADP) to release the energy needed for muscular activity and maintenance of the membrane ionic gradients on which control of muscle contraction relies.

Meanwhile, during absorption from the gut, excess glucose in the circulation is taken up by liver cells for synthesis of liver glycogen, which provides a store of the essential glucose required during fasting by brain cells but not stored by them. Insulin does not directly influence uptake of glucose by brain cells. Indirectly by depressing blood glucose severely, excessive insulin can induce unconsciousness and death.

Very fit active individual

This individual has well developed skeletal muscles and high cardiac stroke volume. Strenuous physical activity is undertaken for some hours each day—either in an occupation requiring such activity (rare now in more developed parts of the world) or in training for and participating in high-level sporting activity. The skeletal muscles will have large glycogen granules and fat droplets able to contain several times as much energy substrate as the sedentary individual. Particularly after a prolonged bout of exercise the energy stores will be depleted. If the individual then takes a substantial meal, the muscle stores will take up glucose and fat at a high rate. Depletion of internal glucose during strenuous activity allows glucose uptake into the muscle without much need for insulin. Indeed, insulin-dependent diabetic sportspeople must reduce their insulin dose before strenuous activity to avoid hypoglycaemia. A major effect of increasing energy use to perhaps twice or three times the sedentary level is that food intake must be increased proportionately. Eating enough food (two to three times the average portion of everything) is a major effort, possibly requiring some struggle with the satiety centres.

When such individuals face major trauma or burns, they come with the advantage not only of a very effective circulatory system, but also large stores of muscle protein which can be mobilized by cortisol for survival during days or weeks of critical care.

Elderly frail individual

This individual is particularly vulnerable to physical stress for a variety of reasons. All the major systems, including the cardiovascular system, have greatly reduced reserves due to aging. Aging reduces organ bulk and tissue flexibility. Protein reserves in the muscles are small, due partly to aging and partly to loss of activity often related to joint stiffness.

Anorexia

Both anorexia nervosa and the relative anorexia seen in some athletes, particularly female ('anorexia athletica') can lead to **severe underweight**. For complex reasons, the appetite/satiety balance is distorted in the opposite direction to obesity and the individual has severely depleted stores of protein and fat. A similar state is produced by wasting illnesses, such as advanced cancer, and in famine conditions. All such severely underweight individuals lack the necessary stores of protein and energy to be mobilized by cortisol in times of stress. In advanced cases they move towards **hypotension** and **hypothermia** and even moderate stress is fatal. Operative mortality is very high in such people.

Energy balance and body weight

Considering the various situations above, ranging from severe obesity to severe wasting—all of which can develop in previously apparently healthy people—it is appropriate to consider briefly a fundamental equation.

Over a period of time:

Change in body mass = dietary energy content minus **energy use**

If dietary energy content exceeds energy use, the change is positive—weight gain; if the reverse is true, the change is negative—weight loss

If a sedentary person uses 2000kcal (8.4MJ) of energy daily and adheres to a reduction diet of 1500kcal (6.3MJ) a reduction of body mass equivalent to 500kcal (2.1MJ) results. This would be equivalent to loss of about 55g of fat (9kcal per gram). Thus the fundamental equation would indicate:

Change in body mass = 6.3MJ minus 8.4MJ = **minus** 2.1MJ = 55g weight **loss**

Dietary and exercise control of body weight

Both over- and underweight pose serious problems in surgery, the risk rising steeply with marked departure from normal in either direction. When some time is available before non-urgent surgery, the overweight patient is advised to combine a reduction diet with increased exercise, following the equation above. Both weight reduction and increased exercise have important general benefits in terms of reduction in risk for surgery. The operation becomes technically more feasible and the risks of complications such as vascular thrombosis are reduced.

Underweight patients pose rather different problems as their underweight may be due to a variety of serious diseases which may reduce appetite. However, a high calorie nutritious and palatable diet may succeed in producing some weight gain and thereby reduce the risks of major surgery. In view of the beneficial effects of exercise, it would be rare to ask these underweight patients to reduce exercise, unless in the relatively rare case of severe weight loss associated with inappropriate prolonged strenuous exercise.

From the above considerations, public health advice on how to avoid obesity is simple—eat less (sensibly) and exercise more—but in recent decades it hasn't worked! At a time when advice and help for maintaining optimal weight have been widely spread, obesity, and to a lesser extent, anorexic undernutrition, have increased worldwide, bearing a strong correlation to wealth of the population, whether in large areas like USA and Europe, or in the wealthier population groups of less developed countries. It seems that the appetite/satiety balance, aided by advertising, social attitudes, and tempting unhealthy foods can overcome public health education—and provide more work for surgeons!

Scenarios

Scenario 1

A 60-year-old man complains of incessant vomiting for 3–4 weeks. The vomitus contains food material that he recognizes as having eaten 2 or 3 days ago—old food. It is not bile stained. He feels early satiety. The upper part of his abdomen feels distended.

In the past he suffered from indigestion intermittently for years for which he took proprietary antacids for relief.

On examination he looks very dehydrated with sunken eyes, dry tongue, and loss of skin turgor. What is going through your mind with regard to the diagnosis?

Scenario 2

A fit 25-year-old man has been extricated from a house fire. His total body surface area (TBSA) burnt has been estimated as 20%. He has been resuscitated. He is breathing normally and he has been made stable. He is now in the burns unit. His burns are in the trunk and lower limbs. He has no head and neck burns and therefore fit for parenteral nutrition.

Outline his enteral nutritional requirements.

Answers

Scenario 1

Please read in detail Fig. 6.16 with the questions and answers in Chapter 6 on imaging.

Scenario 2

I would insert a NG tube to feed the patient. All patients with burns over 15% need to have extra nutrition. Burn injuries are catabolic. Therefore feeding should start within 6 hours of the injury. There are several formulae available. To this patient I would give 25kcl/kg body weight + 70kcl/% total body surface area burnt. Between the 5th and 10th day the greatest nitrogen losses occur. 20% of the kilocalories should be provided by proteins.

The actual composition of the nutritional fluid will be decided upon after consultation with the dietitian. Successful management involves several strategies, nutrition being one of them. Simultaneously excision of the burn and wound coverage should be done and the patient must be kept warm. The patient's nutritional balance is monitored regularly by measuring the weight and nitrogen balance.

Chapter 30 The liver

Introduction

The liver is a four-lobed structure, based on surface features, located just below the diaphragm on the right side of the abdominal cavity. It is the largest gland in the body weighing between 1.4–1.6kg in the adult. It receives its blood supply via the hepatic arteries (25%) and the hepatic portal vein (75%), receiving approximately half of its oxygen supply from the artery and the remainder from the vein. The hepatic portal vein carries venous blood from the spleen and GI tract so that the liver acts as a first-pass filter of digested intestinal contents except those derived from high-molecular-weight lipids which are conveyed from the gut in the lymphatic system. Lymph from the gut is 'milky' compared to that from other organs. Each lobe is composed of numerous lobules which can be imagined as a roughly polygonal-shaped series of vertically arranged plates of heptatocytes one or two cells thick, radiating from a central vein and bathed in blood flowing in the sinusoids from branches of the hepatic artery and hepatic portal vein. The hepatocytes can exchange molecules into, or out of, the blood because a large portion of the hepatocyte's surface will be in intimate contact with blood. Blood is drained out of the lobule via the central vein. Biliary canaliculi lie between adjacent hepatocytes draining bile into the bile ducts (see Fig. 30.1). It is probably logical to assume that the number of 'portal' sinusoids outnumber the 'arterial' sinusoids by approximately 3 to 1 but sinusoidal blood is often mixed. The bile ducts receive their blood supply from the hepatic artery. The 'triads' of hepatic artery, hepatic portal vein, and bile duct are located at each angle of the polygonal lobules.

Functions of the liver

- Synthesis of proteins
- Coagulation of blood
- Lipid metabolism
- Secretion of bile
- As a storage organ
- Breakdown of various endogenous and exogenous chemicals which enter the bloodstream
- Is part of the mononuclear phagocytic system

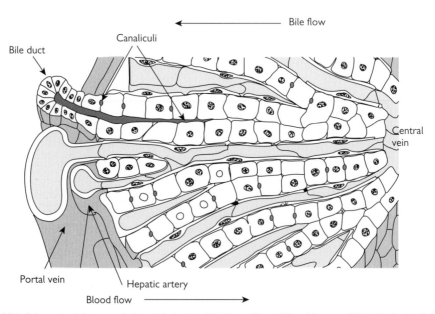

Figure 30.1 Schematized diagram of a liver lobule. (Modified from Bloom W. and Fawcett DW. *A Textbook of Histology*, 12th Edition, (1995), with permission from Elsevier and Dona Fawcett Boggs).

Protein synthesis

The liver synthesizes a large number of proteins which play a major part in maintaining the plasma oncotic pressure allowing capillary fluid exchange with the interstitial fluid to effectively 'wash' the tissue cells of the body, removing products of metabolism and supplying them with nutrients (see Chapter 24). Some of these proteins play a major role in blood coagulation or to prevent its occurrence under inappropriate conditions (as can happen with prolonged periods of sitting down as in long-haul air travel). They can also act as carriers for hormones and metallic ions which latter, in free solution in the plasma, could be extremely dangerous. Some are also hormones or prohormones. It also produces a class of proteins called the apolipoproteins which are essential for transporting dietary fats in the blood. Fats are insoluble in water but the apolipoproteins have a 'detergent-like' action which solubilizes them. These compounds also serve as enzyme cofactors, receptor ligands, and also act to regulate the metabolism of lipoproteins and their tissue uptake. Table 30.1 shows the diversity of proteins synthesized by the liver and their actions. The table is included, not to be memorized, but to illustrate more fully, the broad classes of activity in which they play a role (shown in the left hand column). In the fetus, α-fetoprotein, the equivalent of adult albumin, is produced in the liver; this type of protein virtually disappears within 1–2 years after birth.

Table 30.1 Proteins synthesized by the liver

Activity	Proteins	Function
Plasma	Albumin	Oncotic pressure and carrier
	α-fetoprotein	Fetal albumin
	Soluble plasma fibronectin	Forms blood clot
Coagulation	All factors except VIII	Coagulants
	α2-macroglobulin	Coagulation inhibitor
	α1-antitrypsin	Coagulation inhibitor
	Antithrombin III	Coagulation inhibitor
	Protein S	Coagulation inhibitor
	Protein C	Coagulation inhibitor
	Plasminogen	Fibrinolysis
	α2-plasmin	Inhibits fibrinolysis
Carrier	Ceruloplasmin	Carries Cu^{2+}
	Transcortin	Carries cortisol, aldosterone, and progesterone
	Haptoglobin	Carries free Hb
	Haemopexin	Carries free haem from Hb
	IGF binding protein	Carries insulin-like growth factor
	Retinol binding protein	Carries retinol
	Sex-hormone binding globulin	Carries testosterone and oestradiol
	Thyroxine binding globulin	Carries T_4 and T_3
	Transthyretin	Carries T_4
	Transferrin	Carries Fe^{3+}
	Vitamin D binding protein	Carries vitamin D
Hormones	Insulin-like growth factor 1	Anabolic effects in adults
	Thrombopoetin	Regulates platelet production
Prohormones	Angiotensinogen	Produces angiotensin
Apolipoproteins	All except apo B48	Solubilization of lipids

Table 30.2 Liver proteins involved in the clotting process. Vitamin K-dependent proteins are shown shaded

Function	Name	Half-life (days)	Plasma concentration (mcg/mL)
Contact system proenzymes	XII	2	29
	Prekallikrein		45
	XI	2.5	4
Coagulant proenzymes	VII	0.2	0.5
	IX	1	4
	X	1.5	8
	Prothrombin (II)	3	150
Cofactors	HMW kininogen		70
	V	1.5	7
	VIII	0.5	0.2
	Protein S		25
Factors of fibrin deposition	Fibrinogen (I)	4.5	2500
	XIII	7	8
Inhibitors	Protein C	0.3	4
	Antithrombin III	2.5	150

HMW= high molecular weight.

The production of some of the coagulation proteins depends upon an adequate supply of Vitamin K. The daily requirement of this fat soluble vitamin is some 120mcg which is gained by diet (green vegetables) and by bacterial action in the intestine. Therefore, a deficiency of this vitamin can occur if fat absorption is compromised e.g. patients with terminal ileal resection or those on oral antibiotics. Vitamin K acts as a cofactor for a hepatic enzyme, γ-glutamyl carboxylase. This adds a carboxyl group to glutamic acid residues necessary for their activation to bind to phospholipids in the presence of Ca^{2+}. In the carboxylase reaction, vitamin K is oxidized and is then returned to its former state by vitamin K reductase enzyme. This reductase is blocked by warfarin which decreases the amount of activated clotting factors. The blood clotting factors which are influenced by this vitamin are shown in Table 30.2.

Blood coagulation

The formation of a clot is started by platelets forming a plug at an injury site (primary haemostasis). Low-level dosage of aspirin interferes with this process. The plug formation is accompanied by a coagulation cascade in the blood plasma to form strands of fibrin to strengthen the platelet plug (secondary haemostasis). The coagulation process involves three major steps:

- Generation of prothrombin (Factor II) activators
- Cleavage of prothrombin to thrombin, which together with
- Factor XIIA reacts to convert fibrinogen (Factor I) to insoluble cross-linked polymers of fibrin

All of the clotting factors circulate in plasma as inactive procoagulants. To start the coagulation cascade, factor XII is activated to commence the process in the intrinsic or contact activation pathway and factor VII to initiate the process in the extrinsic or tissue factor pathway. These two pathways come together in the final, common pathway to produce a clot. The entire process is shown in Fig. 30.2, not to be learnt but to show the interactions of the various factors, their functions, and, by their absence, the various ways of producing a coagulopathy. With the exception of the production of activated Factor XI all the other reactions require Ca^{2+} as a cofactor.

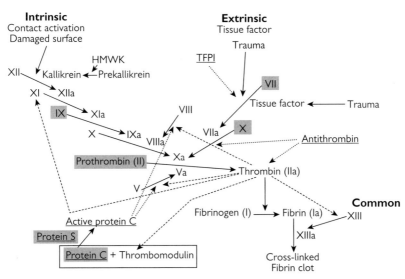

Figure 30.2 The coagulation cascade. The enzymatically active form of the factors are indicated by an 'a'. Factors inhibiting the clotting mechanism are underlined. Linkage of factors to accelerate the process are shown as dotted lines. Vitamin K-dependent factors are highlighted in a grey box. The box in the lower left of the figure represents a negative feedback loop on the reaction. Protein C and thrombin bind to a cell surface protein, Thrombomodulin which, in turn, binds these proteins in a way that activates Protein C. Factors VIII and V are activated by a positive feedback process. HMWK, high-molecular-weight kininogen; TFPI, tissue factor pathway inhibitor.

Normally clots are located to the site of tissue damage and prevented from spreading by the action of the natural anticoagulants in the plasma:

- The vitamin K-dependent **protein C** is a physiological anticoagulant
- **Antithrombin** is constantly active and degrades thrombin, activated factors IXa, Xa, XIa, and XIIa. Its ability to bind with these factors is enhanced by heparins
- **TFPI** limits the action of Tissue Factor
- **Plasmin** is generated by the cleavage of the liver protein plasminogen by plasminogen activator secreted by endothelial cells. It acts to turn the polymolecular fibrin molecules into smaller fragment so inhibiting excessive fibrin production
- **Prostacyclin PGI2** is released by endothelial cells and depresses platelet activation by decreasing the level of calcium ions in their cytosol

Pathological development of blood clots is termed thrombosis. A large thrombus can block venous drainage and cause tissue oedema by increasing the capillary venular pressure and increasing filtration. If the thrombus loses its attachment to a blood vessel wall and circulates in the blood it is called an embolus which may be of a sufficient size to impair tissue perfusion and cause ischaemia.

Eventually the clot will be resorbed by fibrinolysis. As the clot forms, plasminogen becomes trapped in the fibrin mesh. It is the slow activation of plasminogen to plasmin which breaks down the fibrin firstly into smaller polymer chains and then to soluble molecules (see Fig. 30.3). Patients with clots blocking blood vessels (thrombus), e.g. coronary vessel blockage after a heart attack, ischaemic stroke, PE, and DVT may be given streptokinase (thrombolytic) to speed up the degradation of the clot, often with heparin (anticoagulant) to prevent further clotting.

Various tests can be used to assess the function of coagulation in patients. The two commonest are prothrombin time (PT) which measures the efficacy of the extrinsic and common pathways and the activated partial thromboplastin time (aPTT) which measures the intrinsic and common pathways.

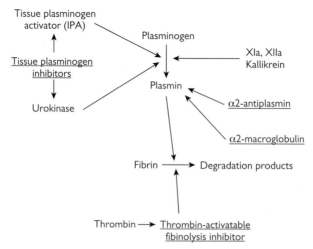

Figure 30.3 Simplified diagram to show the fibrinolytic reactions. Reactions in black aid fibrinolysis and those underlined impede fibrinolysis.

In the **PT** test a sample of plasma is mixed with tissue factor and Ca^{2+} and the time to clot production is measured, normally 12–15 seconds. The result is returned, however, in the form of the international normalized ratio (INR):

$$INR = \frac{(PT_{test})^{ISI}}{(PT_{normal})}$$

ISI is the international sensitivity index for the batch of tissue factor used. The normal range is between 0.8–1.2, patients on warfarin therapy show a value of 2.0–3.0. If the INR has a value of ≤0.5 it indicates a high chance of thrombosis, if ≥5.0 a high chance of bleeding.

In the **aPTT** test the sample of plasma is mixed with a phospholipid, a contact activator such as silica and Ca^{2+} and the time to produce a clot is measured. The normal range is between 25–39 seconds.

Lipid metabolism

The daily intake of lipid, either as fats from meat and animal products or oils from plant products, varies markedly but on average is some 60–100g/day. Most is in the form of neutral triglycerides, the remainder is phospholipids, cholesterol, and its esters. Lipids are insoluble in water so they pose a special problem for the digestive tract. The churning action of the stomach breaks up the immiscible lipid into small droplets. The small amount of simple lipid breakdown in the stomach from lingual lipase and breakdown products from protein digestion act to emulsify these droplets producing even smaller droplets which the lipolytic enzymes of the duodenum can act upon. Since the emulsion floats on water the lipid content of the stomach is the last to empty into the duodenum. The rate of gastric emptying is controlled such that the lipid is passed into the duodenum at a rate which can be digested and absorbed, so as not to overwhelm the system, by duodenal receptors which respond to lipid by releasing GI hormones and initiating neural reflexes that slow stomach emptying. In the duodenum the bile salt–phospholipid–cholesterol micelles interact with the lipids to form other micelles such that the hydrophilic ends of the bile salt molecules become arranged as an outer bile salt shell, facing the aqueous intestinal 'juices', and the hydrophobic ends of the bile salt molecules align themselves to the interior of the micelle, trapping the lipid or its insoluble digestive products in the centre of the shell. This effectively solubilizes the lipids for the absorptive process. In general, triglycerides of long-chain fatty acids, cholesterol esters, and phospholipids are digested by enzymatic hydrolysis (lipases) and micellar solubilization of their products, esters of short-chain fatty acids are dealt with by hydrolysis alone, and the fat soluble vitamins and cholesterol are dealt with by micellar solubilization alone. Figure 30.4 summarizes the digestion and absorption of lipids.

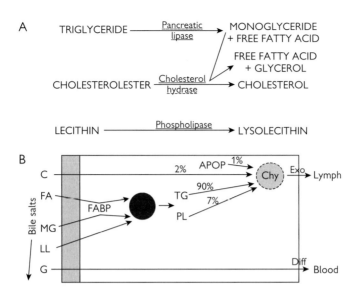

Figure 30.4 A) The major classes of lipases (underlined), their substrates (left-hand side) and breakdown products (right-hand side). B) Schematic diagram of an enterocyte. Lipids are absorbed through the brush border of the enterocyte (shaded portion). The products of digestion, in mixed micelles, are brought into contact with the brush border. Here the low pH microclimate allows proton transfer to the fatty acids which reduces their micellar solubility and they can come into contact with the cell membrane. Because of their lipid solubility they can diffuse into the cell membrane. The cytosol of the cell contains fatty acid binding proteins (**FABP**), with a high affinity for these acids, and they enter the cell. The long chain fatty acids (**FA**) and monoglycerides (**MG**) are then re-synthesized into triglycerides (**TG**) via an energy dependent enzymatic process (dark grey shaded circle). Shorter chain fatty acids diffuse through the cell directly into the bloodstream where they are bound to albumin for transport to various organs. A small fraction of the monoglycerides are converted into phospholipids (**PL**) and lysolethicin (**LL**) is converted back to lecithin (**PL**). Cholesterol (**C**) is absorbed in its free form but most is esterified in the enterocyte. The re-synthesized lipid products and apoproteins (**APOP**) form chylomicrons (**Chy**). These are large lipid-carrying particles ranging in size from 750–6000Å which have a composition indicated by the percentages and are essential for transporting the lipids out of the cell by exocytosis (**Exo**) to enter the lacteals in the villi and thence via lymphatic drainage to reach the bloodstream via the thoracic duct. Chylomicrons are similar to micelles, they have an outer shell composed of the more polar lipids (cholesterol and phospholipids) and the apopprotien surrounding a lipid core. Glycerol (**G**) is water soluble and diffuses through the cell, exiting at is basolateral surface to diffuse (**Diff**) into the capillaries. The bile salts released from the micelles return to the intestinal lumen for re-use. (You are not required to have a detailed knowledge of the biochemical reactions occurring in the dark grey shaded circle so I haven't included it. Those of an inquiring mind can find it in any textbook of— pardon my language—biochemistry).

The liver has the ability to synthesize triglycerides from plasma fatty acids or glucose. These triglycerides are incorporated together with apolipoproteins, plus some cholesterol, to form the very low-density lipoproteins (VLDL), important for the transport of fat-soluble vitamins. Triglycerides and their breakdown products are high-energy substrates for metabolism. Lipoprotein lipase produced by capillary endothelium splits the fatty acids from the chylomicrons and VLDL. Insulin released after a meal activates lipoprotein lipase, which is responsible for the rapid breakdown of dietary triglycerides. However, in the liver the fatty acids are turned back into triglycerides and only a limited amount can be exported as VLDL. This can lead to fat deposition in the liver (fatty liver) if there are excessive amounts of triglycerides.

Liver cells also contain acid lipases which hydrolyses cholesterol esters in chylomicron remnants to give cholesterol. Cholesterol is used in five ways in the body:

- Excreted as cholesterol in bile
- Converted to bile salts
- Incorporated in low-density lipoprotein (LDL) (cholesterol is not very soluble in water, 0.095mg/L, and needs to be solubilized as lipoprotein complexes for transport in the circulation and to take

Table 30.3 Lipoprotein percentage composition. Cholesterol and phospholipids are in the outer shell

Lipoprotein	Triglycerides (%)	Cholesterol (%)	Cholesterol esters (%)	Phospholipids (%)	Protein units (%)
VLDL	53	7	12	18	8
LDL	6	8	42	22	22
HDL	4	4	15	30	47

part in cellular metabolic processes. Lipoproteins with a greater cholesterol content are less dense. See Table 30.3)
- Incorporated in high-density lipoprotein (HDL)
- LDL is the major source of transport of cholesterol to body tissues where its cholesterol component can be used for incorporation into cell membranes (to give correct fluidity and permeability), or for steroid (adrenal and sex hormones) and vitamin-D synthesis

Most of the circulating cholesterol is manufactured in the liver. Typically about 1g of the total body content of 35g is synthesized per day. LDL (the 'bad cholesterol' linked to atherosclerosis) is produced by reducing 3-hydroxy-4methylglutaryl-CoA (HMG-CoA) via an enzyme called HMG-CoA reductase. Statins have a molecular structure similar to HMG-CoA and they can compete as a substrate with the naturally occurring compound in the reductase reaction. This leads to a reduction in cholesterol production with a reduction in the potential to develop atherosclerosis and hence cardiovascular disease. Statins have also been linked to a reduction in prostate cancer and benign prostatic enlargement in some studies. The desirable level of LDL is ≤200mg/dL ≈5.0mmol/L.

Table 30.4 Composition of bile

	Liver	Gallbladder	Units
pH	7.2	6.9	
Na^+	149	209	mmol/L
K^+	4.8	20.4	mmol/L
Ca^{2+}	2.6	3.7	mmol/L
Cl^-	105	66	mmol/L
HCO_3^-	25	19	mmol/L
Bile acids	10	16	g/L
Fatty acids	3	24	g/L
Bilirubin	0.5	2.4	g/L
Phospholipid	2.5	23.5	g/L
Cholesterol	1.8	4	g/L
Proteins	2–20	45	g/L
Osmolality	284	330	

Secretion of bile

Bile produced by the hepatocytes passes into the bile ducts which join up to exit from the liver as the common hepatic duct. This joins with the cystic duct from the gallbladder to form the common bile duct which then joins with the pancreatic duct to empty into the duodenum via the sphincter of Oddi. If this is closed then the bile flows into the gallbladder to be stored and concentrated (see Table 30.4).

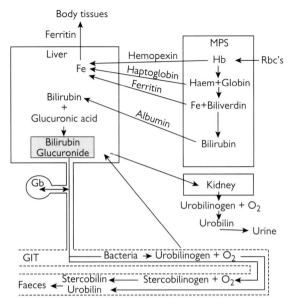

Figure 30.5 Bilirubin production and excretion. For details see text.

Approximately 1L of bile is produced per day. Ninety-five per cent of the bile acids are reabsorbed in the terminal ileum and transported back to the liver via the hepatic portal vein.

Bile pigments

At the end of their lifecycle the membranes of red blood corpuscles change making them capable of adhering to cells of the mononuclear phagocytic system (MPS, alternatively named the reticuloendothelial system; Fig. 30.5). The cells of this system are mainly monocytes and macrophages, in lymph nodes, spleen, Kupffer cells on the walls of the liver sinusoids, and tissue histiocytes which phagocytose and degrade them. Haemoglobin from lysed red blood cells is degraded into haem and globin in the macrophages. The haemoglobin from any red blood cells which lyse elsewhere becomes attached to a plasma protein, haemopexin, for transport into the MPS for disposal. Freed haemoglobin is highly toxic and has to be bound to haemopexin. The macrophages degrade the haem (*heme in American English*) to iron and biliverdin which is then rapidly reduced to bilirubin. Free bilirubin, unlike its name suggests, is a yellow-coloured water-insoluble pigment and is bound to plasma albumin for transport via the bloodstream to the liver. It is the pigment which gives the yellow colour to bruises and the yellow discoloration in jaundice. Excess haem is bound to haptoglobin and transported via the bloodstream to other parts of the MPS for conversion to bilirubin. Iron bound to ferritin is transported to the liver via the bloodstream to be recycled or stored. The globin is reduced to its component amino acids and enters the general amino acid pool for protein synthesis. In the liver bilirubin is separated from its albumin and taken up by hepatocyes, bound to protein, transported to the intracellular microsomes, and conjugated with glucoronic acid, to form a water-soluble conjugated bile pigment. This is then actively transported out of the hepatocytes into the biliary system and ultimately to the common hepatic duct and then to the duodenum (GIT, Fig. 30.5). In the duodenum bacterial action converts the conjugated bile pigment to urobilinogen which is further oxidized, by oxygen in the intestinal fluid, to urobilin to be excreted with the faeces. A small fraction of the urobilinogen is transported back to the liver via the hepatic portal circulation and passed into the bloodstream to the kidney to be excreted. This urobilinogen is then oxidized in the urine and excreted, giving the urine a pale yellow colour. In the colon further bacterial action converts some of the bile pigment conjugate into stercobilinogen which is oxidized to produce stercobilin which is excreted with the faeces.

The normal concentration of bilirubin in the plasma is 3–10mg/L, if this rises to above 18mg/L jaundice develops. First of all the sclera take on a yellow colouration followed by the skin. Jaundice can result from three causes, pre-hepatic, hepatic, and post-hepatic.

- Pre-hepatic causes are an increase in red cell destruction, or haemolysis leading to excess amounts of bilirubin production exceeding the conjugation capability of the liver. In addition some drugs. e.g. sulphonamides, compete with bilirubin to bind with plasma albumin raising its free plasma concentration. In this case unconjugated bilirubin can enter the brain where it is highly toxic
- Hepatic jaundice arises from hepatocyte damage due to poisons (poisonous agaric) or hepatitis which causes decreased albumin production (transport impaired) or decreased conjugation ability. In this condition the concentration of conjugated bilirubin in urine is increased giving it a brown colouration
- Post-hepatic jaundice is caused by any form of obstruction to the bile ducts by gallstones or tumours causing a reflux of conjugated bilirubin into the bloodstream. Normally if the sphincter of Oddi is closed, bile will accumulate in the gallbladder (Gb, Fig. 30.5) giving a normal filling pressure between 10–20mmHg. Pressures above 23mmHg will stop the production of bile and allow counter current diffusional bile interchange in the portal triads so that bile components enter the bloodstream. Alkaline phosphatase (a normal bile constituent) concentrations in blood are elevated which is a diagnostic feature of this type of jaundice. Since no bile enters the intestine the stool will become pale (clay-coloured) with the absence of both urobilin and stercobilin

Bile acids

These are made in the liver by the oxidation of cholesterol to produce the primary bile salts of cholic and chenodesoxycholic acids. These are then conjugated with taurine or glycine to produce taurocholic and glycocholic salts respectively. This conjugation is necessary to increase their water solubility, prevents their passive re-absorption from the intestine, and allows their 'detergent like' action on lipid droplets, i.e. their solubilization by the formation of micelles. In the liver bile they are in salt form (pH 7.5) in the intestine either as acids in the duodenum (pH 6.1–7.20) or, in the lower parts, as salts (pH 7–8). Secondary bile salts are formed in the intestine by bacterial action, mainly the dehydroxylation of cholate acid to desoxycholate. This bacterial action also deconjugates some of the bile salts. Conjugated (water soluble) bile salts are actively re-absorbed whereas the deconjugated salts (lipid soluble) are passively re-absorbed. Ninety-five per cent of the bile salts are reabsorbed and passed back to the liver via the enterohepatic portal system in, mainly, the lower third of the small intestine. This reabsorption means that the bile salts become a mixture of primary and secondary salts. In the liver the deconjugated salts are reconjugated for further use. It is estimated that each molecule of bile salts is re-used some 20 times, multiple times during a single digestive phase. Some 800mg of cholesterol is produced in the liver per day and around half of this is used for bile acid synthesis.

Bile salts are potentially cytotoxic and their concentration is regulated by negative feedback reactions. If the concentration of bile salts in the portal vein rises the liver hepatocyte production of bile salts falls, their secretion is increased which in turn increases bile flow, leading to bile salt-dependent choleresis. The active secretion of the bile salts will drag water osmotically with them into the bile canaliculi, inorganic salts will then follow down this gradient.

This ability of the liver to conjugate molecules is also used to detoxify drugs by combining them with glucuronic acid or glutathione and the same chemical activity is used to remove circulating hormones. These conjugated derivatives are passed out in the urine.

For the production of bile the liver can be considered as a two-component system, comprised of the hepatocytes and the duct cells. The function of the hepatocytes is to absorb bilirubin and bile salts from the blood and actively secrete them into the bile canaliculi with inorganic molecules and water following passively to maintain the osmolality of the bile the same as that in the plasma. The hepatocyte secretion is controlled by a negative feedback mechanism which senses bile salt concentration in the hepatic portal blood. If bile salt concentration rises their production is decreased and their secretion is increased (bile salt-dependent choleresis). The contents of the canaliculi drain into the bile ducts where HCO_3^- ions and water is added. The duct cells are under both vagal and hormonal control (secretin) to increase the volume of fluid produced after a meal. Bile is further modified in its storage organ, the gallbladder. This has a maximum volume of around 60–80ml. With a daily bile production of some 700ml (approximately one-third of the daily outout per meal) there will be a small storage problem. When the sphincter of Oddi is closed the gall-bladder is 'back-filled' via the common bile duct. The stored bile is concentrated by active co-transport of Na^+ and Cl^-, with water following passively into the gallbladder interstitium to be removed via its venous drainage. This reduces the volume of fluid to be stored by some 10–20%. This concentration effect is to ensure: a) that the hydrostatic pressure in the gallbladder does not exceed 23mmHg and damage the liver and b) to increase the concentration of the bile salts so that their detergent action is intensified when they are released into the duodenum. The emptying of the gallbladder is controlled by the hormone CCK.

Cholesterol in the bile is solubilized by bile salts and the phospholipid lecithin. Alterations in the ratios of these bile components can result in the formation of cholesterol crystals producing gallstones. Another cause of gallstone formation is the interaction between Ca^{2+}, bilirubin, and already formed cholesterol crystals which can lead to a precipitation of calcium bilirubinate onto the cholesterol crystals. Gallstones are initially asymptomatic until they grow to about 8mm in diameter. This can lead to inflammation of the gallbladder. If a stone passes out into the bile duct it can cause intense pain located to the upper abdominal region (biliary colic) causing further gallbladder inflammation. If it gets lodged in the duct this can lead to obstructive jaundice. Hopefully the stone will pass, eventually, through the duct into the intestine. If a stone remains stuck then surgical intervention (endoscopic retrograde sphincterectomy) is required to remove it. After one attack of biliary colic has occurred the probability of a further occurrence is highly likely so an open or laparoscopic cholecystectomy will be performed.

Food entering the small intestine is a mixture of simple and complex carbohydrates, simple and complex proteins, and simple water soluble and complex insoluble lipids. It is logical to assume that the simple molecules will be absorbed first and the complex molecules therefore further down the intestine. The evidence that the fats are absorbed last comes from the observation that patients who have a resection of the terminal ileum show the fat malabsorption symptom of steatorrhoea coupled with a propensity to fat soluble vitamin deficiencies. The products of digestion and absorption such as glucose, amino acids, and fatty acids plus glycerol are conveyed to the liver in the hepatic portal vein, triglycerides, fat soluble vitamins, and vitamin B12 are conveyed to the liver, as chylomicrons via the hepatic artery.

Glucose

After a meal the plasma glucose concentration will rise, stimulating the release of insulin which acts, in the liver, to cause the hepatocytes to change soluble glucose into the storage polysaccharide glycogen (glycogenesis). After a meal glucose levels fall and glucagon is secreted, stimulating the liver to produce glucose from glycogen (glycolysis), a process which is also stimulated in exercise by the release of adrenaline and in stress by the release of glucocorticoids. In conditions of anaerobic cellular respiration the lactate produced can be converted to glucose in the liver.

Amino acids

Amino acids are used for the production of liver proteins and passed to all the other tissues in the body also for protein manufacture. Excess amino acids are dealt with by a process of delamination, i.e. the

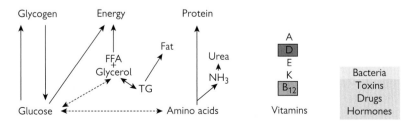

Figure 30.6 Simplified diagram of post-absorptive activity in the liver. For further details see the text.

removal of terminal amino groups. This produces some ammonia, glutamate plus pyruvate and is catalyzed by two enzymes:

- **Alanine transaminase**: α-ketoglutarate + alanine ↔ glutamate + pyruvate, and
- **Aspartate transaminase**: α-ketoglutarate + aspartate ↔ glutamate + oxaloacetate

The pyruvate can enter the Krebs cycle (or citric acid cycle) to be used as an energy substrate or it can be converted into glucose. Any ammonia which is produced will enter the ornithine cycle (or urea cycle) to be converted into urea $(NH_2)_2CO$ by reacting HCO_3^- with the ammonia (NH3). A sudden large influx of amino acid as occurs during transurethral resection of the prostate can lead to excessive production of ammonia (see Chapter 28).

Free fatty acids and triglycerides

Depending upon circumstances, free fatty acids will be recombined with glycerol to produce triglycerides to be transported in the plasma for use by all body tissues or to be stored as fat in adipose tissue. Immediately after a meal insulin will drive the reaction to produce triglycerides and, when hungry, glucagons will produce free fatty acids and glycerol, a reaction which is also driven by adrenaline in exercise or stress conditions. The glycerol can then be converted into glucose. The formation of glucose from short-chain conversion products of amino acids and glycerol is termed gluconeogenesis.

Vitamins

The water-soluble vitamin C is absorbed in the ileum, the other water-soluble vitamins in the jejunum by an active Na^+ co-transport process. They reach the liver via the hepatic portal vein and are conveyed to the body tissues via the hepatic vein. All of the fat-soluble vitamins are absorbed by their incorporation into micelles and transported to the liver in chylomicrons or attached to VLDL via the hepatic artery. Vitamin D is 25 hydroxylated in the liver from calciferol to cholecalciferol. Vitamin K is necessary for the liver's production of vitamin K-dependent coagulation factors (see above). Vitamin B_{12} is bound to a glycoprotein (intrinsic factor) produced in the gastric parietal cells and is absorbed in the ileum where there are specific binding sites, on the luminal surface of the enterocytes, for the B_{12}-intrinsic factor complex. The enterocytes then take up the complex by endocytosis which requires Ca^{2+}. In the plasma it binds with a specific transporter protein (transcobalamine). It is stored in the liver, or if in excess excreted. The store will last for several years in the absence of a dietary intake.

Bacteria

Bacteria transported via the hepatic portal vein are phagocytosed by the Kupffer cells lining the liver sinusoids. Each phagocytosed bacterium (phagosome) fuses with intracellular lysosomes forming a phagolysosome in which it is broken down.

Drugs and hormones

Drugs and hormones are removed from the plasma by conjugation with glucuronic acid or glutathione passing to the kidney for excretion.

The portal circulation

In common with all other circulatory systems this system can become disturbed to produce portal hypertension defined as a >5mmHg difference between portal vein pressure compared to that in the hepatic vein. Causes are:

- Pre-hepatic, e.g. portal vein thrombosis
- Hepatic, e.g. cirrhosis, hepatitis or hepatatoxic drugs
- Post-hepatic, e.g. hepatic vein thrombosis, inferior vena cava thrombosis, and constrictive pericarditis

The dangers of portal hypertension are that it can cause accumulation of free fluid in the peritoneal cavity, hepatic encephalopathy (inability of the liver to convert ammonia to urea), an increased risk of spontaneous bacterial peritonitis (leaky capillary walls), hepatorenal syndrome (altering blood flow in the splanchnic bed leading to a reduction in renal flow and vessel tone causing kidney failure), splenomegaly, and by producing post-caval anastomoses with collateral blood flow through vessels in the stomach and oesophagus can lead to the formation of varices.

Liver function tests

Diseases of the liver (hepatitis) and liver damage (alcohol, paracetamol) are grave conditions and a need for early diagnosis of impending liver failure is important. Various blood constituents can be measured to assess its function:

Albumin	Normal range 3.8–5.0g/dL
Alanine transaminase (ALT)	5–40IU/L often expressed as multiples of the upper limit
Aspartate transaminase (AST)	10–40IU/L not specific but the ratio AST/ALT is useful
Alkaline phosphatase (ALP)	30–120IU/L (enzyme in biliary duct cells)
Total bilirubin (TBIL)	0.1–1.2mg/dL but can change due to pre-, post- or hepatic causes
Direct bilirubin	I.e. unconjugated 0–0.3mg/dL. If total bilirubin is raised then if direct bilirubin is normal it indicates a pre- (haemolysis) or hepatic (failure to conjugate = liver damage) if raised it indicates a failure to excrete (blocked bile duct)
γ-glutamyl transpeptidase (GGT)	0–51IU/L raised in alcohol toxicity

Cirrhosis caused by chronic alcoholism is an escalating problem in the UK. Excessive ingestion can cause an activation of both the Toll-like (TLR4) and CD14 receptors on the Kupffer cell surfaces which normally internalize endotoxin. This leads to transcription of pro-inflammatory cytokines (tumour necrosis factor-α, TNFα) and production of superoxides. TNFα then enters the hepatic stellate cells (hepatic fat-storing cells) leading to collagen synthesis and eventually fibrosis.

Scenarios

Scenario 1

A 50-year-old lady was taken ill on a long-haul flight and has been brought to the hospital from the airport. She is obviously in pain which she localizes in her right iliac fossa. She tells you that she has had an upset tummy for the last 48 hours and because she had a DVT after a previous flight her GP has prescribed Clexane which she injected just before boarding the plane approximately 8 hours previously. On examination she has an elevated core temperature, right iliac fossa tenderness with rebound.

Scenario 2

A 70-year-old male is admitted to the A&E department following referral by his GP. The GP notes state that the patient had woken at 2am with a pain in his belly which got steadily more severe until at 9am his wife phoned the GP. On examination the GP noted that the patient had a steady severe pain in the right upper abdomen and phoned for an ambulance. On examination the patient was in obvious distress showing no signs of jaundice or increased venous pressure with a blood pressure of 135/80, a steady pulse rate of 80, and an aural temperature of 37.2°C. He had his prevailing medication in his pocket (Coracten 10mg, oxybutinin 2.5mg both taken twice daily with ramipril 2.5mg and simvastatin 2.5mg both taken once a day). An ultrasound abdominal scan showed a large collection of stones in the gallbladder.

Scenario 3

A 60-year-old man underwent a Whipple's operation for periampullary carcinoma. On the 2nd postoperative day, while still in the ITU, his urinary output has reduced to 300ml in the previous 12 hours. The catheter is not blocked. What will you suspect and how will you manage him?

Answers

Scenario 1

Diagnosis is of acute appendicitis which will require an immediate operation. The pain will be treated with morphine and the effects of the low-molecular-weight heparin can be partially reversed with protamine. During the operation scrupulous care will have to be taken to cauterize all bleeding points and she should be made to wear compression stockings. Post-operatively checks for bleeding will have to be made and she should be made mobile as quickly as possible.

Scenario 2

The signs suggest that a gallstone has moved into his cystic duct. Treatment is initially to administer morphine to block the pain and then keep him in hospital to watch and wait. The possibility of performing an endoscopic retrograde cholangiopancreatography was suggested but the decision was made to wait another 12 hours in the hope that the stone would pass down the duct. A further dose of morphine was administered at 10pm. The next morning the patient woke and went to the toilet where, in his own words, he had a copious vomit and the pain suddenly stopped! The intra-abdominal pressure changes had possibly forced, or helped to force, the stone through his sphincter of Oddi

The patient was discharged and was referred for an elective laparoscopic cholecystectomy.

Scenario 3

Hepatorenal syndrome.

This can occur following an operation in a patient with obstructive jaundice. There is reduced GFR, circulating endotoxins causing endotoxinaemia. There is absorption of endotoxin produced by the intestinal microflora. In the jaundiced patient there is a relationship between impaired renal function and the presence of circulating endotoxins.

An attempt should be made to counter this condition by:

- Adequate hydration and pre-operative induction of diuresis
- For 12–24 hours pre-operative 5% dextrose saline IV
- Mannitol (osmotic diuretic) or furosemide (loop diuretic) IV at anaesthetic induction
- Catheterize—hourly urine output
- Further diuretics if urine output <40 ml/hr in peri-operative and post-operative period

Some hepatobiliary surgeons do a two-stage operation by inserting a common bile duct stent about 2 weeks prior to the Whipple's operation. This brings the serum bilirubin down thus reducing the chances of hepatorenal syndrome. However, most surgeons do not insert a stent because the procedure may introduce infection and inevitably reduces the diameter of the common bile duct thereby making the biliary-jejunal anastomosis technically difficult.

Chapter 31 **Neurological system in critical care**

Introduction

The neurological system can be divided into the central nervous system (CNS) (brain and spinal cord) and the peripheral nervous system (nerves which link the CNS to the various organs of the body). The CNS is divided into the brain and spinal cord.

The brain

The brain, with its billions of neurons and billions more supporting glial cells, and with many links radiating from the average cell, is immensely complex. Yet major specific functions can be assigned to many parts (e.g. an area in the left motor cortex which controls voluntary movements of the right hand), and many other important functions can be assigned to organized networks which are virtual centres without a specific location (e.g. the exercise centre which ensures appropriate ventilation and cardiac output tailored to specific muscular activities).

We look first at the major naked eye components of the brain. Starting at the bottom, the brainstem links the top of the spinal cord with the four hemispheres—left and right cerebral hemispheres and left and right cerebellar hemispheres. Thus, overall, the CNS consists of a long stem with four outgrowths at the top.

The brainstem

The brainstem shares some properties with the two structures it links—the spinal cord and the rest (higher regions) of the brain. Like the spinal cord, the brainstem is divided into segments—from below upwards, the medulla oblongata, the pons, and the midbrain. Structurally and functionally, these show, from below upwards, gradually decreasing similarity with the spinal cord and increasing similarity with other parts of the brain. Functionally, parts of the brain just above the brainstem, such as the thalamus and hypothalamus, are similar to the brainstem and form a continuum with it in terms of increasingly complex reflexes/drives/instincts.

The medulla oblongata

This carries major ascending sensory and descending motor tracts which are continuous with those in the spinal cord. However, like the brain, it contains more elaborate central control centres than does the spinal cord (with the exception of the sacral region of the spinal cord with its autonomic control centres for the functions of the pelvic organs, including micturition and defecation, and some aspects of the sexual reflexes).

The medulla oblongata contains autonomic and somatic centres for thoracic and abdominal organs and muscles. These include centres for breathing, swallowing, vomiting, and for autonomic control of cardiac function. These centres (like the simpler reflex centres in the spinal cord) are basically reflexes which have important inputs from higher centres in the brain, up to cortical level. Activity from other parts of the brainstem (pons and midbrain) contributes to these reflexes.

Pons, midbrain, and adjoining regions above

Moving up from the medulla oblongata, the pons continues the various tracts linking the spinal cord with the brain, and plays a part in maintaining regular cyclical activity in the inspiratory and expiratory centres of the medulla.

The midbrain and adjoining regions in the base of the brain where the hemispheres have not yet separated are particularly involved with eye and ear reflexes, gathering information from the vestibular system in particular and sending signals to the very precise muscles which move the eyes. In this way, slight movements of the head do not detract from the focus on the maculae of the two eyes of light signals from a particular object, such as a portion of this book which you are currently reading.

A number of relatively simple responses which are regulated in this region are important in the diagnosis of brainstem death as discussed in a subsequent chapter.

In the brainstem generally, the major ascending and descending tracts to and from the cerebral and cerebellar hemispheres gradually diverge to and from their destinations and origins, and communicating tracts from the cerebrum to the cerebellum make their way—a kind of motorway junction region.

Basal regions of the cerebral hemispheres

The region around the junction of the brainstem and the cerebral hemispheres includes the thalamus and hypothalamus. This is where conscious awareness and emotional drives begin to appear, to be more fully evaluated and controlled by the higher centres in the cerebral cortex.

Thalamus and pain

The awareness of pain and its accompanying distress are produced in the thalamus on each side as impulses pour in from the spinothalamic tracts, carrying impulses initiated by damage to body tissues. The source of the pain in a particular part of the body is determined, with varying degrees of precision, by relay of the thalamic inputs to the parietal (sensory) cerebral cortex, where the pain is assigned (referred) to its point or region of origin. In general, the source of pain in the peripheries of the body (face, hand, foot, parietal pleura, and peritoneum) is precisely identified, whereas pain coming from internal organs such as the heart, gall bladder and gut is 'referred' with varying degrees of imprecision.

The severity of pain and a degree of awareness of the serious import of pain in certain regions, such as severe crushing central chest pain, are major factors driving people to seek medical attention. Pain is thus an emotional drive, like those considered below in relation to the hypothalamus.

Hypothalamus, appetite, thirst, and thermal awareness

Just below the thalamus on each side, the hypothalamus receives a major load of information from the peripheries and internal regions. The information ranges from an awareness of gastric emptiness or distension and information on nutritional stores, to the state of local hypothalamic osmoreceptors, and the temperature of the skin.

Food deprivation leads to a sense of hunger, which can become so dominant that it is difficult to ignore, distracting people from normal routine activities. Similarly people in the desert are reputed to be driven mad by thirst. Persistent coldness and chilling can also be severely demoralizing. These **emotional drives** are powerful determinants of behaviour—as they must be for survival—but they are more complicated and more amenable to higher centre control than simpler subconscious reflexes. Thus, structurally and physiologically the basal regions of the cerebral cortices lie between simple reflexes such as the knee jerk and planned activity originating in the thought processes of the cerebral cortex.

In general, the adverse inputs described in the previous paragraph cause discomfort and a strong desire to remove the discomfort. In moderation such sensations can, however, lead to pleasant anticipation in a way which has become part of our language and culture (hunger is the best sauce, a long satisfying drink, coming in from the cold).

Emotions

Regions above the thalamus are particularly concerned with more complex determinants of behaviour, such as excitement, rage, happiness, sadness, and sexual drives. Here the input largely involves the cerebral cortex and the output can determine long-term planning and activity.

Exercise centre

The finding that ventilation and cardiac output are intimately related to level of exercise has given rise to the concept of a virtual centre which receives information from the motor cortex (and also from metaboreceptors in exercising muscle). The emotions of fear and aggression can raise performance

further in escaping danger ('fear lent wings to his feet'), and, by sports psychologists, to enhance performance during competitive sport.

Cerebral hemispheres

We look first at the outer, higher functionally, cerebral cortex covering the two hemispheres. Firstly
general properties will be considered, then the very detailed specific local functions with which specific
cortical areas are associated.

Cerebral cortex

The cerebral cortex, darker (grey matter) than the underlying white matter, is the site of huge numbers
of large cells linked in highly complicated networks. General regions are named from the overlying bones
of the skull—right and left frontal, parietal, temporal, occipital. The cortical cells are permanently active,
day and night, sending out action potentials and receiving chemical transmitters from other neurons.

Activities of cerebral cortical cells

In order to undertake their function, the cerebral cortical neurons are constantly synthesizing **chemical
transmitters** and activating **membrane pumps**. The pumps maintain transcellular ionic gradients to drive
ionic movements when the relevant ion channels open. These ionic movements produce action potentials and excitatory and inhibitory synaptic potentials on which all cerebral activity and ultimately all
human thought and actions depend. A significant proportion of the human genome is concerned with
control of ion channels which these cells share in various forms with most of the body cells.

Cerebral cortical electrical activities and synthesis of transmitters demand elaborate supporting
chemical activities within the cell and an abundant supply of **oxygen** and **glucose**. They normally rely
almost entirely on glucose as substrate, though in prolonged partial or complete starvation they can
adapt moderately to the use of fat products such as ketones. Cortical cells are the first to show evidence of malfunction when the circulating blood glucose level falls. A profound fall in blood glucose
causes coma and death because of irreversible depression of brain function, particularly the cerebral
cortical cells.

Complex demands

For normal function, these highly specialized cerebral cortical cells have very precise environmental
requirements. As well as a supply of glucose and oxygen, which in turn demands a **constant high blood
flow** through the cerebral capillaries in all states and postures of the body, these cells demand a **constant
temperature** within a degree or so of 37°C. 35°C is definite hypothermia and from 39–40°C upwards
thought processes are noticeably slowed. Similar constraints apply to many other requirements—normal
pH, osmolality, and normal levels of a variety of ions. Cerebral cortical cells also cannot function normally
in the presence of a variety of drugs and toxins, including the toxins which accumulate in renal and
hepatic failure. Thus the level of a patient's consciousness is often an indicator of the severity of underlying conditions, such as respiratory failure, hypoglycaemia, hypothermia, renal and hepatic failure, and
excessive levels of drugs and alcohol.

Localized function of the cerebral cortex

Localization occurs in two ways. Firstly, *large areas* of cortex and adjoining tissue share the *same general function*, such as the motor cortex in the posterior part of the frontal region, just in front of the
central sulcus of each hemisphere. The part of the parietal cortex just behind this sulcus is the sensory
cortex; the temporal cortex is concerned with hearing and the occipital cortex with vision. Parts of the
frontal cortex in front of the motor area are particularly concerned with the critical ability of knowing
what is appropriate in given circumstances. This may range from knowing during driving whether it is

safe to overtake in a particular circumstance, to knowing where it is acceptable to micturate or defecate.

Secondly, within the above large areas, *smaller subdivisions* are concerned with particular parts of the body. Thus movements of the face and hand are controlled particularly from the lateral part of the motor area, with lower body parts represented more medially and the feet represented over the top in the sulcus between the two hemispheres. A similar arrangement occurs in the sensory cortex. The hearing and vision areas can be subdivided into areas concerned with particular wavelengths of the different sounds and colours.

It has also been found that localized regions are concerned with such functions as identifying colour patterns and even recognizing the paintings of particular artists.

Subcortical regions of the cerebral hemispheres

Like the brainstem, these large regions contain pathways or radiations diverging from the brainstem to and from the various sensory and motor areas just described. Deep in the hemispheres is where thrombosis or haemorrhage often leads to a major stroke. In severe cases this interrupts function in both motor and sensory pathways, leading to a combination of paralysis, loss of feeling and loss of vision involving the opposite side of the body to the side of the lesion (hemiplegia, hemianaesthesia and hemianopia).

The subcortical regions of the cerebral hemispheres also contain networks for motor control which are more elaborate than the lower reflexes, but still outside voluntary control. This 'automatic pilot' network of unconscious associated movements supports the main voluntary activities. When we decide to sprint from one part of a sporting field to another we do not have to work out which particular muscles to use, or how to maintain balance. These supporting regions of the brain constitute the extrapyramidal system and Parkinsonism is a common disorder of this system.

Cerebellar hemispheres

These two smaller hemispheres also contribute unconscious support to skilled voluntary movements. Their contribution is particularly concerned with maintaining balance, correcting deviations from the required muscle actions, and controlling the extraocular muscle actions which keep vision focused clearly while the head is moving vigorously. Thus features of cerebellar disease include difficulty maintaining balance, intention tremor (during movements) and nystagmus (a kind of tremor of eye fixation).

Spinal cord

Functions here are in general simpler than in the brain and the cells here have less exacting metabolic requirements; spinal reflexes may still be present when adverse conditions have eliminated function in the brain, including the brainstem.

The various spinal cord regions—cervical, thoracic, lumbar, and sacral—distribute and receive impulses to and from specific regions in the arms, thorax, abdomen, and legs. They also provide simple local coordination in these regions with the spinal stretch and withdrawal reflexes having their centres in the spinal cord.

As well as providing a simple example of the physiological components of a reflex arc (Fig. 31.1), the spinal stretch reflexes (knee, ankle jerk, etc.) illustrate the concept of local reflexes which may be inhibited or facilitated by descending impulses from higher centres. The stretch organs are the *intrafusal* fibres in skeletal muscles which run in parallel with the main motor (*extrafusal*) fibres. The sense organs are contained within spindle shaped (fusiform) capsules, hence the terms intrafusal and extrafusal.

Thus for the knee jerk, stretching the quadriceps femoris by striking its attachment to the tibia at the patellar tendon stretches the muscle spindles and thus generates action potentials in the sensory nerves which supply them. The signals are transmitted across a synapse in the anterior horn of grey matter to anterior horn motor neurons. These fire off action potentials to the extrafusal muscle fibres and provoke quadriceps contraction and extension of the knee. This type of reflex is of split-second importance

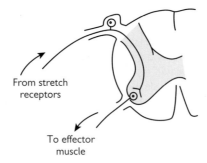

Figure 31.1 A spinal reflex arc

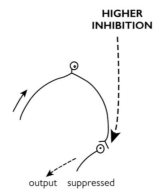

Figure 31.2 Higher centre suppression of a spinal reflex arc

during vigorous running and the axons which serve it are of the fastest type (large, myelinated) so the entire reflex response time is a small fraction of a second.

Routine clinical examination shows stretch reflexes to be depressed or absent if either the sensory or motor neurons involved are impaired in their function, or if the reflex centre is damaged, or if there is strong central inhibition with the knee consciously or subconsciously held stiff.

Similarly the micturition reflex (a much slower autonomic stretch reflex involving unmyelinated nerves) can be impaired by corresponding damage. Also, in normal life, the reflex is held suppressed until the individual wishes to empty the bladder (see Figs. 31.2 and 31.3)

Peripheral nervous system

This consists largely of pathways, but, in places, cell bodies are involved. Many major **somatic nerves**, such as the radial and sciatic, are mixed sensory and motor nerves. The axons are grouped by function and region supplied so when a nerve is cut, accurate suture of the individual nerve bundles is necessary, in order that the severed axons can regrow along their previous path to the appropriate sense organ or muscle fibre.

Autonomic nerves tend to travel independently of the somatic nerves. The major parasympathetic nerves, the left and right vagi, wander around the body, from the neck to the thorax and abdomen where they have various branches. The word *vagus* has the same origin as the word *vagrant,* a tramp, or wanderer. **Sympathetic nerves** often accompany blood vessels to the organs supplied, which may be the blood vessels themselves.

Autonomic nerves, like somatic nerves, consist of sensory and motor axons serving various reflexes. While the reflex centres for the somatic nerves are all in the CNS, organs such as the gut and the bladder have groups of cells (ganglion cells) close to the smooth muscle in these organs. These cells

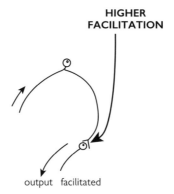

**HIGHER
FACILITATION**

output facilitated

Figure 31.3 Higher centre facilitation of a spinal reflex arc

form a nerve network helping to coordinate actions such as peristalsis of the gut and emptying of the bladder.

Supporting cells in the nervous system

In the brain and spinal cord, billions of nerve cells (neurons) play the leading role in function. However billions of other cells have a supporting role. These cells are generally referred to as **glia**, or glial cells. Throughout the central and peripheral nervous systems, these cells carry out activities which are essential for the function of neurons. There is increasing evidence that abnormality of their function can lead to serious distortions of nervous system function, including inappropriate pain in the absence of the usual painful stimulus, as with 'phantom limb' pain.

These cells produce their own chemicals which help to provide the appropriate environment for normal neuronal function. If they provide too much or too little of their chemicals, nerve function can be adversely affected. Efforts are being made to find drugs to remedy inappropriate activity of glial cells and hence relieve nervous system malfunctions.

A further function of some supporting cells is provided by the Schwann cells which generate myelin sheaths. This insulating function facilitates rapid conduction in myelinated nerves.

Central and local governance in the body

While much of the body's activity is controlled from the brain, many aspects of regional function are locally controlled. The **central governance** resides in the brain, which regulates the body largely by the nervous system, but also by the brain's control of hormones, of which cortisol is a major example. Turning to the brain's governance through the nervous system, the brain's activity can be seen to be concerned particularly with two major functions: control of body movements and regulation of the internal environment, particularly of itself, the brain.

Firstly, the brain controls body movements; those involved in everyday activities, and those required for more unusual activities such as escaping from danger and excelling in sport. Much of the cerebral and cerebellar function is concerned with these skeletal muscle movements.

Secondly, the brain regulates vital aspects of constancy of the internal environment (homeostasis). Ultimately these secure the brain's own highly demanding environment required for normal function and survival. One example of central governance is given by the temperature regulating reflexes. These maintain constancy within narrow limits of the brain's own temperature, together with that of other vital organs such as heart and lungs on which the brain depends for circulation and oxygenation. Control of pulmonary ventilation also regulates the body's carbon dioxide content. This in turn regulates pH. Maintenance of homeostasis is largely effected by the brainstem.

Regulation of body temperature is an example of *central governance taking precedence over local governance.* When a person is in a very challenging chilling environment (low temperature, high wind, and wet conditions so that evaporation favours cooling) the central decision is made in the temperature regulating region of the brainstem to conserve heat in the body's core. This leads to peripheral vasoconstriction, particularly in the hands and feet. The vasoconstriction is caused by sympathetic nerve activity This overrides several aspects of local control, or **local governance**, since not only local cold, but also local lack of oxygen and a rise in local acidity as carbon dioxide accumulates, tend to relax smooth muscle in local arteriolar resistance vessels, causing vasodilation. The consequence is that temperature in the hands falls well below the comfort and functional level, there is peripheral cyanosis, and hand movements become clumsy. If the ambient temperature is below freezing point, there is a risk of ice crystals forming in the peripheries causing tissue damage (frostbite). At his stage, the low temperature may have abolished activity in sensory nerves and numbness may develop. Thus the pain of frostbite may not be experienced at this stage. If the person survives and is rewarmed, return of sensation leads to severe pain from the accumulated products of tissue destruction by freezing.

Peripheral cooling is accentuated (but the core protected) by the fact that in cold environments superficial veins are tightly constricted. Venous return from arms and legs then takes place by deep venae comitantes alongside the main arteries. This leads to **counter-current heat exchange** so that heat is transferred from efferent arteries to afferent veins. Thus much of the heat in the blood is returned to the core and the blood passing to the periphery is pre-cooled. Hence heat loss is minimized and peripheral cooling maximized.

If this peripheral cooling did not occur, core temperature would fall, leading to confusion and inability to take cover from the chilling environment.

Local control of the circulation occurs in most tissues and is often referred to as **autoregulation** (auto = autonomous). The basic mechanism is that the products of metabolism (the metabolites, carbon dioxide, hypoxia, acidosis, increased temperature) act locally on the smooth muscle of resistance vessels to cause vasodilation. Thus during a period of increased skeletal muscular activity, the metabolites produced cause increased flow to meet the metabolic demands. **When flow to an extremity has been abolished** by a ligature to facilitate surgery of an extremity, vasodilator chemicals accumulate in huge amounts. When the ligature is released, a sustained period of intense blood flow (**reactive hyperaemia**) results in the extremity. Release of these chemicals into the general circulation can have adverse cardiac and other effects, the risk increasing with the length of deprivation of blood flow. As this **ischaemic time** is increased, there is also the risk of release into the circulation of products of tissue damage, such as released myoglobin which can cause renal damage.

In organs, such as brain and kidneys, which maintain a fairly constant blood flow in normal resting conditions, autoregulation tends to produce constancy of blood flow. This is how the term **cerebral autoregulation** is understood. It usually refers to maintenance of a constant cerebral blood flow in the face of variations in mean arterial blood pressure (and hence perfusion pressure) in quite a wide range from around 60–160mmHg. Arterial blood pressure tends to vary as we change our posture from lying down to standing up, or the reverse, and systolic pressure rises during muscular exercise. Particularly when aroused from a deep sleep, a sudden leap to the upright posture can overcome the cerebral autoregulation response and lead to fainting.

Some organs have a specific metabolite which predominates in causing local regulation. In the case of the brain this is carbon dioxide. As brain blood flow falls, carbon dioxide rises locally and causes acidosis, which dilates the resistance vessels and restores adequate flow. Abnormal ventilation can distort this effect. If any normal person hyperventilates markedly, the resulting fall in the carbon dioxide level in the cerebral circulation causes vasoconstriction which can impair brain function. Conversely, in patients with carbon dioxide retention due to respiratory failure, brain blood flow increases, causing increased capillary pressure and cerebral oedema.

In the heart, hypoxia is a dominant metabolic change which tends to restore normal blood flow when required.

Stratified complexity of function linked with level of metabolic demands

As already mentioned, various perturbations of the internal environment threaten neurological function. As the disturbance (such as hypothermia or hypoglycaemia) gets worse, a recognizable pattern of change can be seen in the neurological system. Clinically there is increasing **confusion** and, as things get worse, **coma** gradually develops. These **impaired levels of consciousness** are often quantified in the **Glasgow Coma Scale** (GCS). Such quantification is possible because, whatever the cause, impairment of brain function tends to follow the same downward path.

A well-known cause of this downward path is an increasing blood level of ethyl alcohol. The very earliest effects of a rising blood alcohol level are not detectable clinically, but involve potentially fatal impairment of driving skill. (Similar dangers arise with certain drugs and after a major epileptic attack.) As the blood alcohol level rises, behavioural changes occur, with loss of normal inhibitions and the risk of antisocial activities and violence. As the alcohol level rises further, the person becomes quieter and drowsy, gradually passing into coma, respiratory depression and death. This is essentially the same downward path which occurs in many clinical conditions impairing brain function as quantified in the GCS.

Principles of the Glasgow Coma Scale

The scale uses assessment of three basic cerebral functions to score progression towards and through various levels of coma. These tests involve examination of the person's use of the eyes, of speech, and of the motor system. In each case, normal appropriate use scores maximally, with a total of 15 points. With no response (no evidence of cerebral function) the score is 1 at each point, so that 3 is the minimal response. Clinical coma is present from about 7–8 downwards. The value of this scoring system is that fairly repeatable results can be obtained over time by different observers and evidence may thus be obtained of deterioration or gain in the level of consciousness. The results help to determine management.

Space occupying lesions

These provide examples of where the Glasgow coma scale is used. By occupying space in the brain, lesions such as tumours or areas of haemorrhage compress the brain, together with its blood supply. With the brain in an inexpansible cranial box, as the lesion expands, the brain is compressed, its circulation declines, and the function of the hypoxic brain deteriorates. Decompression is urgently required.

Physiological basis of the downward path of progressive deterioration in brain function

This specific downward path of brain function can be explained by a gradient of metabolic requirements from the highly sophisticated and sensitive cortical cells, through the cerebral hemispheres and the brainstem to the spinal cord. Any one of the causes of impairment of cellular function will initially affect the highest level of brain function—the ability to detect and evaluate various factors relevant to a crucial skilled decision. This is the ability used, for example, by a vehicle driver deciding whether it is safe to pass another vehicle on a relatively narrow road, or by a pilot deciding whether a landing has to be aborted. Such decisions involve large areas throughout the cerebral cortex networking to put together spatial information and compare it with known criteria for safety, bearing in mind factors such as engine power, manoeuvrability, wind and rain. The frontal regions appear particularly important in the final decision. Loss of awareness of appropriate behaviour can impinge on patients' clinical states, as with the hypoxic patient pulling off the oxygen mask, or the ketoacidotic patient pulling out the drip.

As deterioration develops, impairment of fine coordination suggests impairment of other parts of the cerebral hemispheres. Emotional lability suggests that the emotional centres in the region adjoining the brainstem are no longer under normal higher control.

Evidence of involvement of the brainstem comes with the early signs of stupor and suppression of ventilation. Inhalation of vomit can result from loss of the normal protective reflexes associated with the vomiting centre in the brainstem.

Thus this progressive deterioration can be seen as a wave of impaired function spreading over the cerebral cortex from the frontal area, then downwards and backwards through the hemispheres and through the brainstem.

Critical care situations

So far we have considered the neurological system the patient brings to critical care. We now look at implications for loss of neurological function during such care. General anaesthesia for major surgery is an example of a planned situation in which the patient is going to require critical care which takes into account the inevitable loss of neurological function during anaesthesia. Such loss also takes place in the unplanned scenario of the life-threatening injuries of the patient admitted as an emergency, where the injuries include brain damage. We now look briefly at the therapeutic basis of general anaesthesia.

General anaesthesia

This has three components –hypnotic, analgesic, and muscle relaxant.

The **hypnotic** component—putting the patient to sleep—involves rapidly acting drugs with widespread depression of brain function. These effects are quite similar to a very high alcohol level, and indeed alcohol was used for centuries for its anaesthetic properties. Anaesthetics act particularly by suppressing the brainstem network which allows stimuli from the outside world to reach cortical level and thereby maintains the alert state. Since pain during surgery is the main such input, it is logical also to use a powerful **analgesic** component to reduce the dose of hypnotic required to keep the patient asleep and unaware (and unable to recall the situation). The third component, a **muscle relaxant,** facilitates surgery by blocking neuromuscular transmission in skeletal muscle and thereby abolishing muscle tone and movements. Because the respiratory muscles are paralysed, artificial ventilation is required.

Local anaesthesia provides a different approach which may also supplement general anaesthesia in some cases. By blocking axonal transmission, it prevents sensation from and movement of (where applicable) a region of the body so that limited surgery can be carried out in that region.

Various forms of **spinal and epidural anaesthesia** are an extension of this, in blocking axonal transmission at spinal cord level, permitting surgery on the lower parts of the body without impairing the patient's consciousness.

Monitoring and managing during anaesthesia

During general anaesthesia, since the functions of the brain are severely suppressed, there is loss of important brainstem reflexes such as those which regulate arterial blood pressure. Ventilation is also suppressed at this site, and, in addition, muscle relaxants paralyse the muscles of ventilation.

Mimicking the brain

During anaesthesia and surgery, the anaesthetist, in collaboration with the surgeon, must mimic the brain in order to replace these vital functions. The basis is similar to the normal control by the neurological system, with natural reflex arcs replaced by monitoring and managing.

For ventilation, this means monitoring the arterial oxygen level and the carbon dioxide level, and adjusting the minute volume upwards if the oxygen level falls below normal, to prevent hypoxia, and adjusting it downwards if the carbon dioxide level falls below normal, to prevent alkalosis. Monitoring may be by arterial line if there are indications for its insertion or by oximeter if the invasive approach is not justified. With oximetry, it is necessary to bear in mind that the reading reflects general arterial oxygen saturation only if the region has a relatively high blood flow. Otherwise the hypoxia detected may be stagnant in variety (due to poor local blood flow) rather than hypoxic (due to inadequate oxygenation in the lungs).

For the **circulation,** arterial blood pressure is monitored. Again this may be invasively via an arterial line, or non-invasively by sphygmomanometry. An arterial line can give more information on the arterial waveform, but carries the risks of invasion of the arterial system and is made ineffective by clots which may block the line. Hypotension when detected may need to be corrected by a vasoconstrictor drug, or hypertension reversed by a vasodilator. In some cases close collaboration with the surgeon may be necessary if hypotension is needed to restrict blood loss, and at times when major blood vessels are being either clamped or released.

In some cases, complex decisions may need to be made. With positive pressure ventilation, airway patency is improved, but venous return and hence cardiac output is reduced. Management decisions need to incorporate the patient's pathological state, physiological monitoring, and knowledge of physiological mechanisms.

The body's suppressed **thermoregulation** reflexes must be replaced by devices which insulate and heat limbs, and by avoidance where possible of rapid cold infusions. Departure from normal body temperature interferes with important protective mechanisms, such as the chemical reactions involved in blood clotting. The dangers of sudden malignant hyperthermia require that core temperature should be closely monitored.

Various **blood constituents** such as glucose and potassium in particular must be monitored when life-threatening abnormalities of these are a serious possibility. As in normal physiology, insulin and glucose can be administered to maintain an appropriate blood glucose, and in some cases to moderate the potassium level by the action of insulin which drives potassium into cells.

Critical care management of life-threatening injuries

As mentioned earlier, these situations need to be monitored and managed using the same principles discussed for general anaesthesia. The problem is that the situation may be complex and evolving, and priorities for treatment need to be established rapidly. It is being realized that where a considerable number of staff are dealing with a life-threatening situation, it may be very helpful to have an experienced person to direct management. This may be seen as a parallel to how the body mechanisms allocate priority to maintaining cerebral and coronary circulation in the face of serious haemorrhage, while sacrificing flow to skin, gut, and kidneys. Patient simulators can be helpful in training, just as for assessment in OSCEs!

Scenarios

Scenario 1

A 25-year-old footballer was injured while heading a ball. He was unconscious for less than a minute and then continued to play. At the end of the game he felt drowsy and has been brought to the A&E department. What would you suspect and outline your management.

Scenario 2

A fit 25-year-old jockey fell off a horse while competing in a race. He has been brought into A&E department, fully conscious and complaining of inability to use any of his four limbs. How will you go about managing this patient—initial examination, investigations, and treatment?

Answers

Scenario 1

Diagnosis
Head injury—extra-dural haematoma.

Clinical features
- Lucid interval
- Deteriorating GCS score
- Temporal haematoma
- Dilated ipsilateral pupil—why?
- Localizing signs

Why?

EDH
↓
Pushes hemisphere to opposite side
↓
Uncus and sharp edge of tentorium
↓
Presses against 3rd nerve
↓
Dilatation of pupil

Overall management
- ABC
- CT scan?—Do not waste time on a CT scan if clinical features are classical and precious time may therefore be lost
- Burr hole—emergency intervention: at the pterion
- Craniotomy—definitive intervention
- Rehabilitation

Scenario 2

Diagnosis
Spinal injury. Traumatic paraplegia.

Immobilization
- Suspected C-spine injury requires continuous immobilization of the entire patient with a semirigid cervical collar, backboard, tape, and straps before and during transfer to the A&E department. This is usually carried out by the pre-hospital care team
- Once the patient's spine is protected, accurate evaluation of spinal injury can be postponed until life-threatening problems are dealt with, e.g. hypotension and hypoxia

Overall management
- Identify and control life-threatening problems
- Immobilization—part of pre-hospital care; this is maintained until C-spine injury is excluded
- X-rays and CT scan
- IV fluids—be careful; over-zealous administration of fluids may cause pulmonary oedema because hypotension is due to vasodilatation; in uncertain cases a Swan–Ganz catheter may be useful. Hypovolaemic shock causes tachycardia and neurogenic shock causes bradycardia. Vasopressors may be indicated.
- Urinary catheter
- NG tube to prevent aspiration
- Medication: methylprednisalone 30mg/kg immediately followed by 5.4mg/kg per hour for the next 23 hours
- Transfer to spinal injuries centre for definitive management
- Rehabilitation—long term

Chapter 32 **Brainstem death and end of life care**

Introduction

The purpose of this chapter is to consider some basic science relating to clinical decisions about death and approaching death. Medical staff and relatives need to decide when death has occurred and further life-sustaining efforts are inappropriate; they need to distinguish effects of the process of dying from effects of processes threatening death. Decisions about immediate treatment, possible organ transplant, and the time of death for legal purposes are based on many inputs, including an understanding of some details of what is happening in the body around the time of death.

Brainstem death

This concept arose some decades ago when cardiac resuscitation and prolonged artificial ventilation became increasingly common. It was developed as a way of deciding when it was appropriate to end these efforts to maintain life in an unresponsive patient. Previously, the absence of detectible heart-beat and breathing provided the diagnosis of death and the patient passed from the hospital ward or home to the mortuary. Even then, however, care had to be taken not to be premature in gradual death, such as that from hypothyroidism or some forms of poisoning. People coming alive in the mortuary or even the coffin highlighted the possibility of premature confirmation of death. For this reason, the basic requirement for diagnosing brainstem death is that the person must not be suffering from a condition such as hypothermia or toxicity which could mimic death but be reversed with time and appropriate treatment.

The orderly process of the death of body cells

Organs and tissues removed after the individual has been pronounced dead by conventional criteria can be shown to have physiological function. Function deteriorates at various rates for different organs. Survival times have been established for organs such as kidneys, livers, and hearts, which can be removed after death and used as effective cadaveric transplants. The interval after death within which the organ is viable tends to decline with the complexity of the organ and hence the level of its metabolic requirements. Corneal transplants with low metabolism can be removed without undue haste for effective function in a recipient. Peripheral arteries can give contractile responses to noradrenaline when removed some hours after the patient's death. In contrast, the brain suffers permanent damage within a few minutes of circulatory arrest.

A wave of death

We have seen in a previous chapter that the metabolic requirements of brain cells are greatest in the cerebral cortex and least in the brainstem; metabolic requirements are less still for cells in the spinal cord. There is a further reduction in requirements as we move from organs such as the heart, liver, and kidneys to less specialized tissues. Thus we can envisage that in death generally, when there is fairly abrupt cessation of heartbeat and breathing, a wave of death of cells begins in the cerebral cortex and moves through the rest of the brain towards the brainstem. The wave then spreads through the complex central organs, finally to reach the peripheral tissues, perhaps some days after death, especially if the body has been kept in cool surroundings.

Significance of brain death

Since all aspects of personality are expressed as a result of brain function, it is reasonable to regard brain death as death of the individual. Since the brain loses its function before the other organs of the body, it is also reasonable to look for signs of brain death as evidence of death of the individual when the rest of the body is still functioning due to artificial maintenance of pulmonary ventilation and, where required, artificial support of the circulation.

Doubts about brain death

The problem with diagnosing brain death is in deciding that it is irreversible, since brain functions, such as coordination of muscle movements, can recover markedly with time after brain damage due to a stroke or trauma. This is recognized by considering the diagnosis of brain death only in the absence of clearly reversible conditions which may suppress normal metabolism. Another pre-requirement for diagnosing brain death is the absence of any detectable electrical activity—even deeply unconscious people can show EEG activity.

Significance of brainstem death

There are at least two reasons why focusing on brainstem activity is helpful in the diagnosis of brain death. Firstly, as already discussed, the brainstem appears to be more resistant to adverse metabolic situations than other parts of the brain, so if it has succumbed, the rest of the brain is likely to have succumbed also.

Secondly, the brainstem has a variety of functions, which are vital for normal life. In the circulation, it controls, via the vagus and sympathetic nerves, the heart rate and arterial blood pressure. It is also essential for pulmonary ventilation and its regulation. It controls swallowing and normal gastric emptying.

Diagnosis of brainstem death

In the present state of knowledge it isn't practicable to study the cells of the brainstem directly. Nor are attempts made to assess the ability of the axonal tracts to conduct impulses. Instead, a number of relatively simple physiological reflexes are tested. These reflexes rely on function in the brainstem for a normal response. If any of these reflexes is present, there is evidence of brainstem life. Only if all the tests are confirmed negative by competent repeated testing can it be assumed that the brainstem is not functioning.

Brainstem physiological reflexes tested

The physiological reflexes to be tested are like the spinal cord stretch and withdrawal reflexes, but tend to be a little more complicated. As with the spinal reflexes, finding a response indicates the integrity of the afferent and efferent pathways, and, crucially, of the reflex centre which controls the response.

The **pupillary light reflex** has the optic nerve as its afferent path and the brainstem centre sends efferent signals, via parasympathetic fibres, to circular fibres in the iris, which constrict the pupil. Similarly, in the **corneal reflex**, afferents from the highly sensitive cornea send signals to the brainstem centre which controls, via somatic efferents, the skeletal muscle fibres which cause blinking. The **gag reflex** reflects the brainstem's control of movements of the upper gut, in this case eliciting retching fragments of the brainstem vomiting reflex.

The **vestibulo-ocular reflex** is an ingenious test, whereby severely cold saline in the outer ear canal induces currents in the vestibular fluid surrounding the hair cells of the semicircular canals and other organs of balance. In the conscious person this would lead to terrible nausea and vertigo, but in the unconscious person, this false information from the inner ear leads to disordered ocular movements, a parody of the normal control of eye fixation on an object during head movements. This control is mediated through the brainstem. Thus the presence of nystagmus is an indication of the presence of brainstem function and the absence of brainstem death.

Control of ventilation of the lungs is an example of brainstem activity which regulates the complex activity of the thoracic muscles and diaphragm in breathing. Basic quiet ventilation depends on cyclical activity in the brainstem controlling centre whereby there is periodic activation of the somatic nerves to the muscles of inspiration, leading to periodic active inspiration, interspersed with periodic relaxation of the inspiratory muscles. As the inspiratory muscles relax, the elastic and surface tension forces in the lung parenchyma cause passive expiration.

The brainstem is also the site of quantitative control of ventilation by afferents from chemoreceptors which detect hypoxia and hypercapnia. In testing the integrity of the brainstem control of ventilation, the aim is to give powerful chemoreceptor stimulation to ensure the maximal chance of observing ventilation in someone who is being ventilated artificially, usually in the intensive care situation. It is quite practical for this purpose to allow the carbon dioxide level to build up in the initially apnoeic person, but it is not appropriate to allow hypoxia to build up, even though the combination of a raised carbon dioxide level and a depressed oxygen level is a much more potent stimulator of ventilation than is a raised carbon dioxide alone. The reason for not allowing hypoxia to develop is that, in the individual's critical state, even a short period of deepening hypoxia could irreversibly impair possible recovery.

Thus hypoxia must be actively avoided. This is done by pre-oxygenation before the patient is disconnected temporarily from the artificial ventilation system. Raising the oxygen concentration in the alveoli by the use of a maximal inspired oxygen concentration can bring the percentage of alveolar oxygen close to 100. For example, if the person has a functional residual capacity of 3L, and the oxygen concentration is 90%, the amount of oxygen in the lungs at the start of the test is around 2.7L. If the person uses 250ml oxygen per minute, then it would be about 9 minutes before the alveolar oxygen fell to around the normal 14%:

- Initial alveolar O_2: 90% of 3L = 2.7L of O_2
- O_2 consumption in 9 minutes = 9 × 250 = 2.25L
- Final alveolar O_2 0.45L = 15% of 3L

By this time the carbon dioxide would have risen to a high level. Clearly in an individual patient close monitoring of this critical test is essential to ensure safety and an accurate result.

End of life care

As with the diagnosis of brainstem death and the associated decision about continued intensive care, an understanding of the physiological situation in other end of life situations can help with decisions about care which have major emotional and ethical aspects.

In patients with some brainstem functions present, and in other patients with serious long-term impairment of brain function where heartbeat and ventilation are proceeding unaided, various situations are possible which are intermediate between brainstem death and the presence of brain function which, however impaired, allows some expression of the original personality.

Persistent vegetative state

This state is, in a sense, a step up from brainstem death. Not only is there evidence of brainstem function, but there may be varying evidence of brain function at a higher level, with, at the same time, absence of any evidence of awareness of and response to the environment.

In the **positive** direction these people have evidence of more elaborate activities associated with subcortical regions of the cerebral hemispheres. Thus a sleep–wake cycle may be observed, with the patient apparently awake, but unable to show evidence of thought processes.

In the **negative** direction there is no manifestation of the personality in terms of cerebral cortical activities.

The term vegetative state then implies that unconscious visceral, or vegetative functions of the body, such as a functioning digestive system, breathing, and circulation are present, to the exclusion of purposive conscious communication and movements.

Timescale is also crucial. Since patients recovering from deep unconsciousness pass through a vegetative state, the vital aspect of diagnosis of the persistent vegetative state is that it is present, without significant change, for a considerable period of time. For example, after 4 weeks without change, the patient may be said to be in a **vegetative state**, without the term 'persistent'. After this time, the term **continuous vegetative state** may be used. After a year, the description **persistent vegetative state** is commonly used. As with brainstem death, criteria and terminology can vary from country to country. The term permanent vegetative state, with its implications of total irreversibility, would be around the borderline of what can be justified on experimental evidence.

The dying patient

The development of the hospice movement has been associated with specialist care of patients with extensive nursing requirements, and a need for relief of pain, nausea, and, as far as possible, other unpleasant aspects of the terminal state, as in terminal cancer, for example. Patients may have similar care in their own homes or communal residences.

An aspect of this treatment is recognition of when a patient has entered the process of dying. This process precedes the identified time of death in contrast to the gradual process of the death of body tissues after death referred to earlier in the chapter. The patient may be failing to eat because he/she is dying, in contrast to dying because of failure to eat.

The physiological basis of this state would seem to be loss of so much of the normal framework of living—in terms of environment, ability to think, and ability of body organs to function—that normal functions such as changing body position and swallowing are literally impossible.

This would seem to be an even less precise state than the vegetative state and notable recovery may in some cases be possible, but in general this situation requires the most sensitive end of life care in terms of providing what the patient needs and not providing what is not needed.

Scenario

Scenario 1

A 25-year-old motor-cyclist, Mr Robert Macdonald, has been comatose for 3 days. Clinically he is suspected to be brain dead. In his wallet, police found an organ donor card indicating that he would wish to donate his organs if ever he were to be brain dead. His parents have acceded to his request. Explain to the actors or examiners (who are acting as the parents) the tests that need to be done and the circumstances.

Answer

Scenario 1

Mr Macdonald, your son Robert has been extremely generous to decide to donate his organs in a situation such as this. He had decided to give the ultimate gift. We are sorry to say Robert fulfils the criteria for brainstem death which are:

- He is cannot breathe on his own (apnoeic) and on a ventilator and in deep coma
- The cause of his brain damage is known
- Hypothermia and drug ingestion are excluded

Tests for brainstem function to be done are:

- Oculocephalic reflex (not done in suspected cervical spine injury)
- Vestibulo-ocular reflex
- Gag reflex
- Cough reflex
- Jaw jerk
- Ciliospinal reflex
- Oculocardiac reflex
- Respiratory function tests—blood gases
- EEG activity

He will be seen by two senior consultants who have nothing to do with the transplant team and assessed independently at 48-hour intervals before he is declared 'brain dead'.

Questions that might be asked without a scenario in 'Applied science and critical care' station

1 What level of Glasgow Coma Scale would be expected in this situation?
2 Would the finding of nystagmus in response to cold saline in the outer ear be compatible with brainstem death?

3 Would the presence of a knee jerk be compatible with brainstem death?

4 What parts of the nervous system may continue to function after brainstem death?

Answers to questions

1 Assessment for brainstem death would only be undertaken in those with none of the evidences of brain function examined in assessment of the Glasgow Coma Score. With no evidence of brain function, the score is 3

2 Nystagmus is evidence of persistent brainstem activity with a brainstem reflex ocular response to stimulation of the balancing system by currents in the endolymph induced by cold saline. It rules out brainstem death

3 Since the knee jerk is a spinal reflex, its presence does not rule out brainstem death

4 The spinal cord may continue to function after death of the brainstem and peripheral nerves would tend to survive and function even longer, due to their greater resistance to hypoxia

Index

Note: *Italic* entries indicate references to a figure, **bold** entries indicate references to a table.